Current Practice of Electroencephalography

Current Practice of Electroencephalography

Editor: Chandler Morris

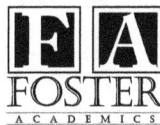

FA FOSTER
ACADEMICS

www.fosteracademics.com

www.fosteracademics.com

FA
FOSTER
ACADEMICS

Cataloging-in-Publication Data

Current practice of electroencephalography / edited by Chandler Morris.
　　p. cm.
Includes bibliographical references and index.
ISBN 978-1-63242-891-2
1. Electroencephalography. 2. Brain--Diseases--Diagnosis. 3. Electrodiagnosis. I. Morris, Chandler.
RC386.6.E43 C87 2020
616.804 754 7--dc23

Foster Academics,
118-35 Queens Blvd., Suite 400,
Forest Hills, NY 11375, USA

ISBN 978-1-63242-891-2 (Hardback)

Contents

Permissions

List of Contributors

Index

Preface

Electroencephalography (EEG) is an electrophysiological monitoring technique which is used to record the electrical activity of the brain. It measures voltage fluctuations generated due to neuronal activity in the brain. The event-related potentials and the spectral content of an EEG are vital for making medical diagnosis. This includes the diagnosis of epilepsy, sleep disorders, coma, encephalopathies, brain death, etc. It can also be used in intensive care units to monitor brain function and the effect of anesthesia/sedation in coma-induced patients, detect any secondary brain damage, and non-convulsive seizures or status epilepticus. EEG has extensive use in cognitive science and psychology, neuroscience, neurolinguistics and psychophysiological studies. This book elucidates new techniques and applications of electroencephalography in a multidisciplinary manner. It includes some of the vital pieces of work being conducted across the world, on various topics related to electroencephalography. As this field is emerging at a rapid pace, the contents of this book will help the readers understand the modern concepts and applications of the subject.

This book is a comprehensive compilation of works of different researchers from varied parts of the world. It includes valuable experiences of the researchers with the sole objective of providing the readers (learners) with a proper knowledge of the concerned field. This book will be beneficial in evoking inspiration and enhancing the knowledge of the interested readers.

In the end, I would like to extend my heartiest thanks to the authors who worked with great determination on their chapters. I also appreciate the publisher's support in the course of the book. I would also like to deeply acknowledge my family who stood by me as a source of inspiration during the project.

Editor

Oscillation Encoding of Individual Differences in Speech Perception

Yu Jin[◑], **Begoña Díaz***[◑], **Marc Colomer, Núria Sebastián-Gallés**

Speech Acquisition and Perception Group, Center for Brain and Cognition, Department of Technology, Pompeu Fabra University, Barcelona, Spain

Abstract

Individual differences in second language (L2) phoneme perception (within the normal population) have been related to speech perception abilities, also observed in the native language, in studies assessing the electrophysiological response mismatch negativity (MMN). Here, we investigate the brain oscillatory dynamics in the theta band, the spectral correlate of the MMN, that underpin success in phoneme learning. Using previous data obtained in an MMN paradigm, the dynamics of cortical oscillations while perceiving native and unknown phonemes and nonlinguistic stimuli were studied in two groups of participants classified as good and poor perceivers (GPs and PPs), according to their L2 phoneme discrimination abilities. The results showed that for GPs, as compared to PPs, processing of a native phoneme change produced a significant increase in theta power. Stimulus time-locked analysis event-related spectral perturbation (ERSP) showed differences for the theta band within the MMN time window (between 70 and 240 ms) for the native deviant phoneme. No other significant difference between the two groups was observed for the other phoneme or nonlinguistic stimuli. The dynamic patterns in the theta-band may reflect early automatic change detection for familiar speech sounds in the brain. The behavioral differences between the two groups may reflect individual variations in activating brain circuits at a perceptual level.

Editor: Manuel S. Malmierca, University of Salamanca- Institute for Neuroscience of Castille and Leon and Medical School, Spain

Funding: This research was supported by grants from the European Community's Seventh Framework Programme (FP7/2007–2013): ERG grant agreement number 323961, the Spanish Ministerio de Economía y Competitividad (PSI 2012 - 34071), and the Catalan Government (SGR 2009-1521) to N. Sebastián-Gallés, and the People Programme (Marie Curie Actions) of the European Union'sSeventh Framework Programme (FP7/2007–2013) under REA grant agreement n° 328671 to B. Díaz. N. Sebastián-Gallés received the "ICREA Acadèmia" Prize for Excellence in Research, funded by the Generalitat de Catalunya. The funders had no role in study design, data collection and analysis, decision to publish, or preparation of the manuscript.

Competing Interests: The authors have declared that no competing interests exist.

* Email: begona.diaz@upf.edu

[◑] These authors contributed equally to this work.

Introduction

A particularly challenging theoretical question in the field of language learning is addressing the large individual differences in second language (L2) mastery. What makes some people more successful non-native language learners than others? Previous research has identified different factors involved in successful learning, such as age of acquisition, amount of previous experience, working memory, attention control, or motivation [1–6]. But even when controlling for all of these variables, substantial individual differences persist, in particular in the perception and production of speech sounds. With the advent of new neurophysiological and imaging methods, the inquiry into individual differences in second language learning has moved to a new level of analysis in terms of how individual brains work [7–14]. One attractive feature of some neural-based methods is the possibility of directly measuring the brain activity, removing the need to ask participants for overt responses and eliminating response-related effects. One of the most widely used measures of second-language speech perception is the event-related response (ERP) mismatch negativity (MMN) that is measured during passive listening and signals auditory discrimination sensitivity. The MMN has been showed to capture differences in individual phoneme discrimination capabilities in healthy populations [7,15]. The present study investigates the oscillatory neural patterns related to

success in phoneme learning by analyzing the spectral dynamics underneath the MMN responses of individuals with different levels of mastery of L2 phonemes.

The MMN is elicited by "deviant" sounds; these are sounds that violate the preceding sound sequence. The MMN is elicited without participants' awareness [16] and even when attending to an unrelated task to the auditory stimulation [17]. The MMN system is considered to operate preattentively. However, the elicitation of MMN *per se* does not imply that all processes leading to the detection of deviants are also attention independent [18,19]. The MMN peaks between 100–250 ms after the auditory change, with a negative fronto-central scalp distribution. The main neural source of the MMN has been located in the supratemporal plane, in or near the primary auditory cortex, with additional contributions from the frontal and parietal lobes [20–31]. The MMN has been proved to be a very useful tool for investigating different aspects of speech perception in normal and pathological populations [32–36]. Relevant to our current goals, the amplitude of the MMN is directly related to the magnitude of the perceived change and, hence, it is considered a measure of individual auditory discrimination accuracy [37,38].

Differences in MMN amplitude are used to characterize individual differences in speech perception. [7] compared two groups of highly skilled bilinguals (Good Perceivers, GPs, and Poor Perceivers, PPs) who differed in their capacity to perceive an L2 vowel contrast. The classification was performed based on their performance on different behavioral tasks [39]. For the two groups of participants, we recorded ERPs responses to nonlinguistic (perception of frequency, duration, and presentation order differences in tones) and speech (perception of spectral frequency differences in native and unknown vowels) changes. Importantly, the unknown vowel did not belong to participants' L2. The results showed larger MMNs over frontal electrodes for GPs when compared to PPs, only for speech sounds, native and unknown. Moreover, the difference in MMN amplitude between the groups was present at the frontal electrodes, but absent at the supratemporal ones. The absence of differences in the acoustic conditions indicated that the perceptual analysis of simple sound features and their neural memory representation were not the cause of the behavioral differences between the GPs and PPs. This indicates that the origin of individual variability in L2 phoneme mastery is rather speech-specific. Furthermore, the similarity of responses in the acoustic conditions (and also at the temporal electrodes for the speech conditions) ruled out any account based on general attention differences between the two groups. In an ERP study testing unknown phonetic contrast (neither L1 nor L2) discrimination abilities in successful versus unsuccessful L2 learners, [15] reported analogous findings. They concluded that unsuccessful L2 learners have a less efficient speech process than successful L2 learners. Together, these findings in different populations suggest a speech-related origin (rather than a perceptual one) underlying individual differences in speech perception.

Although by using EEG signals solely it is not possible to infer the exact location and nature of the neural contributions underlying the MMN, EEG recordings in lesion patients [40], source imaging (EEG combined with fMRI or MEG, [41,42]), dipole sources modelling with EEG [29,43,44] or new approaches to EEG signal analysis, like Independent Component Analysis (ICA, [27]) have consistently revealed the disassociated functions of frontal and temporal MMN generators. These methods have allowed researchers to infer that the temporal MMN generator is closely associated with integrating information from the sensory input streams with memory traces, whereas the frontal (and parietal) generator is in part related to an involuntary attention-switching mechanism responsible for the detection of deviant sounds. Since GPs and PPs differed at frontal electrodes during speech discrimination, whereas no differences were found at temporal sites, [7] concluded that the two groups differed in their attention orienting mechanism involved in speech change-detection. Yet, EEG signals are thought to be the summation of oscillatory activities and reliance on measures of peak amplitude calculated from an average waveform, as the MMN, have a limitation – they could be hiding the underlying oscillatory mechanisms involved in the EEG generation. Therefore, the lack of differences in the MMN amplitude for the speech changes at the temporal electrodes between GPs and PPs could uncover potential differences in the oscillatory modulations at temporal sites. Following the same rationale, oscillatory differences between GPs and PPs during the processing of nonlinguistic changes may not be captured by the MMN. The present study aims to examine the underlying oscillatory responses during the MMN, and whether they contribute to the observed individual differences. This will be assessed by comparing GPs' and PPs' oscillatory responses underlying the MMN responses to nonlinguistic and speech changes.

Several EEG and magnetoencephalography (MEG) studies suggested that the auditory discriminatory process reflected by the MMN is accompanied by phase alignment and power modulation at the theta frequency range [45–48]. Besides auditory discrimination, the theta band is associated to several cognitive functions as working memory processes, attentional processing, spatial navigation and (episodic) long-term memory processes [49]. [45] used time-frequency analysis of single-trial ERPs to demonstrate that the MMN is due to a combination of increased theta power and phase alignment for deviant trials. They also found that amplitude modulation and phase alignment mechanisms depend on the source location of the MMN: event-related spectral modulation was higher for deviants than for standards at frontal, but not at temporal sites. [46] revealed a similar finding in an MEG study: the phase modulation of theta oscillation during a passive oddball paradigm was associated with deviant evoked responses. They identified phase synchronizations between temporal and ipsilateral frontal regions, as well as temporal-temporal and temporal-parietal synchronies. [47] performed single trial analyses of the MMN (subtracting deviant trials from the preceding standard). They found no evidence for event-related spectral power changes, but there was a significant event-related phase alignment in the theta frequency. Relevant for the topic of individual differences, the phase alignment in the theta band was a predictor of behavioral discriminability of a difficult acoustic (i.e. frequency) change. All these previous studies indicate that the MMN response is related to theta power and phase modulations. [48] addressed the question of whether the EEG oscillations underlying the MMN are elicited by acoustic stimuli and/or by the presentation probability, since the MMN is usually measured in oddball paradigms, during which infrequent deviant sounds violate an auditory regularity engendered by frequently presented standard sounds. To eliminate the effect of probability differences, the neural response to the same sounds was compared when presented in an oddball paradigm and in a control paradigm in which the tones were presented with equal probability. In the oddball paradigm, an ERSP and ITC increase in the theta band was associated with the presentation of the deviant stimuli, whereas no significant event-related spectral power changes were detected for the control paradigm. Their results were in broad agreement with previous studies showing that the MMN response in the oddball paradigm is related to theta power and phase modulations. Additionally, this study proved that the oscillatory changes in theta are caused by the violation of auditory regularities, rather than by acoustic changes alone. Based on these findings, we expect that the MMN differences related to phoneme discrimination reported by [7] will be accompanied by differences in spectral modulations in the theta band.

Here, we assessed the differences between GPs and PPs using measures of EEG event-related spectral power (ERSP) and intertrial coherence (ITC). ERSP measures spectral power changes at a given frequency range, time-locked to a stimulus event relative to pre-stimulus baseline. ITC measures the extent to which activity at a given frequency is in phase across different trials in time, and is indicative of event-related phase resetting. Furthermore, we will study the ERSP and ITC changes associated with deviant and standard sounds separately. Taken together the reported involvement of the theta rhythm in the MMN [45–48] and our previous data on individual differences in speech sound perception [7], we hypothesized that differences between GPs and PPs for vowel processing are most likely related to the modulations (amplitude and/or phase-locking) of theta frequency oscillations (4–8 Hz) during the speech conditions, particularly in frontal areas, whereas no differences were expected for the processing of nonlinguistic stimuli.

Materials and Methods

EEG Data Acquisition

We applied EEG spectrum analyses on the same EEG data set studied in [7]. Here, we will describe briefly the data collection procedure (for a detailed description, see [7]). In that study, a relationship between native and non-native phoneme perception capacities was reported in healthy adults. Thus, the researchers first selected two groups of early and highly proficient Spanish (first language, L1) - Catalan (second language, L2) bilinguals differing in their capacity to perceive a difficult vowel contrast in their L2 (the mid-front Catalan vowel contrast/e/-/ɛ/). Sixteen participants were considered good perceivers (GPs) because they scored within the range of natives in three behavioral tasks (a phoneme discrimination task, a gating task and an auditory lexical decision task; see [39] for details). Fifteen participants were considered poor perceivers (PPs) because they did not score within the range of natives in any of the three tasks. The two groups represented exceptionally good and poor L2 perceivers, as approximately, 23% of the original sample of 126 participants was classified as PPs and 12% as GPs. In [7] the data from one PP was excluded because there were not enough EEG epochs free of artifacts (<70%). Following the same exclusion criteria, one GP participant was excluded in the frequency condition and one additional PP participant was excluded in the duration condition. In the present study the same participants as in [7] were included in each condition.

Participants central sound representation was measured for conditions tapping general acoustic perception (duration, frequency, and pattern conditions) and speech perception (native and nonnative phoneme conditions). During the EEG recording, participants were asked to watch a silent movie and to ignore the auditory stimulation.

In the duration condition, the stimuli were four pure tones of 1,000 Hz: the standard tone was 200 ms, and the three deviant tones were 120, 80 and 40 ms. In the frequency condition, stimuli were four pure tones of 50 ms: the standard tone was 1,000 Hz, and the deviant tones were 1,030, 1,060, and 1,090 Hz. In both conditions the presentation probability was 0.8 (1,200 presentations) for the standard and 0.066 (100 presentations) for each deviant. Tones were presented in random order with the restriction that at least one standard tone was presented between two deviants. The stimulus onset asynchrony (SOA) was of 314 ms. In the pattern condition, 400 trains of 50 ms-tones were presented. Each train consisted of six alternating pure tones of either 500 or 1,000 Hz (2,400 tones altogether). Tones were presented at a SOA of 128 ms. Stimulus trains were presented in a predictable way (ABABAB-BABABA-**B**ABABA-ABABAB...), in which A represents the 500 Hz tone and B the 1,000 Hz tone, the hyphen indicates the beginning of the trains, and A and B denote the deviant event (i.e., repetition of the last tone presented in the preceding train).

In the native and unknown phoneme conditions, the same synthesized phonemes used by [35] were presented. The standard stimulus for both native and unknown phoneme conditions was the Spanish vowel/o/with a presentation probability of 0.8. The native deviant phoneme was the Spanish vowel/e/and the unknown deviant phoneme was the Estonian vowel/ö/ (unfamiliar to all participants), with a presentation probability of 0.2 each. As described in [7], the acoustic properties of the Finnish/e/and/o/ vowels employed by [35] were similar to the Spanish/e/and/o/ vowels. Both native and unknown phoneme blocks contained 500 stimuli each (400 standards and 100 deviants) with a constant stimulus onset asynchrony (SOA) of 488 ms. The duration of all

the phonemes was 200 ms. The stimuli were presented at random but there was at least one standard stimulus before a deviant one.

EEG Data Processing

To investigate the neural oscillatory changes associated to the MMN, we applied spectral analyses on EEG data to measure event-related spectral perturbation (ERSP) and intertrial coherence (ITC) for those stimuli that elicited a MMN in [7]: for the duration condition the standard 200 ms-tone vs. the deviant 40 ms-tone (40 ms), for the frequency condition the standard 1,000 Hz-tone vs. the deviant 1,090 Hz-tone, in the pattern condition the standard alternating tones vs. the repeated tones, in the native phoneme condition the standard/o/vs. the deviant/e/, and in the nonnative phoneme condition the standard/o/vs. the deviant/ö/. The EEG data processing is detailed below, as it is different from the previous study [7].

The EEG data was digitized at 500 Hz and band-pass filtered (0.01 to 80 Hz). A 50 Hz notch filter was employed. Eye blinks and other focal artifacts were removed using independent component analysis (ICA) implemented in BrainVision Analyzer software (Brain Products GmbH, Munich, Germany). The data was segmented into 2000 ms epochs, including a pre-stimulus baseline of 500 milliseconds. The epochs were sorted into standard and deviant trials. For all the standard epochs, there were no deviant stimuli presented in the 2000 ms window. Because deviant stimuli were always preceded and followed by standard stimuli, the deviant epochs included the presentation of standard stimuli. In the deviant epochs no other deviant was presented. Therefore, the standard and deviant epochs only differed in the stimuli presented at time 0. The scalp electrode positions included in the analysis were: C3, C4, Cz, F3, F4, F5, F6, F7, F8, Fz, LM, P3, P4, Pz, RM, T3L, and T4L. The EEG spectrum analyses were performed using the EEGLAB software [50].

ERSP and ITC

ERSP and ITC were computed on the individual 2s-epochs using the *newtimef* function of EEGLAB. Spectral decompositions were done from 0 to 50 Hz using Morlet wavelets with a constant 1 cycle length.

ERSP measures average dynamic changes in the amplitude of the EEG frequency spectrum as a function of time relative to the onset of the experimental stimulus. In the current study, ERSP values (dB) were computed using a 500 ms time window relative to a 200 ms baseline period.

The ITC (*newtimef* function) is a measure of consistency of the EEG spectral phase at different frequency ranges and times across epochs. ITC values range from 0 to 1, with values near 1 implying almost perfect phase coincidence across epochs. In the present study, ITC values were computed for a 0–500 ms time window.

Statistical analysis

For the ERSP and ITC statistical analyses we combined the use of time-frequency analysis with more conventional amplitude criteria for identifying periods of significant changes in ERSP and ITC. We compared GPs and PPs for standard and deviant trials separately for the frequency bands theta (4–8 Hz), alpha (8–12 Hz), beta (12–30 Hz), and gamma (30–50 Hz). To control for multiple testing of data points at each electrode, we required a minimum sequence length of 8 consecutive data points (56 ms) to exceed the significance level ($p<0.05$) for an interval of 200 ms [47,51].

Ethics Statement

The experiment was approved by the local ethical committee of the University of Barcelona and it was in compliance with the Code of Ethics of the World Medical Association (Declaration of Helsinki). Written consent was obtained from each participant prior to the experiment. All participants were paid at the end of the experiment for their participation.

Results

The epoch numbers for each condition and stimulus type were not different between the two groups (Table 1), yet there was a trend towards PPs having more epochs than GPs for the phoneme stimuli. Since spectral analyses may depend on the number of epochs, a sub-set of epochs for the PPs that matched the number of segments for GPs were randomly selected to be analyzed for the phoneme stimuli.

ERSP

The analysis of the native deviant trials showed an increase in oscillation power at theta frequency for GPs, when compared to PPs, at the F3 (74–246 ms), F4 (134–228 ms), Fz (168–236 ms), C3 (90–150 ms), C4 (142–202 ms), and Cz (56–152 ms) electrodes. Figure 1 shows the ERSP values for the theta band time-locked to the onset of the native deviant phoneme. For the other frequency ranges, no other effects were observed (except for the alpha band that increased for GPs at F3 between 82–150 ms). No differences were observed for any of the other phoneme stimulus (except for the nonnative deviant phoneme, for which one electrode - Fz - showed an increase in alpha band for PPs when compared to GPs in the 176–254 ms time range).

For the nonlinguistic conditions no significant differences were found between the groups (except for one electrode, F5, that showed an increase for PPs in theta band in the time interval 108–168 ms and in alpha band 98–228 ms).

ITC

The analysis did not yield any significant difference between the groups for any frequency band or stimulus.

Discussion

In the present study, we investigated the oscillatory characteristics of individual differences in the learning of the phonemes of an L2 by applying EEG spectrum analyses. The oscillatory changes related to the processing of several nonlinguistic and speech changes were compared between good and poor perceivers of an L2 speech contrast. The results of the spectral analyses showed a significant increase in the theta band power in GPs when compared to PPs in response to native speech changes at frontal and central electrodes. In line with [7], no differences between groups were found for the processing of nonlinguistic stimuli. The theta band has been repeatedly reported to be the neural oscillatory mechanism of auditory discrimination [45–48]. The analysis of the stimulus time-locked spectral changes revealed that GPs increased the strength of theta oscillation (ERSP) but not the intertrial coherence (ITC). Similar to the results of [7], we found differences between GPs and PPs in the theta power at frontal electrodes, but not at the temporal electrodes.

The EEG data analyzed in the present study was recorded for several tonal and speech changes in paradigms in which one stimulus type was presented frequently (standard) to create a regular context that was violated by a deviant stimulus, with a lower probability to be presented. The event-related potential response evoked by these auditory changes elicited an MMN [7]. The amplitude of the MMN was similar between GPs and PPs for the changes involving tones (nonlinguistic stimuli), but GPs showed larger MMNs for the speech changes. In the present study, when the spectral changes were analyzed, oscillations in the theta band were found to underlie the group differences in the MMN response to native phonemes. This finding is in line with previous studies relating the MMN to changes in the theta band [45,46,48]. As in previous studies, the stimulus time-locked power spectral changes (ERSP) in the theta band were found between 80–240 ms, the time window of the MMN. The lack of ERSP differences between the groups for the nonlinguistic stimuli converges with the similar MMNs found for the two groups in these conditions and supports the claim that PPs and GPs are similar in their skills to process auditory changes.

The analysis of the spectral modulations time-locked to the stimulus revealed that GPs and PPs differed only for the oscillation strength (ERSP), but not in the phase coherence (ITC) in the theta frequency during the MMN interval (50–250 ms) for the deviant

Table 1. Epoch numbers in the different conditions, for the GPs and PPs groups.

	PPs	GPs	t(df), p value
Native phoneme standards	156.86±15.84*	126±4.75	t(28) = 1.97, p = 0.06
Native phoneme deviants	85.29±8.15*	72.94±2.88	t(28) = 1.50, p = 0.15
Unknown phoneme standards	156.71±13.98*	130.94±3.30	t(28) = 1.91, p = 0.07
Unknown phoneme deviants	89.14±7.63*	76.13±1.91	t(28) = 1.76, p = 0.09
Frequency standards	727.57±20.34	731.93±52.26	t(27)<1, p = 0.77
Frequency deviants	98.64±1.82	98.86±6.24	t(27)<1, p = 0.89
Duration standards	749.84±108.87	722.93±36.26	t(27)<1, p = 0.37
Duration deviants	102.69±14.48	98.62±6.50	t(27) = 1.01, p = 0.35
Pattern standards	415.57±54.44	397.12±6.25	t(28) = 1.34, p = 0.22
Pattern deviants	415.71±54.68	397.18±6.30	t(28) = 1.34, p = 0.21

*For the spectral analysis, the number of segments for the PPs was randomly selected to match the number of segments for the GPs: 135.35±7.11 native phoneme standards, 77.35±6.14 native phoneme deviants, 136.14±10.02 unknown phoneme standards and 79.42±4.5 unknown phoneme deviants. There were no differences between the groups in the number of segments for any phoneme stimulus (for all t-tests t<1).

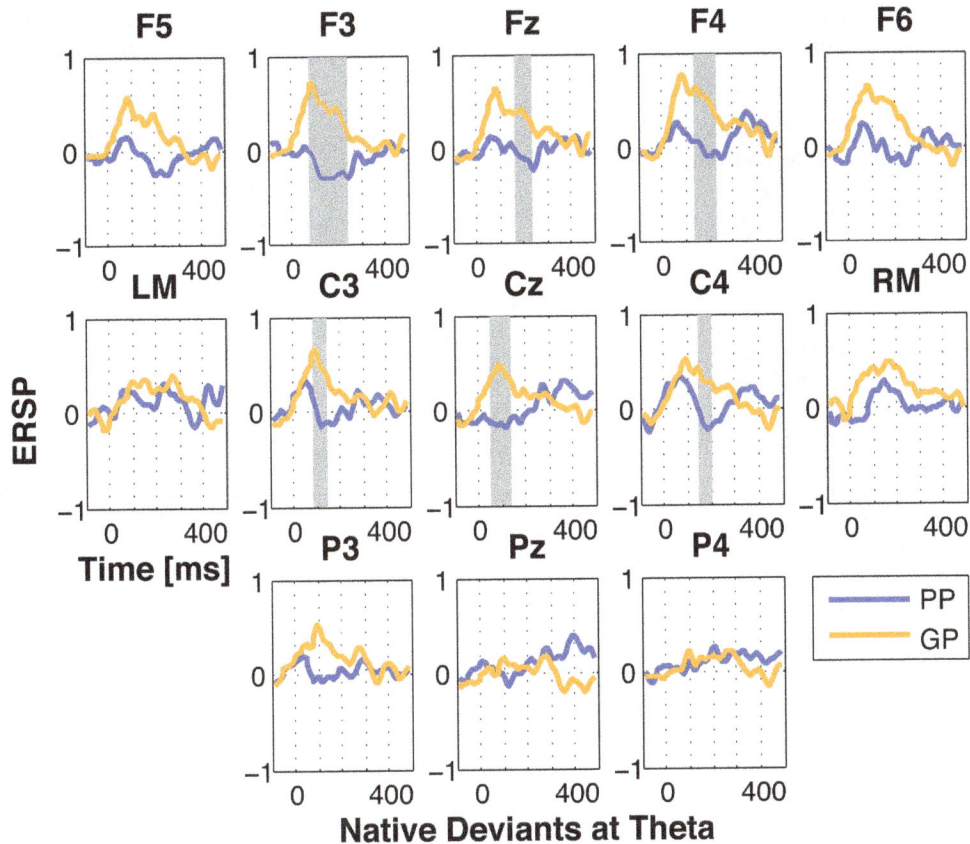

Figure 1. ERSP for the theta band time-locked to the onset of the native deviant phoneme. The grey bars depict the time windows where t-tests yielded significant differences (i.e., $p<0.05$ at least for eight consecutive data points) between the two groups (F3 (74–246 ms), F4 (134–228 ms), Fz (168–236 ms), C3 (90–150 ms), C4 (142–202 ms), and Cz (56–152 ms)).

native phoneme. We analyzed the ERSP and ITC separately for standard and deviant stimuli as previous studies [45,46,48] showed that the elicitation of the MMN is mainly driven by the modulation of theta oscillations for deviant stimuli. However, [47] found no evidence for event-related spectral power changes performing single trial analyses of the MMN (subtracting deviant trials from the preceding standard), but a significant phase-locking at the theta frequency. In the present study, the analysis of ERSP showed again for GPs, in comparison to PPs, an increase in theta power for the native deviant phoneme at central (C3, C4, and Cz) and frontal electrodes (F3, F4 and Fz). For the native standard phoneme, there were no differences between the two groups, suggesting that GPs and PPs process speech sounds similarly, but it is the detection of a change within the auditory context that is different between the groups. The similar pattern of neural oscillations for the unknown vowels suggests that the difference between the two groups lies in the cognitive mechanism responsible for detecting familiar speech changes, rather than the one in charge of speech acoustic analysis.

We did not observe any group difference in the responses to the unknown deviant sound in the theta frequency band. The lack of differences for the unknown phonemes differs from the results in [7]. In this previous study, the MMN elicited by the native and nonnative speech changes were analyzed by means of a single ANOVA. The analysis revealed a significant group effect, indicating that GPs showed larger MMNs than PP for both native and unknown phonemes. Despite the fact that in [7] no interaction was found between group (GP and PP) and phoneme type (native

and unknown), the difference between the groups in their MMN to the unknown phoneme change was quantitatively smaller than the difference for native deviants. The present study, following the analysis procedures from previous studies on oscillatory responses underneath the MMN [45–48], compared the groups separately for each standard and deviant stimulus. Hence, the two groups were compared for each vowel type separately, rather than running a global analysis with the two phoneme conditions as in [7]. When the two phoneme conditions were analyzed separately, differences between the groups were only found for the native vowel. The present group differences only for the native phoneme indicate that the two groups differ mainly in the processing of familiar speech sounds. One possible explanation for this pattern is that GPs have more efficient speech processing capacities in comparison to PPs. Lifelong experience with native contrasts should result in better neural representations for GPs than for PPs, whereas the lack of previous experience with unknown sounds for all participants should diminish (if not abolish) the difference between GPs and PPs in detecting unknown contrasts.

The ERSP group differences between GPs and PPs did not concur with ITC differences. It has been shown that oscillatory phase alignment may not concur with change in power [52]. [45] found that frontal components of the MMN were formed by increases in both ITC and ERSP, whereas temporal components of the MMN were formed by phase alignment alone. However, [47] suggested that the MMN is described best by changes in the ITC. Understanding the distinction between ERSP and ITC is important for understanding the ERP generation. Whether ERPs are generated by phase-locking ongoing neural activities or they originate in additive stimulus-evoked responses is still under debate [53–56].

In the current study, the differences between GPs and PPs in theta oscillations were found mainly at fronto-central electrodes, whereas no difference was found at the temporal electrodes (left and right mastoids, T3L and T4L). Previous studies [45–48] reported the involvement of theta oscillations in both temporal and frontal areas. [45] argued that the different components (i.e. temporal and frontal) of the MMN are driven by changes in the phase alignment and power modulation, to a different extent. They found an enhanced theta ITC, but no ERSP changes at the mastoid electrodes. In contrast to the mastoid electrodes, the fronto-central electrodes showed changes of theta ERSP and ITC in the MMN intervals. These findings support the existence of different MMN sources, with distinct functional roles. Our ERSP and ITC results also showed group differences at the fronto-central electrodes, but not at the mastoid electrodes. In line with our previous findings [7], differences in speech discrimination between GPs and PPs were found at fronto-central electrodes mainly. The frontal differences between GPs and PPs suggest that the origin of individual differences in phoneme learning may be due to a functional difference of the frontal MMN generator. Hence, our analysis strengthens the conclusion that the differences between GPs and PPs may not be related to the encoding and comparison of sensory features (reflected by the temporal component of the MMN), but that they may be linked to differences in the attentive or pre-attentive detection of signal change, supported by the frontal component [30,57].

Our results indicate the existence of differences in the theta oscillatory activity between individuals differing in their capacity to perceive foreign phonemes. The GPs showed an increased theta power and phase alignment for native speech discrimination in fronto-parietal areas, when compared to PPs. The present study provides evidence supporting the use of time-frequency analyses to understand the underlying neural mechanisms of speech processing and provides new insights into brain mechanisms involved in speech learning.

Acknowledgments

We thank Volker Ressel, Anna Basora, Judith Schmitz, Miguel Burgaleta, Kimberly Brink, Cristina Galusca, and Robert Frank de Menezes for useful conversations and for correcting the English manuscript.

Author Contributions

Conceived and designed the experiments: YJ BD NSG. Performed the experiments: BD. Analyzed the data: YJ BD MC. Wrote the paper: YJ BD MC NSG.

References

1. Harrington M, Sawyer M (1992) L2 Working Memory Capacity and L2 Reading Skill. Stud Second Lang Acquis 14: 25–38.

2. Miyake A, Friedman NP (1998) Individual differences in second language proficiency: Working memory as language aptitude. In: Healy AF, Bourne LE, editors. Foreign language learning Psycholinguistic studies on training and retention. Mahwah, NJ: Lawrence Erlbaum Associates. 339–364.

3. Flege JE, Yeni-Komshian GH, Liu S (1999) Age Constraints on Second-Language Acquisition. J Mem Lang 41: 78–104.

4. Moyer A (1999) Ultimate attainment in L2 phonology. Stud Second Lang Acquis 21: 81–108.

5. Guion SG, Pederson E (2007) Investigating the role of attention in phonetic learning. In: Bohn OS, Munro M, editors. Language Experience in Second Language Speech Learning. Amsterdam: John Benjamins. 57–77.

6. Majerus S, Poncelet M, Van der Linden M, Weekes BS (2008) Lexical learning in bilingual adults: The relative importance of short-term memory for serial order and phonological knowledge. Cognition 107: 395–419.

7. Díaz B, Baus C, Escera C, Costa A, Sebastián-Gallés N (2008) Brain potentials to native phoneme discrimination reveal the origin of individual differences in learning the sounds of a second language. Proc Natl Acad Sci U S A 105: 16083–16088.

8. Golestani N, Molko N, Dehaene S, LeBihan D, Pallier C (2007) Brain structure predicts the learning of foreign speech sounds. Cereb Cortex 17: 575–582.

9. Golestani N, Zatorre RJ (2004) Learning new sounds of speech: reallocation of neural substrates. Neuroimage 21: 494–506.

10. Mei L, Chen C, Xue G, He Q, Li T, et al. (2008) Neural predictors of auditory word learning. Neuroreport 19: 215–219.

11. Sebastián-Gallés N, Soriano-Mas C, Baus C, Díaz B, Ressel V, et al. (2012) Neuroanatomical markers of individual differences in native and non-native vowel perception. J Neurolinguist 25: 150–162.

12. Ventura-Campos N, Sanjuán A, González J, Palomar-García M, Rodríguez-Pujadas A, et al. (2013) Spontaneous Brain Activity Predicts Learning Ability of Foreign Sounds. J Neurosci 33: 9295–9305.

13. Wong P, Perrachione T, Parrish T (2007) Neural characteristics of successful and less successful speech and word learning in adults. Hum Brain Mapp 28: 995–1006.

14. Wong P, Warrier C, Penhune V, Roy A, Sadehh A, et al. (2008) Volume of left Heschl's gyrus and linguistic pitch learning. Cereb Cortex 18: 828–836.

15. Jakoby H, Goldstein A, Faust M (2011) Electrophysiological correlates of speech perception mechanisms and individual differences in second language attainment. Psychophysiology 48: 1517–1531.

16. Näätänen R (1979) Orienting and Evoked Potentials. In: Kimme HD, van Olst EH, Orlebeke JF, editors. The orienting reflex in humans. New Jersey: Erlbaum. 61–75.

17. Alho K, Woods DL, Algazi A (1994) Processing of auditory stimuli during auditory and visual attention as revealed by event-related potentials. Psychophysiology 31: 469–479.

18. Takegata R, Brattico E, Tervaniemi M, Varyagina O, Näätänen R, et al. (2005) Preattentive representation of feature conjunctions for concurrent spatially distributed auditory objects. Cogn Brain Res 25: 169–179.

19. Winkler I, Czigler I, Sussman E, Horváth J, Balázs L (2005) Preattentive binding of auditory and visual stimulus features. J Cogn Neurosci 17: 320–339.

20. Aaltonen O, Tuomainen J, Laine M, Niemi P (1993) Cortical differences in tonal versus vowel processing as revealed by an ERP component called mismatch negativity (MMN). Brain Lang 44: 139–152.

21. Sharma A, Kraus N, Carrell T, Thompson C (1994) Neurophysiologic bases of pitch and place of articulation perception: A case study. J Acoust Soc Am 95: 3011.

22. Halgren E, Baudena P, Clarke JM, Heit G, Liegeois C, et al. (1995) Intracerebral potentials to rare target and distracter auditory and visual stimuli. I. Superior temporal plane and parietal lobe. Electroencephalogr Clin Neurophysiol 94: 191–220.

23. Rinne T, Gratton G, Fabiani M, Cowan N, Maclin E, Stinard A (1999) Scalp-recorded optical signals make sound processing in the auditory cortex visible. Neuroimage 10: 620–624.

24. Liasis A, Towell A, Alho K, Boyd S (2001) Intracranial identification of an electric frontal-cortex response to auditory stimulus change: A case study. Cogn Brain Res 11: 227–233.

25. Müller BW, Jüptner M, Jentzen W, Müller SP (2002) Cortical activation to auditory mismatch elicited by frequency deviant and complex novel sounds: a PET study. Neuroimage 17: 231–239.

26. Doeller CF, Opitz B, Mecklinger A, Krick C, Reith W, et al. (2003) Prefrontal cortex involvement in preattentive auditory deviance detection: neuroimaging and electrophysiological evidence. Neuroimage 20: 1270–1282.

27. Marco-Pallarés J, Grau C, Ruffini G (2005) Combined ICA-LORETA analysis of mismatch negativity. Neuroimage 25: 471–477.

28. Molholm S, Martinez A, Ritter W, Javitt DC, Foxe JJ (2005) The neural circuitry of pre-attentive auditory change-detection: An fMRI study of pitch and duration mismatch negativity generators. Cereb Cortex 15: 545–551.

29. Oknina LB, Wild-Wall N, Oades RD, Juran SA, Röpcke B, et al. (2005) Frontal and temporal sources of mismatch negativity in healthy controls, patients at onset of schizophrenia in adolescence and others at 15 years after onset. Schizophr Res 76: 25–41.

30. Garrido MI, Kilner JM, Stephan KE, Friston KJ (2009) The mismatch negativity: A review of underlying mechanisms. Clin Neurophysiol 120: 453–463.

31. Dima D, Frangou S, Burge L, Braeutigam S, James AC (2012) Abnormal intrinsic and extrinsic connectivity within the magnetic mismatch negativity brain network in schizophrenia: A preliminary study. Schizophr Res 135: 23–27.

32. Aaltonen O, Niemi P, Nyrke T, Tuhkanen M (1987) Event-related brain potentials and the perception of a phonetic continuum. Biol psychol 24: 197–207.

33. Kraus N, McGee TJ, Carrell TD, Zecker SG, Nicol TG, et al. (1996) Auditory neurophysiologic responses and discrimination deficits in children with learning problems. Science (80-) 273: 971–973.

34. Dehaene-Lambertz G (1997) Electrophysiological correlates of categorical phoneme perception in adults. Neuroreport 8: 919–924.

35. Näätänen R, Lehtokoski A, Lennes M, Cheour M, Huotilainen M, et al. (1997) Language-specific phoneme representations revealed by electric and magnetic brain responses. Nature 385: 432–434.

36. Sharma A, Dorman M (1999) Cortical auditory evoked potential correlates of categorical perception of voice-onset time. J Acoust Soc Am 106: 1078–1083.

37. Amenedo E, Escera C (2000) The accuracy of sound duration representation in the human brain determines the accuracy of behavioural perception. Eur J Neurosci 12: 2570–2574.

38. Näätänen R (2001) The perception of speech sounds by the human brain as reflected by the mismatch negativity (MMN) and its magnetic equivalent (MMNm). Psychophysiology 38: 1–21.

39. Sebastián-Gallés N, Baus C (2005) On the relationship between perception and production in L2 categories. In: Cutler A, editor. Twenty-first Century Psycholinguistics: Four Cornerstones. New York: Erlbaum. 279–292.

40. Alain C, Woods DL, Knight RT (1998) A distributed cortical network for auditory sensory memory in humans. Brain Res 812: 23–37.

41. Waberski T, Kreitschmann-Andermahr I, Kawohl W, Darvas F, Ryang Y, et al. (2001) Spatio-temporal source imaging reveals subcomponents of the human auditory mismatch negativity in the cingulum and right inferior temporal gyrus. Neurosci Lett 308: 107–110.

42. Opitz B, Rinne T, Mecklinger A, von Cramon DY, Schröger E (2002) Differential contribution of frontal and temporal cortices to auditory change detection: fMRI and ERP results. Neuroimage 15: 167–174.

43. Scherg M, Vajsar J, Picton TW (1989) A source analysis of the late human auditory evoked potentials. J Cogn Neurosci 1: 336–355.

44. Jemel B, Achenbach C, Müller BW, Röpcke B, Oades RD (2002) Mismatch Negativity Results from Bilateral Asymmetric Dipole Sources in the Frontal and Temporal Lobes. Brain Topogr 15: 13–27.

45. Fuentemilla L, Marco-Pallarés J, Münte TF, Grau C (2008) Theta EEG oscillatory activity and auditory change detection. Brain Res 1220: 93–101.

46. Hsiao FJ, Wu ZA, Ho LT, Lin YY (2009) Theta oscillation during auditory change detection: An MEG study. Biol Psychol 81: 58–66.

47. Bishop DVM, Hardiman MJ (2010) Measurement of mismatch negativity in individuals: A study using single-trial analysis. Psychophysiology 47: 697–705.

48. Ko D, Kwon S, Lee G-T, Im CH, Kim KH, et al. (2012) Theta Oscillation Related to the Auditory Discrimination Process in Mismatch Negativity: Oddball versus Control Paradigm. J Clin Neurol 8: 35–42.

49. Sauseng P, Griesmayr B, Freunberger R, Klimesch W (2010) Control mechanisms in working memory: A possible function of EEG theta oscillations. Neurosci Biobehav Rev 34: 1015–1022.

50. Delorme A, Makeig S (2004) EEGLAB: an open source toolbox for analysis of single-trial EEG dynamics including independent component analysis. J Neurosci Methods 134: 9–21.

51. Guthrie D, Buchwald JS (1991) Significance testing of difference potentials. Psychophysiology 28: 240–244.

52. Sauseng P, Klimesch W (2008) What does phase information of oscillatory brain activity tell us about cognitive processes? Neurosci Biobehav Rev 32: 1001–1013.

53. Klimesch W, Hanslmayr S, Sauseng P, Gruber WR (2006) Distinguishing the evoked response from phase reset: A comment to Mäkinen, et al. Neuroimage 29: 808–811.

54. Makeig S, Westerfield M, Jung TP, Enghoff S, Townsend J, et al. (2002) Dynamic brain sources of visual evoked responses. Science (80-) 295: 690–694.

55. Sauseng P, Klimesch W, Gruber WR, Hanslmayr S, Freunberger R, et al. (2007) Are event-related potential components generated by phase resetting of brain oscillations? A critical discussion. Neuroscience 146: 1435–1444.

56. Yeung N, Bogacz R, Holroyd C, Nieuwenhuis S, Cohen J (2007) Theta phase resetting and the error-related negativity. Psychophysiology 44: 39–49.

57. Näätänen R, Paavilainen P, Rinne T, Alho K (2007) The mismatch negativity (MMN) in basic research of central auditory processing: A review. Clin Neurophysiol 118: 2544–2590.

2

Event-Related Brain Potentials during a Semantic Priming Task in Children with Learning Disabilities not Otherwise Specified

Thalía Fernández[1], Juan Silva-Pereyra[2]*, Belén Prieto-Corona[2], Mario Rodríguez-Camacho[2], Vicenta Reynoso-Alcántara[3]

1 Departamento de Neurobiología Conductual y Cognitiva, Instituto de Neurobiología, Universidad Nacional Autónoma de México, Juriquilla, Querétaro, México, 2 Proyecto de Neurociencias, Facultad de Estudios Superiores (FES) Iztacala, Universidad Nacional Autónoma de México, Estado de México, México, 3 Facultad de Psicología, Universidad Veracruzana, Campus Xalapa, Veracruz, México

Abstract

Learning disabilities (LDs) are the most common psychiatric disorders in children. LDs are classified either as "Specific" or "Learning Disorder Not Otherwise Specified". An important hypothesis suggests a failure in general domain process (i.e., attention) that explains global academic deficiencies. The aim of this study was to evaluate event-related potential (ERP) patterns of LD Not Otherwise Specified children with respect to a control group. Forty-one children (8–10.6 years old) participated and performed a semantic judgment priming task while ERPs were recorded. Twenty-one LD children had significantly lower scores in all academic skills (reading, writing and arithmetic) than twenty controls. Different ERP patterns were observed for each group. Control group showed smaller amplitudes of an anterior P200 for unrelated than related word pairs. This P200 effect was followed by a significant early N400a effect (greater amplitudes for unrelated than related word pairs; 350–550 ms) with a right topographical distribution. By contrast, LD Not Otherwise Specified group did not show a P200 effect or a significant N400a effect. This evidence suggests that LD Not Otherwise Specified children might be deficient in reading, writing and arithmetic domains because of their sluggish shifting of attention to process the incoming information.

Editor: J Bruce Morton, University of Western Ontario, Canada

Funding: This research was partially supported by grants IN226001 and IN204103 from PAPIIT UNAM-México, and by grants E59 from CONCYTEQ and 69145 from CONACYT, México. The funders had no role in study design, data collection and analysis, decision to publish, or preparation of the manuscript.

Competing Interests: The authors have declared that no competing interests exist.

* Email: jsilvapereyra@gmail.com

Introduction

Learning disabilities

Learning disabilities (LDs) are the most common psychiatric disorders in children during their school years [1]. Various groups estimate the prevalence of children with specific learning disabilities to be between 4–10% of all school-aged children [2,3,4], but the prevalence of LDs varies widely depending upon operational criteria [5]. According to the American Psychiatric Association [6], LDs are diagnosed when an individual's achievement on individually administered, standardized tests in reading, mathematics, or written expression is substantially below that expected for their particular age, schooling, and level of intelligence. LDs are classified either as "specific" (reading disorder, math disorder, or disorder of written expression) or "learning disorder not otherwise specified" (when the impairments do not satisfy the criteria of any specific learning disability). This latter category includes observed deficiencies in reading, mathematics, and written expression that may significantly interfere with academic performance even if the individual's performance on standardized tests is not substantially below the expected performance for the individual's age, IQ, and grade level.

While efforts have been made to elucidate the underlying cognitive deficits in children with LDs, there is no uniform hypothesis that affords definite knowledge of their causes [7]. Learning disabilities could be due to atypical brain functions, reflected as neurobiological disorders of cognitive processing [8]. There are two main hypotheses with regard to atypical processing patterns underlying LDs [5]. First, the *common deficit hypothesis* postulates that certain patterns of processing are common to all LD children. Second, the *domain-specific cognitive deficit hypothesis* proposes the existence of LD subgroups with specific deficits. Supporting the first hypothesis, Swanson [9] proposed that LD children fail in mechanisms of executive functioning, which also points to working memory (WM) deficits as essential problems in children and adults with LDs [10,11], specifically in Baddeley's proposed phonological loop and central executive [5,12,13,14,15]. Meanwhile, Hari and Renvall [16] postulate sluggish shifting of attention as the source of reading acquisition disorders [17]. Both theoretical frameworks could explain the global deficiencies of LD Not Otherwise Specified.

With respect to the second hypothesis, Siegel [18] contends that there is evidence for independent subgroups of LD children who exhibit distinctive characteristics and existing conditions that consistently predict specific patterns of learning difficulties. For example, children who have reading disabilities have problems with language skills, reading, rapid naming, and spelling. They also have deficiencies in morphological, semantic, and syntactic skills as well as deficits in lexical access, most likely because they have poorer vocabularies [5,7,8,19]. Semantic memory deficiencies arise in this hypothesized subgroup when verbal information is included. Specifically, in LD children and children at risk for dyslexia, some studies that used word pairs or sentences have shown deficiencies in semantic priming tasks [20,21].

Semantic priming and ERP

Priming is a phenomenon that, under certain circumstances, can facilitate stimulus processing given the prior processing of a similar stimulus. Although the evaluation of semantic priming frequently employs lexical decision tasks [22,23], the priming effect can also be evaluated with tasks in which the subject must decide whether two words are semantically related or not. A neurophysiological technique employed to assess different neural processes involved in semantic priming is the method of the Event-Related Potentials (ERPs), which represent brain electrical activity temporally associated with the processing of an event, which can be a sensory, motor, or cognitive process [24]. Among the ERPs studied in Specific LD children are the P200 and N400 components. P200 has been associated with the re-allocation of attentional resources and stimulus evaluation [25]. The P200 amplitude decreases with age [26] but increases with task difficulty [26,27]. Recent studies have related P200 to an attentional state in preparation for linguistic stimuli that can be anticipated from the sentence context [28,29]. The N400 ERP component is consistently associated with semantic priming. The N400 is a negative wave that occurs approximately 400 milliseconds after the stimulus in adults [30]. It is elicited during the processing of both written and spoken words. The amplitude of the N400 is modulated as a function of the ease with which a word can be integrated within a higher-order representation of a preceding word or sentence context [31]. Although N400 is sensitive to higher-level factors that have an effect on meaning processing, in some circumstances, it can also be sensitive to lower-level factors (i.e., pre-lexical factors). Typically, the amplitude of the N400 is augmented in response to words that are semantically unprimed (semantically unexpected), i.e., for target words that are not preceded by a related word.

ERP studies analyzing individuals with LDs have also shown contradictory results. Some of these studies showed delayed and attenuated N400 effects during sentence reading [32] and during semantic word priming [27]. A combined functional Magnetic Resonance Image (fMRI) and ERP study revealed reduced N400 effects in dyslexics compared with a control group [33]. In contrast, other studies have found no differences from controls, which could suggest entirely different cognitive profiles in children with LDs. For example, Silva-Pereyra et al. [34] observed normal N400 priming effects in children with reading disorders, and Russeler, Probst, Johannes, and Münte [35] also observed normal N400 effects in adults with reading disorders. Semantic priming seems relatively intact in reading-disabled children; however, neural responses to contextual incongruence are delayed [36].

Surprisingly, ERP studies that include different subtypes of LD children are scarce. Distinct cognitive profiles were observed in LD reading- and arithmetic-disabled children in one ERP semantic priming study [37]. These subgroups were defined by deficient performance on tests of reading and spelling (Group RS) and arithmetic (Group A). Children had to attend to and name pictures and words that varied in their degree of semantic relatedness. In Group RS, children exhibited reduced N400

amplitudes relative to controls, whereas their ERPs in response to pictures were normal, pointing to specific deficiencies in linguistic processing. By contrast, Group A did not exhibit reliable early frontal negative waves, an effect potentially related to a selective attention deficit in these children. These early processing differences were also evidenced by N400 waves of smaller amplitude.

The present study

Most studies of children with LD have focused on the specific type, especially in those children with reading disorders, which could explain why there is no cognitive or neurobiological profile that describes children with LD Not Otherwise Specified, although they are more prevalent than those with Specific LDs [38]. Previous studies on LD suggest that general deficiencies of children with LD Not Otherwise Specified do involve different cognitive areas related to their school activities (i.e., reading, writing, and arithmetic), because alteration of a general domain process could influence almost every aspect of learning, which would be consistent with the common deficit hypothesis. If results from studies of a Specific LD show deficiencies of semantic processing that are reflected in a decrease of N400 amplitude, it is very probable that children with LD Not Otherwise Specified will also display a pattern of N400 that is different from a control group and probably also from that of children with a specific LD. But more important, if we think that deficiencies of children with LD Not Otherwise Specified are due to a failure in a general domain process or process in common, this fact would be reflected in a different amplitude pattern of the P200, because this ERP component has been associated with the attention process [25]. Therefore, the aim of this study was to assess the ERP pattern of children with LD Not Otherwise Specified during a semantic judgment task.

Materials and Methods

Participants

Forty-one children participated in this study. All of the children were volunteers selected from groups of third and fourth graders at two elementary schools. The children had no major cultural disadvantages (in all cases, the mother had at least a primary education, and the family per capita income was above the minimum wage level), all were right-handed, and their neurological exams were normal. All children were assessed with the Child Neuropsychological Assessment (Evaluación Neurológica Infantil, ENI) [39] standardized for the Mexican population, the Wechsler Intelligence Scale for Children – Revised (WISC-R) [40], and the Conners' Rating Scales – Revised [41]. The children did not show evidence of any psychiatric disorders beyond their LDs, and none met the criteria to be diagnosed with ADHD. Only three domains of the Child Neuropsychological Assessment ENI were evaluated: writing, reading, and arithmetic. Within each domain, we evaluated three variables: accuracy, comprehension, and speed of reading; accuracy, composition and speed of writing as well as counting, numbering (i.e., number comparison), and arithmetic calculations.

Twenty-one children (5 females) with Learning Disabilities Not Otherwise Specified were selected; they had an average age of 9.46±.98 years and an intelligence quotient [40] greater than 80 (Verbal scale 88.29±17.93; Performance scale: 96.29±16.15; Total IQ: 91.52±17.14). These children were referred by a social worker because they had academic performance issues and ranked below the 11th percentile at least on two domains of the Children's Neuropsychological Evaluation [39].

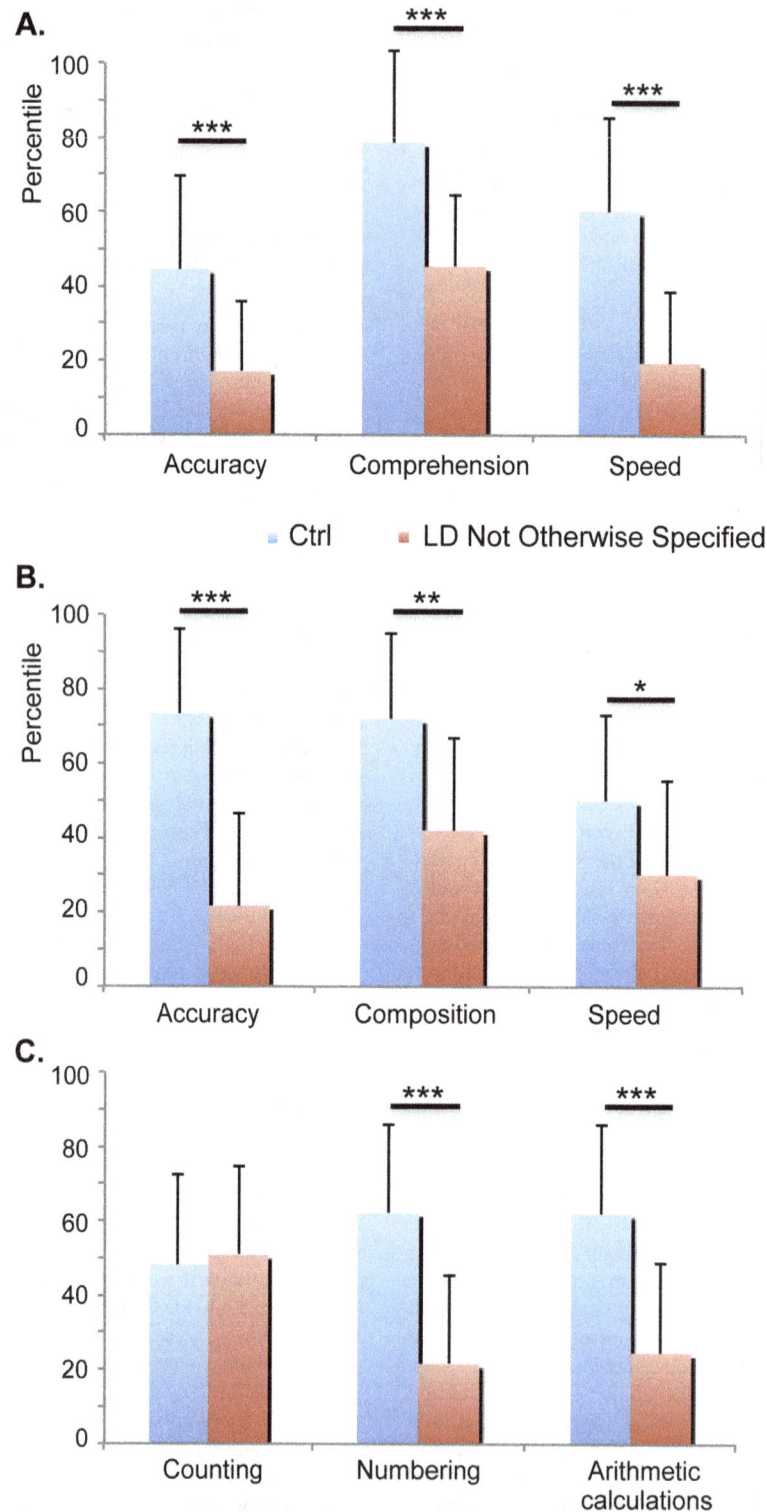

Figure 1. Mean percentile values of groups from subtests of the reading, writing, and arithmetic tests. A. Reading: The LD group showed lower scores than Ctrl group in all measurements. **B. Writing:** The LD group mainly showed lower scores for accuracy and composition than the Ctrl group. **C. Arithmetic:** The LD group showed much lower scores on the arithmetic calculations and numbering than and Ctrl group. Significant differences are marked with asterisks: *p<.05, **p<.01, ***p<.001.

Twenty right-handed children (11 females) participated in the study as controls (Ctrl). Their ages ranged from 7 to 12 years old (mean 9.18, standard deviation ±1.25), and each of them had a total intelligence quotient that was within the normal range or higher than average (Verbal scale, 107.7±13.67; Performance scale, 106.45±13.25; Total IQ, 107.7±11.95; evaluated with the

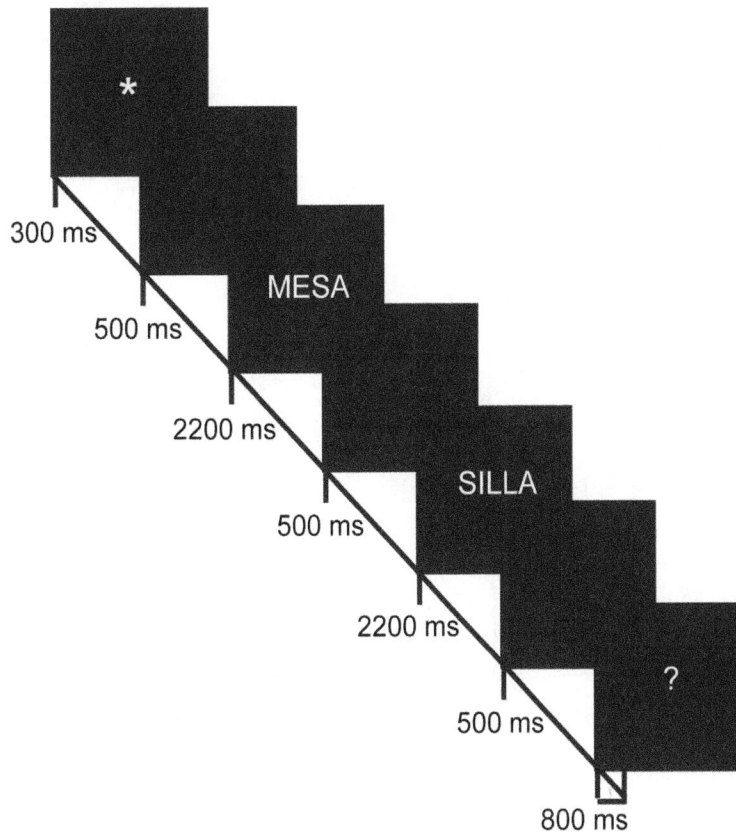

Figure 2. The timing and presentation sequence of stimuli in each trial.

Wechsler Intelligence Scale for Children-Revised [40]. The children scored within the normal limits in subtests of the Children's Neuropsychological Evaluation.

Groups did not differ significantly with respect to age (F<1). However, the groups differed in total IQ (F(1,39) = 12.17, p = .001) and if verbal and executive IQ were included as within-subject factor, a Group by IQ subscales interaction was significant (F(1,39) = 4.03, p = .052). The LD Not Otherwise Specified group had lower IQ scores than the Ctrl group (Tukey's honest significant difference test, MD$_{HSD}$ = 19.41, p<.001 for verbal IQ and MD$_{HSD}$ = 10.16, p = .034 for performance IQ). No child presented with mental retardation. A three-way ANOVA was performed to assess differences between groups across academic skills (i.e., reading, writing, and arithmetic) in the three different measurements of each skill (i.e., accuracy, precision and comprehension-composition for writing-, counting, numbering and arithmetic calculations) and differences are shown in Figure 1.

Significant Group by Academic skills by Measurement interaction (F(4,156) = 7.22, p<.001, epsilon = .989) shows greater scores of Ctrl group than LD for every variable in the reading, writing, and arithmetic domains with the exception of the Counting subtest, where no differences between groups were observed.

Ethics statement

All the procedures were in line with the Declaration of Helsinki for human research [42]. The Ethics Committee of the Institute of Neurobiology, National Autonomous University of Mexico, approved the experimental protocol. Parents and children provided written informed consent for their participation in this study. Legally, on behalf of children enrolled, parents as their legal guardians signed written informed consent forms.

Stimuli

A list of 120 pairs of words, including 60 related and 60 unrelated word pairs, were obtained from children's literature sources [43,44,45,46,47,48,49,50]. All words had a single meaning (according to the Dictionary of the Royal Spanish Academy, 2003). A word pair was considered related if the words belonged to the same semantic category. Unrelated word pairs did not belong to the same semantic category. Word pairs had to meet the criterion that the second word could not begin or end with the same phoneme as the first. We included several semantic categories: animals, toys, furniture, food, clothing, body parts, musical instruments, professions, places, and tools. All words were singular nouns with one to three syllables, written in Spanish, with no umlauts. Words were displayed in 1-cm uppercase letters in the center of a 14-inch computer monitor (white letters on a black screen). At the viewing distance employed, each letter subtended a visual angle of 0.573×0.573 degrees.

Procedure

Word pairs were randomly presented. Participants were instructed to respond by pressing one button of a mouse if the second word of the pair was related and a different button if it was not. Because the subjects naturally took the mouse in both hands and used their thumbs to press the buttons, the use of the mouse button was counterbalanced across left- and right-handed subjects.

The stimuli were delivered through Mind Tracer software (Neuronic S.A., México D.F., México). Each trial began with the

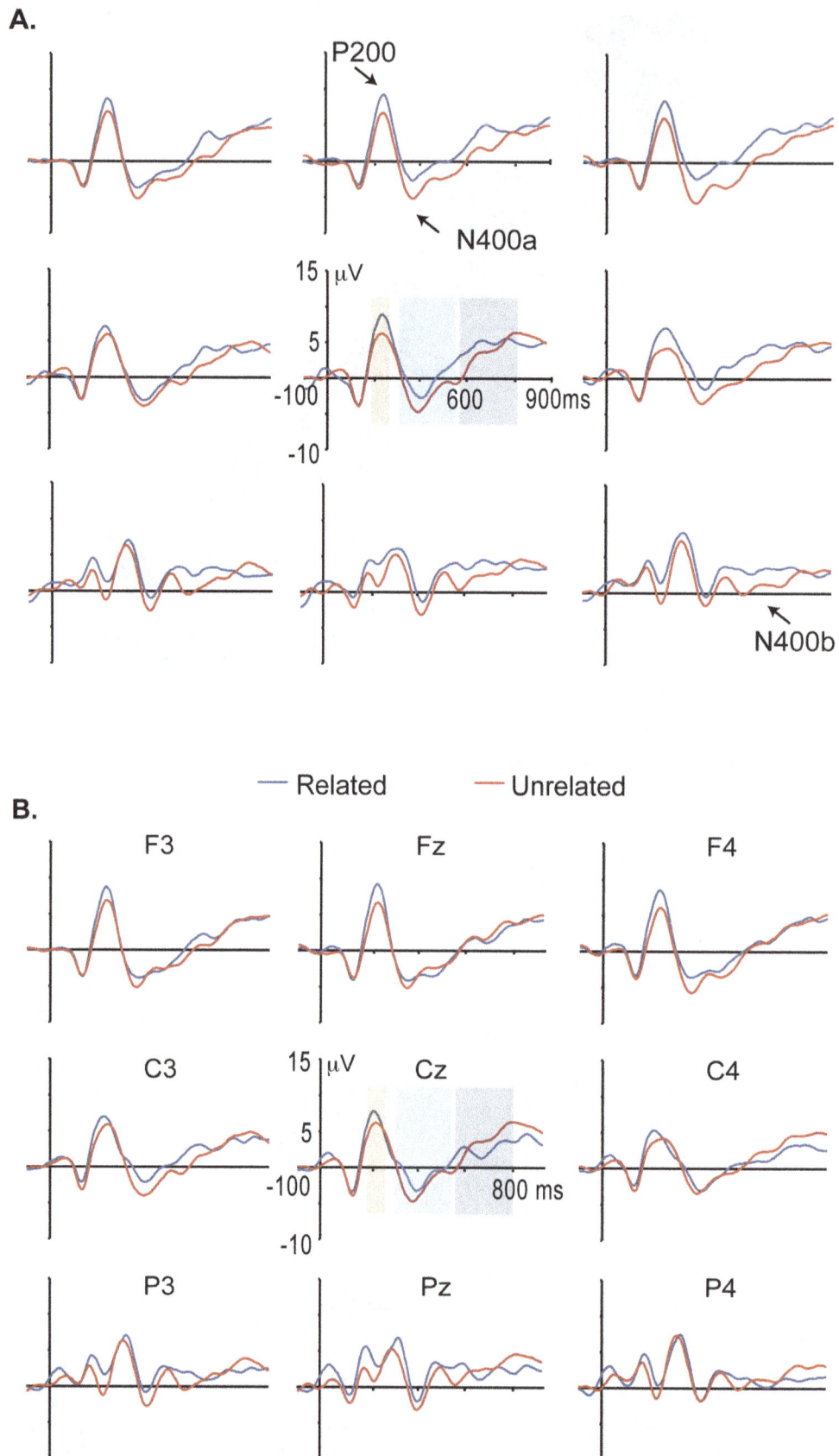

Figure 3. ERP wave grand averages across nine electrode sites of A. Ctrl children and B. LD Not Otherwise Specified children.
Responses to related and unrelated word pairs are represented by the blue and red lines respectively. Negativity is plotted downwards. A P200 effect in anterior regions was observed in the Ctrl (i.e., greater amplitudes to related pairs). Unrelated word pairs elicited greater amplitudes of N400a than those elicited by related pairs on anterior right regions in the Ctrl group but this effect was not significant in the LD group.

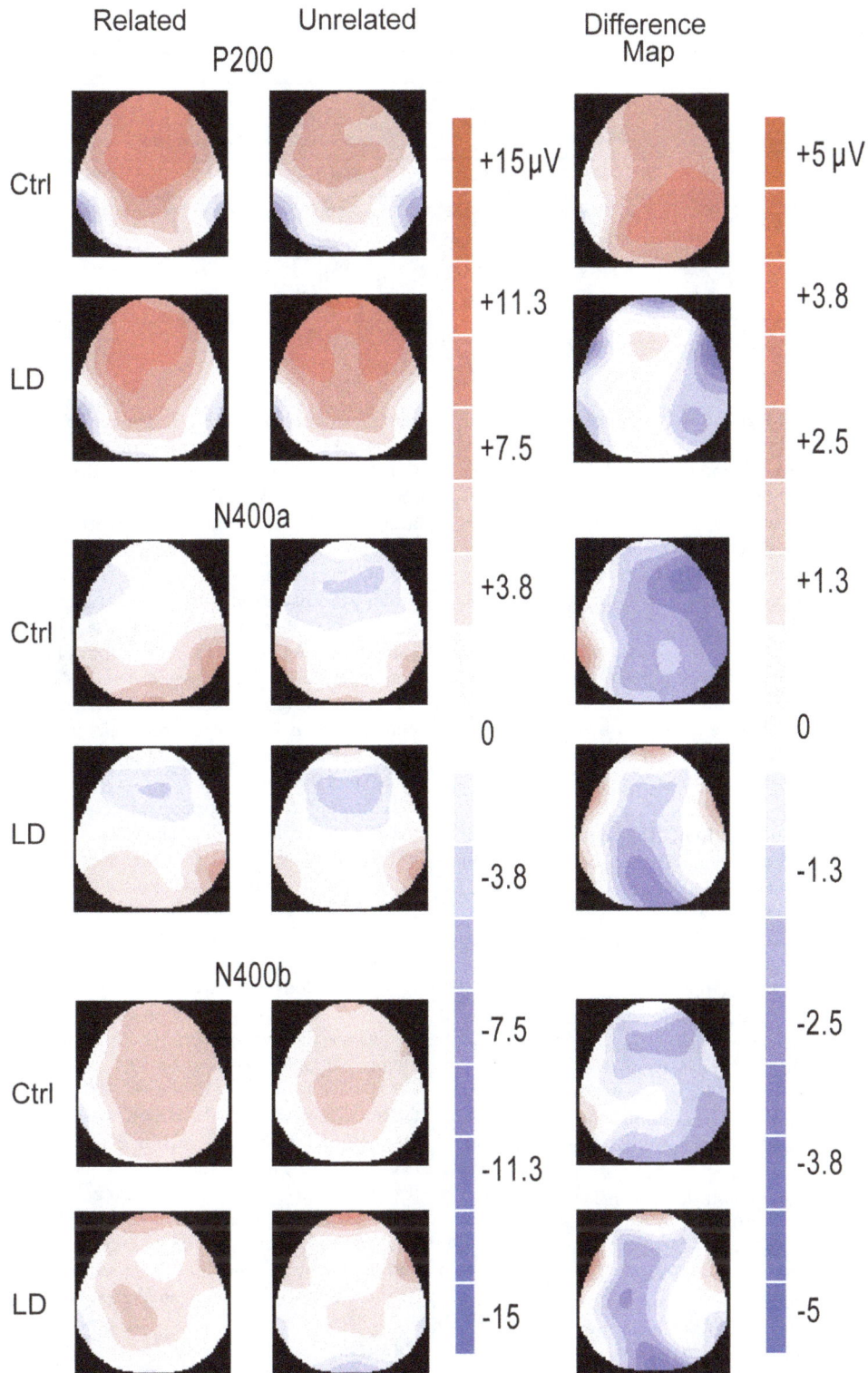

Figure 4. Amplitude Maps per experimental condition and Maps of difference waves for each ERP component in each group. Unrelated word pairs elicited an amplitude effect at approximately 400 ms with right distribution in the Ctrl group.

presentation of a warning signal (an asterisk) for 300 ms at the center of a computer monitor. Next, after 500 ms of dark screen, the first word of the pair was presented for 2200 ms; 500 ms later, the second word was presented for 2200 ms. Finally, 500 ms later, a question mark (?) was presented for 800 ms, and an additional 1200 ms was allowed for answering. The children were instructed to respond as rapidly and accurately as possible to each stimulus, but they had to wait to respond until after the question mark appeared. If a child took more than 2 seconds to respond, the trial was considered to be a "no response", and the presentation of a

Table 1. Behavioral data by Group of children.

		Groups			
		Control		LD Not Otherwise Specified	
		Mean	SD	Mean	SD
RT	Related pairs	522.40	188.50	595.52	167.51
	Unrelated pairs	549.25	192.60	667.29	182.64
% CR	Related pairs	85.74	10.94	74.76	16.72
	Unrelated pairs	88.92	8.47	75.45	13.20

RT = reaction time; % CR = Percentage of Correct responses; SD = standard deviation.

new sequence was initiated. Figure 2 shows the stimuli presentation sequence.

Before performing the experimental task, each participant was given a short test to verify that he/she understood the task and was familiar with the activity. The subject was comfortably seated in front of the computer monitor at a distance of 50 cm for stimulus presentation. The task was divided into 4 blocks of 30 word pairs each. Each block lasted approximately 4 minutes. A short break was given to the children between blocks. To determine the time stimulus parameters, a pilot study was conducted with 12 adults and then with another sample of 8 elementary school children. From this study, we estimated that the time of presentation of the word needed to be at least 2200 ms to be read by young readers and children with reading disorders.

ERP recording

EEGs were recorded with a MEDICID-4 system (Neuronic S.A., México D.F., México) from 19 leads of the 10–20 International System (Fp1, Fp2, F3, F4, C3, C4, P3, P4, O1, O2, F7, F8, T3, T4, T5, T6, Fz, Cz, and Pz) in a standard electrocap (Electro-Cap International Inc., Ohio, USA) referenced to the short-circuited earlobes (A1–A2). The amplifier bandwidth was set between 0.05 and 30 Hz. All electrode impedances were at or below 5 k Ohms, and the signal was amplified with a gain of 20,000. The EEG was digitized at a sampling rate of 200 Hz and stored on a hard disk for further analysis. Blinking and eye movements were monitored from a supra-orbital electrode and from an electrode placed at the external canthus of the right eye. Trials with artifacts due to eye movements or excessive muscle activity were eliminated off-line before averaging. A pre-stimulus time of 100 ms was used to establish the baseline.

Artifact-free EEG segments 1000-ms in length with a 100-ms pre-stimulus time were selected and synchronized with the second word of the pair. At least 25 segments were required from each of the two experimental conditions (i.e., related and unrelated word pairs). Segments were selected only when the answer was correct. Approximately equal numbers of EEG segments were included in the averages for each experimental condition across subjects.

Data analysis

For behavioral data, the median reaction time (RT) for correct responses was calculated for each subject, and the data were used to perform a two-way ANOVA. The variables included were Group (Ctrl and LD) and Semantic judgment (related and unrelated). The percentages of correct responses were transformed using an ARCSIN [SQRT (percentage/100)] transformation, and these data were used to perform a two-way ANOVA with the same factors used in the RT analysis. Tukey's honest significant difference post hoc tests were completed after the ANOVA.

ERPs from correct responses were obtained for each group (Ctrl and LD) and each experimental condition. Figure 3 shows grand average ERPs and Figure 4 displays the voltage maps of related and unrelated word pairs. Visual inspection reveals that in control group, at approximately 200 milliseconds on frontocentral regions, brainwaves associated with unrelated pairs were smaller (i.e., less positive) than those associated with the related pairs. This effect is commonly referred to as a P200 and this finding is very similar to that reported by Silva-Pereyra et al. [34]. The P200 effect was followed by a typical N400 effect, showing larger amplitudes for unrelated than for related word pairs (i.e., more negative). This effect started at approximately 300-ms and was maintained for more than 500 ms.

According to their appearance in the grand average waveforms, the P200 was considered for analysis as mean amplitude within the interval of 180–250 ms. Due to the long duration of the N400, we decided to divide it into two time windows as others have done [36], thus the N400a was considered the mean amplitude within the interval of 300–550 ms, and the N400b was defined as the mean amplitude within the interval of 555–800 ms.

Separate four-way ANOVAs were performed on amplitude data for each ERP component without midline electrodes using Group as between-subject factor, and Semantic judgment, Hemisphere (left and right) and Electrode site (Fp1, Fp2 F3, F4, C3, C4, P3, P4, F7, F8, T3, T4, T5, T6, O1, O2) as within-subject factors. Three-way ANOVAs were performed on amplitude data for each ERP component with midline electrodes using Group as between-subject factor, and Semantic judgment and Electrode site (Fz, Cz, Pz) as within-subject factors. The Huynh-Feldt epsilon was applied to the degrees of freedom of those analyses with more than one degree of freedom in the numerator. Corrected p-values and epsilon were reported. Tukey's honest significant difference (HSD) post-hoc tests were completed after the ANOVA.

Results

Behavioral data

There was no significant main effect of Group on reaction times (F(1, 39) = 2.91, p = .096) but there was a significant Group by Semantic judgment interaction (F(1, 39) = 4.14, p = .049). Tukey's HSD post hoc analyses showed priming effects (i.e., faster responses to related than to unrelated pairs) for the LD group (mean of differences: MD_{HSD} = 71.76 ms, p<.001) but not for Ctrl (MD_{HSD} = 26.85 ms, p = .097) group (see Table 1). Reaction time differences between groups were for unrelated pairs (MD_{HSD} = 118.04 ms, p = .05). Transformed percentages of cor-

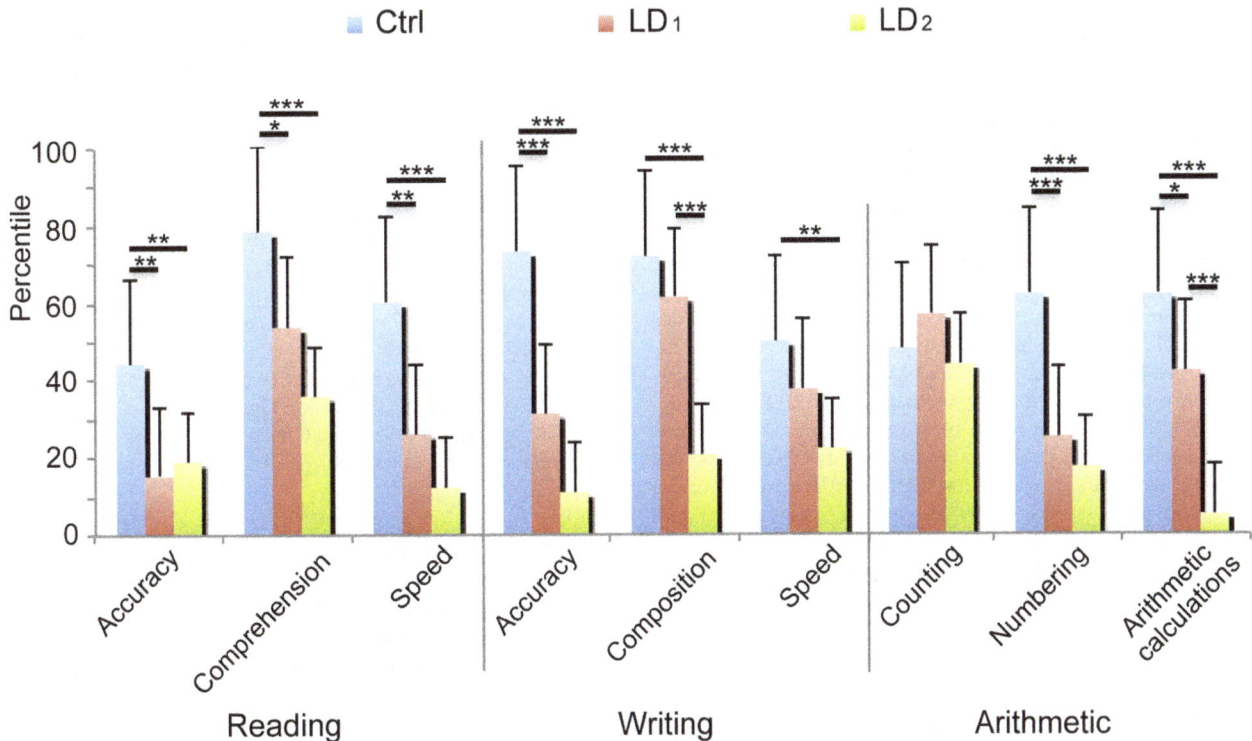

Figure 5. Mean percentile values of three groups (Ctrl, LD₁ and LD₂) from all subtests of the reading, writing, and arithmetic tests. LD₁ group shows greater scores than LD₂ group only in Composition subtest from Writing and Arithmetic calculations subtest from Arithmetic. Significant differences are marked with asterisks: *p<.05, **p<.01, ***p<.001.

rect responses were employed to perform a two-way ANOVA with the same factors used in the RT analysis. This analysis showed greater percentage of correct responses for the Ctrl group (Mean = 87.33%) than for the LD group (75.11%) (F(1, 39) = 11.78, p = .001), but there was no significant Group by Semantic judgment interaction (F(1, 39) = 1.86, p = .18).

ERP data

P200 (180−250 ms). In this time window, for the analysis without midline electrodes there was a significant Group by Semantic judgment interaction (F(1, 39) = 5.8, p = .021), which indicated smaller amplitudes of the P200 to Ctrl than LD group for unrelated word-pairs experimental condition (MD$_{HSD}$ = − 2.43 μV, p = .03). This interaction also showed smaller amplitudes for unrelated than for related word pairs in the Ctrl group (MD$_{HSD}$ = 1.81 μV, p = .04) but no differences for LD group (MD$_{HSD}$ = −1.08 μV, p = .21). Such P200 effect was lateralized (Group × Semantic judgment × Hemisphere, F(1, 39) = 4.38, p = .043) to the right hemisphere for Ctrl group (MD$_{HSD}$ = 2.3 μV, p = .01). There were no significant Group × Semantic judgment × Electrode site (F<1) and Group × Semantic judgment × Hemisphere × Electrode site interactions (F(7, 273) = 1.22, p = .304, epsilon = .579), and there was no significant main effect of Group (F(1,39) = 1.463, p = .234).

For the ANOVA using midline electrodes, there was no significant main effect of Group (F<1), nor Group by Semantic judgment (F(1, 39) = 2.28, p = .139) and Group by Semantic judgment by Midline electrodes interactions (F<1).

N400a (300−550 ms). For the ANOVA without midline electrodes there was a significant Group by Semantic judgment by Hemisphere interaction (F(1, 39) = 5.41, p = .025). This interaction showed greater amplitudes for unrelated than for related word

pairs on the right hemisphere in the Ctrl group (MD$_{HSD}$ = 2.36 μV, p = .036) but no differences for LD group (MD$_{HSD}$ = .235 μV, p = .83). This ANOVA also revealed no other significant interactions (Group × Semantic judgment interaction F<1; Group × Semantic judgment × Electrode site interaction F(7, 273) = 1.12, p = .341, epsilon = .372; Group × Semantic judgment × Hemisphere × Electrode site interaction F(7, 273) = 1.733, p = .127, epsilon = .733). No main effect of Group (F<1) was observed.

For the analysis using midline electrodes, there was no significant main effect of Group (F<1), and Group by Semantic judgment (F<1) and Group by Semantic judgment by Midline electrodes interactions (F(2, 78) = 1.837, p = .171, epsilon = .88).

N400 b (555−800 ms). In this time window, there was no significant main effect of Group (F<1) and there were no significant interactions (Group × Semantic judgment interaction F<1; Group × Semantic judgment × Electrode site F<1; Group × Semantic judgment × Hemisphere F(1,3 9) = 1.722, p = .197; Group × Semantic judgment × Hemisphere × Electrode site interaction F<1).

For the analysis using midline electrodes there was a marginal main effect of Group (F(1, 39) = 3.58, p = .066), but no significant interactions (Group × Semantic judgment F<1; Group × Semantic judgment × Midline electrodes F<1).

Data reanalysis separating LD Not Otherwise Specified into two groups

A hierarchical cluster analysis was applied to identify possible homogeneous subgroups of children with LD Not Otherwise Specified. Percentiles from three tests of the neuropsychological battery ENI (reading comprehension, writing composition, and arithmetic calculations) were used in this analysis, which was completed using the Ward method with a measure of squared Euclidean distance. Once the clusters were obtained, a one-way ANOVA was performed to assess differences between groups in academic skills (reading, writing, and arithmetic) as shown in Figure 5. The Huynh-Feldt epsilon was applied to the degrees of freedom of those analyses with more than one degree of freedom in the numerator and it was reported. Tukey's honest significant difference (HSD) post-hoc tests were completed after the ANOVA.

A visual inspection of the dendrogram revealed two independent clusters almost equal in size and with different characteristics. The following two groups were obtained: LD_1: n = 11 (4 female, age 9.36±.77; total IQ: 99.36±10.41; verbal IQ: 95.36±18.53; performance IQ: 103.82±17.53); and LD_2: n = 10 (1 female, age 9.57±1.2; total IQ: 82.9±10.89; verbal IQ: 80.5±14.31; performance IQ: 88±9.63). As it can be seen at Figure 5, there were differences between LD subgroups in several subscales of the neuropsychological test (F(8, 152) = 4.64, p<.001, epsilon = .975). LD_2 group showed lower scores in writing composition, and arithmetic calculations than LD_1 who showed lower scores in reading accuracy, reading speed, reading comprehension, writing accuracy, numbering and arithmetic calculations than the Ctrl group. The LD_2 group showed lower scores in reading accuracy, reading comprehension, reading speed, writing accuracy, writing composition, writing speed, numbering, and arithmetic calculations than the Ctrl group.

Groups (Ctrl, LD_1 LD_2) did not differ significantly with respect to age (F<1), however, the groups differed in total IQ (F(2, 38) = 10.86, p<.001), Ctrl had greater IQ scores than LD_2 (MD_{HSD} = 24.8, p<.001), LD_1 also had significantly greater IQ scores than LD_2 (MD_{HSD} = 16.464, p = .009), but there were no differences between Ctrl and LD_1 (MD_{HSD} = 8.336, p = .114). ANOVA results including verbal and performance IQ scores as within-subject factor showed also differences between groups (F(2, 38) = 11.156, p<.001) as the previous result only using total IQ scores as variable. There was no Group by Verbal and Performance IQ scores interaction (F(2, 38) = 1.98, p = .153).

Behavioral data

A two-way ANOVA was performed with the behavioral data using the two groups obtained from cluster analysis and our Ctrl group (Ctrl, LD_1, and LD_2) as between-subject factor and Semantic judgment (related and unrelated) as within-subject factor. There were no significant main effect of Group on reaction times (F(2, 38) = 1.525, p = .23) neither significant Group by Semantic judgment interaction (F(2, 38) = 2.06, p = .14). However, there was a significant main effect of Group regarding percentage of correct responses (F(2, 38) = 8.34, p = .001). This result indicates a greater percentage of correct responses for the Ctrl group relative to the LD_2 group (MD_{HSD} = .24, p<.001), LD_1 also displayed greater percentage than LD_2 group (MD_{HSD} = .134, p = .05), but there were no significant differences between Ctrl and LD_1 (MD_{HSD} = .11, p = .071). The Group by Semantic judgment interaction was not significant for the percentage of correct responses (F<1).

ERP data

Three time windows were used as in the previous analysis (i.e., P2: 180–250 ms, N400a: 300–550 ms, and N400b: 555–800 ms) and Group factor now included: Ctrl, LD_1 and LD_2.

P200

ANOVA without midline electrodes showed a significant Group by Semantic judgment interaction (F(2,38) = 6.64, p = .003),

showing smaller amplitudes of the P200 to Ctrl than LD_2 group for unrelated word-pairs experimental condition (MD_{HSD} = −3.59 µV, p = .008). This interaction also shows smaller amplitudes for unrelated than for related word pairs in the Ctrl group (MD_{HSD} = 1.81 µV, p = .03), in contrast, LD_2 group displayed the inverse pattern (MD_{HSD} = −3.19 µV, p = .008) and LD_1 showed no differences between conditions (MD_{HSD} = .85 µV, p = .44). Results also showed no significant Group by Semantic judgment by Electrode site (F<1), Group by Semantic judgment by Hemisphere (F(2, 38) = 2.14, p = .13) and Group by Semantic judgment by Hemisphere by Electrode site (F(14, 266) = 1.19, p = .308, epsilon = .567) interactions, and there was no significant main effect of Group (F<1).

For the analysis using midline electrodes there was no significant main effect of Group (F<1), nor Group by Semantic judgment (F(2, 38) = 2.12, p = .135) and Group by Semantic judgment by Midline electrodes interactions (F<1).

N400a

Analysis without including midline electrodes showed that Group by Semantic judgment by Hemisphere interaction was marginally significant (F(2, 38) = 2.9, p = .067). This interaction shows greater amplitudes for LD_1 than LD_2 in unrelated word pairs on the left hemisphere (MD_{HSD} = −3.203 µV, p = .045). This effect also shows greater amplitudes for unrelated than related word pairs for Ctrl group on the right hemisphere (MD_{HSD} = 2.36 µV, p = .033) in contrast to LD_1 (MD_{HSD} = 1.72 µV, p = .24) and LD_2 (MD_{HSD} = −1.40 µV, p = .36) where no differences were observed. This ANOVA also revealed no other significant interactions (Group × Semantic judgment interaction F(2, 38) = 1.95, p = .16; Group × Semantic judgment × Electrode site interaction F(14, 266) = 1.11, p = .363, epsilon = .382; Group × Semantic judgment × Hemisphere × Electrode site interaction F(14, 266) = 1.35, p = .203, epsilon = .74). No main effect of Group (F<1) was observed.

For the analysis using midline electrodes there was no significant main effect of Group (F<1), nor Group by Semantic judgment (F<1) and Group by Semantic judgment by Midline electrodes (F(4, 76) = 1.88, p = .131, epsilon = .89).

N400b

There was no significant main effect of Group (F<1) and there were no significant interactions for ANOVA without midline electrodes (Group × Semantic judgment interaction F<1; Group × Semantic judgment × Electrode site interaction F<1; Group × Semantic judgment × Hemisphere interaction F<1; Group × Semantic judgment × Hemisphere × Electrode site interaction F(14, 266) = 1.36, p = .22, epsilon = .566).

For the analysis using midline electrodes there was no significant main effect of Group (F(2, 38) = 1.93, p = .16) nor significant interactions (Group × Semantic judgment F<1; Group × Semantic judgment × Midline electrodes F<1).

Discussion

The present study aimed to compare the ERP pattern of children with LD Not Otherwise Specified to that of a control group during a semantic judgment task, because there are no studies considering this type of LD. We think that general deficiencies across cognitive areas in LD Not Otherwise Specified are due to a general domain process failure, so first we expected children with LD and controls would show different P200 pattern and second, this attention problem (i.e., without any evidence of Attention Deficit Disorder) would probably also be reflected in a different N400 pattern, all of this in way similar to findings in Specific LD. Our results support this idea. LD Not Otherwise Specified children showed no differences in the P200 between related and unrelated word pairs. By contrast Ctrl group displayed larger P200 amplitudes in response to related than to unrelated word pairs, which was mainly observed over the frontal regions, as found previously in normal readers [34]. This group difference at P200 has been found in other studies using children with Specific LD i.e., reading disabled children [37]. Enhanced P200 responses have often been observed for words in constraining sentence contexts, perhaps reflecting a preparatory attentional response elicited by language contexts that generate a strong expectation for particular upcoming stimuli [28,29,51]. The formation of strong context-based expectations for upcoming words seems to change how the perceptual processing system allocates attention and analyzes subsequent stimuli [52]. Thus, a P200 amplitude pattern in children with LD Not Otherwise Specified or children with Specific LD that differs from the Ctrl group could reveal an attention deficit, i.e., a deficit in a general domain process. In fact, a previous study showed reduced P200 activation of the right superior parietal region (BA7) in poor readers relative to normal readers in cue condition trials during a visual continuous performance task [53]. Such P200 amplitude pattern in LD children with reading disabilities could support the common deficit hypothesis. So, differences in P200 found between groups suggest important attention differences when children include a word in a semantic category (as Federmeier's studies have indicated).

Probably these P200 ERP differences are reflected in important cognitive profile differences between groups; whereas the LD Not Otherwise Specified group showed severe deficiencies in all areas evaluated (i.e., reading speed and comprehension, writing accuracy and composition, numbering and arithmetic), the Ctrl group showed normal scores, and in fact, reflects differences at other ERP components related to later cognitive processes such as lexical and semantic processes. Thus, this study shows that Ctrl group displayed N400 effects (i.e., larger amplitudes for unrelated than related pairs) at 300 to 550 ms in contrast to our LD Not Otherwise Specified children who displayed no significant effect, as many others have shown with semantic priming tasks [34,36] but in children with Specific LD. At 555 to 800 ms however, there were no differences between groups. Here, N400 topographic differences between the groups were shown at plots of ERP grand averages where the Ctrl group showed an N400 effect on frontal sites, in line with previous studies performed with normal subjects [34,36]; however significant statistical differences were only observed on the right hemisphere.

Our findings certainly support the common deficit hypothesis, which is compatible with the Working Memory deficits [9] and Sluggish Attentional Shifting (SAS) [16] frameworks because it clusters all Specific LDs, and we would include here children with LD Not Otherwise Specified, into a common cognitive impairment. For example, according to SAS, when LD Not Otherwise Specified children deal with the stimulus sequences or word pairs, first, they have to efficiently read each stimulus presented, and after that, children have to judge if the pair belongs to the same semantic category, so their automatic attention system cannot disengage fast enough from one item to the next one, yielding slow and degraded processing. SAS is assumed to distort cortical networks such as those that support sublexical auditory-phonological and visual-orthographic representations. Consequently, it is possible to suggest that the global deficits in LD Not Otherwise Specified can be linked to a generally inefficient multi-sensory processing of perceptual stimulus. However, our findings cannot discard the idea that there is a failure in mechanisms of executive

functioning of working memory in children with LD Not Otherwise Specified [9], but it would be necessary to design an experiment ad hoc to link children's deficiencies to working memory mechanisms.

The altered attention pattern in children with LD Not Otherwise Specified may be due to multiple factors such as a great heterogeneity in their brain maturation. In fact, it has been suggested that the neurobiological maturation of cognition is reflected by the long time brain specialization areas take to mature [54]. The last brain area to mature is the frontal lobe, which is the region where one component of the P200 has its source [53]. Thus, these lower scores in the LD Not Otherwise Specified group probably reflect a lag in prefrontal maturation [55]. In fact, a large percentage of children with LD show EEG-delayed maturation [56,57], characterized by an excess of theta activity in frontal regions [58].

Now, small differences in the amplitude in the window of N400 found between groups may be due to other factors that arise as a consequence of an alteration in the attention process. That is, an initial deficiency in the attention mechanism may broadly directly influence other processes, such as lexical access and semantic judgment required to execute the task. Although statistically significant differences have not been shown between groups and between experimental conditions regarding behavioral results, in general children with LD Not Otherwise Specified show a lower number of correct answers. One explanation that would account for the bare differences in the N400 effect in this study and even others [35,36,40] whose results are not consistent [37,39], may be that the greater amplitude of P200 to unrelated stimuli makes it remain above the baseline that would be the beginning of N400. Therefore, by comparing both conditions (related vs. non-related), differences in amplitude would be reduced between the conditions of this latter component. One possibility that may be added to the above would be that the IQ scores may be an important marker of disadvantage of the LD Not Otherwise Specified, since statistically significant differences have been observed in scores in the verbal scale of IQ between groups of children. More so, upon dividing the LD into two groups according to the neuropsychological profile of ENI, group LD_2 that had lower IQ scores and more severe cognitive deficit presented an inverse pattern of P200 (i.e., greater amplitude for unrelated pairs than related ones) regarding controls, a fact that may influence in the N400 effect, as mentioned above, since LD_1 displayed a greater amplitude than LD_2 for unrelated pairs. These results suggest that, regardless of whether the LD is a type not otherwise specified or specific, the degree of deterioration in children's skills becomes most important, since it is clear that LD_2 group elicits a worst brain response than LD_1 in this semantic priming task.

In summary, children with LD Not Otherwise Specified showed an altered P200 that is similar to that reported in children with Specific LD (i.e., reading disabled). It is probable that the alteration in the N400 effect in these children is due to the lack of attention that is previous to semantic judgment required in the priming task. It is also feasible that differences in the N400 effect are due to a wave overlapping with the previous P200, a heterogeneity in the maturation of the frontal lobe, or even a low IQ.

Conclusions

According to the definition provided by the DSM-IV [6], children with LD evaluated in this study can be characterized as "Not Otherwise Specified". This kind of LD probably shows an important deficit in preparatory attention provoked by context and generating a strong expectation for the stimuli that are to appear. Similar to that reported for Specific LD, lack of attention in children with LD Not Otherwise Specified may be common to all LDs and affect, in a snowball effect, other cognitive processes such as lexical access and, later, semantic judgment. It will be necessary to obtain ERPs during writing and arithmetic tasks to further test the hypothesis of common deficit.

Acknowledgments

The authors are grateful for the participants' cooperation in this study. The authors also acknowledge the technical assistance of Javier Sánchez-López, Leonor Casanova, Lourdes Lara, Héctor Belmont and Rodrigo Silva Fernández, and Dorothy Pless for revising English style.

Author Contributions

Conceived and designed the experiments: TF JSP BPC MRC VRA. Performed the experiments: TF BPC VRA. Analyzed the data: TF JSP BPC MRC. Contributed reagents/materials/analysis tools: BPC VRA. Contributed to the writing of the manuscript: TF JSP BPC MRC VRA.

References

1. Handler SM, Fierson WM (2011) Learning disabilities, dyslexia, and vision. Pediatrics 127: e818–856.
2. Fletcher TV, Kaufman de Lopez CK (1995) A Mexican perspective on learning disabilities. J Learn Disabil 28: 530–534, 544.
3. Lagae L (2008) Learning disabilities: definitions, epidemiology, diagnosis, and intervention strategies. Pediatr Clin North Am 55: 1259–1268, vii.
4. Sotelo-Dynega M, Flanagan D, Alfonso V (2010) Overview Of Specific Learning Disabilities. In: Flanagan D, Alfonso V, editors. Essentials of Specific Learning Disability Identification. Hoboken, New Jersey: John Wiley & Sons, Inc. 1–20.
5. Landerl K, Fussenegger B, Moll K, Willburger E (2009) Dyslexia and dyscalculia: two learning disorders with different cognitive profiles. J Exp Child Psychol 103: 309–324.
6. American Psychiatric Association (2002) Manual Diagnóstico y Estadístico de los trastornos mentales, DSM-IV-TR. Barcelona: Masson.
7. Büttner G, Hasselhorn M (2011) Learning Disabilities: Debates on definitions, causes, subtypes, and responses. International Journal of Disability, Development and Education 58: 75–87.
8. Silver CH, Ruff RM, Iverson GL, Barth JT, Broshek DK, et al. (2008) Learning disabilities: the need for neuropsychological evaluation. Arch Clin Neuropsychol 23: 217–219.
9. Swanson HL (1987) Information processing theory and learning disabilities: a commentary and future perspective. J Learn Disabil 20: 155–166.
10. Berninger V (2008) Defining and differentiating dysgraphia, dyslexia, and language learning disability within a working memory model. In: Mody M, Silliman E, editors. Brain, behavior, and learning in language and reading disorders. New York: The Guilford Press. 103–134.
11. Swanson HL, Siegel L (2001) Learning disabilities as a working memory deficit. Issues Educ Contrib Educ Psychol: 1–48.
12. Fletcher J (1985) Memory for verbal and nonverbal stimuli in learning disability subgroups: analysis by selective reminding. J Exp Child Psychol 40: 244–259.
13. Maehler C, Schuchardt K (2011) Working Memory in Children with Learning Disabilities: Rethinking the criterion of discrepancy. International Journal of Disability, Development and Education 58: 5–17.
14. Swanson HL (2012) Cognitive profile of adolescents with math disabilities: are the profiles different from those with reading disabilities? Child Neuropsychol 18: 125–143.
15. Swanson HL, Stomel D (2012) Learning Disabilities and Memory. In: Wong B, Butler D, editors. Learning about learning disabilities. USA: Elservier.
16. Hari R, Renvall H (2001) Impaired processing of rapid stimulus sequences in dyslexia. Trends Cogn Sci 5: 525–532.
17. Lallier M, Tainturier MJ, Dering B, Donnadieu S, Valdois S, et al. (2010) Behavioral and ERP evidence for amodal sluggish attentional shifting in developmental dyslexia. Neuropsychologia 48: 4125–4135.
18. Siegel L (2003) Learning Disabilities. In: Reynolds WM, Miller, G.E, Weiner, I.B., editor. Handbook of Psychology, Educational Psychology. Hoboken, New Jersey: John Wiley & Sons, Inc. 455–486.
19. Shafrir U, Siegel LS (1994) Subtypes of learning disabilities in adolescents and adults. J Learn Disabil 27: 123–134.
20. Rodríguez M, Prieto B, Bernal J, Marosi E, Yáñez G, et al. (2006) Language Event-Related Potentials in Poor Readers. In: Randall SV, editor. Learning disabilities New research. New York, USA: Nova Science, Publishers, Inc. 187–217.
21. Torkildsen JvK, Syversen G, Simonsen HG, Moen I, Lindgren M (2007) Electrophysiological correlates of auditory semantic priming in 24-month-olds. Journal of Neurolinguistics 20: 332–351.
22. Meyer DE, Schvaneveldt RW (1971) Facilitation in recognizing pairs of words: evidence of a dependence between retrieval operations. J Exp Psychol 90: 227–234.
23. Neely J (1991) Semantic priming effects in visual Word recognition: a selective review of current findings and theories; Besner D, Humphreys G, editors. Hillsdale, New Jersey: Lawrence Erlbaum Associates.
24. Picton TW, Bentin S, Berg P, Donchin E, Hillyard SA, et al. (2000) Guidelines for using human event-related potentials to study cognition: recording standards and publication criteria. Psychophysiology 37: 127–152.
25. Johnson R Jr (1989) Developmental evidence for modality-dependent P300 generators: a normative study. Psychophysiology 26: 651–667.
26. Taylor MJ, Khan SC (2000) Top-down modulation of early selective attention processes in children. Int J Psychophysiol 37: 135–147.
27. Stelmack RM, Saxe BJ, Noldy-Cullum N, Campbell KB, Armitage R (1988) Recognition memory for words and event-related potentials: a comparison of normal and disabled readers. J Clin Exp Neuropsychol 10: 185–200.
28. Federmeier KD, Mai H, Kutas M (2005) Both sides get the point: hemispheric sensitivities to sentential constraint. Mem Cognit 33: 871–886.
29. Wlotko EW, Federmeier KD (2007) Finding the right word: hemispheric asymmetries in the use of sentence context information. Neuropsychologia 45: 3001–3014.
30. Kutas M, Federmeier KD (2011) Thirty years and counting: finding meaning in the N400 component of the event-related brain potential (ERP). Annu Rev Psychol 62: 621–647.
31. Kutas M, Federmeier KD (2000) Electrophysiology reveals semantic memory use in language comprehension. Trends Cogn Sci 4: 463–470.
32. Brandeis D, Vitacco D, Steinhausen HC (1994) Mapping brain electric micro-states in dyslexic children during reading. Acta Paedopsychiatr 56: 239–247.
33. Schulz E, Maurer U, van der Mark S, Bucher K, Brem S, et al. (2008) Impaired semantic processing during sentence reading in children with dyslexia: combined fMRI and ERP evidence. Neuroimage 41: 153–168.
34. Silva-Pereyra J, Rivera-Gaxiola M, Fernandez T, Diaz-Comas L, Harmony T, et al. (2003) Are poor readers semantically challenged? An event-related brain potential assessment. Int J Psychophysiol 49: 187–199.
35. Russeler J, Probst S, Johannes S, Munte T (2003) Recognition memory for high- and low-frequency words in adult normal and dyslexic readers: an event-related brain potential study. J Clin Exp Neuropsychol 25: 815–829.
36. Jednorog K, Marchewka A, Tacikowski P, Grabowska A (2010) Implicit phonological and semantic processing in children with developmental dyslexia: evidence from event-related potentials. Neuropsychologia 48: 2447–2457.
37. Greenham SL, Stelmack RM, van der Vlugt H (2003) Learning disability subtypes and the role of attention during the naming of pictures and words: an event-related potential analysis. Dev Neuropsychol 23: 339–358.
38. Dirks E, Spyer G, van Lieshout EC, de Sonneville L (2008) Prevalence of combined reading and arithmetic disabilities. J Learn Disabil 41: 460–473.
39. Matute E, Rosselli M, Ardila A, Ostrosky-Solís F (2008) Evaluación Neuropsicológica Infantil (ENI). México D.F: Manual Moderno.
40. Weschler D (2001) Escala de inteligencia de Weschler para niños-revisada (WISC-R). México D.F: Manual Moderno.
41. Conners K (1997) Conners' rating Scales-Revised. Technical Manual. New York: Multi-health system. Inc.
42. World Medical Association (2004) Declaration of Helsinki: ethical principles for medical research involving human subjects. J Int Bioethique 15: 124–129.
43. Ahumada R, Montenegro A (1990) Juguemos a leer: libro de lectura y manual de ejercicios. México, D.F: Trillas.
44. Ahumada R, Montenegro A (2007) Juguemos a leer: libro de lectura y manual de ejercicios. México, D.F: Trillas.
45. Mondada A (1992) Prácticas de ortografía, 3.Ortografía funcional para el tercer grado de enseñanza primaria con base en cuadros ortográficos. México D.F: Fernández Editores.
46. Mondada A (1992) Prácticas de ortografía, 2.Ortografía funcional para el segundo grado de enseñanza primaria con base en cuadros ortográficos. México, D.F: Fernández Editores.
47. Mondada A (1992) Prácticas de ortografía, 4.Ortografía funcional para el cuarto grado de enseñanza primaria con base en cuadros ortográficos. México, D.F: Fernández Editores.
48. Mondada A (1992) Prácticas de ortografía, 5.Ortografía funcional para el quinto grado de enseñanza primaria con base en cuadros ortográficos. México, D.F: Fernández Editores.
49. Mondada A (1992) Prácticas de ortografía, 6.Ortografía funcional para el sexto grado de enseñanza primaria con base en cuadros ortográficos. México, D.F: Fernández Editores.
50. Pestum J (1996) Maya y el truco para hacer la tarea. México D.F: Fondo de Cultura Económica.

51. Federmeier KD, Kutas M (2002) Picture the difference: electrophysiological investigations of picture processing in the two cerebral hemispheres. Neuropsychologia 40: 730–747.

52. Huang HW, Lee CL, Federmeier KD (2010) Imagine that! ERPs provide evidence for distinct hemispheric contributions to the processing of concrete and abstract concepts. Neuroimage 49: 1116–1123.

53. Silva-Pereyra J, Bernal J, Rodriguez-Camacho M, Yanez G, Prieto-Corona B, et al. (2010) Poor reading skills may involve a failure to focus attention. Neuroreport 21: 34–38.

54. Silva-Pereyra J, Rivera-Gaxiola M, Kuhl PK (2005) An event-related brain potential study of sentence comprehension in preschoolers: semantic and morphosyntactic processing. Brain Res Cogn Brain Res 23: 247–258.

55. Segalowitz SJ, Wagner WJ, Menna R (1992) Lateral versus frontal ERP predictors of reading skill. Brain Cogn 20: 85–103.

56. Harmony T, Marosi E, Diaz de Leon AE, Becker J, Fernandez T (1990) Effect of sex, psychosocial disadvantages and biological risk factors on EEG maturation. Electroencephalogr Clin Neurophysiol 75: 482–491.

57. John ER, Prichep L, Ahn H, Easton P, Fridman J, et al. (1983) Neurometric evaluation of cognitive dysfunctions and neurological disorders in children. Prog Neurobiol 21: 239–290.

58. Fernandez T, Harmony T, Fernandez-Bouzas A, Silva J, Herrera W, et al. (2002) Sources of EEG activity in learning disabled children. Clin Electroencephalogr 33: 160–164.

3

Relationship between Optical Coherence Tomography and Electrophysiology of the Visual Pathway in Non-Optic Neuritis Eyes of Multiple Sclerosis Patients

Prema Sriram[1], Chenyu Wang[2], Con Yiannikas[3], Raymond Garrick[4], Michael Barnett[2], John Parratt[5], Stuart L. Graham[1,6], Hemamalini Arvind[1,6], Alexander Klistorner[1,6]*

1 Australian School of Advanced Medicine, Macquarie University, Sydney, Australia, 2 Brain and Mind Research Institute, University of Sydney, Sydney, Australia, 3 Concord Hospital, Sydney, Australia, 4 St Vincent's Hospital, Sydney, Australia, 5 Royal North Shore Hospital, Sydney, Australia, 6 Save Sight Institute, Department of Ophthalmology, University of Sydney, Sydney, Australia

Abstract

Purpose: Loss of retinal ganglion cells in in non-optic neuritis eyes of Multiple Sclerosis patients (MS-NON) has recently been demonstrated. However, the pathological basis of this loss at present is not clear. Therefore, the aim of the current study was to investigate associations of clinical (high and low contrast visual acuity) and electrophysiological (electroretinogram and multifocal Visual Evoked Potentials) measures of the visual pathway with neuronal and axonal loss of RGC in order to better understand the nature of this loss.

Methods: Sixty-two patients with relapsing remitting multiple sclerosis with no previous history of optic neuritis in at least one eye were enrolled. All patients underwent a detailed ophthalmological examination in addition to low contrast visual acuity, Optical Coherence Tomography, full field electroretinogram (ERG) and multifocal visual evoked potentials (mfVEP).

Results: There was significant reduction of ganglion cell layer thickness, and total and temporal retinal nerve fibre layer (RNFL) thickness ($p<0.0001$, 0.002 and 0.0002 respectively). Multifocal VEP also demonstrated significant amplitude reduction and latency delay ($p<0.0001$ for both). Ganglion cell layer thickness, total and temporal RNFL thickness inversely correlated with mfVEP latency ($r = -0.48$, $p<0.0001$ respectively; $r = -0.53$, $p<0.0001$ and $r = -0.59$, $p<0.0001$ respectively). Ganglion cell layer thickness, total and temporal RNFL thickness also inversely correlated with the photopic b-wave latency ($r = -0.35$, $p = 0.01$; $r = -0.33$, $p = 0.025$; $r = -0.36$, $p = 0.008$ respectively). Multivariate linear regression model demonstrated that while both factors were significantly associated with RGC axonal and neuronal loss, the estimated predictive power of the posterior visual pathway damage was considerably larger compare to retinal dysfunction.

Conclusion: The results of our study demonstrated significant association of RGC axonal and neuronal loss in NON-eyes of MS patients with both retinal dysfunction and post-chiasmal damage of the visual pathway.

Editor: Pablo Villoslada, Institute Biomedical Research August Pi Sunyer (IDIBAPS) - Hospital Clinic of Barcelona, Spain

Funding: Funding was provided by Sydney Medical Foundation (AK), Glaucoma Australia (PS), and Novartis, Save Neuron Study (AK). The funders had no role in study design, data collection and analysis, decision to publish, or preparation of the manuscript.

Competing Interests: Two authors received funding from Novartis.

* Email: sasha@eye.usyd.edu.au

Introduction

Susceptibility of the visual system to damage in multiple sclerosis (MS) is well documented. Apart from acute inflammation of the optic nerve, which is often the first manifestation of the disease, all other elements of the visual pathway from outer-retina to visual cortex are frequently involved.

Hierarchical organization of the visual system coupled with recent technological advances makes visual pathway an ideal model to study mechanisms of MS. Retinal Ganglion Cells (RGC) are of particular interest since their unique position and accessibility to direct *in vivo* measurement by high resolution spectral domain OCT allows study of MS-related neurodegeneration including the possible effect of pathological changes in neighboring cellular elements, which are yet to be characterised.

It is well recognised that axonal transection during acute inflammation of the optic nerve (optic neuritis) is a major cause of RGC axonal and neuronal loss in MS. Correlation of RNFL thickness with stage of MS, brain atrophy, degree of disability and

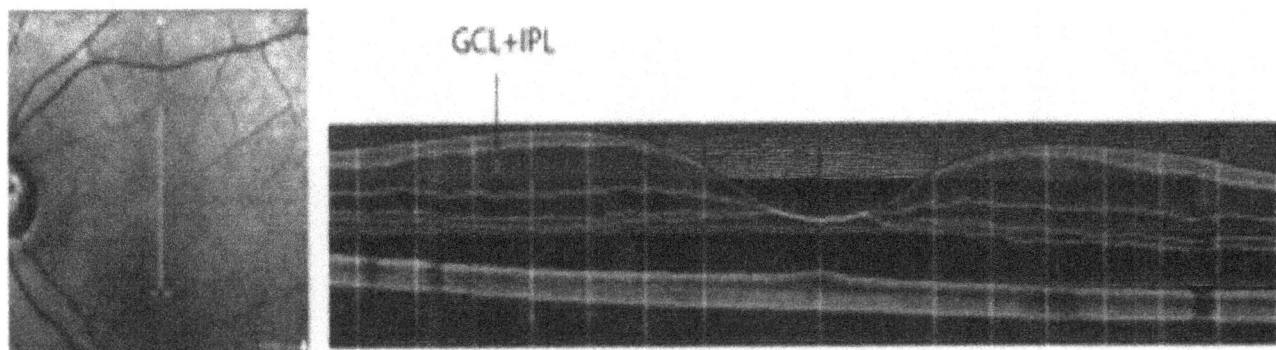

Figure 1. OCT scanning pattern (left) and segmentation of retinal layers (right).

disease duration found in a number of cross-sectional studies incited considerable interest in using assessment of the anterior visual pathway as a structural marker of CNS neurodegeneration in MS [1–8] and was even suggested as a possible outcome for future neuroprotection trials. [4,9,10] Recently, however, loss of RGC has also been demonstrated in non-optic neuritis (NON) eyes. A meta-analyses published by Petzold et al [11] showed significant thinning of RGC axons (so called retinal nerve fiber layer-RNFL) in MS-NON eyes. However, the pathological basis of this loss at present is not clear.

In the current study we performed functional assessment of the visual pathway in NON-eyes of MS patients using clinical (high and low contrast visual acuity) and electrophysiological (electro-retinogram and multifocal Visual Evoked Potentials) measures and its relationship with RGC. We hypothesized that studying potential associations of functional measures with neuronal and axonal loss of RGC may advance our understanding of the nature of this loss.

Methods

Sixty-two patients with relapsing remitting multiple sclerosis with no previous history of optic neuritis in at least one eye were enrolled. Patients with any other systemic or ocular disease that

Table 1. Comparison of functional and structural measurements in controls and MS-NON eyes.

	Control (n = 25)	MS-NON eyes (n = 58)	MS-NON eyes (n = 58)
	Mean±SD	Mean±SD	p value*
Global RNFL (μ)	99.2±7.5	93.6±9.9	0.002
Temp RNFL (μ)	70.8±7.8	64.2±9.3	0.0002
GCL (μ)	86.5±5.5	81.4±7.1	<0.0001
mfVEP amplitude (μV)	238.1±36.1	151.6±42.9	<0.0001
mfVEP latency (μV)	149.3±5.1	161.5±9.2	<0.0001
Dim white b-wave amplitude (μV)	354.4±134.8	353.7±90.7	0.92
Dim white b-wave latency (ms)	97.7±8.9	97.3±7.9	0.89
Dark max 3 a-wave amplitude (μV)	−268.3±48.4	−287.0±58.8	0.11
Dark max 3 a-wave latency (ms)	16.6±1.4	16.8±0.6	0.37
Dark max 3 b-wave amplitude (μV)	490.9±103.8	524.5±104.6	0.10
Dark max 3 b-wave latency (ms)	53.1±3.6	53.9±4.0	0.26
Dark max 12 a-wave amplitude (μV)	−325.5±52.4	−342.5±64.6	0.20
Dark max 12 a-wave latency (ms)	13.5±1.1	13.7±0.9	0.43
Dark max 12 b-wave amplitude (μV)	511.9±109.2	537.0±111.1	0.27
Dark max 12 b-wave latency (ms)	52.9±1.9	53.4±1.5	0.17
Photopic a-wave amplitude (μV)	−41.4±18.1	−46.3±10.9	0.15
Photopic a-wave latency (ms)	15.1±0.8	15.4±0.6	0.06
Photopic b-wave amplitude (μV)	174.7±35.5	185.3±41.4	0.21
Photopic b-wave latency (ms)	29.8±0.8	30.4±0.8	0.004

*p value calculated using student t-test.

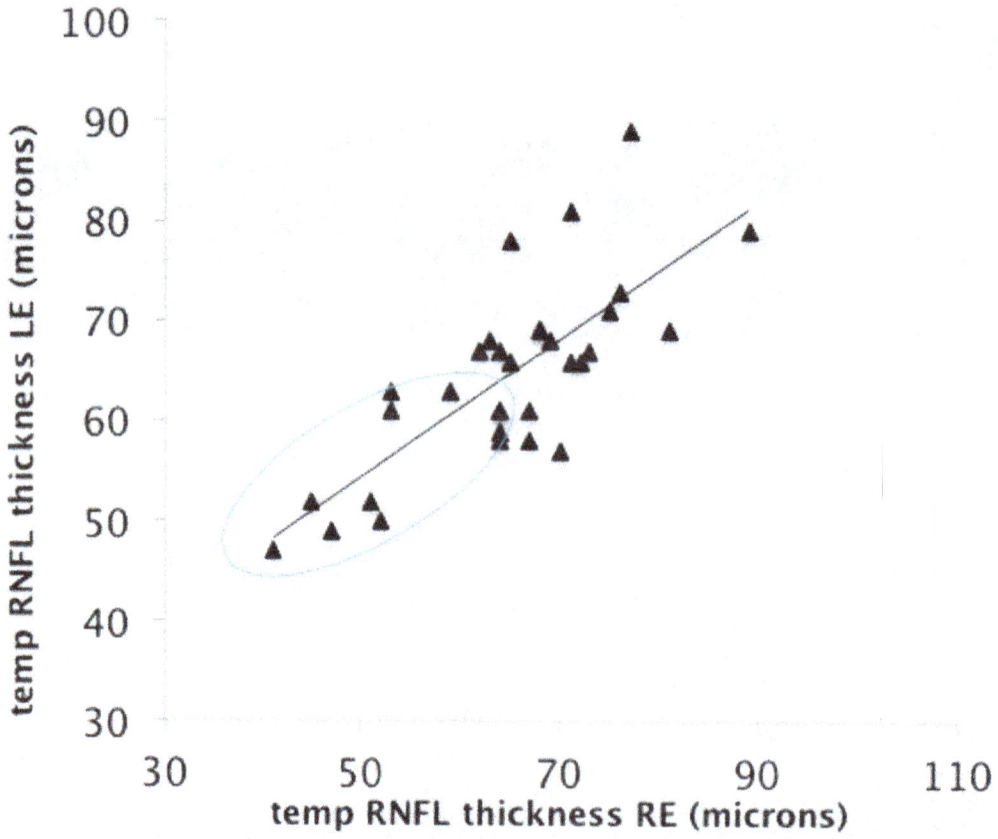

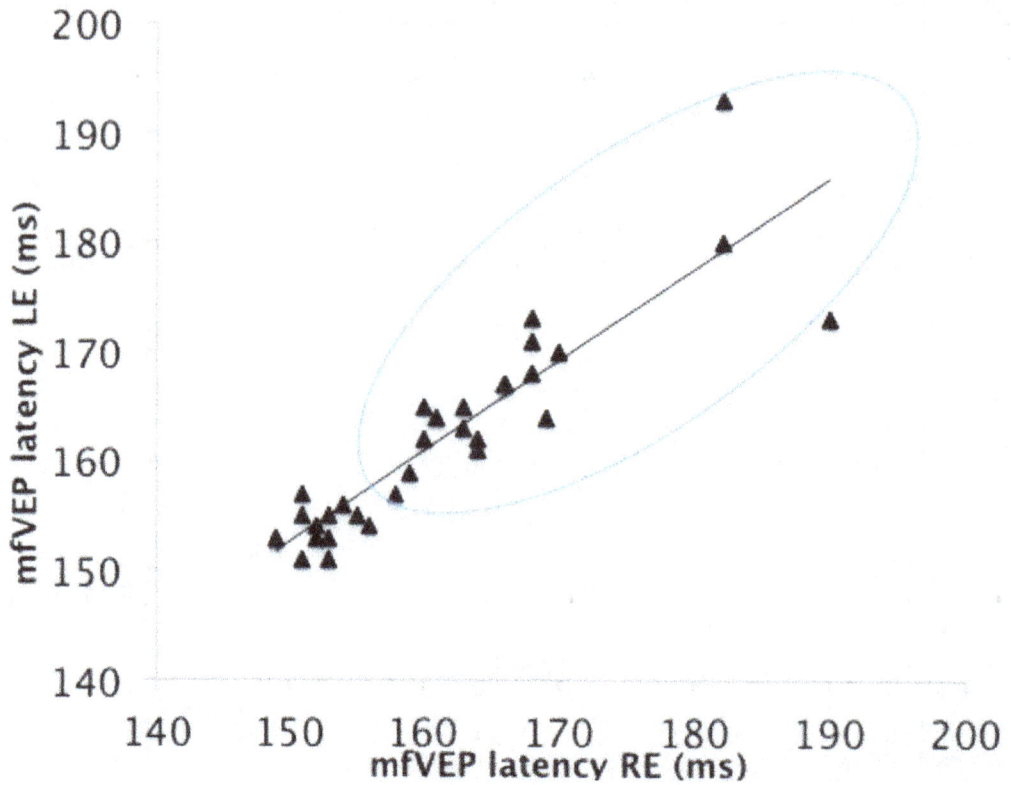

Figure 2. Figure 2a: Correlation of temporal RNFL thickness between the right and left eyes in MS patients without ON in either eye. Figure 2b: Correlation of mfVEP latency between the right and left eyes in MS patients without ON in either eye.

could confound results, such as diabetes, retinal lesions or glaucoma, were excluded.

Latency of the mfVEP demonstrated significant inverse correlation with GCL thickness, global and temporal RNFL thickness ($r = -0.48$, $p < 0.0001$; $r = -0.53$, $p < 0.0001$ and $r = -0.59$, $p < 0.0001$ respectively) (Fig. 3a–c).

Ethics statement

The Institutional Review Board of University of Sydney and Macquarie University approved the study. Procedures followed the tenets of the Declaration of Helsinki and written informed consent was obtained from all participants.

Clinical assessments

Best-corrected visual acuity (VA) was measured using Sloan high contrast (100%) and low contrast letter acuity charts (LCVA) (2.5% and 1.25%) at 4 m. Snellen VA equivalents (documented in LogMAR notation) were determined from 100% contrast charts. For LCVA, the numbers of letters correctly identified (maximum 60/chart) were recorded for each eye. A detailed ophthalmological examination was also performed.

In addition, amplitude of the mfVEP significantly correlated with tRNFL and RGC layer thickness ($r = 0.44$, $p = 0.002$ and $r = 0.32$, $p = 0.026$) and displayed tendency for association with total RNFL ($r = 0.26$, $p = 0.057$) (Fig. 4a–c).

GCL thickness, global and temporal RNFL thickness also inversely correlated with the photopic b-wave latency ($r = -0.35$, $p = 0.01$; $r = -0.33$, $p = 0.025$; $r = -0.36$, $p = 0.008$ respectively) (Fig. 5a–c). No correlation with other ERG parameters was noted.

mfVEP recording and analysis

Multifocal VEP testing was performed using the Accumap (ObjectiVision Pty. Ltd., Sydney, Australia) employing standard stimulus conditions that entailed recordings from 58 segments of the visual field. Monocular recordings were completed for 10 to 12 runs until a sufficient signal to noise ratio was reached. Four gold cup electrodes were placed around the inion and used for bipolar recording from four channels: superior and inferior; left and right, and obliquely between horizontal and inferior electrodes. Data were analysed using Opera V1.3 software. For amplitude analysis the largest peak-trough amplitude within the interval of 70–200 ms was determined. The second peak of the wave of

maximum amplitude for each segment in the visual field was used for latency analysis. Averaged (across entire stimulated field) amplitude and latency were used for analysis. mfVEP measurements were compared to values of 25 age and gender matched controls.

Full-field ERG

Full-field ERG was performed according to the ISCEV standard [12] using ESPION system (Diagnosys LLC, Lowell, MA, USA). Amplitude and latency of dark-adapted rod response, dark-adapted mixed rod/cone response at 2 levels of flash intensity and light adapted cone response were analysed.

Optical coherence tomography (OCT)

Optical Coherence Tomography was performed on a Spectralis scanner (Heidelberg Engineering). Global RNFL (gRNFL) thickness and temporal quadrant RNFL (tRNFL) thickness were assessed using the RNFL protocol. In addition, a radial protocol using a star-like pattern of line scans centered on the macula with resolution of 1536 pixels was used for measurement of thickness of retinal layers. Analysis was performed on vertical scan only. One hundred scans were averaged for each line scan. Thirty degrees of visual angle (15 degrees of eccentricity) were scanned, but only the central 14 degrees (7 degrees of eccentricity) were used for analysis, since the definition of layers becomes much less distinct beyond that. Retinal layers were segmented automatically using a custom designed algorithm, which applied vessel detection and removal, multiple size median filtering, and Canny edge detection to identify borders of retinal layers [13].

The Ganglion Cell Layer and Inner Plexiform layer were combined together (for brevity this layer will be called GCL) (see example in Fig. 1). The thickness of this layer was measured at seven points for each hemifield, which were equally distributed between 1.75 and 7 degrees of eccentricity. OCT measurements were compared to values of 50 age and gender matched controls.

Statistical Analyses

Statistical analyses were performed using IBM SPSS 20. Pearson correlation coefficient was used for bivariate correlation, while Student's t-test was used to compare means. Significance was determined at 0.05 level.

Table 2. Correlation with LCVA.

	LCVA 2.5% contrast	LCVA 2.5% contrast	LCVA 1.25% contrast	LCVA 1.25% contrast
	Correlation (r)	p value	Correlation (r)	p value
Global RNFL	0.44	0.003	0.4	0.008
Temporal RNFL	0.39	0.01	0.32	0.03
mfVEP amplitude	0.47	0.002	0.36	0.02
mfVEP latency	−0.39	0.01	−0.41	0.007

Fig 3a

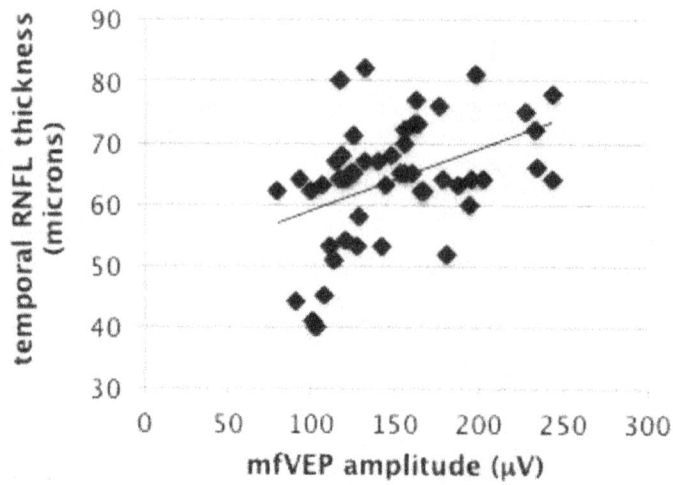

Fig 3b

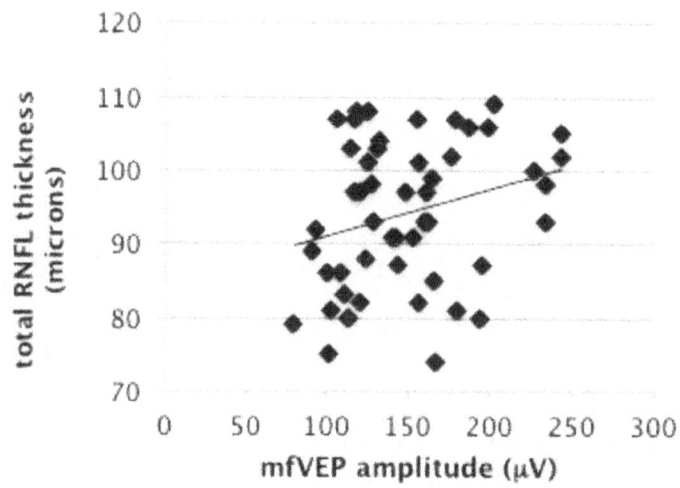

Fig 3c

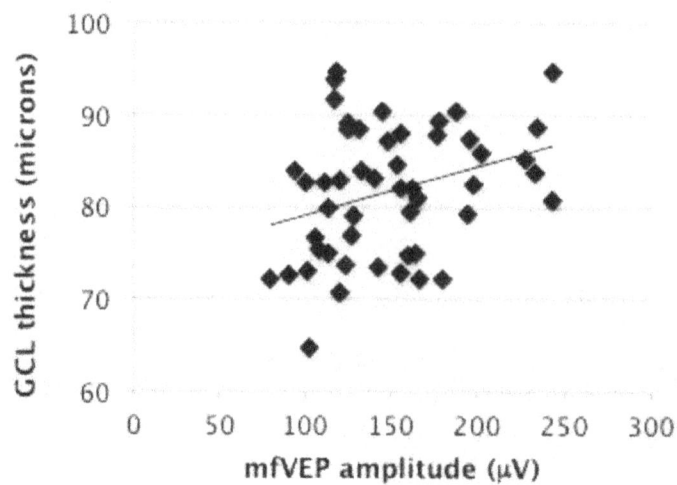

Figure 3. Figure 3a: Correlation of mfVEP latency with temporal RNFL thickness. Figure 3b: Correlation of mfVEP latency with total RNFL thickness. Figure 3c: Correlation of mfVEP latency with GCL thickness.

For the multivariate linear regression model, a backward elimination variable selection procedure in which all variables are entered into the equation and then sequentially removed based on removal criteria, was employed. Probability of F = 0.05 was used as entry criteria, while F = 0.1 was used as removal criteria.

All procedures followed the tenets of the Declaration of Helsinki and written informed consent was obtained from all participants.

Results

In total 62 RRMS patients were recruited. Four patients had high myopia and had to be excluded from analysis. One patient had an extremely large optic disc and hence his temporal RNFL was not included in analysis. Therefore, data from 58 patients (39.9±11.3 years, 18 Males/40 Females) were analyzed. Average time from diagnosis of MS was 4.7±2.9 years (1–14 years). Twenty-five patients had a previous history of optic neuritis in one eye only. Thirty-three patients did not have a history of optic neuritis in either eye. One eye of these patients was randomly selected and analysed together with the fellow eyes of optic neuritis patients.

There was significant reduction of GCL thickness as well as total and temporal RNFL in the NON-eyes of MS patients (Table 1). All three measures correlated between each other (p<0.001 for all pairs). In relation to normal controls tRNFL demonstrated by far the largest thinning as compared to gRNFL and RGC thickness (10%, 5.9% and 6.3% for tRNFL, gRNFL and GCL respectively).

In patients without history of ON in either eye RNFL and RGC thinning, where present, tended to be binocular (see example of tRNFL in Fig. 2a, oval includes points below 5th percentile (1.96 SD) of tRNFL thickness in normal controls). To quantify binocular nature of RGC axonal and neuronal loss we performed correlation between study eye and non-study eye for tRNFL, gRNFL and RGC thickness. To avoid effect of individual inter-eye correlation only eyes with significantly thinner retinal layers (below 5th percentile of thickness value of the normal controls) were included. Correlation was highly significant (p<0.001 for all).

Multifocal VEP demonstrated significant amplitude reduction and latency delay in the MS-NON eyes as compared to normal controls (p<0.0001 for both) (Table 1).

In patients without ON in either eye the mfVEP latency delay, where present, also displayed tendency for being binocular (Fig. 2b, oval indicates points above 5% (1.96 SD) of mfVEP latency in normal controls).

The b-wave latency of the photopic ERG was significantly delayed in the MS-NON eyes in comparison to the normal controls (p = 0.03). No other ERG parameters were affected (Table 1).

LCVA (both 2.5% and 1.25% contrast) significantly correlated with global and temporal RNFL thickness as well as mfVEP amplitude and inversely correlated with mfVEP latency (Table 2). No correlation between high contrast visual acuity and any of the measures was found.

There were no correlations between ERG and mfVEP parameters.

Multivariate linear regression model

Since RNFL and RGC layer thinning correlated with both photopic ERG latency and mfVEP latency we used multivariate linear regression model to assess combined predictive power and relative strength of those association. GCL thickness, gRNFL and tRNFL were used as dependent variables in individual models. The latency of mfVEP, the photopic b-wave latency of ERG, age, gender and disease duration were entered into each model.

Individual models explained 47% of tRNFL thickness variability, 36% of gRNFL thickness variability and 30% of GCL thickness variability. Multifocal VEP latency was significant in all models, while the photopic b-wave latency contributed significantly to tRNFL and GCL models. No other variables were retained by any of the models. According to Standardized Beta coefficient, the mfVEP latency was a much stronger predictor of RNFL and RGC layer thinning compared to the photopic ERG b-wave latency (Table 3).

Discussion

In the current study we assessed functional measures of the visual pathway in NON-eyes of MS patients and its association with axonal and neuronal loss of RGC.

Our result confirms previous reports of RNFL and RGC layer thinning in NON-eyes of MS patients as compared to normal controls. While this reduction was significant, it was considerably less then the loss typically reported in ON eyes. Association of thinner RNFL and RGC thickness with worse LCVA score demonstrated potential functional significance of this loss. It has been shown that conventional measures of the visual function suffer only after RNFL loss reaches a certain threshold (<70 μ). [14] Our study, however, shows that even minor losses of RGC and their axons may result in measurable deterioration of vision, provided sensitive means for the assessment of the visual function, such as LCLA, are used [15].

Correlation of RNFL and RGC thickness with amplitude of the mfVEP, which is regarded as an objective marker of the visual function, also supports functional significance of RGC neurodegeneration in NON-eyes.

RNFL thinning in NON eyes has previously been attributed to several factors, such as sub-clinical inflammation of the optic nerve, primary retinal degeneration or trans-synaptic transmission of the damage from the posterior visual pathway. [2,4,16,17] Therefore, it is of interest that in the patients without history of ON in either eye, reduction of both RNFL and RGC thickness displayed binocular nature. Due to the fact that ON fibers are partially crossing at the chiasm, this may suggest retro-chiasmal origin of the loss.

On a potential abnormality of the retro-chiasmal pathway in our cohort also pointed out binocular nature of mfVEP delay. While VEP latency delay in NON-eyes of MS patients has been reported in numerous studies, binocular character of this delay has only recently been noticed. [17] Correlation performed between eyes with delayed latency only, performed in the current study, confirmed binocular character of the delay even when inter-subject variability was minimized.

Fig 4a

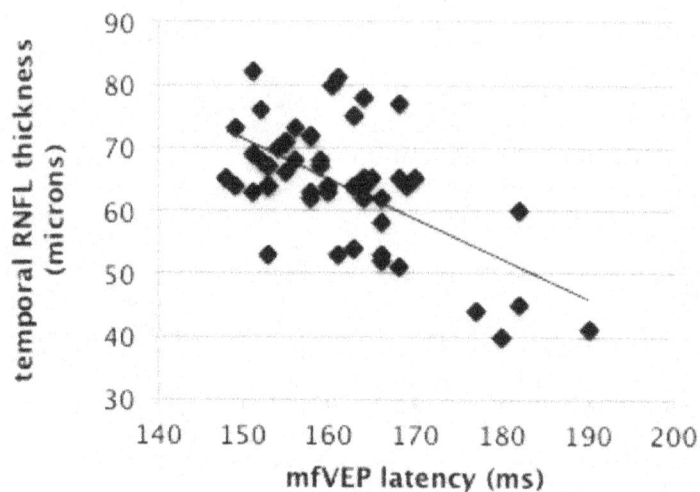

Fig 4b

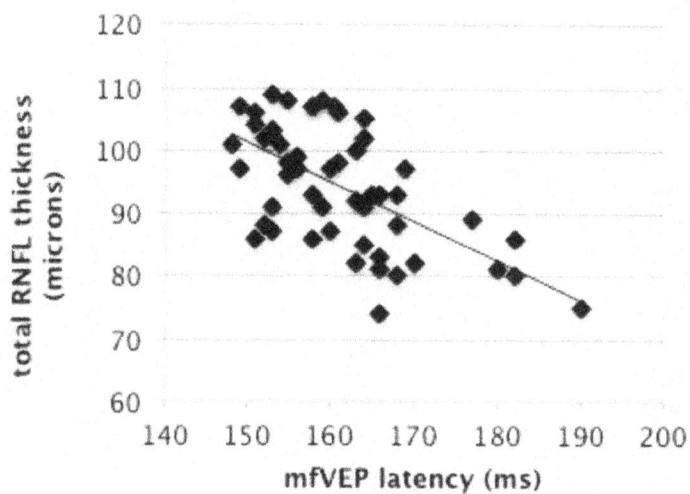

Fig 4c

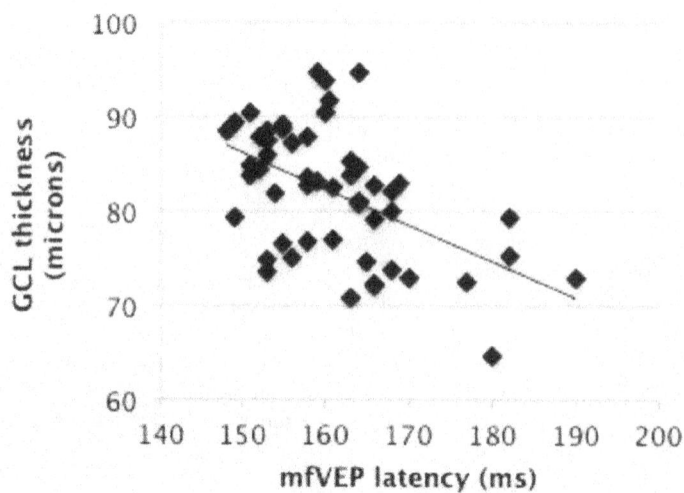

Figure 4. Figure 4a: Correlation of mfVEP amplitude with temporal RNFL thickness. Figure 4b: Correlation of mfVEP amplitude with total RNFL thickness. Figure 4c: Correlation of mfVEP amplitude with GCL thickness.

VEP delay not only showed similar pattern of binocular abnormality in patients without episode of ON in either eye, but more importantly, it demonstrated significant correlation with RNFL and RGC layer thinning in entire study cohort.

It is believed that VEP is generated at the level of striate cortex by the combined activity of post-synaptic potentials. [18,19] Therefore, VEP latency may be affected by demyelinating process along the retro-chiasmal part of the visual pathway, namely optic tract (OT) and optic radiation (OR). Since the OT represents continuation of the RGC axons after chiasmal crossing, the lesions of the OT can cause RNFL and RGC layer thinning via the mechanism of retrograde degeneration. While there are reported cases of optic tract lesions in MS (which typically presented with homonymous visual field defect), those lesions are rare. [20,21] In contrast, the OR, which is formed by axons of neighboring, more proximal neurons located in the lateral geniculate nucleus (LGN), is known to be a frequent site of MS-related inflammatory demyelination. [22] However, for lesions confined to the optic radiations it would require trans-neuronal transmission to reach RGC axons.

Compelling evidence of retrograde trans-neuronal degeneration in the visual pathway has emerged from animal and human studies recently [23,24] Mehta and Plant [25] reported topographically accurate reduction of RNFL thickness in patients with long-standing occipital lesions, while Cowey et al demonstrated transneuronal retinal ganglion cell degeneration following cortical lesions in both primate species and humans using MRI. [26] Jindahra et al recently demonstrated trans-synaptic retrograde degeneration in the visual system in acquired lesions of occipital cortex [27] and Bridge et al showed that RNFL thinning presents after post-striate lesions. [28] There is also some evidence that trans-neuronal degeneration may cause axonal loss in MS. [29,30] In 2012 Inigo et al presented data supporting trans-neuronal degeneration in the visual system of MS patients using Diffusion Tensor Imaging. [31] However, while it is tempting to speculate that trans-neuronal transmission of damage from LGN to RGC may play a part in the observed loss of RGC axons, the cross-sectional nature of the study prevents us from drawing definite conclusions.

It deserves mention that a possible causative association between OR lesions and RGC axonal loss is consistent with the preferential damage of tRNFL fibers supplying the central part of the visual field found in MS patients previously [1,7,22,32,33] and confirmed by the current study. Horton and Hoyt demonstrated that more than 50% of visual cortex is dedicated to central 10 degrees of the retina. [34] This overrepresentation of the central visual field is largely formed at the retinal level and preserved in the OR. [35] Assuming uniform distribution of lesions within the OR, it is likely that OR fibers sub-serving central vision are damaged more extensively, which, in turn, may cause larger damage of the central (temporal) RNFL.

Another key finding of this study is related to the functional assessment of the outer-retina and its association with RNFL and RGC layer thinning. We demonstrated significant delay of the photopic ERG b-wave in our MS cohort and its correlation with RGC axonal and neuronal deficit. While various ERG abnormalities have previously been reported in MS patients, [36,37] the finding of a significant association between ERG delay and thinning of RGC layer and RNFL is novel.

Delay of the photopic ERG b-wave found in this study is particularly intriguing considering the recent report by Green et al who identified significant neuronal loss and focal reduction of cell density in the inner nuclear layer of MS patients. [36] Since it is believed that delay of the photopic ERG b-wave indicates impaired response of retinal bipolar cells (which constitute major cellular component of the inner nuclear layer), our finding may represent functional counterpart of the inner nuclear layer structural damage found in that study.

Regarding the correlation of the photopic ERG b-wave delay with thinning of RNFL and RGC layer, several potential explanations can be suggested. Both bipolar and RGC may simultaneously be subjected to MS-related primary retinal process of inflammatory or neurodegenerative nature. Alternatively, since bipolar and ganglion cells are in direct contact with each other, primary injury of one cellular layer can cause damage to the neighboring cellular layer via the mechanism of trans-synaptic degeneration. Our recent study suggests that the spread of retrograde trans-synaptic degeneration from RGC to bipolar cells is unlikely. [13] This is also in line with studies of experimental optic nerve axotomy, which failed to show damage of outer-retina. [38,39] Therefore, it remains to be seen whether a primary damage to bipolar cells initiates anterograde degeneration of RGC or primary retinal process affects both neuronal layers simultaneously.

To quantify relative association of outer retinal dysfunction and posterior visual pathway damage with RNFL and RGL thinning we have also performed multivariate linear regression analysis, which confirmed significant relationship of RGC axonal and neuronal loss in NON-eyes of MS patients with both measures. However, estimated predictive power of the posterior visual pathway damage was considerably larger compare to retinal dysfunction, implying on potentially more important role of MS-related optic radiation damage in RGC loss.

In addition, even for the best correlating tRNFL thickness the model explained less then 50% of the variability. Therefore, other factors may be involved in RGC neurodegeneration. Thus, for instance, while binocular nature of RGC axonal and neuronal loss advocates its retro-chiasmal origin, the possibility of sub-clinical ON at least in some cases cannot be fully excluded. Alternatively, moderate correlation may be related to the fact that the degree of the initial inflammation in the posterior visual pathway (and, as a consequence, the level of the chronic demyelination measured by the latency of the mfVEP), does not fully define the extent of the acute lesional axonal loss.

In conclusion, the results of our study demonstrated association of RGC axonal and neuronal loss in NON-eyes of MS patients with both outer retinal dysfunction and post-chiasmal visual pathway damage. However, only longitudinal study, which is now underway, may help to reveal causative relationship between investigated measures.

Fig 5a

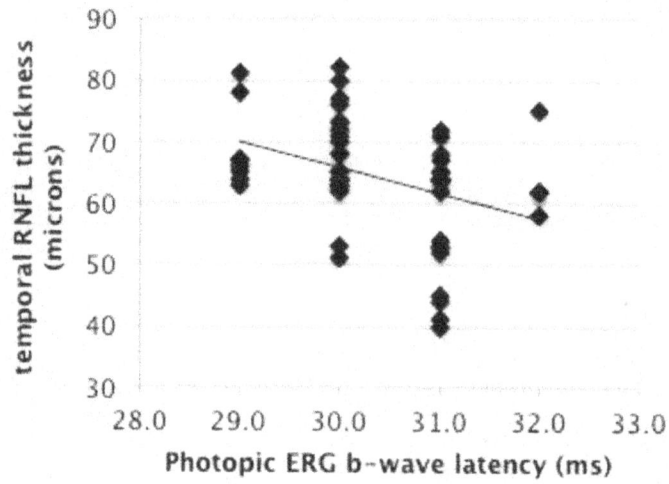

Fig 5b

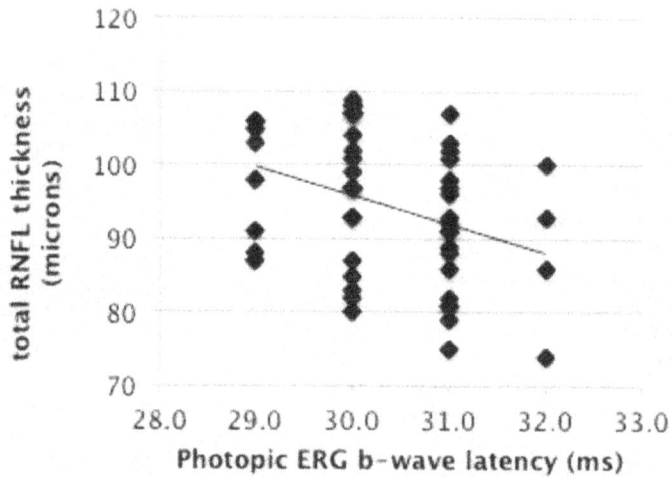

Fig 5c

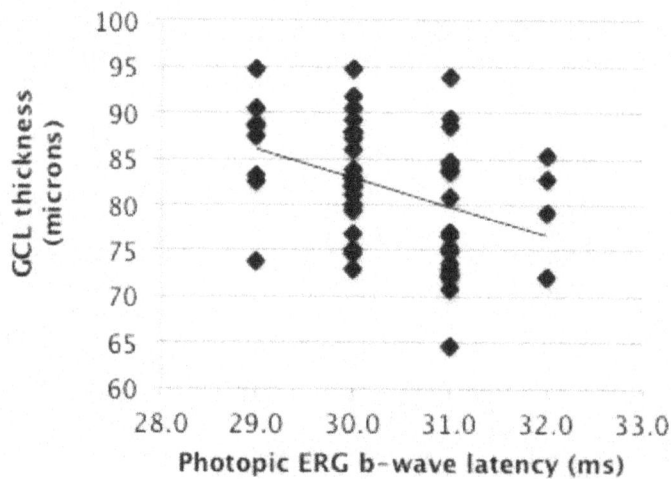

Figure 5. Figure 5a: Correlation of photopic ERG b-wave latency with temporal RNFL thickness. Figure 5b: Correlation of photopic ERG b-wave latency with total RNFL thickness. Figure 5c: Correlation of photopic ERG b-wave latency with GCL thickness.

Table 3. Linear Regression Model.

Variables	GCL Stand Beta	GCL Sig	Global RNFL Stand Beta	Global RNFL Sig	Temporal RNFL Stand Beta	Temporal RNFL Sig
mfVEP latency	−0.46	<0.001	−0.61	<0.001	−0.56	<0.001
Photopic b-wave ERG latency	−0.25	0.04			−0.24	0.03

Author Contributions

Conceived and designed the experiments: CY RG SLG AK. Performed the experiments: PS CW. Analyzed the data: PS AK. Contributed reagents/materials/analysis tools: CY RG MB JP HA. Contributed to the writing of the manuscript: PS CY SLG HA AK. Designed the software used in analysis: CY.

References

1. Pueyo V, Martin J, Fernandez J, Almarcegui C, Ara J, et al. (2008) Axonal loss in the retinal fiber layer in patients with multiple sclerosis. Mult Scler 14: 609–14.
2. Sepulcre J, Murie-Fernandez M, Salinas-Alaman A, Garcia-Layana A, Bejarana B, et al. (2007) Diagnostic acuracy of retinal abnormalities in predicting disease activity in MS. Neurology 66: 1488–94.
3. Gordon-Lipkin E, Chodkowski B, Reich DS, Smith SA, Pulicken M, et al. (2007) Retinal nerve fiber layer is associated with brain atrophy in multiple sclerosis. Neurology 69: 1603–9.
4. Siger M, Dziegiewski K, Jasek L, Bieniek M, Nicpan A, et al. (2008) Optical coherence tomography in multiple sclerosis: thickness of the retinal nerve fibre layer as a potential measure of axonal loss and brain atrophy. J Neurol 255: 1555–60.
5. Costello F, Hodge W, Pan YI, Freedman M, DeMeulemeester C. (2009) Differences in retinal nerve fiber layer atrophy between multiple sclerosis subtypes. J Neurol Sci 281(1–2): 74–9.
6. Pulicken M, Gordon-Lipkin E, Balcer LJ, Frohman EM, Cutter GR, et al. (2007) Optical coherence tomography and disease subtype in multiple sclerosis. Neurology 69: 2085–92.
7. Frohman EM, Dwyer M, Frohman T, Cox JL, Salter A, et al. (2009) Relationship of optic nerve and brain conventional and non-conventional MRI measures and RNFL, as assessed by OCT and GDx: a pilot study. J Neurolog Sci 15: 96–105.
8. Grazioli E, Zivadinov R, Weinstock-Guttman B, Lincoff N, Baier M, et al. (2008) Retinal nerve fiber layer thickness is associated with brain MRI outcomes in multiple sclerosis. J Neurolog Sci 268: 12–7.
9. Gordon GE, McCulloch DL. (1999) A VEP investigation of parallel visual pathway development in primary school age children. Doc Ophthalmol 99(1): 1–10.
10. Frohman EM, Fujimoto JG, Frohman TC, Calabresi PA, Cutter GR, et al. (2008) Optical coherence tomography: a window into the mechanisms of multiple sclerosis. Nat Clin Pract Neurol 4: 664–75.
11. Petzold A, de Boer JF, Schippling S, Vermersch P, Kardon R, et al. (2010) Optical coherence tomography in multiple sclerosis: a systematic review and meta-analysis. Lancet Neurol 9: 921–32.
12. Marmor MF, Fulton AB, Holder GE, Miyake Y, Brigell M, et al. (2009) ISCEV Standard for full-field clinical electroretinography. Doc Ophthalmol 118: 69–77.
13. Sriram P, Graham SL, Wang C, Yiannikas C, Garrick R, et al. (2012) Transsynaptic retinal degeneration in optic neuropathies: optical coherence tomography study. Invest Ophthalmol Vis Sci 53: 1271–1275.
14. Costello F, Hodge W, Pan YI, Eggenberger E, Coupland S, et al. (2008) Tracking retinal nerve fiber layer loss after optic neuritis: a prospective study using optical coherence tomography. Mult Scler 14: 893–905.
15. Balcer LJ, Frohman EM. (2010) Evaluating loss of visual function in multiple sclerosis as measured by low-contrast letter acuity. Neurology 74: S16–23.
16. Dasenbrock HH, Smith SA, Ozturk A, Farrell SK, Calabresi PA, et al. (2011) Diffusion Tensor Imaging of the Optic Tracts in Multiple Sclerosis: Association with Retinal Thinning and Visual Disability. J Neuroim 21: e41–e9.
17. Klistorner A, Garrick R, Barnett MH, Graham SL, Arvind H, et al. (2013) Axonal loss in non-optic neuritis eyes of patients with multiple sclerosis linked to delayed visual evoked potential. Neurology 15: 242–5.
18. Bridge H, Jindahra P, Barbur J, Plant GT. (2011) Imaging reveals optic tract degeneration in hemianopia. Invest Ophthal Vis Sci 52: 382–8.
19. Evangelou N, Konz D, Esiri MM, Smith S, Palace J, et al. (2001) Size-selective neuronal changes in the anterior optic pathways suggest a differential susceptibility to injury in multiple sclerosis. Brain 124: 1813–20.
20. Hornabrook RS, Miller DH, Newton MR, MacManus DG, du Boulay GH, et al. (1992) Frequent involvement of optic radiation in patients with acute isolated optic neuritis. Neurology 42: 77–9.
21. Lehoszky T (1954) Pathologic changes in the optic system in disseminated sclerosis. Acta Morphol Acad Sci Hung 4: 395–408.
22. Gundogan FC, Demirkaya S, Sobaci G (2007) Is optical coherence tomography really a new biomarker candidate in multiple sclerosis? Invest Ophthalmol Vis Sci 48: 5773–81.
23. Johnson H, Cowey A (2000) Transneuronal retrograde degeneration of retinal ganglion cells following restricted lesions of striate cortex in the monkey. Exp Brain Res 132: 269–75.
24. Weller RE, Kaas JH (1989) Parameters affecting the loss of ganglion cells of the retina following ablation of striate cortex in primates. Vis Neurosci 3: 327–49.
25. Mehta JS, Plant GT (2005) Optical coherence tomography findings in congenital/long-standing homonymous hemianopia. Am J Ophthalmol 140: 727–9.
26. Cowey A, Alexander I, Stoerig P (2011) Transneuronal retrograde degeneration of retinal ganglion cells and optic tract in hemianopic monkeys and humans. Brain 134: 2149–57.
27. Jindahra P, Petrie A, Plant GT. (2009) Retrograde trans-synaptic retinal ganglion cell loss identified by optical coherence tomography. Brain 132: 628–34.
28. Bridge H, Jindahra P, Barbur J, Plant GT (2011) Imaging reveals optic tract degeneration in hemianopia. Invest Ophthal Vis Sci 52: 382–8.
29. Evangelou N, Konz D, Esiri MM, Smith S, Palace J, et al. (2001) Size-selective neuronal changes in the anterior optic pathways suggest a differential susceptibility to injury in multiple sclerosis. Brain 124: 1813–20.
30. Reich DS, Smith SA, Gordon-Lipkin EM, Ozturk A, Caffo BS, et al. (2009) Damage to optic radiation in multiple sclerosis is associated with retinal injury and visual disability. Arch Neurol 66: 998–1006.
31. Gabilondo I, Saiz A, Martinez E, Fraga E, Llufriu S, et al. (2012) Retinal atrophy and brain damage in MS: a model for trans-synaptic neuronal degeneration? Mult Scler 18 (4 Suppl): 9–53.
32. Henderson AP, Trip SA, Schlottmann PG, Altmann DR, Garway-Heath DF, et al. (2008) An investigation of the retinal nerve fibre layer in progressive multiple sclerosis using optical coherence tomography. Brain 131: 277–87.
33. Gelfand JM, Goodin DS, Boscardin WJ, Nolan R, Cuneo R, et al. (2012) Retinal Axonal Loss Begins Early in the Course of Multiple Sclerosis and Is Similar between Progressive Phenotypes. PloS ONE 7: e36847.
34. Horton JC, Hoyt WF (1991) The representation of the visual field in the human striate cortex. Arch Ophthalmol 109: 816–24.
35. Chaplin TA, Yu HH, Rosa MG (2013) Representation of the visual field in the primary visual area of the marmoset monkey: magnification factors, point-image size, and proportionality to retinal ganglion cell density. J Comp Neurol 521: 1001–19.
36. Green IJ, McQuaid S, Hauser SL, Allen IV, Lyness R (2010) Ocular pathology in multiple sclerosis: retinal atrophy and inflammation irrespective of disease duration. Brain 133: 1591–601.
37. Forooghian F, Sproule M, Westall C, Gordon L, Jirawuthiworavong G, et al. (2006) Electroretinographic abnormalities in multiple sclerosis: possible role for retinal autoantibodies. Doc Ophthalmol 113: 123–32.
38. Komaromy AM, Brooks DE, Kallberg ME, Dawson WW, Szel A, et al. (2003) Long-term effect of retinal ganglion cell axotomy on the histomorphometry of other cells in the porcine retina. J Glaucoma 12: 307–15.
39. Hollander H, Bisti S, Maffei L, Hebel R (1984) Electroperinographic responses and retrograde changes of retinal morphology after intracranial optic nerve section. Exp Brain Res 55: 483–93.

4

A Dynamic Selection Method for Reference Electrode in SSVEP-Based BCI

Zhenghua Wu[1,2]*, Sheng Su[1]

1 School of Computer Science and Engineering, University of Electronic Science and Technology of China, ChengDu, China, 2 Key Laboratory for NeuroInformation of Ministry of Education, School of Life Science and Technology, University of Electronic Science and Technology of China, ChengDu, China

Abstract

In SSVEP-based Brain-Computer Interface (BCI), it is very important to get an evoked EEG with a high signal to noise ratio (SNR). The SNR of SSVEP is fundamentally related to the characteristics of stimulus, such as its intensity and frequency, and it is also related to both the reference electrode and the active electrode. In the past, with SSVEP-based BCI, often the potential at 'Cz', the average potential at all electrodes or the average mastoid potential, were statically selected as the reference. In conjunction, a certain electrode in the occipital area was statically selected as the active electrode for all stimuli. This work proposed a dynamic selection method for the reference electrode, in which all electrodes can be looked upon as active electrodes, while an electrode which can result in the maximum sum relative-power of a specific frequency SSVEP can be confirmed dynamically and considered as the optimum reference electrode for that specific frequency stimulus. Comparing this dynamic selection method with previous methods, in which 'Cz', the average potential at all electrodes or the average mastoid potential were selected as the reference electrode, it is demonstrated that the SNR of SSVEP is improved significantly as is the accuracy of SSVEP detection.

Editor: Bin He, University of Minnesota, United States of America

Funding: The authors have no support or funding to report.

Competing Interests: The authors have declared that no competing interests exist.

* Email: wzhzxwz@sina.com

Introduction

SSVEP-based BCI system possesses many advantages compared to other types of BCI system [1,2,3,4,5,6], and one of the most prominent properties is its high transfer rate [7,8,9]. To get a high transfer rate, besides using a valid method for SSVEP extraction, it is most important to get an evoked EEG with a high signal to noise ratio (SNR). In an SSVEP-based BCI system, a widely used method for SSVEP extraction is to compute the SSVEP relative-power by FFT [4,10,11], and this method is referred to Power Spectrum (PS) Method. In fact, the relative-power of SSVEP can be seen as the SNR of SSVEP in a specific frequency band. In the Power Spectrum Method, a reference electrode (for example, 'Cz') is firstly selected, and then one or a few active electrodes (for example, 'O1' and/or 'O2') are selected [10,12]. The relative-power of a certain frequency in spontaneous EEG at the active electrode is computed to build a threshold, and the relative-power of the corresponding frequency in evoked EEG at the active electrode is computed within a short period, such as 2 s or 3 s, then compared with the threshold. If the relative-power of that frequency is higher than the corresponding threshold, it can be concluded that this frequency SSVEP is included in this span, in other words, it can be detected that the subject is staring at the button with this frequency flicker inside and decides to select that button.

The BCI system which uses PS method is simple to build, because only one reference and one or a few active electrodes are employed [4,8,10,13,14,15,16]. However, because of the inter-subject difference of the SSVEP power [17,18,19,20,21], a certain active electrode may be very effective at a known frequency stimulus for a few subjects, while not so valid for the other subjects [22,23,24,25]. Alternatively, even for the same subject, because of the traveling property of SSVEP [26], a certain active electrode may be very effective for a certain frequency stimulus while not so effective for the other frequency stimuli. In other words, the most effective active electrode can vary between subjects or different stimulus frequencies. To statically select only one or a few active electrodes, we cannot cover all of the most effective active electrodes, and thus must limit improvements to the SNR of SSVEP for all frequency stimuli.

Consider inter-subject differences and the traveling property of SSVEP. If all the electrodes on the scalp are selected as the active electrodes and the relative-power of SSVEP at these electrodes are summed together as an SSVEP indicator, the drawback of only utilizing one or a few active electrodes can be overcome to some extent. Although different frequency SSVEPs can come to their maximum power at different electrodes, these maximum powers can all be included in the sum relative-power. The signal at each electrode can make contributions to the recognition of SSVEP frequency, so the detection accuracy can be improved for all stimuli.

For a certain frequency SSVEP, the sum relative-power of SSVEP can vary with different reference electrodes [17]. In order to get the maximum sum relative-power, a suitable reference electrode should be confirmed dynamically for each frequency, and this reference electrode is referred to the optimum reference. The selection of the optimum reference electrode is conducted for every stimulus automatically. The optimum reference electrode can vary between subjects and different stimulus frequencies. The sum relative-power under the optimum reference is used as an indicator of SSVEP. The method of dynamically selecting an optimum reference electrode under the situation of selecting all electrodes as active electrodes is proposed for the first time in this work, and is referred to as the Dynamic Selection (DS) Method.

In this study, six frequencies in different bands were selected as the stimulus frequency, a 129 channel EEG system was used to record EEG signals, and 100 s length spontaneous EEG and evoked EEG were collected separately and then divided into 2 s length segments. For the evoked EEG segments, the sum relative-power of SSVEP for each frequency was computed according to the DS method, and compared to the sum relative-power under 'Cz' reference, the reference of the average potential at all electrodes, or the reference of the average mastoid potential, respectively. The results indicate that the sum relative-power under the optimum reference is significantly higher than the sum relative-power under other three kinds of reference; accordingly, the detection accuracy under the optimum reference is higher than that under the other three kinds of reference. Although the optimum reference electrodes for a certain frequency or a certain subject can be different from each other, most of them locate at the occipital lobe.

There are many other kinds of BCI system except for SSVEP-based BCI, such as P300-based BCI [27], sensorimotor rhythm (SMR)-based BCI [28]. The singal used for classfication in BCI can mainly be recorded over the scalp, over the cortical surface, and within the brain [29]. A new classification method of BCI which is simliar to the communication system is proposed recently [29], according to this method, the BCI system can be sorted into five types: TDMA, FDMA, CDMA, SDMA, and HMA. SSVEP-based BCI is the kind of FDMA, while P300-based BCI is the kind of TDMA. In these different kinds of BCI system, although the signal extraction methods are different, for example, FFT method is often used in SSVEP-based BCI, while the superposition method is often used in P300-based BCI, it is very important to get an evoked EEG with a high SNR. Although the method proposed in this study is based on the property of SSVEP, it can be extended to other type BCIs. For example, in a motor imagery based BCI, the ERP amplitude is related to the reference electrode. To select dynamically an optimum reference can lead to a high ERP amplitude, which can improve the classfication accuracy of the BCI system.

Methodology

2.1 Ethics Statement

This study was approved by the Human Research and Ethics Committee of the University of Electronic Science and Technology of China. Before the experiment, all the subjects were told the purpose and procedure of the experiment in detail and signed a consent form. These forms were approved by the University of Electronic Science and Technology of China Ethics Committee Data Acquisition.

2.2 Data Acquirement

Eleven subjects were chosen to take part in this experiment, having either normal sight or corrected normal sight. Six subjects were male, and five subjects were female. The mean age was 24 (range 24 ± 2) years old. The subjects were seated in a dark room, 60 cm from the stimulator. A high luminance focused LED was used as the SSVEP stimulator, driven by a pulse generator, and the duty-cycle of the pulse was set to 1:1. The cycle of the pulse can only be adjusted in 1 ms step, and six cycles were selected, i.e.

30, 40, 60, 80, 120, and 160 ms, the corresponding six frequencies were 33.33, 25, 16.67, 12.5, 8.33, and 6.25 Hz, located at β, α, and θ band, respectively. This frequency arrangement can be used to study the validity of DS method for the fundamental frequency and the harmonics extraction. The order of these six stimuli was random for different subject, and this can cancel the probable influence resulted by the stimuli order. A 129-channel EEG system was used to collect the spontaneous EEG and evoked EEG. Electrode impedance was kept below 10 kΩ, and salt water dropped into the electrode periodically in order to retain good contact with the subjects scalp. Fig. 1 shows the location of the electrodes in this system. In the EEG recording stage, 'Cz' electrode (No. 129) was selected as the reference. In order to avoid power line interference, the cutoff frequency of the EEG system was set to 49 Hz. For each stimulus, 100 s length spontaneous EEG was collected first, and then 100 s length evoked EEG was collected. This spontaneous EEG was used to build the threshold for each frequency SSVEP.

2.3 Computation Method

Because the SSVEP has relative immunity to noise such as eye or body movement [2,18], no pre-process method, such as removing eye movement was adopted in this work.

2.3.1 SSVEP Gain Under Different Kinds of Reference. The original EEG was referenced at 'Cz' electrode. For 100 s length spontaneous EEG, FFT was applied directly, then a spectrum was attained at each electrode with a frequency resolution of 0.01 Hz. For a specific frequency 'f' Hz and the electrode L_1, L_2, ... L_n, the relative-power of 'f' Hz at any electrode 'm' can be computed as follows:

$$R_{fm} = P_{fm}/\mathbf{mean}(P_{(f-1)m}, P_{(f+1)m}) \qquad (1)$$

Where 'm' is from '1' to 'n', 'R_{fm}' stands for the relative-power of 'f' Hz at electrode 'm', 'P_{fm}' stands for the absolute-power of 'f' Hz at electrode 'm', '$\mathbf{mean}(P_{(f-1)m}, P_{(f+1)m})$' stands for the average absolute-power from 'f–1' Hz to 'f+1' Hz at electrode 'm'. The sum relative-power of 'f' Hz can be stated as:

$$R_f = R_{f1} + R_{f2} + ...R_{fn} \qquad (2)$$

Where 'R_f' stands for the sum relative-power of 'f' Hz at all electrodes in spontaneous EEG, this sum relative-power is looked as SNR of this frequency in spontaneous EEG, and it is used as the baseline of this frequency. In this work, 'n' equals to 129, and 'f' equals to 33.33, 25, 16.67, 12.5, 8.33, and 6.25 Hz, respectively.

For evoked EEG, the same method as that for spontaneous EEG was adopted, and the sum relative-power of SSVEP was obtained which is looked as SNR of this frequency in evoked EEG. This sum relative-power of SSVEP was divided by the corresponding baseline in spontaneous EEG and the quotient referred to as the SSVEP gain under 'Cz' reference:

$$G_f = SR_f/R_f \qquad (3)$$

Where 'G_f' stands for SSVEP gain at 'f' Hz, 'SR_f' stands for the sum relative-power of SSVEP at 'f' Hz in the evoked EEG, i.e. the SNR of SSVEP in evoked EEG, and the computation of 'SR_f' in evoked EEG is the same as that of 'R_f' in spontaneous EEG. This SSVEP gain under 'Cz' reference is compared to the next computed SSVEP gain under the optimum reference.

To compute the SSVEP gain under the other kinds of reference, the spontaneous EEG and evoked EEG at each electrode were

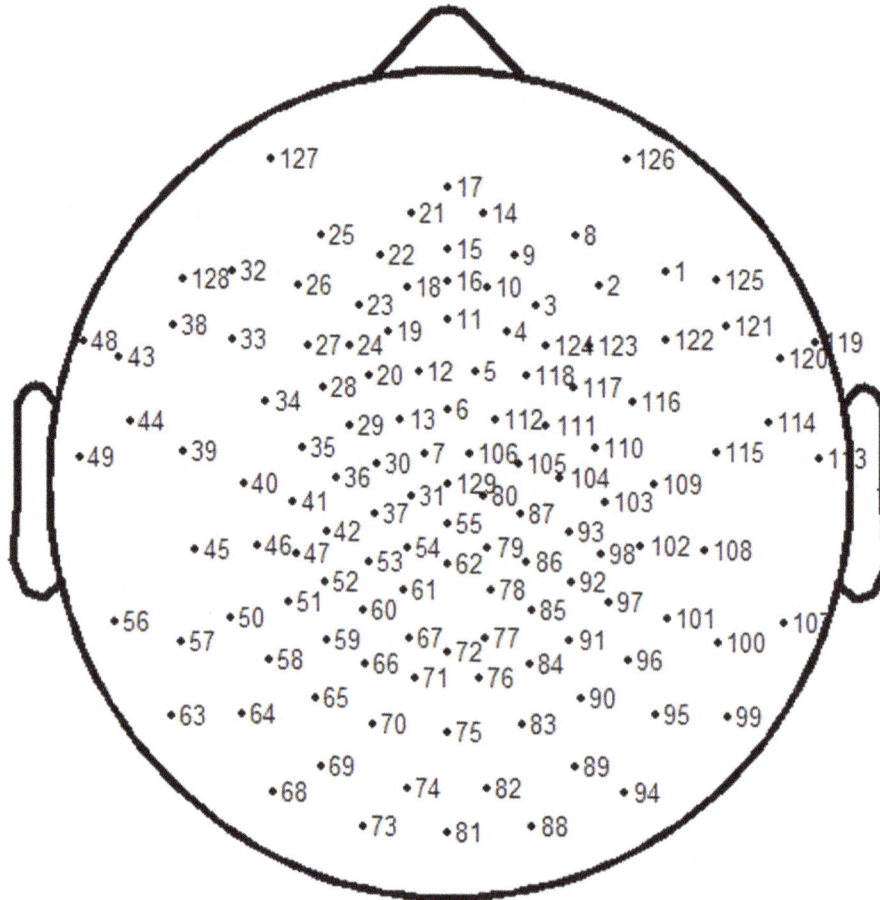

Figure 1. Electrodes location of 129 channel EEG system.

firstly re-refrenced at the average potential at all electrodes and the average potential at both mastoids, respectively. The average potential at electrode No. 56 and 107 was viewed as the average mastoid potential. The computation of SSVEP gain under these two kinds of references is the same as that under the 'Cz' reference.

2.3.2 Selecting the Optimum Reference. For 100 s length evoked EEG of a known frequency, firstly the channel No. 1 is selected as the reference and the original signal at each electrode re-computed under this reference to get a new evoked EEG. FFT is applied on the new evoked EEG. The sum relative-power of SSVEP is computed using the same method as in 2.3.1. Following this, channel No. 2 is selected as the reference, and the same method as above applied. These steps are repeated until all channels have been selected as the reference once.

For the 129 channel EEG system, a total of 129 sum relative-power is computed and the maximum within them chosen as the optimum sum relative-power of SSVEP. The corresponding electrode is then selected as the optimum reference for the known frequency.

2.3.3 SSVEP Gain Under the Optimum Reference. For spontaneous EEG, the sum relative-power of each stimulus frequency is re-computed under the corresponding optimum reference, and viewed as the baseline of each frequency under the optimum reference.

For evoked EEG, the sum relative-power of stimulus frequency is computed under the optimum reference, and this sum relative-power is divided by the corresponding baseline to get SSVEP gain under the optimum reference. The sum relative-power of the other five frequencies, which can be viewed as noise under the known stimulus, are computed under the corresponding optimum reference also, and divided by the corresponding baseline under the optimum reference to get noise gain. Noise gain is used to evaluate, while improving the SSVEP gain significantly under the optimum reference, whether the noise gain had improved appreciably or not.

2.3.4 Detection Accuracy Under Different Kinds of Reference. Spontaneous EEG and evoked EEG were divided into segments of 2 s length separately. For each segment, '0' series were added with a length of 2 s to get a whole 4 s length segment. The technique of adding '0' series is utilized to improve the frequency resolution of FFT, and is widely applied in BCI studies [10,11,30]. In this work, if applying FFT directly on the 2 s length signal, the frequency resolution is 0.5 Hz. After appending '0' series, the frequency resolution can be improved to 0.25 Hz. Then the four kinds of reference, i.e. 'Cz' reference, the reference of the average potential at all electrodes, the reference of average potential at mastoid, and the optimum reference, are applied to this 4 s length segment respectively to compute the sum relative-power. The sum relative-powers extracted from each spontaneous EEG segment is used to build a threshold for each frequency. An estimated threshold is used to check the sum relative-power of a certain frequency in spontaneous EEG segments, and adjusted continually until the detection accuracy equaled 90%. This means that the relative-power in 90% spontaneous EEG segments is smaller than this threshold and the adjusted value can be seen as the threshold of the corresponding frequency under a kind of reference. As a result, six thresholds can be confirmed under each type reference, respectively.

Under different kinds of reference, the sum relative-power in evoked EEG segments is compared to the corresponding threshold to check whether the SSVEP is included. First, only the first harmonic is utilized for detecting SSVEP with the checking standard being as follows: For an evoked EEG segment including a known frequency SSVEP, if the sum relative-power of the first harmonic exceeded its threshold, while the sum relative-powers of other frequencies except the second harmonic are all below the corresponding thresholds, the detection for this segment is correct. Secondly, for the high frequency stimuli such as 33.33 and 25 Hz, only the first harmonic is used for detecting, while for other middle and low frequency stimuli, both the first and second harmonics are utilized for detecting SSVEP. The checking standard used was as follows: For an evoked EEG segment including a known frequency SSVEP, if the sum relative-power of the first harmonic or the second harmonic exceeded the corresponding threshold, while the sum relative-powers of other frequencies are all below the corresponding thresholds, then the detection for this segment is correct.

For the results obtained via these steps, in order to test the significance of difference between methods, one-way Analysis of Variance (ANOVA) was applied. Significance level 'p' was selected as 0.05. If 'p' is smaller than 0.05, it suggests that there is a significant difference between the compared situations.

Results

3.1 Optimum Reference Distribution

For the total 11 subjects, everyone took 6 SSVEP-frequency tests, so there were.

66 optimum reference electrodes chosen and most of these electrodes were located at the occipital area. For a certain subject, the optimum reference for different frequencies can be different. For a certain stimulus frequency, the optimum reference for different subjects can vary. Table 1 shows the optimum reference for different subjects at different stimuli. Fig. 2 shows the optimum reference distribution topography for all subjects under all stimuli.

3.2 SSVEP's SNR Improvement Under the Optimum Reference

Under a 33.33 Hz stimulus, the SNR of SSVEP under the optimum reference is significantly higher than that under 'Cz' reference ($F(1,20) = 4.45$, $p = 0.04$), the average mastoid reference ($F(1,20) = 6.8$, $p = 0.03$) and the commom average reference ($F(1,20) = 5.47$, $p = 0.03$), while for the other 5 frequencies which can be looked at as noise, the ANOVA results 'p' are far bigger than 0.05. This suggests that there is no significant improvement of the SNR for noise under the optimum reference. The SSVEP's SNR improvement under the optimum reference can be seen from the average SSVEP gain across all subjects. For the stimulus frequency 33.33 Hz, the SSVEP gain under the optimum reference is 1.65 times of that under 'Cz' reference, 1.57 times of that under the average mastoid reference, and 1.7 times of that under the common average reference, while for other noise frequencies, this ratio is 1.0 or so, which means that the noise power in evoked EEG is the same level as that in spontaneous EEG under the optimum reference.

Under a 25 Hz stimulus, the comparison results between the optimum reference and the other kinds of reference were similar to

Table 1. The optimum reference for different subject under different stimuli.

Subject	S1	S2	S3	S4	S5	S6	S7	S8	S9	S10	S11
Stimulus frequency (Hz)											
33.33	76	72	85	76	77	76	75	70	61	78	123
25	76	75	75	71	67	85	55	72	76	75	77
16.67	72	74	91	62	76	76	75	77	71	61	75
12.5	72	76	76	70	71	75	69	60	76	72	76
8.33	71	75	100	72	75	75	72	17	79	66	75
6.25	72	76	96	78	83	76	72	17	75	75	126

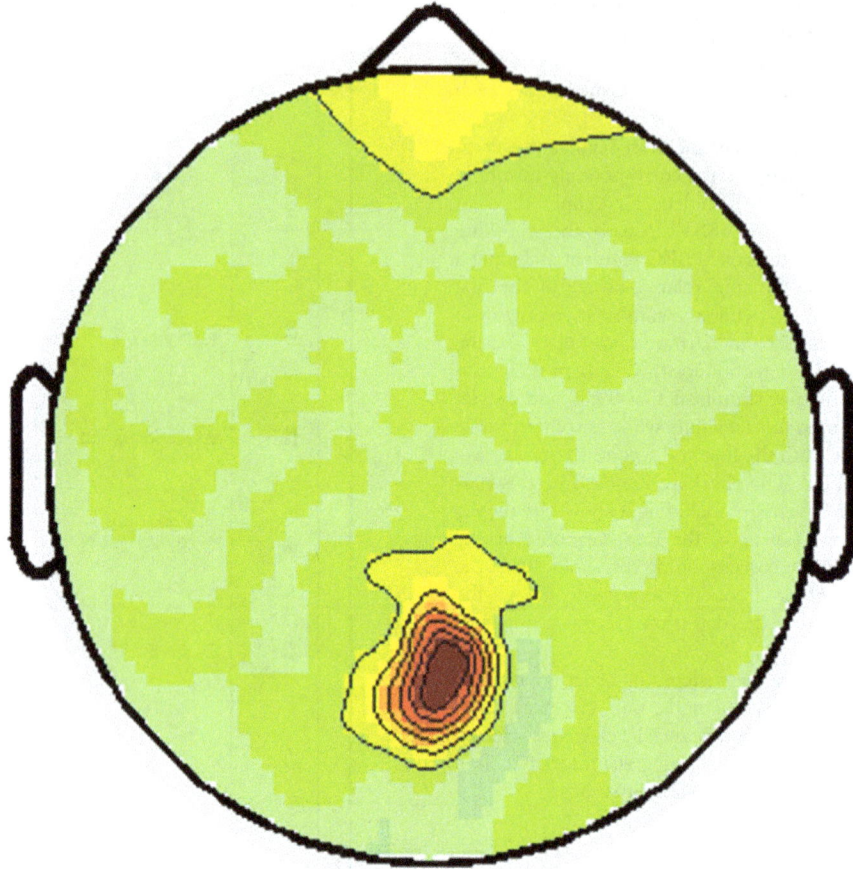

Figure 2. Optimum reference distribution topography. The deep color means more reference electrodes located in this area.

that under 33.33 Hz stimuli. Under other middle or low frequency stimuli, i.e 16.67, 12.5, 8.33, and 6.25 Hz, the comparison results between the optimum reference and other three kinds of reference were similar to that under 33.33 Hz stimulus except that of the second harmonic. When stimulated at middle or low frequency, sometimes the second harmonic becomes stronger than the first harmonic under 'Cz' reference, or the average mastoid reference, or the common average reference, and the SNR of the second harmonic can be improved significantly when utilizing the optimum reference. Table 2 lists the average sum relative-power (SNR) across all subjects and the ANOVA results under every stimulus.

3.3 Detection Accuracy Under Different Kinds of Reference

When only taking the first harmonic into account, the average detection accuracy across all subjects and stimuli is low under all kinds of references, i.e. 31.2% under 'Cz' reference, 34.4% under the average mastoid reference, 33.2% under the common average reference and 42.9% under the optimum reference. However, the average detection accuracy across all stimuli under the optimum reference is significantly higher than that under 'Cz' reference $(F(1, 20) = 8.19, p = 0.01)$, the average mastoid reference $(F(1, 20) = 6.3, p = 0.01)$, and the common average reference $(F(1, 20) = 10.2, p = 0.01)$. For all subjects, the detection accuracy of different frequencies is different. Normally, the detection accuracy of middle and low frequencies such as 16.67, 12.5, 8.33, and 6.25 Hz is lower than that of high frequencies such as 33.33 and 25 Hz.

Fig. 3 illustrates the average detection accuracy across all stimuli for every subject when only taking the first harmonic into account.

When taking the first harmonic into account for high frequency stimuli such as 33.33 and 25 Hz (due to not recording the second harmonic), and taking the first and second harmonic into account for middle and low frequency stimuli, such as 16.67, 12.5, 8.33, and 6.25 Hz, the average detection accuracies across all stimuli can be improved significantly under all kinds of reference. Furthermore, the average detection accuracies across all subjects and stimuli are 62.2% under 'Cz' reference, 61.8% under the average mastoid, 61.6% under the common average and 73.7% under the optimum reference, respectively. In this situation, the average detection accuracy across all stimuli under the optimum reference is significantly higher than that under 'Cz' reference $(F(1,20) = 11.3, p = 0.0)$, the average mastoid reference $(F(1, 20) = 9.52, p = 0.0)$, and the common average $(F(1, 20) = 8.3, p = 0.0)$. For all subjects, the detection accuracy of different frequencies is different. Normally, the detection accuracy of middle and low frequency stimuli such as 16.67, 12.5, 8.33, and 6.25 Hz is higher than that of high frequency stimuli such as 33.33 and 25 Hz. Fig. 4 illustrates the average detection accuracy across all stimuli for every subject when taking both the first and second harmonic into account.

Table 3 lists the average detection results across all subjects under different stimulus frequencies. From this table, it can be seen that when using middle or low frequency stimuli, the second harmonic is very important for SSVEP detection. Under any situation, the ANOVA 'p' is far smaller than 0.05, which suggests

A Dynamic Selection Method for Reference Electrode in SSVEP-Based BCI

Table 2. Average SNR across all subjects and ANOVA results under every stimulus.

Frequency (Hz)			33.33	25	16.67	12.5	8.33	6.25
Spontaneous EEG	SNR under Cz reference		216.3	208.9	211.7	209.8	201.5	211.4
	SNR under average mastoid reference		211.5	212.3	213.1	214.7	210.2	207.8
	SNR under common average reference		214.2	209.4	215.1	211.7	213.8	200.9
	SNR under optimum reference		212.4	213.6	209.2	215.6	210.8	203.9
Stimulus frequency 33.33 Hz	Cz reference	SNR	720.5	211.7	208.9	215.4	198.7	223.2
		SSVEP/noise gain	3.33	1.01	0.99	1.03	0.99	1.06
	mastoid reference	SNR	710.8	209.3	210.5	211.1	210.8	215.9
		SSVEP/noise gain	3.36	0.99	0.99	0.98	1	1.04
	common reference	SNR	726.4	214.2	207.8	211.9	204.3	217.6
		SSVEP/noise gain	3.39	1.02	0.97	0.98	0.96	1.08
	Optimum reference	SNR	1167	220.2	219.3	211.1	194.7	203.1
		SSVEP/noise gain	5.49	1.03	1.05	0.98	0.92	1
	ANOVA 'p' (optimum vs Cz)		0.04	0.82	0.42	0.18	0.65	0.54
	ANOVA 'p' (optimum vs mastoid)		0.03	0.57	0.69	0.32	0.48	0.59
	ANOVA 'p' (optimum vs common)		0.03	0.72	0.33	0.46	0.63	0.37
Stimulus frequency 25 Hz	Cz reference	SNR	201.2	615.6	211.4	216.3	200.8	203.6
		SSVEP/noise gain	0.93	2.95	1	1.03	1	0.96
	mastoid reference	SNR	210.8	633.1	216.9	208.7	209.8	211.4
		SSVEP/noise gain	1	2.98	1.02	0.97	1	1.02
	common reference	SNR	212.3	617.2	211.8	210.9	217.5	215.9
		SSVEP/noise gain	0.99	2.95	0.98	1	1.02	1.07
	Optimum reference	SNR	211.3	904.9	215.6	203.3	186.7	205.6
		SSVEP/noise gain	0.99	4.24	1.03	0.94	0.89	1.01
	ANOVA 'p' (optimum vs Cz)		0.73	0.02	0.55	0.67	0.48	0.56
	ANOVA 'p' (optimum vs mastoid)		0.46	0.03	0.27	0.44	0.59	0.34
	ANOVA 'p' (optimum vs common)		0.66	0.01	0.35	0.57	0.32	0.64
Stimulus frequency 16.67 Hz	Cz reference	SNR	377.6	207.8	597.6	203.7	210.5	211.3
		SSVEP/noise gain	1.75	0.99	2.82	0.97	1.04	1
	mastoid reference	SNR	389.5	211.7	603.8	210.7	211.3	208.3
		SSVEP/noise gain	1.84	1	2.83	0.98	1.01	1
	common reference	SNR	373.7	209.8	612.9	213.7	219.2	204.8
		SSVEP/noise gain	1.74	1	2.85	1.01	1.03	1.02
	Optimum reference	SNR	464.4	224.4	974.1	215.9	218.9	213.4
		SSVEP/noise gain	2.19	1.05	4.66	1	1.04	1.05
	ANOVA 'p' (optimum vs Cz)		0.06	0.47	0.01	0.74	0.66	0.28

Table 2. Cont.

Frequency (Hz)			33.33	25	16.67	12.5	8.33	6.25
ANOVA 'p' (optimum vs mastoid)			0.05	0.35	0.01	0.47	0.52	0.63
ANOVA 'p' (optimum vs common)			0.1	0.57	0.02	0.33	0.72	0.35
Stimulus frequency 12.5 Hz	Cz reference	SNR	210.9	497.8	208.5	995.6	223.4	205.6
		SSVEP/noise gain	0.98	2.38	0.98	4.75	1.11	0.97
	mastoid reference	SNR	215.7	512.3	213.5	1004.8	216.7	210.4
		SSVEP/noise gain	1.02	2.41	1	4.68	1.03	1.01
	common reference	SNR	216.9	503.5	215.7	987.4	215.6	214.3
		SSVEP/noise gain	1.01	2.4	1	4.66	1.01	1.07
	Optimum reference	SNR	208.8	682.1	212.7	1503	225.6	224.1
		SSVEP/noise gain	0.98	3.19	1.02	6.97	1.07	1.1
	ANOVA 'p' (optimum vs Cz)		0.77	0.06	0.41	0.01	0.63	0.45
	ANOVA 'p' (optimum vs mastoid)		0.56	0.04	0.52	0.01	0.28	0.67
	ANOVA 'p' (optimum vs common)		0.44	0.04	0.38	0.01	0.39	0.55
Stimulus frequency 8.33 Hz	Cz reference	SNR	223.5	256.7	602.5	207.5	561.8	210.3
		SSVEP/noise gain	1.03	1.23	2.85	0.99	2.79	0.99
	mastoid reference	SNR	215.6	237.8	595.6	210.8	593.5	211.9
		SSVEP/noise gain	1.02	1.12	2.79	0.98	2.82	1.02
	common reference	SNR	227.4	232.8	606.9	210.9	600.3	215.4
		SSVEP/noise gain	1.06	1.11	2.82	1	2.81	1.07
	Optimum reference	SNR	239.1	269.5	927.9	193.1	870.8	216.6
		SSVEP/noise gain	1.13	1.26	4.44	0.9	4.13	1.06
	ANOVA 'p' (optimum vs Cz)		0.65	0.42	0.03	0.57	0.02	0.49
	ANOVA 'p' (optimum vs mastoid)		0.47	0.33	0.02	0.39	0.01	0.66
	ANOVA 'p' (optimum vs common)		0.39	0.55	0.02	0.47	0.02	0.27
Stimulus frequency 6.25 Hz	Cz reference	SNR	209.7	225.9	211.4	747.4	209.8	523.8
		SSVEP/noise gain	0.97	1.08	1	3.56	1.04	2.48
	mastoid reference	SNR	214.4	209.5	217.8	699.8	213.2	540.3
		SSVEP/noise gain	1.01	0.99	1.02	3.26	0.99	2.6
	common reference	SNR	211.3	214.5	216.4	726.5	211.9	535.9
		SSVEP/noise gain	0.99	1.02	1.01	3.43	0.99	2.67
	Optimum reference	SNR	201.3	239.5	226.2	1129	214.1	890.5
		SSVEP/noise gain	0.95	1.12	1.08	5.23	1.02	4.38
	ANOVA 'p' (optimum vs Cz)		0.59	0.44	0.23	0.03	0.76	0.01
	ANOVA 'p' (optimum vs mastoid)		0.43	0.38	0.41	0.02	0.59	0.01
	ANOVA 'p' (optimum vs common)		0.63	0.27	0.56	0.02	0.51	0.01

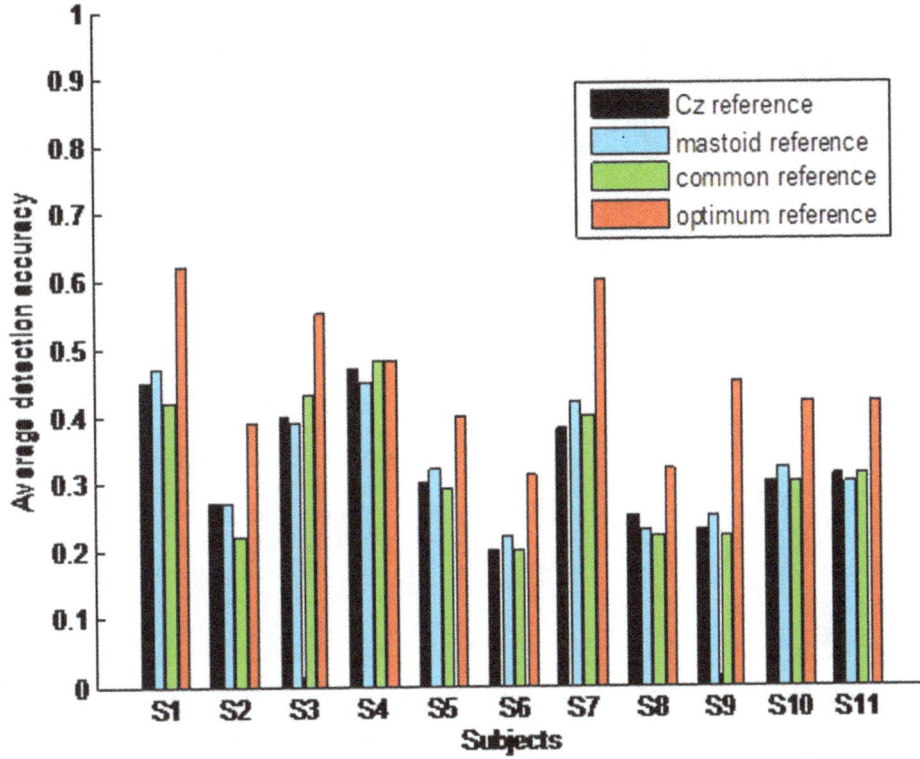

Figure 3. Average detection accuracy across all stimuli for every subject when only taking the first harmonic into account.

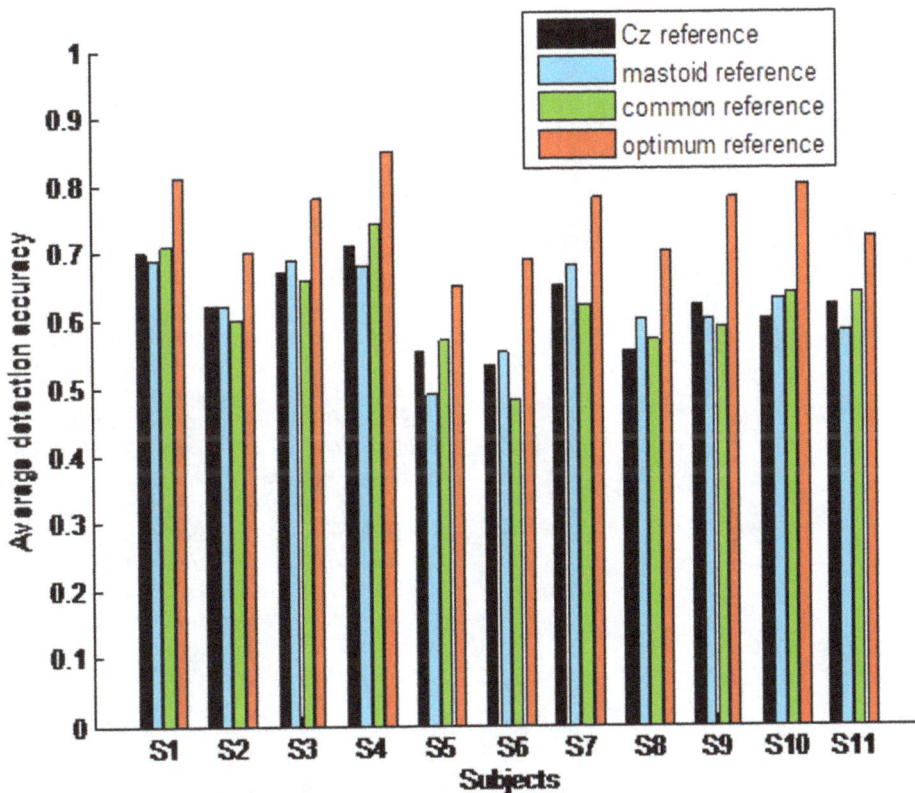

Figure 4. Average detection accuracy across all stimuli for every subject when taking the first and second harmonic into account.

Table 3. Average detection accuracy across all subjects under different situations.

Stimulus Frequency (Hz)	33.33	25	16.67	12.5	8.33	6.25
Detection using the first harmonic						
Accuracy (Cz reference)	0.49	0.39	0.3	0.27	0.22	0.2
Accuracy (mastoid average reference)	0.46	0.4	0.29	0.28	0.22	0.2
Accuracy (common average reference)	0.47	0.4	0.31	0.27	0.23	0.21
Accuracy (optimum reference)	0.63	0.5	0.44	0.42	0.27	0.32
ANOVA 'p' (optimum vs Cz)	0.01	0.01	0.01	0.02	0.04	0.02
ANOVA 'p' (optimum vs mastoid)	0.01	0.01	0.01	0.03	0.03	0.01
ANOVA 'p' (optimum vs common)	0.01	0.02	0.01	0.01	0.02	0.01
Detection using the first and second harmonic						
Accuracy (Cz reference)	0.49	0.39	0.7	0.68	0.72	0.75
Accuracy (mastoid average reference)	0.46	0.4	0.71	0.7	0.71	0.75
Accuracy (common average reference)	0.47	0.4	0.7	0.72	0.72	0.73
Accuracy (optimum reference)	0.63	0.5	0.79	0.83	0.85	0.82
ANOVA 'p' (optimum vs Cz)	0.0	0.0	0.01	0.0	0.0	0.01
ANOVA 'p' (optimum vs mastoid)	0.01	0.01	0.01	0.0	0.0	0.01
ANOVA 'p' (optimum vs common)	0.0	0.01	0.01	0.0	0.01	0.01

that the detection accuracy under optimum reference is significantly higher than that under other three kinds of reference.

Discussion

In this work, even in the consideration of the second harmonic, the detection accuracy for some subjects is still low compared to other works [10,11], this is resulted by the experiment itself. SSVEP power is related to factors such as stimulus intensity, frequency, modulation depth and to the subjects themselves. This work shows that there is considerable intra-difference for the same subject between different frequency stimuli, and there is great inter-difference between subjects even under the same stimuli. These differences lead to the different detection accuracy ratios between subjects. The experiment in this work can lead to more inter-subject or intra-subject differences. Although every subject was asked to be seated in the same location, we have not confirmed whether the subject evoked a maximum SSVEP. Because a focused LED was used as the stimulator of SSVEP in this study, if the subject did not stare at the flicker from the correct vision angle, the light projecting into the eyes decreased acutely and the maximum SSVEP was not evoked. In fact, we have studied the spectrum of the 100 s length evoked EEG, in some trials, the peak is not clear, which suggests that the SSVEP is very weak. Therefore, detection accuracy in this work is not as high as that in the other real BCI experiments [10,11]. However, this does not matter for the comparison between the methods for reference electrode selection. In a real SSVEP-based BCI, the experiment design is very important. Firstly, suitable frequency arrangements can lead to a high SSVEP power and reduce the interference between stimuli. For example, normally selecting a middle or low frequency can evoke a large SSVEP, and a certain stimulus frequency should be far enough from other stimuli and their harmonics. Secondly, stimulator selection is also very important. We have compared the influence on SSVEP power by different stimulators [31]. When using a CRT monitor or emanative LED, the subject can receive almost the same strength light in a wide range, so a little shift of the vision angle does not affect SSVEP power. However, when using a focused LED as the stimulator, the light concentrates in a narrow area, the shift of the vision angle has a great influence on SSVEP power. So, in a multi-target BCI system, because of the vision angle shifting significantly, the focused LED should be avoided.

In order to check the influence on the second harmonic by the dynamic selection method, the SNR of the second harmonic was also computed Firstly, only the first harmonic was used to detect SSVEP. Then the first and second harmonic were used together to detect SSVEP. The results show that, when stimulating at a middle or low frequency, the SNR of the second harmonic can be improved significantly when using the optimum reference, accordingly the detection accuracy using the first and second harmonic together is significantly higher than when only using the first harmonic. In order to avoid the power line interference of 50 Hz, the cutoff frequency of the recording system is set 49 Hz, so a high frequency harmonic of stimulus such as 25 and 33.33 Hz was not collected. In consequence, the detection accuracy for these stimuli is smaller than that of the low frequency stimuli. In an SSVEP-based BCI, the harmonics are very important for improving detection accuracy, so the first and second harmonics, sometimes even the third harmonic, should be taken into account even under the optimum reference. In fact, some works have discussed the usefulness of harmonics in detail [4,10].

In past SSVEP-based BCI systems, often one or a few active electrodes were chosen from the electrodes located at the occipital area [1,10,11,13,32]. There are some drawbacks to doing this. For the same frequency, the optimum active electrode in the occipital area may be different because of inter-subject differences. In order to get the highest detection accuracy for each subject, it should be tested first to confirm the optimum active electrode before detecting targets. This however, is a waste of manpower and time [11,24,33]. Although the occipital area is considered the source of SSVEP [25], suggesting SSVEPs in this area are normally higher than those in other areas, for different frequencies, the location of the maximum SSVEP in the occipital area is different. In a multi-targets SSVEP-based BCI system, there are normally many frequencies applied, it is impossible to find an electrode in the occipital area which is optimum for all frequencies. So, all the electrodes are selected as the active electrode in this work. Under this selection, for any subject and any stimulus frequency, there is no need to confirm the optimum active electrode before detection. The SSVEP power in different areas can all be collected as an indicator of SSVEP, and this indicator includes more information than that for only one or a few active electrodes selected. Therefore, the detection accuracy for all stimuli is improved significantly.

When selecting all electrodes as the active electrode, it is important to find an optimum reference under which the sum relative-power of SSVEP is at a maximum. Under the optimum reference, the SNR of SSVEP is improved significantly compared to the other kinds of reference. While using the optimum reference to improve the SSVEP gain, if the noise gain is improved the same level as SSVEP gain, optimum reference makes no improvement for SSVEP detection accuracy. Fortunately, except for the second harmonic, the other noise relative-power is not increased under optimum reference. Consequentially, when using the first and second harmonic together to detect SSVEP under the optimum reference, a higher detection accuracy compared to the other kinds of reference can be attained.

Although the optimum references for different subjects or different stimulus frequencies can differ, most of them are located at the occipital area. This can be understood through the following analysis. The SSVEP is a response to the visual stimulus mainly by the primary visual cortex, and the occipital area is the source of SSVEP. Here we hypothesize an ideal situation, i.e. there is an ideal reference, which is not related to EEG at any electrode, and only one electrode 'E_0' at the occipital area is the SSVEP source. Furthermore, the SSVEP at electrodes 'E_1',... 'E_m'... 'E_n' are transferred from 'E_0' via the scalp. The SSVEP between the ideal reference and electrode 'E_0', 'E_1',... 'E_m'... 'E_n' are expressed:

$$A_0 * \sin(\omega * t + \phi_0)$$
$$A_1 * \sin(\omega * t + \phi_1)$$
$$...$$
$$A_m * \sin(\omega * t + \phi_m) \qquad (4)$$
$$...$$
$$A_n * \sin(\omega * t + \phi_n)$$

A_0, A_1,.A_m...A_n are the SSVEP amplitude at different electrodes compared to the ideal reference, 'ω' is the SSVEP frequency, Φ_0, Φ_1, ...Φ_m... Φ_n are the initial phase of SSVEP at different electrodes. Because of the travelling property of SSVEP and the attenuation characteristics of the scalp, the amplitude A_0, A_1, ... A_m, ... A_n can be different and A_0 is the biggest among

these amplitudes, the initial Φ_0, Φ_1, ... Φ_m... Φ_n can be different also.

When using electrode 'E_0' as the reference, the relative SSVEP at other electrodes 'E_1',... 'E_m'... 'E_n' can be stood by:

$$S_1 = A_1 * \sin(\omega * t + \phi_1) - A_0 * \sin(\omega * t + \phi_0)$$
$$...$$
$$S_m = A_m * \sin(\omega * t + \phi_m) - A_0 * \sin(\omega * t + \phi_0) \qquad (5)$$
$$...$$
$$S_n = A_n * \sin(\omega * t + \phi_n) - A_0 * \sin(\omega * t + \phi_0)$$

And the sum power 'P_0' of these signals is:

$$P_0 = \frac{1}{T} * \int_0^T ([A_1 * \sin(\omega * t + \phi_1) - A_0 * \sin(\omega * t + \phi_0)]^2 + ... \qquad (6)$$
$$+ [A_n * \sin(\omega * t + \phi_n) - A_0 * \sin(\omega * t + \phi_0)]^2) dt$$

Where 'T' is the cycle of the frequency 'ω'.

When using electrode 'E_m' as the reference, the relative SSVEP at other electrodes is represented:

$$S_0 = A_0 * \sin(\omega * t + \phi_0) - A_m * \sin(\omega * t + \phi_m)$$
$$S_1 = A_1 * \sin(\omega * t + \phi_1) - A_m * \sin(\omega * t + \phi_m)$$
$$... \qquad (7)$$
$$S_n = A_n * \sin(\omega * t + \phi_n) - A_m * \sin(\omega * t + \phi_m)$$

And the sum power 'P_m' of these signals is.

$$P_m = \frac{1}{T} * \int_0^T ([A_0 * \sin(\omega * t + \phi_0) - A_m * \sin(\omega * t + \phi_m)]^2 + ... \qquad (8)$$
$$+ [A_n * \sin(\omega * t + \phi_n) - A_m * \sin(\omega * t + \phi_m)]^2) dt$$

The 'P_0' and 'P_m' can be computed, and the difference of the sum power under reference 'E_0' and 'E_m' is illustrated as:

$$P_0 - P_m = \frac{(n-1) * A_0^2}{2} - \frac{(n-1) * A_m^2}{2}$$
$$- A_1 * A_0 * \cos(\phi_1 - \phi_0)$$
$$- A_2 * A_0 * \cos(\phi_2 - \phi_0) - ...$$
$$- A_n * A_0 * \cos(\phi_n - \phi_0) \qquad (9)$$
$$+ A_0 * A_m * \cos(\phi_0 - \phi_m)$$
$$+ A_1 * A_m * \cos(\phi_1 - \phi_m) + ...$$
$$+ A_n * A_m * \cos(\phi_n - \phi_m)$$

This difference is related to SSVEP amplitude and initial phase at every electrode. The different attenuation properties of a subject's scalp can lead to a different distribution of SSVEP. Even for the same subject, the distribution of SSVEP amplitude and initial phase can be different for different stimulus frequencies. It is impossible to prove 'P_0-P_m' is bigger or smaller than zero using mathematical methods. In order to understand this, a group data including 129 amplitudes and 129 initial phases are simulated randomly 100,000 times in a computer to compute equation (9). Except for assuming the source electrode 'E_0' with the maximum amplitude, there is no other limitation for other amplitudes and all initial phases, this suggests these simulant data can include all the real SSVEP amplitude and initial phase. The results show that the difference 'P_0-P_m' is bigger than zero in more than an average probability of 98%. In other words, even using the real amplitudes and initial phases in place of those in equation (9), 'P_0' is bigger than 'P_m' in most situations. This suggests that, if using SSVEP source as the reference, a maximum sum relative-power can be attained. Therefore, in the dynamic selection method, most optimum references locate at the occipital area.

There is a very great difference between the method proposed in this work and the method in which the average potential at all electrodes in the time domain are selected as the reference. When selecting the average potential at all electrodes in the time domain as a reference, although the background noise can be canceled to some extent, more amplitude information of SSVEP has been canceled on average because of the traveling features of SSVEP, and thus cannot lead to the maximum sum relative-power of SSVEP. In this work, the sum relative-power at all electrodes in the frequency domain is selected as the indicator of SSVEP. The phase of SSVEP has not been taken into account, and the SSVEP amplitude information at all electrodes remains in the sum relative-power. Maximum sum relative-power of SSVEP can be identified.

The cost of the dynamic selection method is the increased complexity of the system because more electrodes can be fixed. Except for this drawback, the procedures using the dynamic selection method are easy to apply. During the stage of building a threshold for each stimulus, the spontaneous EEG within a time period is first obtained, then each stimulus frequency is used once to evoke SSVEP for a period of length the same as for the spontaneous EEG. Ultimately, the optimum reference for each stimulus is confirmed automatically, and the threshold under this optimum reference is computed automatically also. Therefore, time consumption in this stage is minimal. Alternatively, with the other reference selection method, normally finding a suitable active electrode for all stimuli and confirming the threshold is very time consuming. In the formal detection stage, the procedure is similar to that of the power spectrum method, i.e. the power of every adopted frequency under the corresponding optimum

reference is computed and compared to the corresponding threshold. If every power is smaller than its corresponding threshold, then there is no button selected. If there is only one power bigger than its corresponding threshold, the button with the corresponding frequency flicker inside is selected. If there are more powers bigger than their corresponding thresholds, other techniques are applied to confirm which button is valid, for example, taking the results as invalid, or selecting the frequency, which has the highest SSVEP gain as the target frequency.

Too many electrodes adopted in the DS method can limit the popularization of this method. In order to understand the influences of the number of electrodes for the detection accuracy, we reduce the electrode density, for example, only selecting one third electrodes in each lobe, the results show the optimum reference concentrates mostly at the occipital lobe. Although the detection accuracy under situation of lower intensity electrode is sometimes a little lower than that under all electrodes, compared to the other three kinds of reference, the detection accuracy of DS method is still the highest. In consideration of the optimum reference concentrating mostly at the occipital lobe, in order to decrease the complexity of BCI system, we can use only the electrodes in occipital area for EEG recording, and select the optimum reference from these electrodes for SSVEP detection.

Conclusion

Compared to other SSVEP extraction methods, in which one reference is selected statically and one or a few electrodes in the occipital area are chosen as the active electrode, Dynamic Selection Method uses more active electrodes, and thus can increase the complexity of the system. The method of Dynamic Selection Method improves SSVEP's SNR and detection accuracy significantly and is easy to employ by decreasing the number of electrodes, thus being applicable in a real time SSVEP-based BCI.

Acknowledgments

The authors are grateful to Mr. Kong Lu for completing the experiment and Dr. Lin for English proofreading.

Author Contributions

Conceived and designed the experiments: ZH. Performed the experiments: ZH. Analyzed the data: ZH SS. Contributed reagents/materials/analysis tools: ZH SS. Contributed to the writing of the manuscript: ZH. Designed the software used in analysis: ZH SS.

References

1. Luo A, Sullivan TJ (2010) A User-friendly SSVEP-based brain–computer Interface Using a Time-domain Classifier. J. Neural Eng. 7: 1–10.
2. Allison BZ, Wolpaw EW, Wolpaw JR (2007) Brain-computer Interface Systems: Progress and Prospects. Expert Review of Medical Devices 4(No.4): 463–474.
3. Vialatte FB, Maurice M, Dauwels J, Cichocki A (2010) Steady-state Visually Evoked Potentials: Focus on Essential Paradigms and Future Perspectives. Progress in Neurobiology 90: 418–438.
4. Muller-Putz GR, Scherer R, Brauneis C, Pfurtscheller G (2005) Steady-state Visual Evoked Potential (SSVEP)-based Communication: Impact of Harmonic Frequency Components. J. Neural Eng. 2: 123–130.
5. Ghaleb I, Davila CE, Srebro R (1996) Detection of Near Threshold Contrast Visual Evoked Potentials Using Coherent Detection Techniques. Biomedical Engineering Conference 121–124.
6. Wolpaw JR, Birbaumer N, McFarland DJ, Pfurtscheller G, Vaughan TM (2002) Brain-computer Interfaces for Communication and Control. Clinical Neurophysiology 113: 767–791.
7. Lopez MA, Pelayo F, Madrid E, Alberto P (2009) Statistical Characterization of Steady-State Visual Evoked Potentials and Their Use in Brain–Computer Interfaces. Neural Process Lett 29: 179–187.
8. Middendorf M, Mcmillan G, Calhoun G, Jones KS (2008) Brain-Computer Interfaces Based on the Steady-state Visual-Evoked Response. IEEE Transactions on Rehabilitation Engineering 8(No.2): 211–214.
9. Sami S, Nielsen KD (2004) Communication speed enhancement for visual based Brain Computer Interfaces 9th Annual Conference of the International FES Society 475–480.
10. Cheng M, Gao XR, Gao SK, Xu DF (2002) Design and Implementation of a Brain-Computer Interface with High Transfer Rates. IEEE Trans. BME VOL. 49(No.10): 1181–1186.
11. Gao XR, Xu DF, Cheng M, Gao SK (2003) A BCI Based Environmental Controller for the Motion-Disabled. IEEE Transactions on Neural System and Rehabilitation Engineering 11(No.2): 137–140.
12. Hwang HJ, Lim JH, Jung YJ, Choi H, Lee SW, et al. (2012) Development of an SSVEP-based BCI spelling system adopting a QWERTY-style LED keyboard. Journal of Neuroscience Methods 208: 59–65.
13. Lopez MA, Praetor A, Playa F (2010) Use of Phase in Brain–Computer Interfaces Based on Steady-State Visual Evoked Potentials. Morillas Neural Process Lett 32: 1–9.
14. Molina GG, Tsoneva T, Nijholt A (2013) Emotional brain–computer interfaces. Int. J. Autonomous and Adaptive Communications Systems 6: 1–9.

15. Rosario AO, Adeli H (2013) Brain-computer interface technologies: from signal to action. Reviews in the Neurosciences 24: 455–562.
16. McCullagh P, Galway L, Lightbody G (2013) Investigation into a Mixed Hybrid Using SSVEP and Eye Gaze for Optimising User Interaction within a Virtual Environment. Lecture Notes in Computer Science 8009: 530–539.
17. Herrmann CS (2001) Human EEG Responses to 1–100 Hz Flicker: Resonance Phenomena in Visual Cortex and Their Potential Correlation to Cognitive Phenomena. Exp Brain Res.137: 346–353.
18. Carlos ED, Alireza A, Alireza K (1994) Estimation of Single Sweep Steady-State Visual Evoked Potentials by Adaptive Line Enhancement. IEEE Trans. BME 41(No. 2): 197–200.
19. Cheng M, Gao XR, Gao SK, Wang BL (2005) Stimulation Frequency Extraction in SSVEP-based Brain-computer Interface. 2005 First International Conference on Neural interface and Control Proceeding 64–67.
20. Kelly SP, Lalor EC, Reilly RB, Foxe JJ (2005) Visual Spatial Attention Tracking Using High-Density SSVEP Data for Independent Brain-Computer Communication. IEEE Transactions on Neural System and Rehabilitation Engineering 13(No. 2): 172–178.
21. Lin ZL, Zhang CS, Wu W, Gao XR (2007) Frequency Recognition Based on Canonical Correlation Analysis for SSVEP-Based BCIs. IEEE Trans. BME 54(No. 6): 1172–1176.
22. Birbaumer N, Cohen LG (2007) Brain-computer Interfaces: Communication and Restoration of Movement in Paralysis. The Journal of Physiology 579: 621–636.
23. Lee PL, Sie JJ, Liu YJ (2010) An SSVEP-Actuated Brain Computer Interface Using Phase-Tagged Flickering Sequences: A Cursor System. Annals of Biomedical Engineering 38: 2383–2397.
24. Wang RP, Zhang ZG, Gao XR (2005) Electrode Selection for SSVEP-based Binocular Rivalry. 2005 First International Conference on Neural Interface and Control Proceeding 75–78.
25. Wang YJ, Zhang ZG, Gao XR (2004) Electrode Selection for SSVEP-based Brain-computer Interface. Proceeding of the 26th Annual International Conference of the IEEE EMBS 4507–4510.
26. Burkitt GR, Silberstein RB, Cadusch PJ, Wood AW (2000) Steady-state Visual Evoked Potentials and Travelling Waves. Clinical Neurophysiology 111: 246–258.
27. Yin E, Zhou Z, Jiang J, Chen FL, Liu YD, et al. (2013) A novel hybrid BCI speller based on the incorporation of SSVEP into the P300 paradigm. Journal of Neural Engineering 10: 1–10.
28. Yan H, He B (2014) Brain-Computer Interfaces Using Sensorimotor Rhythms: Current State and Future Perspectives. BME VOL.61(No. 5): 1425–1435.
29. Gao SK, Wang YJ, Gao XR, Hong B (2014) Visual and Auditory Brain-Computer Interfaces. IEEE Trans. BME VOL.61(No. 5): 1436–1447.
30. Wu ZH, Yao DZ (2008) Frequency detection with stability coefficient for SSVEP based BCIs. J. Neural Eng. 5: 36–43.
31. Wu ZH, Lai YX, Xia Y, Wu D, Yao DZ (2008) Stimulator selection in SSVEP-based BCI. Medical Engineering & Physics 30: 1079–1088.
32. Friman O, Volosyak I, Graser A (2007) Multiple Channel Detection of Steady-State Visual Evoked Potentials for Brain-Computer Interfaces. IEEE Trans. BME 54(No. 4): 742–750.
33. Ridder WH, McCulloch D, Herbert AM (1998) Stimulus Duration, Neural Adaptation, and Sweep Visual Evoked Potential Acuity Estimates. Invest Ophthalmol. Vis. Sci. 39: 2759–2768.

5

Functional Connectivity in the First Year of Life in Infants at Risk for Autism Spectrum Disorder

Giulia Righi[1], Adrienne L. Tierney[2], Helen Tager-Flusberg[3], Charles A. Nelson[4,5,6]*

1 Department of Psychology, University of Massachusetts at Amherst, Amherst, Massachusetts, United States of America, 2 Harvard College Writing Program, Harvard University, Cambridge, Massachusetts, United States of America, 3 Department of Psychological and Brain Sciences, Boston University, Boston, Massachusetts, United States of America, 4 Division of Developmental Medicine, Boston Children's Hospital, Boston, Massachusetts, United States of America, 5 Department of Pediatrics, Harvard Medical School, Boston, Massachusetts, United States of America, 6 Harvard Graduate School of Education, Cambridge, Massachusetts, United States of America

Abstract

In the field of autism research, recent work has been devoted to studying both behavioral and neural markers that may aide in early identification of autism spectrum disorder (ASD). These studies have often tested infants who have a significant family history of autism spectrum disorder, given the increased prevalence observed among such infants. In the present study we tested infants at high- and low-risk for ASD (based on having an older sibling diagnosed with the disorder or not) at 6- and 12-months-of-age. We computed intrahemispheric linear coherence between anterior and posterior sites as a measure of neural functional connectivity derived from electroencephalography while the infants were listening to speech sounds. We found that by 12-months-of-age infants at risk for ASD showed reduced functional connectivity compared to low risk infants. Moreover, by 12-months-of-age infants later diagnosed with ASD showed reduced functional connectivity, compared to both infants at low risk for the disorder and infants at high risk who were not later diagnosed with ASD. Significant differences in functional connectivity were also found between low-risk infants and high-risk infants who did not go onto develop ASD. These results demonstrate that reduced functional connectivity appears to be related to genetic vulnerability for ASD. Moreover, they provide further evidence that ASD is broadly characterized by differences in neural integration that emerge during the first year of life.

Editor: Vincent M. Reid, Lancaster University, United Kingdom

Funding: Funding was provided by grant from National Institute on Deafness and Other Communication Disorders (NIDCD) R21 DC 08637 and Autism Speaks to HTF. Funding was provided by grant NIDCD RO1 DC 10290 and the Simon's Foundation to CAN and HTF. The agencies/funders had NO role in design data analysis or publication.

Competing Interests: The authors have declared that no competing interests exist.

* Email: charles_nelson@harvard.edu

Introduction

Autism spectrum disorder (ASD) is a developmental syndrome primarily characterized by deficits in social communication and interactions, and repetitive/restricted patterns of behaviors, interests, and/or activities, which are present, at least in part, from early in development [1]. The presentation of ASD is very heterogeneous, and changes depending on a child's intellectual abilities, language proficiency, and age [2]. The phenotypic complexity of ASD has been associated with a variety of differences in both functional and anatomical neural substrates [3]. The multitude of neural atypicalities identified in individuals with ASD coupled with recent findings showing significant generic heterogeneity [4] have contributed to conceptualizing ASD as a syndrome characterized by differences in brain-wide neural circuitry that emerge across development. On the basis of this evidence, ASD is hypothesized to be a "disconnection syndrome", one in which the anatomical and functional integration of neural circuits is disrupted [5]. Neural integration processes are reflected in various frequency domains of an individual's EEG. High frequency activity in the gamma range, for example, is thought to bind neural information from different networks, a process that is

required for a number of perceptual and cognitive tasks and that is disrupted in several neurocognitive disorders including ASD [6]. Disruptions in the binding function of gamma activity may explain a wide range of language and social communication deficits that characterize ASD [7]. More specifically, behaviors that require the coordinated function of several brain regions may not be sufficiently integrated without the appropriate amount of gamma frequency activity.

One question that has motivated recent research in this area is how early in development differences in gamma frequency metrics of neural integration arise. To investigate issues related to very early development, studies rely on infants with an older sibling with ASD [8,9]. These infants are termed "high-risk" for ASD because they have an increased predisposition to develop ASD, estimated to be around fifteen to twenty times higher than infants with no family history of ASD [10,11]. Studies of this population present several advantages to understanding ASD generally and to neural integration specifically [12]. First, we can ask questions about the developmental trajectories in biological and cognitive factors as they relate to the emergence of typical or atypical outcomes. Second, we can ask questions about which factors are specific to individuals who go on to develop ASD and which factors are more generally observed family members of those who have ASD. These latter factors are generally observed with greater frequency in family members of affected individuals are commonly referred to as endophenotypes or intermediate phenotypes. They form a bridge between the two ends of the causal sequence – genes and behavior [13]. Endophenotypes are particularly important to understanding ASD in that they will likely help sort through the heterogeneity that exists at each level of functionality–genetic, neural, cognitive, and behavioral [14].

With respect to neural integration as an early endophenotype, differences in gamma frequency activity have been identified in several studies of infants at high risk. For example, Elsabbagh et al. [15] found higher baseline but lower induced gamma power in response to an eye gaze paradigm in 10-month-old infants. Tierney et al. [16] found lower gamma power at 6 months and flattened developmental trajectories in high-risk infants between 6 and 24 months. Both findings are consistent with a disruption in the integration of neural networks, although the exact nature of the timing and direction of differences in baseline power still needs to be resolved. Evidence of differences in gamma power in infants at high-risk for ASD would not only provide support for the idea that ASD is a disorder of neural integration but would also provide evidence that differences of gamma activity are candidate endophenotypes.

Spectral power, however, is a limited measure of neural integration because it primarily reflects synchronized activity within the specific region in which it is measured. Other transformations of neurophysiological signals provide a better assessment of neural integration. For example, linear coherence is an index of synchronization across regions rendering it a better-suited measure of neural integration–or connectivity as it is referred to in this literature. Linear coherence assesses the correlation between the phase and power information of two EEG signals and can be applied to any frequency range. The higher the correlation, the more synchronized, and therefore integrated, the signals are interpreted to be. Indeed, studies of EEG coherence as a measure of neural connectivity have found that children and adults with ASD showed lower coherence compared to age- and IQ-matched typically developing controls [17,18,19]. These findings of lower coherence have contributed to the proposal that one characteristic of ASD is that there is underconnectivity between distant regions of the brain. More recent coherence studies indicate a more complex pattern of connectivity in children with ASD, finding perturbations in the proportion of long- and short-range connectivity in the theta and alpha frequency ranges [20].

Systematic studies of coherence in gamma activity in high-risk infants have not yet been conducted. If atypical patterns of neural connectivity are responsible for the symptomatology of ASD in older individuals, they are likely to emerge very early in development either before behavioral and cognitive differences emerge or concurrently with the divergence in behavior and cognitive development. If these biological indices are present early in development, they could either be biomarkers of the disorder, or like many of the other measure of neural integration, endophenotypes that are found among individuals with a high genetic load for ASD. Thus, the goal of the present study was to investigate functional connectivity in infants high-risk for ASD in order to evaluate it as a potential endophenotype or biomarker of ASD. Using coherence of gamma frequency activity as a metric of connectivity, we examined whether differences emerge during the first year of life, a period of development that precedes the onset of ASD symptoms, in infants at high or low risk for ASD as well as in the subset of those who go on to develop the disorder.

We assessed functional connectivity in the EEG signal acquired as infants were presented with speech sounds and evaluated differences in coherence in response to hearing these sounds. We employed a task that involved language relevant sounds, given that: (1) language impairments are a common feature of ASD and of the broader phenotype [21,22] and (2) previous studies of toddlers and older children with ASD identified differences in measures of connectivity, specifically as they relate to language-based tasks [23–26]. This paradigm has been used to evaluate speech perception in infants [27] and previous studies of infant siblings using this task have found that there are ASD risk-related differences in the ERPs [28]. Overall we hypothesized that risk for ASD will be associated with reduced functional connectivity in response to speech sounds, which might be a manifestation of disrupted neural integration processes.

Materials and Methods

The study reported here is part of a comprehensive and ongoing longitudinal project on the neurocognitive development of infants at risk for ASD conducted at Boston Children's Hospital/Harvard Medical School and Boston University. All components of the study were approved by the IRB review boards at both institutions and are covered under IRB guidelines approved by both institutions. Written, informed consent was provided by the parents or guardians prior to their child's the participation in the study.

Participants

Participants were assigned to one of two groups in this study. If they had an older sibling with an ASD diagnosis (not due to a known genetic disorder; e.g. Fragile X syndrome), they were categorized as high-risk for ASD (HRA). The older siblings all had expert clinical community diagnoses, which were confirmed by a member of the study staff using the Social Communication Questionnaire (SCQ) [29] or the Autism Diagnostic Observation Schedule Generic (ADOS-G) [30]. Infants in the low-risk group (LRC) had at least one typically developing older sibling and no first-degree relatives with a known developmental disorder, based on a screening questionnaire. All infants had a gestational age of 36 weeks or greater, no history of prenatal or postnatal medical or neurological problems and no known genetic disorder. Furthermore, all infants were from monolingual English-speaking households (English spoken more than 80% of the time) and had no prior exposure to Bengali or Hindi.

In the present paper we report on data from 28 HRA infants and 26 LRC infants. Of the 28 HRA infants, 19 provided usable data at both the 6- and 12-month visits, 3 provided data only at the 6-month visit, and 6 only at the 12-month visit. Of the 26 LRC infants, 17 provided usable data at both the 6- and 12-month visits, 7 provided data only at the 6-month visit, and 2 only at the 12-month visit. Of the 44 infants who contributed data at 12 months of age, 38 of them were assessed using the ADOS at 36 months of age (16 LRC and 22 HRA). None of the 16 LRC infants met criteria for ASD on the ADOS (negative outcomes) whereas, 5 out of the 22 HRA infants met ASD criteria on the ADOS (positive outcomes). Expert clinical impression confirmed a diagnosis of ASD for the 5 infants with positive ADOS outcomes.

Sample demographics are presented in Table 1, displaying means for each group on characteristics of the infants and their families. There were no group differences on any demographic factors. Infants' cognitive abilities were assessed using the Mullen Scales of Early Learning [31] at 6 and 12 months. No significant group differences were detected at 6 months of age. At 12 months

Table 1. Mean demographic characteristic of the LRC and HRA infants (SD).

	n	LRC	n	HRA	t(df)	p
Infant's birth weight	26	7.9(1.2)	28	7.9(0.9)	0.10(52)	0.92
Mother's age at infant's birth	26	33.6(4.4)	28	34.9(4.8)	−1.05(52)	0.3
Father's age at infant's birth	26	36.3(4.5)	28	38.2(5.9)	−1.34(52)	0.19
Mother's education level	19	6.5(1.43)	24	5.7(1.6)	1.63(41)	0.11
Father's education level	19	5.9(1.51)	22	5.1(2.04)	1.50(39)	0.14
Family income	19	7.4(1.61)	24	7.4(1.25)	−0.11(41)	0.91

Note that not all families provided all demographic data.

of age the LRC group obtained significantly higher scores than the HRA on the Expressive Language ($t(40) = 2.39$, $p<0.03$), and Gross Motor ($t(40) = 2.57$, $p<0.02$) subscales, however the scores on these subscales for both groups were within the normal range. See Table 2 for a complete summary of Mullen scores.

Stimuli

The experimental stimuli consisted of three consonant-vowel pairs: a voiced, unaspirated, retroflex stop (/da/), native to English that represented the *standard* condition; a voiceless, aspirated retroflex palatal stop (/ta/), native to English that represented the *deviant native* condition; and a voiced, unaspirated dental stop (/dha/) not found in the English language that represented the *deviant non-native* condition. In order to allow for the matching of low level acoustic characteristics, these syllables were synthesized using STRAIGHT [32], such that all stimuli were matched on total duration (300 ms), and the two voiced, unaspirated syllables were also matched on energy, spectral components, and fundamental frequency of the vowel segment. See Seery et al. [28] for a more detailed description of the experimental stimuli.

These language-relevant stimuli have been used in previous studies examining speech perception in the first year of life. For example, it has been demonstrated that that 6 to 12 months of age is an important period in this process wherein infants become particularly skilled at recognizing speech sounds that are represented in their native language (and are thus more familiar with) while also becoming less able to recognizing speech sounds that are not represented in their native language [33,34]. This phenomenon has been studied using ERP measures, but because it may require the coordination of auditory and higher level language areas, we investigated whether gamma coherence was sensitive to the developmental trajectories in selectively responding to native and non-native phonemes.

Procedure

The testing session took place in a sound attenuated room. Auditory stimuli were presented using E Prime (Psychological Software Tools, PA) over two bilateral speakers while the infant sat on a parent's lap. Each stimulus was presented for 300 ms, followed by a variable inter-stimulus interval (700–1000 ms). The experimental paradigm consisted of a double-oddball design, modeled after Rivera-Gaxiola and colleagues' [27]. The standard stimulus was presented 80% of the time, while the two deviants were each presented 10% of the time. The experiment consisted of a maximum of 600 trials. In order to facilitate the infants' cooperation during testing an experimenter was present in the testing room during each session. The role of the experimenter was to blow bubbles throughout the procedure, which is standard practice used to maintain the infants' interest and increase their

Table 2. Cognitive characteristics of the LRC and HRA infants at 6 and 12 months.

	LRC	HRA	Contrast
	Mean(sem)	Mean(sem)	p-value(df)
6 month-olds			
Visual Reception	48.6(1.8)	48(1.8)	0.816(43)
Receptive Language	49(1.3)	49.9(1.3)	0.637(43)
Expressive Language	47.1(1.1)	46.8(1.1)	0.867(43)
Gross Motor	49.1(1.7)	47.2(1.7)	0.426(43)
Fine Motor	48.2(1.6)	52.2(1.6)	0.081(43)
12 month-olds			
Visual Reception	58.8(1.9)	55.6(1.8)	0.232(40)
Receptive Language	49.6(1.8)	47.7(1.6)	0.419(40)
Expressive Language	52.3(2.1)	45.6(1.9)	**0.022**(40)
Gross Motor	48.4(2.6)	39.3(2.4)	**0.014**(40)
Fine Motor	64.5(2.1)	62.8(1.9)	0.557(40)

The scores provided are t-scores from the Mullen Scales of Early Learning. Note that a total of 4 infants did not provide data.

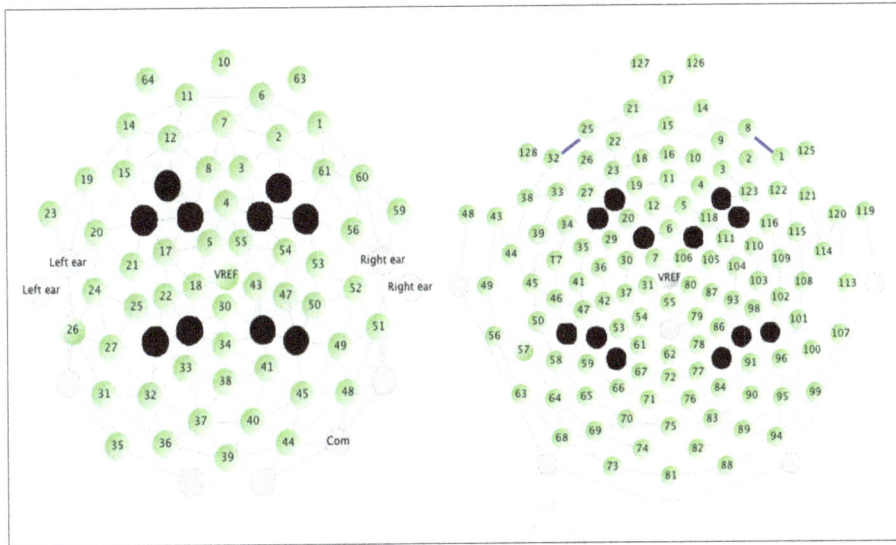

Figure 1. Locations of electrodes used for analysis in the 64-channel and 128-channel nets (electrodes chosen are colored in blue). Linear coherence was calculated between anterior and posterior electrode groupings within each hemisphere.

tolerance for the electrodes [35]. No other visual stimuli were present.

Recording and processing of electrophysiological data

Continuous EEG was recorded using 64- and 128-channel Geodesic Sensor Nets connected to a DC-coupled amplifier (Net Amp 200, Electrical Geodesic Inc.). Data were collected from 62 of 64 and 124 of 128 possible channel locations because EOG electrodes (64-channel: 63, 64; 128-channel: 125, 126, 127, 128) that are placed on the infants face were removed from the nets to decrease fussiness. The signal was amplified with a 0.1–100 Hz bandpass filter, digitized at 250 Hz, and referenced online to a single vertex electrode (Cz). The use of two different net sizes was due an equipment upgrade that took place about two years into the longitudinal study.

Data was sampled at 250 Hz and referenced to the vertex electrode (Cz). Preprocessing of the data was performed using NetStation 4.4.2 (Electrical Geodesic Inc.). In order to prepare the data for a time-frequency analysis, the continuous EEG was segmented to 800 ms, with a baseline period beginning 100 ms before stimulus onset, and 700 ms of post stimulus onset. Automated artifact detection tools were applied to all data segments, in order to identity segments and specific channels that contained movement artifacts, eye movements, eye blinks, and off-scale activity that exceeded ± 200 μV. Epochs were rejected if they contained (1) eye blinks, (2) eye movements, and (3) if more than 10% of channels in a segment were marked bad. The results of the automated artifact detection were visually inspected by a research assistant trained in the analysis of infant EEG data to confirm the presence of artifacts and ensure that all rejection criteria were applied properly. Subsequently, bad channels in all accepted segments were replaced by an automated algorithm that uses spherical spline interpolation. Finally, the data were re-referenced to the average reference.

The data were exported from NetStation into EEGLAB [36] for further processing and analysis. A 58–62 Hz notch filter was applied to remove noise created by electronic equipment present in the testing room. Subsequently, an average reference was applied to all data segments. Functional connectivity in the gamma

band (30–50 Hz) was quantified as linear coherence computed using the *newcrossf* function in EEGLAB. Signal decomposition was achieved with a Morlet wavelet transform that applied 3 cycles per frequency across the frequency spectrum available in the signal.

Linear coherence was calculated between electrode sites covering the frontal and temporo-parietal regions in the left and right hemispheres, and averaged across the 150 ms to 300 ms post-stimulus onset time window. This time window was chosen based on previous ERP studies that have used similar paradigms and identified components relevant to the processing of speech sounds (P150) [28]. Electrodes of interest were chosen a priori to encompass some of the anterior and posterior sites used in prior studies that have used similar paradigms [27,28] and ensure (1) location correspondence between net types, (2) comparable skull area coverage between net types, (3) and comparable number of electrode pairs to compute average coherence between net types. The electrodes we used for each net are as follows (with the corresponding 10–10 system sites noted in parentheses). In the 64-channel net, the left frontal region contained electrodes 13 (F3), 9 (FC1), 16 (FC5); the right frontal region contained electrodes 62 (F4), 58 (FC2), 57 (FC6); the left temporo/parietal region included electrodes 29 (P1–P3), 28 (P5); the right temporo/parietal region included electrodes 42 (P2), 46 (P4–P6). In the 128-channel net the left frontal region included electrodes 24 (F3), 13, (FC1), 28 (FC5); the right frontal region includes electrodes 124 (F4), 112 (FC2), 117 (FC6); the left temporo/parietal region included electrodes 60 (P1), 52 (P3), 51 (P5); the right temporo/parietal region included electrodes 85 (P2), 92 (P4), 97 (P6). These were roughly equidistant across net types, as measured on a mannequin's head (see figure 1).

Results

Analyses were conducted cross-sectionally by age (6 months and 12 months) because not all infants contributed data at both time points. Repeated measures mixed-model factorial ANOVAs were used to compare group differences in linear coherence. The models included group (LRC and HRA) as the between-subject factor; hemisphere (right and left), and condition (standard, native deviant, non-native deviant) as within-subject factors; subject was treated as a random effect. Given that the number of subjects was not equivalent across the two groups, the restricted maximum likelihood (REML) method was used. The dependent measure was linear coherence. Because of the change in equipment, we also evaluated the influence of net type (64-channel, 128-channel) but found no effects; therefore this factor was excluded from the analyses reported below. Additionally, we conducted a preliminary analysis in order to compare the differences in the 12-month data between the subset of infants who at 36 months met criteria for ASD and those who did not. See tables 3 and 4 for a complete summary of the statistical analyses.

Coherence at 6 months of age

Analyses of data from 6-month-old infants revealed two significant main effects. Due to the nature of the statistical model used, effect sizes for significant model effects were calculated using Cohen's f. There was a significant effect of hemisphere $(F(1,44.78) = 5.42, p<0.03;$ Cohen's $f = 0.3)$, showing higher linear coherence in the right hemisphere as compared to the left. There was also a significant effect of condition $(F(2,88) = 47.46, p< 0.0001;$ Cohen's $f = 1.4)$, showing significantly higher linear coherence for both deviant conditions as compared to the standard (native vs. standard: t(45) = 8.90, $p<0.0001$, two-tailed, Cohen's $d = 1.3$; non-native vs. standard: t(45) = 8.47, $p<0.0001$, two-tailed, Cohen's $d = 1.3$), but no difference between deviant conditions (t(45) = 1.3, $p<0.2$; Cohen's $d = 0.2$). There was no significant effect of group at this age. See table 3 for a complete summary of all results.

Coherence at 12 months of age

Analyses of 12-month-old data produced two significant effects. Most notably, we found a significant main effect of group $(F(1,42) = 7.77, p<0.005;$ Cohen's $f = 0.4)$, such that LRC infants displayed higher linear coherence that HRA infants (see Fig. 1). As in the 6-month data, there was a significant main effect of condition $(F(2,84) = 77.33, p<0.0001;$ Cohen's $f = 1.8)$. For both

groups, both deviant conditions elicited significantly more linear coherence than the standard condition (native vs. standard: t(43) = 12.79, $p<0.0001$, two-tailed, Cohen's $d = 1.8$; non-native vs. standard: t(43) = 10.09, $p<0.0001$, two-tailed, Cohen's $d = 1.7$), but no difference was found between the two deviant conditions (t(43) = 0.8, $p<0.5$, Cohen's $d = 0.1$). The analyses did not reveal any significant difference between hemispheres, and no significant interactions among the factors. See table 3 for a complete summary of all results.

Summary of coherence findings according to risk level

To summarize, we found that differences between HRA and LRC were not present at 6 months of age, but by 12 months LRC infants showed overall greater coherence compared to HRC across all experimental conditions (see figure 2). Furthermore, at both ages and for both groups there was evidence of sensitivity to the deviant phonemes. Finally, 6-month olds showed higher linear

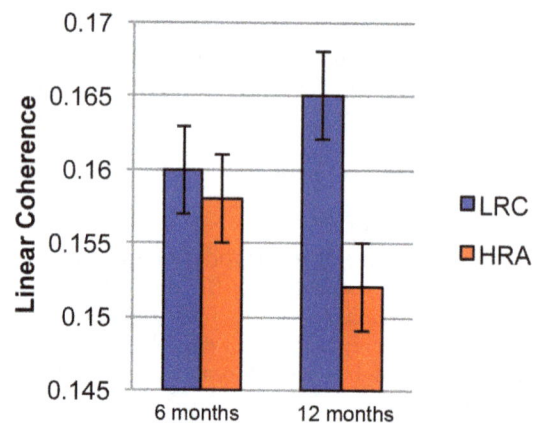

Figure 2. Average linear coherence for LRC (infants at low risk for ASD) and HRA (infants at risk for ASD) infants at 6 and 12 months. Error bars represent standard error.

Table 3. Full results of repeated measures ANOVA for 6-month-old infants and 12-month-old infants.

6 months	F(df)	p
Group	0.07(1)	0.79
Condition	47.46(2)	**<0.0001**
Hemisphere	5.42(1)	**0.02**
Group×Condition	2.71(1)	0.07
Group×Hemisphere	0.52(1)	0.47
Condition×Hemisphere	0.96(2)	0.39
Group×Condition×Hemisphere	0.74(2)	0.48
12 months		
Group	7.77(1)	**0.008**
Condition	77.33	**<0.0001**
Hemisphere	1.92(1)	0.17
Group×Condition	2.01(2)	0.14
Group×Hemisphere	0.01(1)	0.91
Condition×Hemisphere	2.07(2)	0.13
Group×Condition×Hemisphere	0.02(2)	0.98

coherence in the right hemisphere compared to the right, but no lateralization differences were found at 12 months of age.

Differences according to ASD outcome–a preliminary analysis

To determine whether the differences observed at 12 months between HRA and LRC infants are primarily associated with genetic risk for ASD or with the emergence of ASD we conducted a follow-up analysis on a subset of infants who had been assessed using the Autism Diagnostic Observation Schedule (ADOS) at 36 months of age. Out of the 44 infants (19 LRC and 25 HRA) who contributed data at 12 months of age, 38 of them had 36-month outcome data (16 LRC and 22 HRA). None of the 16 LRC infants met criteria for ASD on the ADOS, whereas 5 out of the 22 HRA infants met ASD criteria on the ADOS. For this analysis, we used the same statistical approach described above with the exception that group, which is the between subjects factors, became a three-way variable: LRC infants with negative ADOS outcomes (LRC−; n = 16), HRA infants with negative ADOS outcomes (HRA−; n = 17), and HRA infants with positive ADOS outcomes (HRA+; n = 5). This analysis revealed a significant main effect of group $(F(2,35) = 5.8; p < 0.01;$ Cohen's $f = 0.5)$. Follow up t-tests revealed higher linear coherence in the LRC− group compared to both the HRA− and HRA+ groups (LRC− vs. HRA−: $t(31) = 2.42, p < 0.03$, two-tailed, Cohen's $d = 0.9$; LRC− vs. HRA+: $t(19) = 2.67$, $p < 0.02$, two-tailed, Cohen's $d = 1.4$). A marginally significant difference was observed between HRA− and HRA+ infants $(t(20) = 1.74, p < 0.1$; two-tailed, $p < 0.05$, one-tailed, Cohen's $d = 0.8)$ with higher coherence in the HRA− group As in the results presented in the previous section, there was a main effect of condition $(F(2,70) = 52.2\ p < 0.0001;$ Cohen's $f = 1.5)$. Follow-up t-tests showed that both deviant conditions elicited significantly more linear coherence than the standard condition (native vs. standard: $t(37) = 9.14, p < 0.0001$, two-tailed, Cohen's $d = 1.2$; non-native vs. standard: $t(37) = 8.5$, $p < 0.0001$, two-tailed, Cohen's $d = 1.1$), but no difference was found between the two deviant conditions $(t(37) = 0.6, p < 0.6$, two-tailed, Cohen's $d = 0.1)$. No other differences were observed between these three groups (see table 4 for full ANOVA results). See figure 3 for illustration of the observed effects.

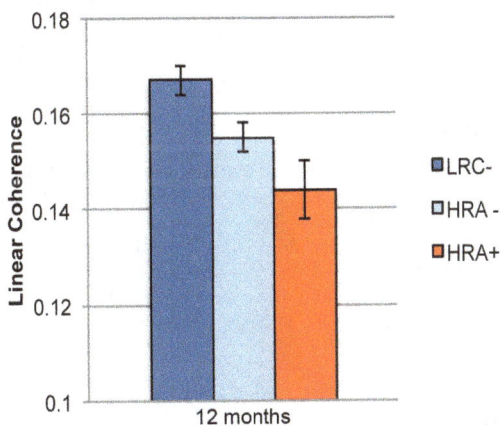

Figure 3. Average linear coherence at 12 months of age for LRC− (low risk infants who did not meet criteria for ASD at 36 months), HRA− (infants at risk for ASD who did not meet criteria for ASD at 36 months), HRA+ (infants at risk who met criteria for ASD at 36 months). Error bars represent standard error.

Discussion

The goal of the present study was to examine whether there are differences in functional connectivity between infants at high- and low- risk for ASD by the first year of life. First, our results show that by 12 months of age, infants at high-risk of developing ASD display significantly lower functional connectivity between frontal and parietal sites compared to infants at low-risk for ASD. Second, infants at high-risk for ASD showed lower functional connectivity compared to low-risk infants, irrespective of ASD outcome. Third, coherence appears to be lowest in those high-risk infants who go on to develop ASD, compared to high-risk infants who do not (see figure 3), but a larger sample is needed to confirm this result. Finally, our results did not show any group differences with regard to the sensitivity to native and non-native phonetic contrast or hemispheric lateralization.

The present results are consistent with a growing body of literature showing the emergence of risk-related differences in electrophysiological responses that emerge over the course of the first year of life [16,37,38]. More specifically, our findings of reduced functional connectivity associated with risk for ASD are consistent with recent studies of infants and toddlers that have used fNIRS [39], DTI [40], and fMRI [23]. Taken together, these results confirm the emerging trend toward atypical developmental patterns in measures of neural integration and anatomical connectivity associated with risk for ASD.

Our findings are the first to demonstrate the presence of reduced functional connectivity as indexed by linear coherence in gamma frequency activity in infants at high-risk for ASD. Furthermore, this is an endophenotype of ASD because reduced functional connectivity between our low-risk group and our high-risk group was present even after infants who went on to develop ASD were excluded from the analyses. Together with recent findings reporting abnormalities in white matter structures in the children with ASD and their unaffected siblings [41], our results provide evidence for a neural architecture that is both anatomically and functionally different from the early stages of development in individuals who are genetically vulnerable to ASD. It is likely that many qualitative and quantitative differences in neural connectivity can account for the heterogeneous phenotypic variations observed in individuals at risk for ASD. Our preliminary results suggest that quantitative differences in functional connectivity might be present between infants at-risk for ASD who later develop ASD and those who do not. This result is not surprising giving the strong evidence of reduced functional and anatomical connectivity in individuals ASD [42]. Nevertheless, it is remarkable that such differences can be detected as early as 12-months-of-age.

The stimuli used in this study derive from a paradigm designed to examine phonetic perception in relation to the perceptual content that infants are exposed to [27,28]. A recent study carried out with the same sample of infants using ERP showed that both low- and high-risk infants displayed experience-dependent changes in their responses to native and non-native phonemes over the first year of life, such that by 12 months of age there were no differences in the ERP responses to a non-native phonetic contrast [28]. Here we demonstrate that linear coherence between frontal and parietal sites is a neural measure sensitive to differences between native and non-native contrasts in both 6-month and 12-month old infants irrespective of risk status, as evidenced by significant differences between the standard condition and both deviant conditions. This pattern is somewhat similar to some of the ERP findings by Seery and colleagues [28] in which, irrespective of risk status, at 6 months and 9 months the P150 amplitude in the

Table 4. Full results of repeated measures ANOVA on the group of infants who have been assessed using the Autism Diagnostic Observation Schedule (ADOS) at 36 months of age.

	F(df)	p
	5.8(2)	**0.007**
Condition	52.17(2)	<0.001
Hemisphere	1.08(1)	0.3
Group×Condition	1.4(2)	0.24
Group×Hemisphere	0.05(1)	0.95
Condition×Hemisphere	1.51(2)	0.22
Group×Condition×Hemisphere	0.64(2)	0.63

'Group' is a three-way between-subject variable: LRC infants with negative ADOS outcomes (LRC−, $n = 16$), HRA infants with negative ADOS outcomes (HRA−, $n = 17$), and HRA infants with positive ADOS outcomes (HRA+, $n = 5$).

frontal region showed a main effect of condition with the two deviant conditions different from the standard, but no differences between the deviants. Nevertheless, Seery and colleagues [28] found that at 12-months-of-age the P150 amplitude in the frontal region was no longer different between non-native deviant and standard conditions. It is important to point out that there are some key methodological differences between the two studies that could account for the differences in results at 12 months. First, linear coherence in the gamma frequency band and ERP used non-overlapping portions of the EEG signal: whereas we focused our analyses on frequencies from 30 to 50 Hz, the ERP signal contains information only from frequencies below 30 Hz. Second, linear coherence, as an index of synchronized activity across sites, is not dependent on morphological attributes of the localized EEG signal across trials, but rather on the relationship in phase and power of the EEG signal between 2 locations. In contrast, ERPs reflect localized activity and are primarily sensitive to the presence of specific morphological characteristics within the EEG signal that are consistent across experimental trials. Third, in Seery et al. [28] these effects were found only in the frontal region, whereas the linear coherence reported on here assesses the connection between frontal and parietal regions.

Previous electrophysiological research on infant siblings has also found evidence of differences in hemispheric lateralization in ERP responses to speech sounds between low- and high-risk infants [28]. Similarly atypical patterns of hemispheric lateralization have also been found using fMRI in tasks that involved language processing [43,44]. In the present study we failed to find any differences in hemispheric lateralization of linear coherence, regardless of risk status or ASD outcome. As discussed above, linear coherence is an index of synchronized activity between regions and does not reflect the absolute amount of activation in response to specific stimuli, in contrast to ERP and fMRI. As such, it is possible that over the first year of life the left and right hemisphere networks sampled by the electrodes chosen in this study are comparably synchronous, irrespective of any differences in absolute activation.

Limitations

The present study has several limitations, primarily related to the nature of the infant sibling studies methodology. First, the combination of the available sample size and the fact that not all infants contributed data points at all ages deemed these data ill-suited for longitudinal analyses that could have shed light to developmental trajectories, Second, given that only a small number of infants met ASD criteria at 36 months (5 infants), our analyses cannot speak directly to the potential for reduced functional connectivity as a neurobiological marker of ASD. Third, it has been suggested that high frequency signals in the EEG are vulnerable to myogenic artifacts [45] and eye movement artifacts [46]. Nevertheless, it is unlikely that these artifacts would have any group- or condition-specific effects.

Conclusions

To conclude, the present study demonstrated that reduced functional connectivity during speech processing is a trait associated with family risk status, and can therefore be considered an endophenotype. While the present study cannot speak directly to the relationship between clinical outcome and functional connectivity, it provides preliminary evidence suggesting that functional connectivity at 12 months is lowest in those infants who do go onto develop ASD. This provides further evidence that ASD is broadly characterized by differences in neural integration. In the future it will be important to determine how the emergence of atypical task-related functional connectivity by the first year of life contributes to a cumulative risk model, which can lead to further understanding of the factors that lead to the development of an ASD diagnosis [12,47].

Acknowledgments

We would like to thank the families for their invaluable contribution to the Infant Sibling Project. We would also like to thank the Infant Sibling Project staff – Vanessa Vogel-Farley, Tara Augenstein, Kristen Concannon, Nicole Coman, Kerri Downing, Nina Leezenbaum, Vanessa Loukas, Stephanie Marshall, Anne Seery, and Meagan Thompson – for their assistance in data acquisition and data processing. Finally we would like to thank Brandon Keehn, Jennifer Wagner, and Rhiannon Luyster – for many helpful conversations.

Author Contributions

Conceived and designed the experiments: HTF CN. Analyzed the data: GR AT. Contributed to the writing of the manuscript: GR AT HTF CN.

References

1. American Psychiatric Association. (2013) Diagnostic and statistical manual of mental disorders (5th ed.). Arlington, VA: American Psychiatric Publishing.
2. Tager-Flusberg H, Joseph RM (2003) Identifying neurocognitive phenotypes in autism. Philos Trans R Soc Lond B Biol Sci 358: 303–14.
3. Amaral DG, Schumann CM, Nordahl CW (2008) Neuroanatomy of autism. Trends Neurosci 31: 137–45.
4. Murdock JD, State MW (2013) Recent development in the genetics of autism spectrum disorders. Curr Opin in Genet Dev 23: 310–15.
5. Geschwind DH, Levitt P (2007) Autism spectrum disorders: Developmental disconnection syndromes. Curr Opin Neurobiol 17: 103–11.
6. Uhlhaas PJ, Singer W (2006) Neural synchrony in brain disorders: Relevance for cognitive dysfunctions and pathophysiology. Neuron 52: 155–68.
7. Brock J, Brown CC, Boucher J, Rippon G (2002) The temporal binding deficit hypothesis of autism. Dev Psychopathol 14: 209–24.
8. Zwaigenbaum L, Thurm A, Stone W, Baranek G, Bryson S, et al. (2007) Studying the emergence of autism spectrum disorders in high-risk infants: Methodological and practical issues. J Autism Dev Disord 37: 466–80.
9. Zwaigenbaum L, Bryson S, Lord C, Rogers S, Carter A, et al. (2009) Clinical assessment and management of toddlers with suspected autism spectrum disorder: Insights from studies of high-risk infants. Pediatrics 123: 1383–91.
10. Rogers SJ (2009) What are infant siblings teaching us about autism in infancy? Autism Res 2: 125–37.
11. Ozonoff S, Young GS, Carter A, Messinger D, Yirmiya N, et al. (2011) Recurrence risk for autism spectrum disorders: A baby siblings research consortium study. Pediatrics 128: 488–95.
12. Jones E, Gliga T, Bedford R, Charman T, Johnson MH (2014) Developmental pathways to autism: A review of prospective studies of infants at risk. Neuroscience and Biobehavioral Reviews 39: 1–33.
13. Gottesman II, Gould TD (2003) The endophenotype concept in psychiatry: Etymology and strategic intentions. Am J Psychiatry 160: 636–45.
14. Viding E, Blakemore SJ (2007) Endophenotype approach to developmental psychology: Implications for Autism research. Behav Genet 37: 51–60.
15. Elsabbagh M, Volein A, Csibra G, Holmboe K, Garwood H, et al. (2009) Neural correlates of eye gaze processing in the infant broader autism phenotype. Biol Psychiatry 65: 31–8.
16. Tierney AL, Gabard-Durnam L, Vogel-Farley V, Tager-Flusberg H, Nelson CA (2012) Developmental trajectories of resting EEG power: An endophenotype of autism spectrum disorder. PLoS ONE 7: e39127.
17. Catarino A, Andrade A, Churches O, Wagner AP, Baron-Cohen S, et al. (2013) Task-related functional connectivity in autism spectrum conditions: An EEG study using wavelet transform coherence. Mol Autism 4: 1–14.
18. Coben R, Clarke AR, Hudspeth W, Barry RJ (2008) EEG power and coherence in autistic spectrum disorder. Clin Neurophysiol 119: 1002–9.
19. Murias M, Webb SJ, Greenson J, Dawson G (2007) Resting state cortical connectivity reflected in EEG coherence in individuals with autism. Biol Psychiatry 62: 270–3.
20. Peters JM, Taquet M, Vega C, Jeste SS, Fernández IS, et al. (2013) Brain functional networks in syndromic and non-syndromic autism: A graph theoretical study of EEG connectivity. BMC Med 11: 54–70.
21. Lindgren KA, Folstein SE, Tomblin JB, Tager-Flusberg H (2009) Language and reading abilities of children with autism spectrum disorders and specific language impairment and their first-degree relatives. Autism Res 2: 2: 22–38.
22. Toth K, Dawson G, Meltzoff AN, Greenson J, Fein D (2007) Early social, imitation, play, and language abilities of young non-autistic siblings of children with autism. J Autism Dev Disord 37: 145–57.
23. Dinstein I, Pierce K, Eyler L, Solso S, Malach R, et al. (2011) Disrupted neural synchronization in toddlers with autism. Neuron 70: 1218–25.
24. Harris GJ, Chabris CF, Clark J, Urban T, Aharon I, et al. (2006) Brain activation during semantic processing in autism spectrum disorders via functional magnetic resonance imaging. Brain Cogn 61: 54–68.
25. Just MA, Cherkassky VL, Keller TA, Minshew NJ (2004) Cortical activation and synchronization during sentence comprehension in high-functioning autism: Evidence of underconnectivity. Brain 127: 1811–21.
26. Knaus TA, Silver AM, Lindgren KA, Hadjikhani N, Tager-Flusberg H (2008) FMRI activation during a language task in adolescents with ASD. J Int Neuropsychol Soc 14: 967–79.
27. Rivera-Gaxiola M, Silva-Pereyra J, Kuhl PK (2005) Brain potentials to native and non-native speech contrasts in 7- and 11-month-old American infants. Dev Sci 8: 162–72.
28. Seery AM, Vogel-Farley V, Tager-Flusberg H, Nelson CA (2012) Atypical lateralization of ERP response to native and non-native speech in infants at risk for autism spectrum disorder. Dev Cogn Neurosci 5C: 10–24.
29. Rutter M, Bailey A, Lord C (2003) Social Communication Questionnaire. In: Los Angeles, CA: Western Psychological Services.
30. Lord C, Risi S, Lambrecht L, Cook EHJ, Leventhal BL, et al. (2000) The autism diagnostic observation schedule-generic: A standard measure of social and communication deficits associated with the spectrum of autism. J Autism Dev Disord 30: 205–23.
31. Mullen E (1995) *Mullen Scales of Early Learning*. Circle Pines, MN: American Guidance Services Inc.
32. Kawahara H, Masuda-Kasuse I, de Cheveigne A (1999) Restructuring speech representations using a pitch-adaptive time-frequency smoothing and an instantaneous-frequency-based F0 extraction: Possible role of a repetitive structure in sounds. Speech Commun 27: 187–207.
33. Kuhl P, Williams KA, Lacerda F, Stevens KN, Lindblom B (1992) Linguistic experience alters phonetic perception in infants by 6 months of age. Science 255: 606–608.
34. Cheour M, Ceponiene R, Lehtokoski A, Luuk A, Allik J, et al. (1998) Development of language-specific phoneme representations in the infant brain. Nat Neurosci 1: 351–353.
35. Hoehl S, Wahl S (2012) Recording infant ERP data for cognitive research. Dev Neuropsychol 37: 187–209.
36. Delorme A, Makeig S (2004) EEGLAB: An open source toolbox for analysis of single-trial EEG dynamics including independent component analysis. J Neurosci Methods 134: 9–21.
37. Bosl W, Tierney A, Tager-Flusberg H, Nelson C (2011) EEG complexity as a biomarker for autism spectrum disorder risk. BMC Med 9: 18–32.
38. Gabard-Durnam L, Tierney AL, Vogel-Farley V, Tager-Flusberg H, Nelson CA (2013) Alpha asymmetry in infants at risk for autism spectrum disorders. J Autism Dev Disord: 1–8.
39. Keehn B, Wagner JB, Tager-Flusberg H, Nelson CA (2013) Functional connectivity in the first year of life in infants at-risk for autism: A preliminary near-infrared spectroscopy study. Front Hum Neurosci 7: 444.
40. Wolff JJ, Gu H, Gerig G, Elison JT, Styner M, et al. (2011) Differences in white matter fiber tract development present from 6 to 24 months in infants with autism. Am J Psychiatry 169: 589–600.
41. Barnea-Goraly N, Lotspeich LJ, Reiss AL (2010) Similar white matter aberrations in children with autism and their unaffected siblings: A diffusion tensor imaging study using tract-based spatial statistics. Arch Gen Psychiatry 67: 1052–60.
42. Just MA, Keller TA, Malave VL, Kana RK, Varma S (2012) Autism as a neural systems disorder: A theory of frontal-posterior underconnectivity. Neurosci Biobehav 36: 1292–313.
43. Eyler LT, Pierce K, Courchesne E (2012) A failure of left temporal cortex to specialize for language is an early emerging and fundamental property of autism. Brain 135: 949–60.
44. Redcay E, Courchesne E (2008) Deviant functional magnetic resonance imaging patterns of brain activity to speech in 2-3-year-old children with autism spectrum disorder. Biol Psychiatry 64: 589–98.
45. Goncharova II, McFarland DJ, Vaughan TM, Wolpaw JR (2003) EMG contamination of EEG: Spectral and topographical characteristics. Clin Neurophysiol 114: 1580–93.
46. Yuval-Greenberg S, Tomer O, Keren AS, Nelken I, Deouell LY (2008) Transient induced gamma-band response in EEG as a manifestation of miniature saccades. Neuron 58: 429–41.
47. Tager-Flusberg H (2010) The origins of social impairments in autism spectrum disorder: Studies of infants at risk. Neural Netw 2010; 23: 1072–6.

6

Dissociable Genetic Contributions to Error Processing: A Multimodal Neuroimaging Study

Yigal Agam[1,2], Mark Vangel[2], Joshua L. Roffman[1], Patience J. Gallagher[3], Jonathan Chaponis[3], Stephen Haddad[3], Donald C. Goff[1], Jennifer L. Greenberg[1], Sabine Wilhelm[1], Jordan W. Smoller[1,3], Dara S. Manoach[1,2]*

1 Department of Psychiatry, Massachusetts General Hospital, Harvard Medical School, Boston, Massachusetts, United States of America, 2 Athinoula A. Martinos Center for Biomedical Imaging, Harvard Medical School, Charlestown, Massachusetts, United States of America, 3 Center for Human Genetics Research, Massachusetts General Hospital, Harvard Medical School, Boston, Massachusetts, United States of America

Abstract

Background: Neuroimaging studies reliably identify two markers of error commission: the error-related negativity (ERN), an event-related potential, and functional MRI activation of the dorsal anterior cingulate cortex (dACC). While theorized to reflect the same neural process, recent evidence suggests that the ERN arises from the posterior cingulate cortex not the dACC. Here, we tested the hypothesis that these two error markers also have different genetic mediation.

Methods: We measured both error markers in a sample of 92 comprised of healthy individuals and those with diagnoses of schizophrenia, obsessive-compulsive disorder or autism spectrum disorder. Participants performed the same task during functional MRI and simultaneously acquired magnetoencephalography and electroencephalography. We examined the mediation of the error markers by two single nucleotide polymorphisms: dopamine D4 receptor (*DRD4*) C-521T (rs1800955), which has been associated with the ERN and methylenetetrahydrofolate reductase (*MTHFR*) C677T (rs1801133), which has been associated with error-related dACC activation. We then compared the effects of each polymorphism on the two error markers modeled as a bivariate response.

Results: We replicated our previous report of a posterior cingulate source of the ERN in healthy participants in the schizophrenia and obsessive-compulsive disorder groups. The effect of genotype on error markers did not differ significantly by diagnostic group. *DRD4 C-521T* allele load had a significant linear effect on ERN amplitude, but not on dACC activation, and this difference was significant. *MTHFR* C677T allele load had a significant linear effect on dACC activation but not ERN amplitude, but the difference in effects on the two error markers was not significant.

Conclusions: *DRD4 C-521T*, but not *MTHFR* C677T, had a significant differential effect on two canonical error markers. Together with the anatomical dissociation between the ERN and error-related dACC activation, these findings suggest that these error markers have different neural and genetic mediation.

Editor: Bart Rypma, University of Texas at Dallas, United States of America

Funding: This work was supported in part by NIH grants F32 MH088081 (YA); K24MH094614 (JWS); and R01 MH67720 (DSM). The funders had no role in study design, data collection and analysis, decision to publish, or preparation of the manuscript.

Competing Interests: The authors have declared that no competing interests exist.

* Email: dara@nmr.mgh.harvard.edu

Introduction

Adaptive, flexible behavior depends on the ability to recognize errors and adjust responses to improve outcomes. Deficits in these abilities characterize several neuropsychiatric disorders including schizophrenia, obsessive-compulsive disorder (OCD) and autism spectrum disorder (ASD) and may contribute to maladaptively rigid and repetitive behavior [1]. Accordingly, illuminating the neural and genetic mediation of error processing is important for both basic and clinical neuroscience. Neuroimaging studies have identified two highly reliable neural correlates of errors: the error-related negativity (ERN), an event-related potential that peaks

~100 ms following an error, and functional MRI (fMRI) activation of the dorsal anterior cingulate cortex (dACC) for erroneous compared with correct responses (see [2]). Although both of these error markers have been extensively characterized, their exact functions and how they are related remain a topic of debate. While influential models postulate that ERN is generated by the dACC [2–4], a review of source localization studies and recent evidence instead support a posterior cingulate cortex (PCC) generator of the ERN [5]. Monkey single-unit recordings confirm increased neuronal firing in the PCC after error commission [6]. This anatomical dissociation suggests that error-related dACC activation, rather than being a hemodynamic reflection of the

Table 1. Breakdown of study sample by allele load for each SNP.

	MTHFR C677T			DRD4 C-521T		
	C/C (0)	C/T (1)	T/T (2)	T/T (0)	C/T (1)	C/C (2)
Healthy participants	16 (41%)	13 (32%)	4 (31%)	10 (37%)	15 (32%)	8 (44%)
Schizophrenia	12 (31%)	13 (32%)	3 (23%)	9 (33%)	14 (30%)	5 (28%)
OCD	7 (18%)	7 (18%)	4 (31%)	4 (15%)	11 (23%)	3 (17%)
ASD	4 (10%)	7 (18%)	2 (15%)	4 (15%)	7 (15%)	2 (11%)
Totals	39	40	13	27	47	18

Allele load (0,1,2) refers to the number of risk alleles: *677T* for *MTHFR C677T* and *521C* for *DRD4 C-521T*.

ERN, indexes a different process. Here, we tested the hypothesis that dACC activation and the ERN also have different genetic mediation, which, if confirmed, would further the evidence of distinct underlying mechanisms. We measured both error markers in the same individuals performing the same task and examined the contributions of two single nucleotide polymorphisms (SNPs): dopamine D4 receptor (*DRD4*) *C-521T* (rs1800955), which has been associated with the ERN [7] and methylenetetrahydrofolate reductase (*MTHFR*) *C677T* (rs1801133), which has been associated with dACC activation [8,9]. No study has compared their influence on both phenotypes.

Converging lines of evidence support a role for dopamine (DA) in error processing [4]. ERN amplitude shows strong heritability among twin pairs [10] and several DA-related genetic polymorphisms have been variably associated with the ERN (for review see [11]). These include *DRD2-TAQ-1A* [12] but see [13] for a negative result; *COMT Val158Met* [14] but see [15]; *DAT1 3'-UTR* variable number of tandem repeats (VNTR) [12] but see [16,17]; and *DRD4 exon 3 VNTR* [17]. The present study examined *DRD4 C-521T*, a SNP in the promoter region of the gene encoding the DA D4 receptor protein, based on evidence of its association with schizophrenia [18,19,20] and the observation that *T*-homozygotes have a larger ERN amplitude than *C*-homozygotes [7].

Two prior studies from our group have examined the effects of *MTHFR C677T* on error-related dACC activation [8,9]. The hypofunctional *677T* allele was associated with reduced error-related dACC activation in three independent samples, one comprising healthy individuals and the other two comprising schizophrenia patients. *MTHFR C677T* may influence several steps in the DA lifecycle by regulating methylation reactions. Each copy of the *677T* allele reduces MTHFR activity by 35% [21] and in two samples, error-related dACC activation was linearly related to the number of *677T* alleles [9]. The *677T* allele is also associated with increased risk for schizophrenia [20], and with increased severity of negative symptoms [22], worse executive function [23] and reduced dorsolateral prefrontal activation during working memory performance [24] in patients with schizophrenia.

We investigated the hypothesis of a double dissociation in genetic mediation of these error markers. We expected each *MTHFR C677T* allele to reduce error-related dACC activation but not affect the ERN, and each *DRD4 C-521T* allele to increase ERN amplitude, but not affect dACC activation. Participants performed an antisaccade paradigm during both fMRI and simultaneous electroencephalography (EEG) and magnetoencephalography (MEG). Antisaccades require inhibition of the prepotent response of looking toward a suddenly appearing stimulus and the substitution of a gaze in the opposite direction. Antisaccade errors

(i.e., looking toward the stimulus) reliably elicit both dACC activation [25,26] and the ERN [27,28,29]. We compared the effects of each polymorphism on the two error markers modeled as a bivariate response, and also examined the source of the ERN using anatomically-constrained EEG/MEG.

Methods

Participants

A total of 144 participants enrolled in a clinical study of error processing. Of these, 105 completed both the fMRI and EEG sessions and 13 were excluded for not having at least 10 usable error trials in each modality. The final sample of 92 (62 male; age 36±13 years) comprised 33 healthy participants, 28 participants diagnosed with schizophrenia, 18 with OCD and 13 with ASD. Fifty of these participants (23 healthy; 27 schizophrenia) were included in a previous analysis of *MTHFR C677T* effects on error-related dACC activation [9]. Participants in each group were divided by *MTHFR C677T* and *DRD4 C-521T* genotype (Table 1).

Healthy participants were screened to exclude a personal history of neurological or psychiatric disorder (SCID-Non-patient edition) [30] and a family history of anxiety disorder, OCD, schizophrenia spectrum disorder or ASD. Clinical diagnoses of schizophrenia and OCD were confirmed by medical records review and the Structural Clinical Interview for DSM-IV (SCID) [31]. OCD participants were also required to have a Yale-Brown Obsessive Compulsive Scale (Y-BOCS) [32,33] total score >16. Clinical diagnoses of ASD were confirmed with the Autism Diagnostic Interview-Revised [34] and the Autism Diagnostic Observation Schedule Module 4 [35] administered by research personnel with established reliability. Patients were all either unmedicated or on stable doses of medication for at least eight weeks. All participants were screened to exclude substance abuse or dependence within the preceding six months and any independent condition that might affect brain function. Participants gave written informed consent and the protocol was approved by the Partners Human Research Committee.

Genotyping

A saliva sample was acquired with an Oragene self-collection kit (DNA Genotek, Ottawa). *MTHFR C677T* and *DRD4 C-521T* genotyping used allele-specific probes in an assay combining Polymerase chain reaction (PCR) and the 5' nuclease (Taqman) technique. The specific primers and probes for *MTHFR C677T* were based on published data [23] and synthesized by Applied Biosystems. PCR for DRD4 C-521T genotyping was performed in a 9.0 ul PCR reaction that contained 15 ng of DNA, 1X PCR Buffer, 11% DMSO, 0.55 uMol each dATP, dCTP and dTTP,

0.27 uMol dGTP, 0.55 uMol 7-deaza-2'deoxyguanosine 5'-triphosphate, 2.5 mM MgCl$_2$, 2.5 pmol of forward (labeled) and reverse primer (5'-GACCGCGACTACGTGGTCTACTC-3' and 5'-CTCAGGACAGGAACCCACCGAC-3'), and 0.5 U Amplitaq Gold. The thermocycling conditions consisted of initial denaturation for 15 mins at 95°C, 35 cycles of denaturation at 94°C for 30 seconds, annealing 66°C for 30 seconds and extension at 72°C for 45 seconds with a final extension at 72°C for 10 minutes.

Multi-Dimensional Scaling Analysis

To control for population stratification, a subset of the analyses were restricted to a Caucasian-only sample. This group was defined based upon both self-report and a multi-dimensional scaling analysis (MDS) performed using an ancestry informative marker set (AIMs) of SNPs. The AIMs panel contains a set of markers that best differentiate and cluster individuals in a dataset into continental populations. Multi-dimensional scaling (MDS) analysis was performed in PLINK (population-based linkage; http://pngu.mgh.harvard.edu/~purcell/plink/0 [36] combining the HapMap Phase 3 (HapMap3) data set with this dataset in order to visualize sample clustering by race/ethnicity in a two-dimensional scatter plot and help assist in measuring genetic distance. In MDS analysis, PLINK assigns an Identity by State (IBS) score for each sample pair at each marker. Using these IBS scores, PLINK performs an algorithm to reduce the IBS information to fewer dimensions. We created a scatter plot using the first two dimensions or axes of variation to determine where the samples in this study fell relative to the HapMap3 samples and then compared those results to the self-reported racial/ethnicity data. Of the 92 samples, 74 samples self-reported Caucasian and also fell within the HapMap3 European/Caucasian cluster.

Antisaccade paradigm

The antisaccade paradigm (Fig. 1) was programmed in Matlab Psychtoolbox (Mathworks, Natick, MA), and consisted of three types of antisaccade trials: Hard (40%), Easy (50%), and Fake-Hard (10%). Hard trials introduced a distraction during the gap – a 3 dB luminance increase of the peripheral squares that mark the location of stimulus appearance. Fake-Hard trials started with a cue indicating a hard trial, but were otherwise identical to Easy trials (i.e., there was no luminance change). They were included as a control condition to allow an examination of the effects of a hard vs. easy cue on fMRI activation unconfounded by the change in luminance that characterizes hard trials. In the present study, error and correct trials were combined across all three trial types for analysis.

Antisaccade trials were balanced for right and left stimuli. Randomly interleaved with the saccadic trials were fixation epochs lasting 2, 4, or 6 s, which provided a baseline and introduced "temporal jitter" to optimize the analysis of rapid presentation event-related fMRI data [37–39]. The schedule of events was determined using a technique to optimize the statistical efficiency of event-related designs [40]. Each task run lasted 5 min 16 s and generated an average of 64 antisaccade trials and 20 fixation epochs. Participants performed six runs in fMRI and eight runs in EEG/MEG. The order of fMRI and EEG/MEG sessions was counterbalanced.

Prior to the first scanning session, participants practiced in a mock MRI scanner, were encouraged to respond as quickly and accurately as possible, and were told that in addition to the base rate of pay, they would receive 5¢ for each correct response.

Recording and scoring of eye movement data

The ISCAN fMRI Remote Eye Tracking Laboratory (ISCAN, Burlington, MA) recorded eye position during fMRI using a 120 Hz video camera. During EEG, eye movements were monitored using two pairs of bipolar EOG electrodes, one vertical (above and below the left eye) and one horizontal. Horizontal EOG activity recorded during a brief calibration allowed an estimate of gaze position for scoring antisaccades [29,41].

Eye movement data were scored in MATLAB (Mathworks, Natick, MA) using a partially automated program. Saccades were identified as horizontal eye movements with velocities exceeding 47°/s. The onset of a saccade was defined as the point at which the velocity of the eye first exceeded 31°/s. Trials with initial saccades in the direction of the stimulus were scored as errors. Reaction time (RT) was defined as the onset time of the initial saccade relative to the appearance of the stimulus. Error rates were logit-transformed before analysis to normalize their distribution. Group differences in error rates and saccadic RT on correct trials were assessed with ANOVA. Since error rates were similar in the EEG and fMRI sessions, they were averaged across modalities for further analysis.

MRI acquisition

Images were acquired with a 3T Siemens Trio whole body high-speed imaging device (Siemens Medical Systems, Erlangen, Germany), equipped for echo planar imaging (EPI). Eighty-two participants were scanned with a 12-channel head coil and 10 healthy participants with a 32-channel head coil. A high-resolution structural scan was acquired in the sagittal plane using 3D rf-spoiled magnetization prepared rapid gradient echo (MP-RAGE) sequences (12-channel: TR/TE/Flip = 2530 ms/3.39 ms/7°; FOV = 256 mm, 176 1.33×1×1.33 mm in-plane slices; 32-channel: TR/TE/Flip = 2530 ms/1.61+1.78 n, $n = 0$–3/7°; iPAT = 3; FOV = 256 mm, 176 1×1×1 mm in-plane slices). To construct the boundary-element model surface for each participant's MEG/EEG source estimation, we acquired a multi-echo multi flip angle (5°) fast low-angle shot (FLASH) pulse sequence (610 Hz/pixel, TR = 20 ms, TE = (1.89+2 n) ms, $n = 0$–7, 128 1×1.33 mm in-plane sagittal slices, 1.33 mm thickness).

Functional images were acquired using a gradient echo T2* weighted sequence (12-channel: TR/TE/Flip = 2000 ms/30 ms/90°, 32 contiguous horizontal slices parallel to the inter-commissural plane, voxel size: 3.1×3.1×3.7 mm, interleaved; 32-channel: TR/TE/Flip = 2000 ms/28 ms/77°, iPAT = 3, 41 contiguous horizontal slices parallel to the inter-commissural plane, voxel size: 3.1×3.1×3.1 mm, interleaved). The functional sequences included prospective acquisition correction (PACE) for head motion [42].

fMRI Analysis

Analyses were conducted on each participant's inflated cortical surfaces reconstructed from the MP-RAGE scan using FreeSurfer (http://surfer.nmr.mgh.harvard.edu) segmentation, surface reconstruction, and inflation algorithms [43,44]. Functional and structural scans were spatially normalized to a template brain consisting of the averaged cortical surface of an independent sample of 40 adults (Buckner laboratory, Washington University, St. Louis, MO) using Freesurfer's surface-based spherical coordinate system, which employs a non-rigid alignment algorithm that explicitly aligns cortical folding patterns and is relatively robust to inter-individual differences in the gyral and sulcal anatomy of the cingulate cortex. Cortical activation was localized using automated surface-based parcellation software [45]. To facilitate comparison with other studies, approximate Talairach coordinates were

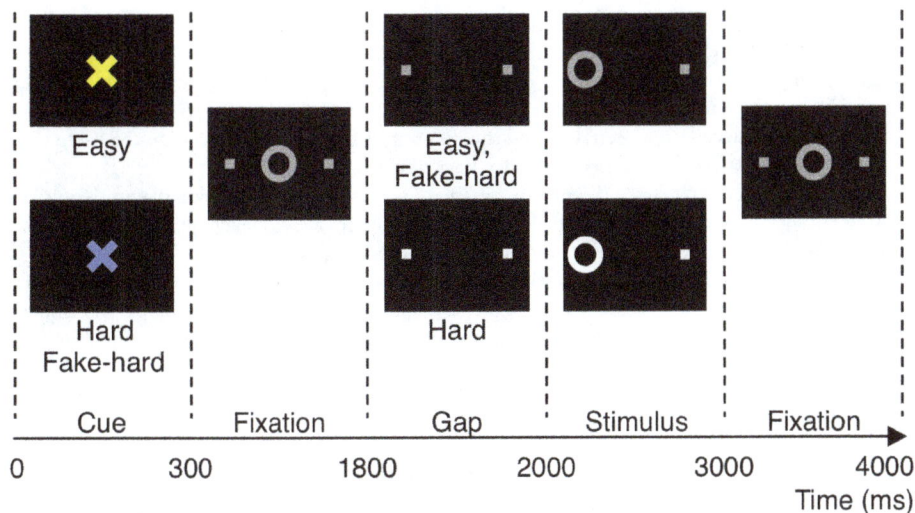

Figure 1. Antisaccade paradigm. Schematic and timeline of the three conditions: easy, hard, and fake-hard. Each trial lasted 4 s and began with an instructional cue (300 ms), either a blue or yellow "X" that indicated whether the trial was hard or easy. The mapping of cue color to trial type was counterbalanced across participants. The cue was horizontally flanked by two white squares of 0.4° width that marked the potential locations of stimulus appearance, 10° left and right of center. The squares remained visible for the duration of each run. At 300 ms, the instructional cue was replaced by a white fixation ring of 1.3° diameter at the center of the screen. At 1800 ms, the fixation ring disappeared (200 ms gap). At 2000 ms, the fixation ring reappeared at one of the two stimulus locations, right or left with equal probability. This was the imperative stimulus to which the participant responded by making a saccade in the opposite direction. The ring remained in the peripheral location for 1000 ms and then returned to the center, where participants were instructed to return their gaze for 1000 ms before the start of the next trial. Fixation epochs were simply a continuation of this fixation display. Hard trials were distinguished by a 3 db increase in luminance of the peripheral squares starting during the gap. Except for the hard cue, fake-hard trials were identical to easy trials.

derived by mapping surface-based coordinates back to the original structural volume for each of the individuals whose brains were used to create the template brain, registering the volumes to the Montreal Neurological Institute (MNI305) atlas [46] and averaging the corresponding MNI305 coordinates. These coordinates were transformed to standard Talairach space (http://imaging.mrc-cbu.cam.ac.uk/imaging/MniTalairach).

In addition to prospective motion correction (PACE), functional scans were retrospectively corrected for motion using the AFNI algorithm [47], intensity normalized, and smoothed using a 3D 8 mm FWHM Gaussian kernel. Functional images were aligned to the MP-RAGE scan for each participant.

Finite impulse response (FIR) estimates [38,39] of the event-related hemodynamic responses were calculated for error and correct trials for each participant. This involved using a linear model to provide unbiased estimates of the average signal intensity at each time point without making *a priori* assumptions about the shape of the hemodynamic response. Estimates were computed at 12 time points with an interval of 2 s (corresponding to the TR) ranging from 4 s prior to the start of a trial to 18 s after the start. Temporal correlations in the noise were accounted for by prewhitening using a global estimate of the residual error autocorrelation function truncated at 30 s [39].

The dACC was defined using automated surface-based parcellation software [45] that delineated cingulate cortex, which was then divided into dACC, rACC, and PCC [48]. Using this anatomical definition, error-related dACC activation was measured at the maximal vertex in each hemisphere for each participant in the error vs. correct contrast at 6 s, the time of maximal error-related activation in the group and in a prior antisaccade study [26]. Because error-related activation in the left and right dACC was strongly correlated (r = .89) we averaged activation across the hemispheres to simplify the model.

MEG/EEG Acquisition and Analysis

EEG and MEG ware acquired simultaneously in a magnetically shielded room (IMEDCO, Hagendorf, Switzerland). MEG was recorded using a dc-SQUID Neuromag VectorView system (Elekta-Neuromag, Helsinki, Finland) comprising 306 sensors arranged in triplets of two orthogonal planar gradiometers and a magnetometer, distributed at 102 locations around the entire scalp. EEG was recorded using a 70-channel electrode cap. Electrode impedances were brought below 20 KOhm at the start of each recording session. All signals were identically filtered to 0.1–200 Hz bandpass and digitized at 600 Hz.

To allow registration of EEG/MEG and MRI data and to record head position relative to the sensor array, the locations of three fiduciary points (nasion and auricular points) defining a head-based coordinate system, the sites of four head position indicator (HPI) coils, and a set of points from the head surface were digitized using a 3 Space Fastrak digitizer (Polhemus, Colchester, VT, USA) integrated with the Vectorview system. At the beginning of each MEG acquisition, currents were fed to the HPI coils and their magnetic fields were used to calculate the relative location of the head with respect to the MEG sensor array.

After excluding noisy EEG channels by visual inspection of the raw data, EEG data were re-referenced to the grand average. MEG channels were processed using the signal-space separation method [49]. Each participant's continuous MEG and EEG data were low-pass filtered at 40 Hz. Trials with eye blinks were defined by a difference between the maximum and minimum voltage of 150 µV or greater at the vertical EOG channel and excluded from analysis. EEG data, time-locked to the onset of the saccade, were baseline-corrected by subtracting the mean signal during the 100 ms preceding the saccade from the 500 ms that followed the saccade. Data for each of trial type (correct and error) were averaged for each participant.

The ERN was derived using the average signal across the following 10/20 locations: FC1, FCz, FC2, C1, Cz, C2, CP1, CPz, CP2 for each participant. An average was used so as not to exclude participants with bad channels. The peak ERN for the entire sample was identified within the 200 ms following saccadic initiation as the time point of maximal difference for the error vs. correct waveforms (140 ms). The peak ERN for each participant was identified as the point of maximal difference within 50 ms on either side of the group peak [5].

MNE software (www.martinos.org/martinos/userInfo/data/sofMNE.php) was used to derive current source estimates of the difference waveform (error-correct) from the combined EEG and MEG group data. The reconstructed cortical surfaces for each participant, which comprised approximately 100,000 vertices per hemisphere, were decimated to a subset of approximately 3,000 dipole locations (vertices) per hemisphere. The forward solution was calculated using a three-compartment boundary-element model [50] with the inner and outer skull surfaces and the scalp surface segmented from the FLASH images. The head position information from the start of each run was used in the calculation of a forward solution for each run, which were averaged together. The amplitudes of the dipoles at each cortical location were estimated every 4 ms using the anatomically constrained linear estimation approach [51]. The orientations of the dipoles were tightly constrained to the cortical normal direction by setting source variances for the transverse current components to be 0.1 times the variance of the currents normal to the cortical surface [52]. Individual source estimate data were mapped to the template cortical surface. This resulted in a set of source estimates at each time point that were spatially aligned across participants.

To localize the ERN source, we used the source estimate of the difference waveform at the time of the peak ERN for each participant. We employed a t-test in each diagnostic group to determine whether the averaged amplitudes of the source estimates differed from zero at each vertex on the cortical surface. Correction for multiple comparisons was based on a permutation analysis, which approximated the null distribution (i.e., no difference between correct and error trials) by randomly swapping the error and correct conditions for each participant (i.e., by multiplying each individual source estimate by either 1 or −1). This procedure was repeated 10,000 times. We then measured the area of the largest cluster of vertices with a significant non-zero current estimate (p≤.05) in each permuted dataset, resulting in a distribution of cluster sizes. This null distribution was then used to determine the probability that the observed cluster size would occur by chance.

Analysis of genotype effects

We assessed the effects of genotype on our primary outcome variables, dACC activation and ERN amplitude, using linear regressions with allele load (0, 1 or 2) as a covariate for each SNP. Because our hypotheses were directional (i.e., reduced error markers with larger risk-allele load), we conducted one-tailed tests. We also examined the effects of genotype on error rate and on correct trial RTs.

To test the hypothesis that each genotype had significantly different effects on dACC activation and the ERN (i.e., the magnitude of activation and ERN amplitude had different slopes as a function of allele load) we modeled the two error markers as a bivariate response and employed multivariate regression analyses using the "R" statistical computing environment [53]. To consider the error markers as a bivariate response it was necessary to standardize each measure (i.e., to have a zero mean and a standard deviation of 1) since they have different units of measurement. Allele load (0, 1, 2) refers to the number of *677T* alleles for *MTHFR C677T* and the number of *-521C* alleles for *DRD4 C-521T* and was treated as a linear covariate. The effect of each allele load is described by four slopes (two SNPs x two error markers) and the differences between slopes were tested using one-tailed tests to reflect our *a priori* hypotheses.

Secondary analyses considered models with diagnosis and its interaction with genotype as covariates, excluded non-Caucasians, and used a dominant model of allele load (*677T* carriers vs. C homozygotes and 521C carriers vs. T homozygotes). We assessed the effect of the interaction of diagnosis with genotype on response by comparing models with and without covariates for diagnosis using ANOVA.

Results

Antisaccade performance

As error rates did not differ significantly in fMRI and MEG/EEG (t(90) = −1.20, p = .23), the results are averaged across modalities (Table 2). The overall antisaccade error rate was 20±16% (mean ± SD) and almost all errors were self-corrected (96%). Error rates differed by diagnosis (F(3,88) = 5.26, p = .002) reflecting that participants with schizophrenia made more errors than healthy (t(59) = 3.42, p = .001) and OCD participants (t(44) = 2.72, p = .009). Error rates were associated (trend) with allele load for *MTHFR C677T* (p = .07; Table 3), but not for *DRD4 C-521T* (p = .80). When diagnosis was included as a factor in the model, the relation of error rate with allele load became significant for *MTHFR C677T* (F(1,87) = 4.14, p = .045) but not *DRD4 C-521T*. The interaction of *MTHFR C677T* with diagnosis was not significant (F(3,84) = 0.43, p = .73) indicating that diagnosis did not substantially affect the results.

Error-related dACC Activation

Relative to correct trials, errors were associated with increased dACC activation (Fig. 2A; Talairach locations of maximal activation: left x = −7, y = 24, z = 23 and right 9, 23, 25), which did not differ by diagnostic group (F(3,88) = 1.03, p = .39, Table 2). Error-related dACC activation was associated with *MTHFR C677T* but not *DRD4 C-521T* allele load (Fig. 3, Table 3). When diagnosis and its interaction with allele load was added to the models, the interaction was not significant for either *MTHFR C677T* (p = .72) or *DRD4 C-521T* (p = .14), indicating that diagnosis did not substantially affect the results.

ERN

The group ERN was observed as a robust negative deflection in the difference waveform for error vs. correct trials that peaked 140 ms after the saccadic response (Fig. 2B). The ERN differed by diagnosis (F(3,88) = 4.19, p = .008, Table 2). Post-hoc t-tests indicated that schizophrenia participants had a smaller amplitude ERN than healthy (t(59) = 2.89, p = .005) and OCD (t(44) = 2.62, p = .01) participants. *DRD4 C-521T* was significantly associated with the amplitude of the ERN (t(90) = −1.75, p = .04, Fig. 4, Table 3), but *MTHFR C677T* was not (t(90) = −0.74, p = .23). When divided by diagnosis, the association with *DRD4 C-521T* allele load reached significance in the schizophrenia group (t(26) = −1.66, p = .05), and approached significance in healthy participants (t(31) = −1.34, p = .09). When diagnosis and its interaction with allele load was added to the models, the interaction was not significant for either *DRD4 C-521T* (p = .92) or *MTHFR C677T* (p = .53) indicating that diagnosis did not substantially affect the results.

Table 2. Outcome measures divided by diagnosis.

	HC (n = 33)	SZ (n = 28)	OCD (n = 18)	ASD (n = 13)	Combined (n = 92)
Error rate (%)[1]	16±10	30±19	16±8	20±11	21±15
Error-related dACC activation (% change)	.11±.07	.13±.10	.10±.07	.15±.13	.12±.09
ERN (μV)	3.7±1.6	2.4±2.1	4.2±2.7	2.7±1.5	3.3±2.1

[1]Collapsed across fMRI and EEG sessions. Note that participants with fewer than 10 usable error trials per modality were excluded from the study.

Our prior finding of a PCC source for the ERN in 30 of the present 33 healthy participants [5] was replicated in the schizophrenia and OCD groups (Fig. S1, Table S1). In both groups, there was a significant cluster of dipole sources in the PCC bilaterally. The PCC cluster in the smaller ASD group did not reach significance, but the source localization was similar to the other groups.

Bivariate Analyses

These analyses tested for differential effects of genotype on error markers. The results were similar in the primary model, which included the entire group and a linear effect of allele load, and in the other models that included either the entire group or Caucasians only, did or did not include diagnosis as a covariate, or did or did not use a dominant model of allele load (Fig. 5, Table 4).

Regardless of the model used, *DRD4 C-521T* genotype had a significantly stronger effect on the ERN than on error-related dACC activation. The interactions of diagnosis with genotype were not significant in any of the four models (i.e., dominant/non-dominant, all data/Caucasians only; all p's ≥.19) suggesting the effects were similar across diagnostic groups.

For *MTHFR C677T*, the difference in the effect of allele load on the two error markers did not reach significance in any model. Nor were the interactions of diagnosis with genotype significant in any of the four models (p's ≥.11).

Discussion

We tested the hypothesis that two canonical neural markers of errors, the ERN and error-related dACC activation have distinct genetic mediation. We previously reported a PCC source for the

ERN in healthy individuals [5] and now, using identical anatomically-constrained EEG/MEG source localization methods, we have replicated this finding in schizophrenia and OCD. This reinforces the anatomical dissociation between error-related dACC activation and the ERN. We now also report evidence of different genetic mediation. First, we replicated the finding that *DRD4 C-521T* is associated with increased ERN amplitude [7], here in a linear model of allele load. This effect was significantly greater than the *DRD4 C-521T* effect on dACC activation, which was not significant. In contrast, we did not find a significant differential effect of *MTHFR C677T* on error markers. *MTHFR C677T* was associated with blunted error-related dACC activation, as previously reported in an independent sample [8] and in subset of the present sample [9]. Although *MTHFR C677T* did not significantly affect ERN amplitude, the difference in the slopes of the relation of allele load with each error marker was not significant. While these findings support the hypothesis of differential genetic mediation of these error markers (i.e., *DRD4 C-521T* showed a significantly stronger effect on ERN than dACC activation), they do not support the hypothesis of a double-dissociation since *MTHFR C677T* did not show a significantly greater effect on dACC activation than the ERN. Together with the anatomical dissociation between the ERN and error-related dACC activation, these findings suggest that these error markers have different neural and genetic mediation. These findings challenge theories that these two error markers reflect the same underlying neural process measured by different techniques.

This study replicated the finding that *DRD4 C-521T* is associated with increased ERN amplitude [7] and extended it by showing linear effect of allele load. Moreover, the *DRD4 C-521T* effect on ERN amplitude was significant in the schizophrenia group alone, making this the first report of this effect in

Table 3. Results of the univariate analyses examining the effect of each SNP on each outcome measure.

	C/C	C/T	T/T	*Regression Result*
	MTHFR C677T			
Error rate (%)	18±13	22±16	24±15	t(90) = 1.85 p = .07[1]
dACC activation (% change)	.10±.10	.04±.09	.04±.08	t(90) = −1.75, p = .04*
ERN (μV)	2.6±2.0	2.2±2.1	2.2±2.9	t(90) = −0.74, p = .23
	DRD4 C-521T			
Error rate (%)	20±11	21±15	22±19	t(90) = −0.26; p = .80
dACC activation (% change)	.08±.08	.07±.10	.06±.11	t(90) = 1.04, p = .85
ERN (μV)	3.3±1.9	2.1±2.1	1.8±2.5	t(90) = −1.75, p = .04*

[1]When diagnosis was included as a factor in the model this effect became significant (p = .045).
*significant at p≤.05.

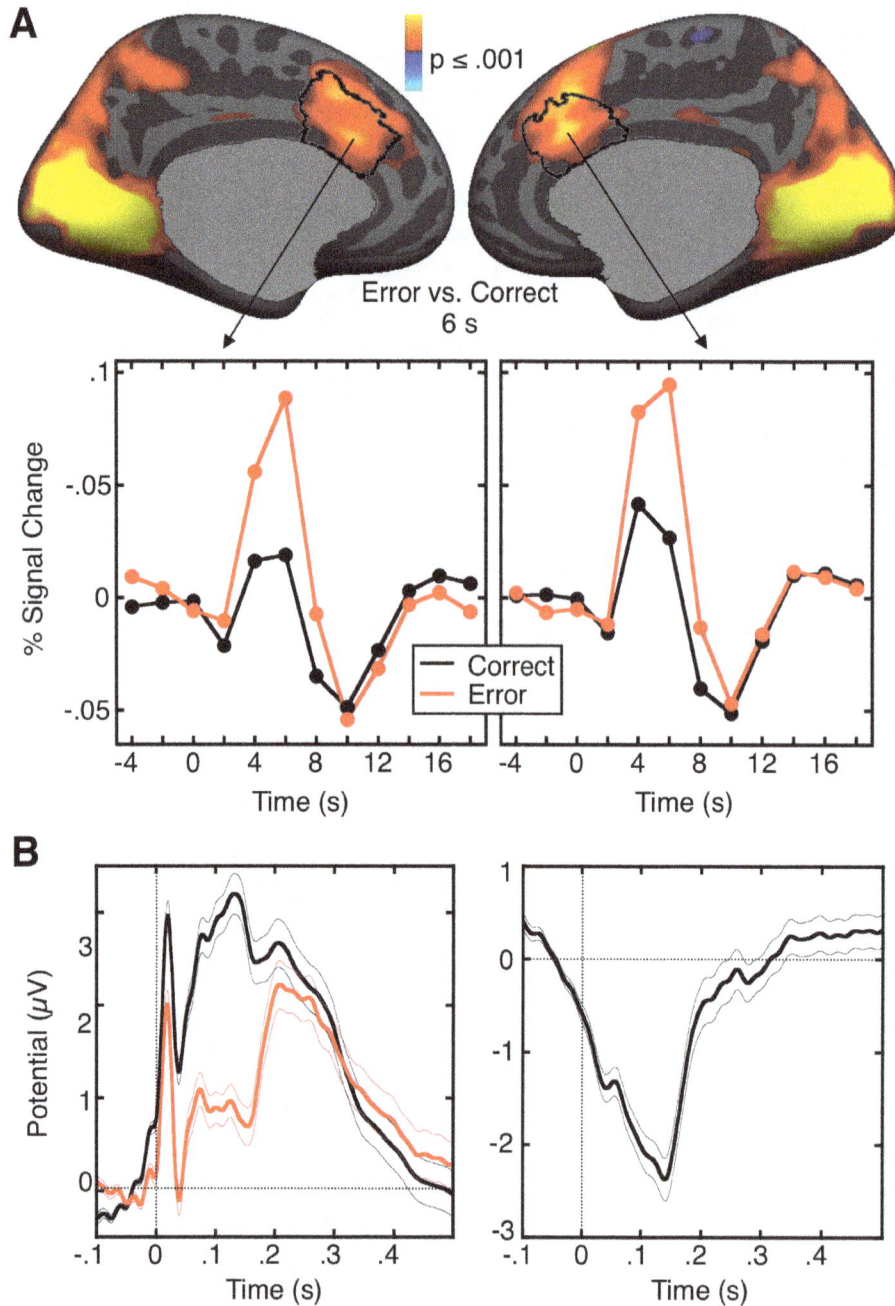

Figure 2. fMRI and EEG error markers. A. Error-related dACC activation. Statistical maps of activation at 6 s in the contrast of error vs. correct are displayed on the inflated medial cortical surfaces. The dACC ROI is outlined in black. Warm colors indicate stronger activation on errors. The gray masks cover subcortical regions in which activity is displaced in a surface rendering. Line graphs show hemodynamic response functions for correct and error trials in the vertices with maximal error-related activation in the dACC. B. The ERN. The left panel shows grand average waveforms for correct (black) and error (red) trials, time locked to the onset of the saccade. The right panel shows the difference waveform, obtained by subtracting the correct waveform from the error waveform. The thin lines on either side of the waveforms represent the standard error of the mean at each time point.

schizophrenia. There is strong evidence of a role for DA in mediating the ERN. ERN amplitude is affected by pharmacological agents that affect DA [54–56] and by Parkinson's Disease, which is associated with a loss of midbrain DA neurons [57–59]. The effect of *DRD4 C-521T* on DA receptor availability is controversial, with one study reporting a 40% decrease in transcriptional efficiency [18], but another finding no effect [60]. In an influential model, the ERN is generated when a mismatch between the intended (correct) versus actual (error) outcome (i.e., prediction error) leads to a phasic decrease in mesencephalic DA release that disinhibits dACC neurons (or, in a revised model, PCC neurons – though DA innervation of the PCC is less than that in the ACC [61,62]), which give rise to the ERN [4]. If *521T* leads to reduced DA receptor availability, one might expect reduced, not increased, ERN amplitude as is seen with the dopamine antagonist haloperidol [56]. DRD4 knockout mice,

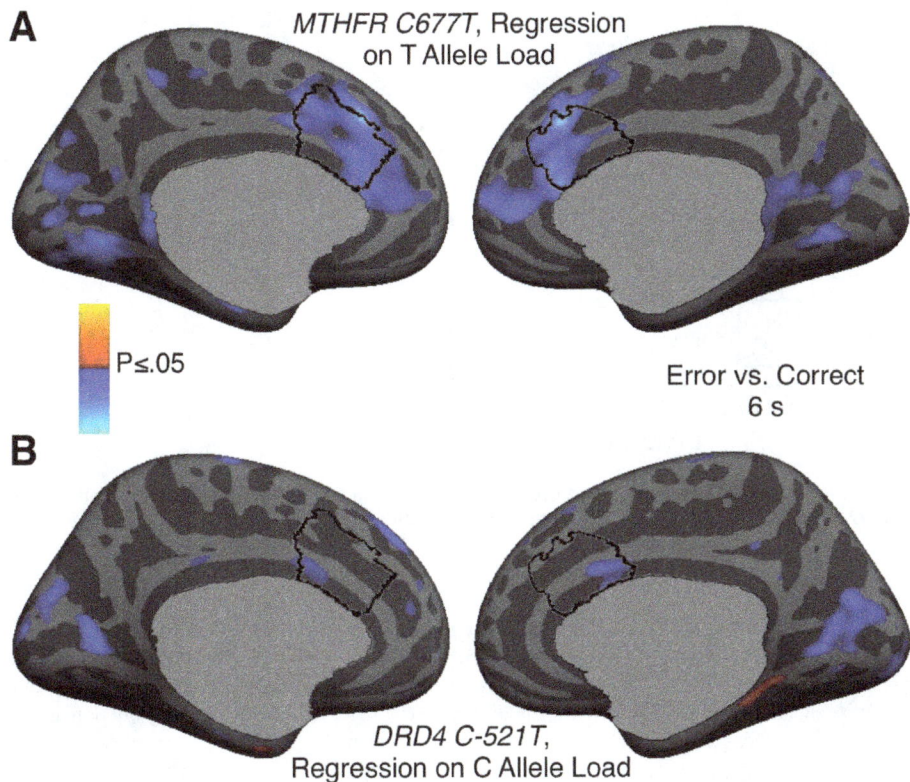

Figure 3. Genetic modulation of error-related dACC activation. A: *MTHFR C677T*. B: *DRD4 C-521T*. Statistical maps show regressions of activation in the error vs. correct contrast on allele load. Blue colors represent a negative correlation, i.e., stronger activation associated with more 677T (A) or -521C (B) alleles. The gray masks cover subcortical regions in which activity is displaced in a surface rendering.

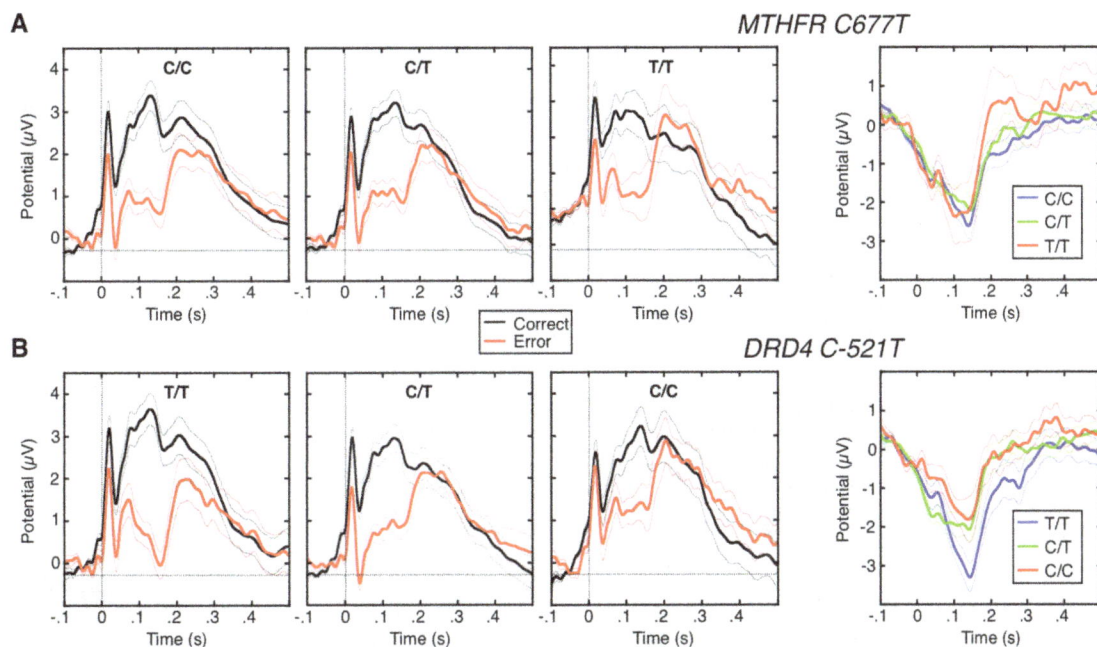

Figure 4. Genetic modulation of the ERN. A: *MTHFR* C677T. B: *DRD4* C-521T. Correct and error trial waveforms are shown for every allele combination of each polymorphism. The error-correct difference waveforms for each allele combination is shown on the right column. The thin lines on either side of the waveforms represent the standard error of the mean at each time point.

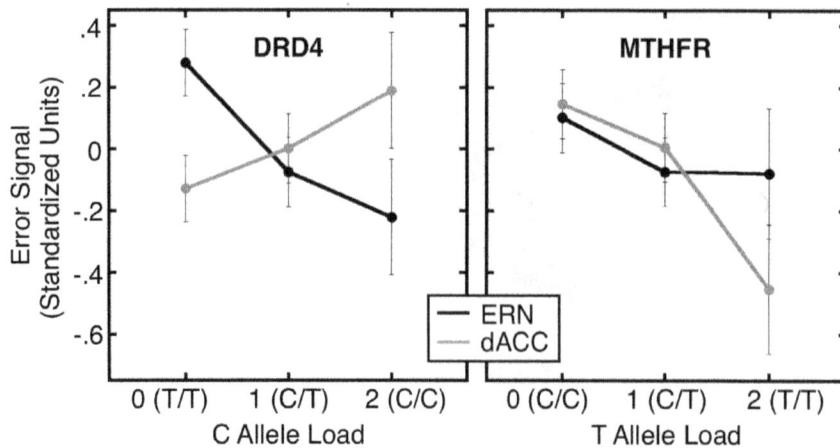

Figure 5. Genetic dissociation between error-related dACC activation and the ERN. Both error markers are shown in standardized units as a function of risk allele load (677T for *MTHFR C677T*, -521C for *DRD4 C-521T*). Error bars represent within subject confidence intervals [75] for each allele combination.

however, show increased DA synthesis and turnover in the basal ganglia [63]. While it is possible that the putative reduction in D4 receptor availability in human *521T*-carriers could indirectly lead to stronger error signaling by some compensatory mechanism, the basis of this effect is unknown. Important caveats to the DA theory of ERN generation [4] include that DA is thought to largely play a modulatory or inhibitory role in the cortex, including in the cingulate [64], that its effects lack the temporal precision to generate a phasic error signal and that glutamate, which is thought to be co-released with DA, may instead transmit error signals [65].

Given that the ERN is localized to the PCC, one might ask whether DRD4 also affects error-related fMRI activation of the PCC. As seen in Figure 3B, there was no significant DRD4 effect on PCC activation. This may reflect that there is no compelling fMRI correlate of the ERN in the PCC. As seen in Figure 2A, although there are small clusters of error-related activation in bilateral PCC, they do not survive correction for multiple comparisons despite the sample size of 92. This lack of error-related PCC activation is consistent with most, but not all [66,67], prior fMRI studies of error processing and may reflect the different sources of fMRI vs. MEG/EEG signals. If the ERN, as has been theorized, arises from disinhibition of cingulate neurons [4], this might not lead to an increase in the BOLD signal [68]. Another possibility is that if the ERN arises due to synchronization of constantly active, but otherwise asynchronous neural populations, this would affect MEG/EEG signals but not necessarily hemodynamic activity. For these reasons, fMRI may not show the ERN.

For *MTHFR C677T*, we previously reported a linear effect of *677T* on error-related dACC activation in a prior analysis of a subset the present healthy and schizophrenia samples [9]. The mechanism of *MTHFR C677T* effects on dACC function is not clear, but in addition to reduced global DNA methylation [69], *677T* may affect the activity of other genes, including those more directly involved in DA function and related to executive function. Consistent with this possibility, *MTHFR C677T* has an epistatic effect with *COMT Val^{158}Met*, on dorsolateral prefrontal fMRI activation during working memory performance in schizophrenia [70]. It is possible that *MTHFR 677T* could decrease methylation in the COMT promoter, which could lead to reduced expression of COMT and higher DA availability in the synapse [23].

Despite strong evidence of genetic mediation of neural error markers, there was only weak evidence of genetic mediation of error rate by *MTHFR C677T*. This is not surprising given the limited sample size and that behavior is usually a less sensitive and specific index of genetic effects than brain activity. Behavior may reflect not only the integrity of the brain system of interest, but also of other systems, including the motor output systems that are required to produce the behavior. For example, in the present study, antisaccade error rate is unlikely to be solely determined by the use of errors to improve performance, but may also reflect other factors including inattention, failure to maintain the task set, and failures of response inhibition.

In summary, we report that a genetic polymorphism, previously associated with error processing, differentially modulates neural

Table 4. Results of the bivariate analyses testing the differential effects of each SNP on error markers.

	MTHFR C677T		DRD4 C-521T	
	Diagnosis as covariate?		**Diagnosis as covariate?**	
	no	**Yes**	**no**	**yes**
Entire sample (n = 92)	t(89) = 0.83 p = .21	t(86) = 0.92 p = .26	t(89) = 2.05 p = .02*	t(86) = 2.43 p = .01*
Caucasians only (n = 74)	t(71) = 0.89 p = .19	t(68) = 1.25 p = .11	t(71) = 1.92 p = .03*	t(68) = 2.30 p = .01*
Whole sample, dominant model	t(89) = 0.49 p = .31	t(86) = .75 p = .23	t(89) = 1.86 p = .03*	t(86) = 2.23 p = .01*

The primary analysis included the entire sample, allele load, and no covariate for diagnosis.
*significant at p≤.05.

error markers. The test of differential modulation reached significance for *DRD4 C-521T* but not for *MTHFR C677T*. The lack of a double dissociation may reflect that error-related dACC activation and the ERN are functionally related, although we cannot rule out Type II error given the relatively small sample size. In a previous study, we reported that the dACC region showing error-related activation and the PCC region that was the source of the ERN were functionally connected during antisaccade performance in healthy participants, and also during rest in a separate sample from a large, publically available dataset of resting state fMRI scans [5]. This suggests that the PCC and dACC are constituents of a functional circuit. We previously proposed that the PCC detects errors, giving rise to the ERN and relays this information to the dACC to implement corrective behavior [5]. This was based on our finding that the structural integrity of the cingulum bundle, which connects dACC and PCC [71], predicts the latency to initiate a corrective saccade, as well as other evidence from the literature of a dACC role in behavioral adjustment [72–74]. If this model is correct, the strength of the ERN could have downstream effects on error-related dACC activation. Despite evidence of a functional relationship, the present findings support models that view the ERN and error-related dACC activation as anatomically and mechanistically distinct error markers.

Supporting Information

Figure S1   Combined EEG/MEG Source estimate of the ERN in each diagnostic group, displayed on the inflated medial cortical surfaces. The statistical maps show vertices where the current estimate at the time of peak ERN was significantly different from zero. Positive (red) and negative (blue) values indicate currents flowing out and into the cortex, respectively.

Table S1   ERN source localization based on combined EEG/MEG data. ERN source localization based on combined EEG/MEG data. Maxima and locations of clusters where dipole sources were significantly different from zero. Clusterwise probabilities (CWP) are based on correction for the entire cortical surface. P-values are provided for the most significant dipole source in each cluster. Current direction in all clusters outwards from the cortical surface.

Author Contributions

Conceived and designed the experiments: YA JLR JSW DSM. Performed the experiments: YA PJG JC SH DSM. Analyzed the data: YA MV JLR PJG JC SH. Contributed reagents/materials/analysis tools: MV DCG JLG SW JWS. Contributed to the writing of the manuscript: YA MV PJG JWS DSM. Patient characterization: DCG JLG SW.

References

1. Manoach DS, Agam Y (2013) Neural markers of errors as endophenotypes in neuropsychiatric disorders. Front Hum Neurosci 7: 350.
2. Taylor SF, Stern ER, Gehring WJ (2007) Neural systems for error monitoring: recent findings and theoretical perspectives. Neuroscientist 13: 160–172.
3. Ridderinkhof KR, Ullsperger M, Crone EA, Nieuwenhuis S (2004) The role of the medial frontal cortex in cognitive control. Science 306: 443–447.
4. Holroyd CB, Coles MG (2002) The neural basis of human error processing: reinforcement learning, dopamine, and the error-related negativity. Psychol Rev 109: 679–709.
5. Agam Y, Hamalainen MS, Lee AK, Dyckman KA, Friedman JS, et al. (2011) Multimodal neuroimaging dissociates hemodynamic and electrophysiological correlates of error processing. Proc Natl Acad Sci U S A 108: 17556–17561.
6. Heilbronner SR, Platt ML (2013) Causal Evidence of Performance Monitoring by Neurons in Posterior Cingulate Cortex during Learning. Neuron 80: 1384–1391.
7. Kramer UM, Cunillera T, Camara E, Marco-Pallares J, Cucurell D, et al. (2007) The impact of catechol-O-methyltransferase and dopamine D4 receptor genotypes on neurophysiological markers of performance monitoring. J Neurosci 27: 14190–14198.
8. Roffman JL, Brohawn DG, Friedman JS, Dyckman KA, Thakkar KN, et al. (2011) MTHFR 677C>T effects on anterior cingulate structure and function during response monitoring in schizophrenia: a preliminary study. Brain Imaging Behav 5: 65–75.
9. Roffman JL, Nitenson AZ, Agam Y, Isom M, Friedman JS, et al. (2011) A hypomethylating variant of MTHFR, 677C>T, blunts the neural response to errors in patients with schizophrenia and healthy individuals. PLoS ONE 6: e25253.
10. Anokhin AP, Golosheykin S, Heath AC (2008) Heritability of frontal brain function related to action monitoring. Psychophysiology 45: 524–534.
11. Manoach DS, Agam Y (2013) Neural markers of errors as endophenotypes in neuropsychiatric disorders. Frontiers in Human Neuroscience 7: 350.
12. Meyer A, Klein DN, Torpey DC, Kujawa AJ, Hayden EP, et al. (2012) Additive effects of the dopamine D2 receptor and dopamine transporter genes on the error-related negativity in young children. Genes, Brain, and Behavior 11: 695–703.
13. Althaus M, Groen Y, Wijers AA, Mulder LJ, Minderaa RB, et al. (2009) Differential effects of 5-HTTLPR and DRD2/ANKK1 polymorphisms on electrocortical measures of error and feedback processing in children. Clinical Neurophysiology 120: 93–107.
14. Osinsky R, Hewig J, Alexander N, Hennig J (2012) COMT Val158Met genotype and the common basis of error and conflict monitoring. Brain Research 1452: 108–118.
15. Frank MJ, D'Lauro C, Curran T (2007) Cross-task individual differences in error processing: neural, electrophysiological, and genetic components. Cognitive, affective & behavioral neuroscience 7: 297–308.
16. Althaus M, Groen Y, Wijers AA, Minderaa RB, Kema IP, et al. (2010) Variants of the SLC6A3 (DAT1) polymorphism affect performance monitoring-related cortical evoked potentials that are associated with ADHD. Biological Psychology 85: 19–32.
17. Biehl SC, Dresler T, Reif A, Scheuerpflug P, Deckert J, et al. (2011) Dopamine transporter (DAT1) and dopamine receptor D4 (DRD4) genotypes differentially impact on electrophysiological correlates of error processing. PLoS ONE 6: e28396.
18. Okuyama Y, Ishiguro H, Toru M, Arinami T (1999) A genetic polymorphism in the promoter region of DRD4 associated with expression and schizophrenia. Biochem Biophys Res Commun 258: 292–295.
19. Xing QH, Wu SN, Lin ZG, Li HF, Yang JD, et al. (2003) Association analysis of polymorphisms in the upstream region of the human dopamine D4 receptor gene in schizophrenia. Schizophr Res 65: 9–14.
20. Allen NC, Bagade S, McQueen MB, Ioannidis JP, Kavvoura FK, et al. (2008) Systematic meta-analyses and field synopsis of genetic association studies in schizophrenia: the SzGene database. Nat Genet 40: 827–834.
21. Frosst P, Blom HJ, Milos R, Goyette P, Sheppard CA, et al. (1995) A candidate genetic risk factor for vascular disease: a common mutation in methylenetetrahydrofolate reductase. Nat Genet 10: 111–113.
22. Roffman JL, Weiss AP, Purcell S, Caffalette CA, Freudenreich O, et al. (2008) Contribution of methylenetetrahydrofolate reductase (MTHFR) polymorphisms to negative symptoms in schizophrenia. Biol Psychiatry 63: 42–48.
23. Roffman JL, Weiss AP, Deckersbach T, Freudenreich O, Henderson DC, et al. (2007) Effects of the methylenetetrahydrofolate reductase (MTHFR) C677T polymorphism on executive function in schizophrenia. Schizophr Res 92: 181–188.
24. Roffman JL, Weiss AP, Deckersbach T, Freudenreich O, Henderson DC, et al. (2008) Interactive effects of COMT Val108/158Met and MTHFR C677T on executive function in schizophrenia. Am J Med Genet B Neuropsychiatr Genet.
25. Klein TA, Endrass T, Kathmann N, Neumann J, von Cramon DY, et al. (2007) Neural correlates of error awareness. Neuroimage 34: 1774–1781.
26. Polli FE, Barton JJ, Cain MS, Thakkar KN, Rauch SL, et al. (2005) Rostral and dorsal anterior cingulate cortex make dissociable contributions during antisaccade error commission. Proc Natl Acad Sci U S A 102: 15700–15705.
27. Belopolsky AV, Kramer AF (2006) Error-processing of oculomotor capture. Brain Res 1081: 171–178.
28. Nieuwenhuis S, Ridderinkhof KR, Blom J, Band GP, Kok A (2001) Error-related brain potentials are differentially related to awareness of response errors: evidence from an antisaccade task. Psychophysiology 38: 752–760.
29. Endrass T, Reuter B, Kathmann N (2007) ERP correlates of conscious error recognition: aware and unaware errors in an antisaccade task. Eur J Neurosci 26: 1714–1720.
30. First MB, Spitzer RL, Gibbon M, Williams JBW (2002) Structured Clinical Interview for DSM-IV-TR Axis I Disorders, Research Version, Nonpatient Edition. New York: Biometrics Research, New York State Psychiatric Institute.

31. First MB, Spitzer RL, Gibbon M, Williams JBW (1997) Structured Clinical Interview for DSM-IV Axis I Disorders, Research Version, Patient Edition with Psychotic Screen (SCID-I/P W/PSY SCREEN). New York: Biometrics Research, New York State Psychiatric Institute.

32. Goodman WK, Price LH, Rasmussen SA, Mazure C, Delgado P, et al. (1989) The Yale-Brown Obsessive Compulsive Scale. II. Validity. Arch Gen Psychiatry 46: 1012–1016.

33. Goodman WK, Price LH, Rasmussen SA, Mazure C, Fleischmann RL, et al. (1989) The Yale-Brown Obsessive Compulsive Scale. I. Development, use, and reliability. Arch Gen Psychiatry 46: 1006–1011.

34. Rutter M, Le Couteur A, Lord C (2003) Autism Diagnostic Interview-Revised. Los Angeles, CA: Western Psychological Services.

35. Lord C, Rutter M, DiLavore PC, Risi S (1999) Autism Diagnostic Observation Schedule - WPS (ADOS-WPS). Los Angeles, CA: Western Psychological Services.

36. Purcell S, Neale B, Todd-Brown K, Thomas L, Ferreira MAR, et al. (2007) PLINK: a toolset for whole-genome association and population-based linkage analysis. American Journal of Human Genetics: 81.

37. Buckner RL, Goodman J, Burock M, Rotte M, Koutstaal W, et al. (1998) Functional-anatomic correlates of object priming in humans revealed by rapid presentation event-related fMRI. Neuron 20: 285–296.

38. Miezin FM, Maccotta L, Ollinger JM, Petersen SE, Buckner RL (2000) Characterizing the hemodynamic response: effects of presentation rate, sampling procedure, and the possibility of ordering brain activity based on relative timing. Neuroimage 11: 735–759.

39. Burock MA, Dale AM (2000) Estimation and detection of event-related fMRI signals with temporally correlated noise: a statistically efficient and unbiased approach. Hum Brain Mapp 11: 249–260.

40. Dale AM (1999) Optimal experimental design for event-related fMRI. Hum Brain Mapp 8: 109–140.

41. Endrass T, Franke C, Kathmann N (2005) Error awareness in a saccade countermanding task. J Psychophysiol 19: 275–280.

42. Thesen S, Heid O, Mueller E, Schad LR (2000) Prospective acquisition correction for head motion with image-based tracking for real-time fMRI. Magn Reson Med 44: 457–465.

43. Dale AM, Fischl B, Sereno MI (1999) Cortical surface-based analysis. I. Segmentation and surface reconstruction. Neuroimage 9: 179–194.

44. Fischl B, Sereno MI, Dale AM (1999) Cortical surface-based analysis. II: Inflation, flattening, and a surface-based coordinate system. Neuroimage 9: 195–207.

45. Fischl B, van der Kouwe A, Destrieux C, Halgren E, Segonne F, et al. (2004) Automatically parcellating the human cerebral cortex. Cereb Cortex 14: 11–22.

46. Collins DL, Neelin P, Peters TM, Evans AC (1994) Automatic 3D intersubject registration of MR volumetric data in standardized Talairach space. J Comput Assist Tomogr 18: 192–205.

47. Cox RW, Jesmanowicz A (1999) Real-time 3D image registration for functional MRI. Magn Reson Med 42: 1014–1018.

48. Desikan RS, Segonne F, Fischl B, Quinn BT, Dickerson BC, et al. (2006) An automated labeling system for subdividing the human cerebral cortex on MRI scans into gyral based regions of interest. Neuroimage 31: 968–980.

49. Taulu S, Kajola M (2005) Presentation of electromagnetic multichannel data: The signal space separation method. J Appl Phys 97: 124905–124901.

50. Hämäläinen MS, Hari R, Ilmoniemi R, Knuutila J, Lounasmaa O (1993) Magnetoencephalography-Theory, instrumentation, and applications to noninvasive studies of the working human brain. Rev Modern Phys 65: 413–497.

51. Hämäläinen MS, Ilmoniemi R (1984) Interpreting measured magnetic fields of the brain: estimates of current distribution. Helsinki: University of Technology, Dept. of Technical Physics Report. TKK-F-A559 p.

52. Lin FH, Belliveau JW, Dale AM, Hämäläinen MS (2006) Distributed current estimates using cortical orientation constraints. Hum Brain Mapp 27: 1–13.

53. Kriegeskorte N, Simmons WK, Bellgowan PS, Baker CI (2009) Circular analysis in systems neuroscience: the dangers of double dipping. Nature neuroscience 12: 535–540.

54. de Bruijn ER, Hulstijn W, Verkes RJ, Ruigt GS, Sabbe BG (2004) Drug-induced stimulation and suppression of action monitoring in healthy volunteers. Psychopharmacology 177: 151–160.

55. de Bruijn ER, Sabbe BG, Hulstijn W, Ruigt GS, Verkes RJ (2006) Effects of antipsychotic and antidepressant drugs on action monitoring in healthy volunteers. Brain Res 1105: 122–129.

56. Zirnheld PJ, Carroll CA, Kieffaber PD, O'Donnell BF, Shekhar A, et al. (2004) Haloperidol impairs learning and error-related negativity in humans. J Cogn Neurosci 16: 1098–1112.

57. Falkenstein M, Hielscher H, Dziobek I, Schwarzenau P, Hoormann J, et al. (2001) Action monitoring, error detection, and the basal ganglia: an ERP study. Neuroreport 12: 157–161.

58. Ito J, Kitagawa J (2006) Performance monitoring and error processing during a lexical decision task in patients with Parkinson's disease. J Geriatr Psychiatry Neurol 19: 46–54.

59. Willemssen R, Muller T, Schwarz M, Falkenstein M, Beste C (2009) Response monitoring in de novo patients with Parkinson's disease. PLoS One 4: e4898.

60. Kereszturi E, Kiraly O, Barta C, Molnar N, Sasvari-Szekely M, et al. (2006) No direct effect of the -521 C/T polymorphism in the human dopamine D4 receptor gene promoter on transcriptional activity. BMC molecular biology 7: 18.

61. Miller MW, Powrozek TA, Vogt BA (2009) Dopamine systems in the cingulate gyrus: Organization, development, and neurotoxic vulnerability. In: Vogt BA, editor. Cingulate Neurobiology and Disease. New York: Oxford University Press. 163–187.

62. Berger B, Trottier S, Verney C, Gaspar P, Alvarez C (1988) Regional and laminar distribution of the dopamine and serotonin innervation in the macaque cerebral cortex: a radioautographic study. J Comp Neurol 273: 99–119.

63. Rubinstein M, Phillips TJ, Bunzow JR, Falzone TL, Dziewczapolski G, et al. (1997) Mice lacking dopamine D4 receptors are supersensitive to ethanol, cocaine, and methamphetamine. Cell 90: 991–1001.

64. Goldman-Rakic PS, Leranth C, Williams SM, Mons N, Geffard M (1989) Dopamine synaptic complex with pyramidal neurons in primate cerebral cortex. Proc Natl Acad Sci U S A 86: 9015–9019.

65. Seamans JK, Yang CR (2004) The principal features and mechanisms of dopamine modulation in the prefrontal cortex. Prog Neurobiol 74: 1–58.

66. Fassbender C, Murphy K, Foxe JJ, Wylie GR, Javitt DC, et al. (2004) A topography of executive functions and their interactions revealed by functional magnetic resonance imaging. Brain Res Cogn Brain Res 20: 132–143.

67. Wittfoth M, Kustermann E, Fahle M, Herrmann M (2008) The influence of response conflict on error processing: evidence from event-related fMRI. Brain Res 1194: 118–129.

68. Logothetis NK (2008) What we can do and what we cannot do with fMRI. Nature 453: 869–878.

69. Friso S, Choi SW, Girelli D, Mason JB, Dolnikowski GG, et al. (2002) A common mutation in the 5,10-methylenetetrahydrofolate reductase gene affects genomic DNA methylation through an interaction with folate status. Proc Natl Acad Sci U S A 99: 5606–5611.

70. Roffman JL, Gollub RL, Calhoun VD, Wassink TH, Weiss AP, et al. (2008) MTHFR 677C⇒T genotype disrupts prefrontal function in schizophrenia through an interaction with COMT 158Val⇒Met. Proc Natl Acad Sci U S A 105: 17573–17578.

71. Schmahmann JD, Pandya DN, Wang R, Dai G, D'Arceuil HE, et al. (2007) Association fibre pathways of the brain: parallel observations from diffusion spectrum imaging and autoradiography. Brain 130: 630–653.

72. Magno E, Foxe JJ, Molholm S, Robertson IH, Garavan H (2006) The anterior cingulate and error avoidance. J Neurosci 26: 4769–4773.

73. Modirrousta M, Fellows LK (2008) Dorsal medial prefrontal cortex plays a necessary role in rapid error prediction in humans. J Neurosci 28: 14000–14005.

74. Williams ZM, Bush G, Rauch SL, Cosgrove GR, Eskandar EN (2004) Human anterior cingulate neurons and the integration of monetary reward with motor responses. Nat Neurosci 7: 1370–1375.

75. Loftus GR, Masson ME (1994) Using confidence intervals in within-subject designs. Psychon Bull Rev 1: 476–490.

7

Might Cortical Hyper-Responsiveness in Aging Contribute to Alzheimer's Disease?

Michael S. Jacob[1,2], Charles J. Duffy[1]*

1 Department of Neurology and the Center for Visual Science, The University of Rochester Medical Center, Rochester, New York, United States of America, **2** Department of Psychiatry, The University of California San Francisco Medical Center, San Francisco, California, United States of America

Abstract

Our goal is to understand the neural basis of functional impairment in aging and Alzheimer's disease (AD) to be able to characterize clinically significant decline and assess therapeutic efficacy. We used frequency-tagged ERPs to word and motion stimuli to study the effects of stimulus conditions and selective attention. ERPs to word or motion increase when a task-irrelevant 2nd stimulus is added, but decrease when the task is moved to that 2nd stimulus. Spectral analyses show task effects on response power without 2nd stimulus effects. However, phase coherence shows both 2nd stimulus and task effects. Thus, power and coherence are dissociably modulated by stimulus and task effects. Task-dependent phase coherence successively declines in aging and AD. In contrast, task-dependent spectral power increases in aging, only to decrease in AD. We hypothesize that age-related declines in signal coherence, associated with increased power generation, stresses neurons and contributes to the loss of response power and the development of functional impairment in AD.

Editor: Donatella Spinelli, University of Rome "Foro Italico", Italy

Funding: This work was supported by National Eye Institute (R01-EY022062, P30-EY01319), National Institute on Aging (R01-AG17596), Office of Naval Research (N000141110525), and University of Rochester Center for Translational Science (RR024135). The funders had no role in study design, data collection and analysis, decision to publish, or preparation of the manuscript.

Competing Interests: The authors have declared that no competing interests exist.

* Email: Charles_Duffy@urmc.rochester.edu

Introduction

Aging is the #1 risk factor for AD, although mechanisms linking those conditions have long remained obscure [1]. The hypothesis that aging induced heightened activation may trigger the transition to early AD [2] has recently found support in neuro-imaging [3,4] and molecular studies [5,6,7].

We previously found evidence of visual cortical hyper-responsiveness in aging [8], consistent with cellular studies in aged animals which found increased neuronal excitability and diminished selectivity [9,10]. We consider that age-related cortical hyper-responsiveness may reflect a variety of contributing factors: local disinhibition from intra-cortical (e.g., loss of GABAergic neurons) or cortico-cortical (e.g., fronto-posterior de-afferentation) [11,12,13], and over-activation as a consequence of, or in compensation for, signal degradation [14,15].

We have now examined these hypotheses by assaying competitive attentional control of the dorsal and ventral extrastriate cortical visual systems in aging and AD. These parallel systems partition signals for object and motion processing [16,17]. The relative activity of these pathways is shaped by selective attention's biasing their competitive interactions [18,19,20] to implement behavioral priorities and optimize function [21,22,23].

We have explored the attentional control of visual motion and object processing in monkeys and humans. In monkey single neurons, we found competitive attentional control between pattern and object motion [24]. In human studies, we found that this competition uniquely disrupts perception in early AD [25]. Such

attentional control of sensory processing has been seen in ERP amplitudes [26,27], evoked power [28,29,30], and phase coherence [31,32].

We have found that ERPs reflect attentional and perceptual impairments in AD [33,34] and now focus on how those changes may distinguish aging and AD. We find that aging degrades response coherence with a paradoxical increase in response power. This cortical hyper-responsiveness is absent in AD, leading us to consider whether aging may stress posterior cortical neurons and contribute to neurodegenerative processes in AD.

Methods

Subject Groups

Young normal subjects (YNs, n = 18) were undergraduates at the University of Rochester. Older normal subjects (ONs, n = 17) were from elderly wellness programs or were the spouses of ADs. ADs (n = 14) were from clinical programs at the University of Rochester Medical Center, diagnosed by a neurologist or psychiatrist specializing in dementia within two years of these studies. Written Informed consent, including screening for competency to grant consent, was obtained before subject enrollment. All procedures are approved by the University of Rochester RSRB. That approval covers this work and ongoing studies applying similar neurophysiological methods in human subjects.

All subjects had normal range Snellen visual acuity (monocular at least 20/40) and contrast sensitivity (5 spatial frequencies, 0.5 to

18 cycles/°, VisTech Consultants, Inc., Dayton, OH). AD patients met DSM-IVR criteria for probable AD including: significant memory impairment with signs and symptoms of either aphasia, agnosia, apraxia, inattention, disorganization, or executive dysfunction [35]. All patients would also meet DSMV criteria, whereas no non-patents would satisfy those criteria.

Diagnostic classification was supported by: the Mini-Mental State Examination of global function [36], WMS-Revised (WMS-R) [37] verbal paired associates (immediate and delayed recall), animal naming verbal fluency, money road map test of topographic orientation [38], WMS-R figural and facial memory tests of visual recognition, and line orientation test of spatial relations [39]. These tests yielded scores consistent with group membership (Table S1). We note the relatively mild impairment of our AD subjects on the MMSE, suggesting mild or early Alzheimer's, corresponding with more pronounced executive impairment at this stage in the disease as indexed by Trails B scores [40,41,42].

Neurophysiological Recordings

Scalp recorded EEG was obtained using a 32-channel Neuroscan system with electrodes in the international 10–20 configuration at impedances <5 kΩ. Activity was low pass filtered at 100 Hz and a high pass filtered at 0.1 Hz and sampled at 500 Hz/32-bit resolution creating MATLAB files. Subjects maintained centered visual fixation (+/−10°) on a centered spot screen during recording. Eye position was monitored using infrared oculometry (ASL, Inc.). EEGLAB created independent components for each subject and recording session to remove eye blinks in one or two components.

Visual Stimuli

Subjects sat facing a rear-projection tangent screen's 60°×40° image. We presented streams of flow and words to activate dorsal and ventral processing, respectively. Flow alternated with random motion masks, words with pound sign masks, with a 50/50 duty-cycle at 1.11 Hz or 1.57 Hz. Target stimuli (25%) were randomly interspersed with non-targets (75%). (Figure 1A).

Optic flow stimuli contained 2000 white dots on a dark background (Michelson contrast = 0.83 at 60 Hz frame rate). Non-target, optic flow contained a screen centered focus-of-expansion with dot speed increasing with distance from the center. The masking, random motion stimulus contained dots moving at the same average speeds with direction and position randomized to yield 0% pattern coherence. Target optic flow was the same as non-target optic flow, except the focus of expansion was shifted to the left or to the right by 20°.

Word stimuli contained 3 letters occupying the central 4°×12° and alternated with 3 similarly sized modified pound signs (mask). Target word stimuli consisted of 2 letters from a 3-letter word with the first (left) or last (right) letter replaced by the mask. The task required that subjects press the button on the side of the hash mark. For superimposed stimuli, the region between letters was transparent and dot motion was visible. Flow and word stimuli were matched for total number of pixels, luminance, and contrast.

Behavioral Paradigm

All subjects completed five recording blocks. The first block was two minutes to, "Rest quietly and remain fixated on the screen." The other blocks engaged subjects in the motion/word task (Figure 1B). Task blocks presented ~120 target stimuli with subjects told to use the flow or word stimuli to guide left/right button presses which were followed by a beep tones if the correct side, and boops if incorrect. False negatives (no response to targets)

and false positives (responses to non-targets) did not yield tones. Error intervals were omitted from the analysis, including false positive responses to non-target stimuli and false negative failures to respond to target stimuli.

Event-related Potentials Analysis

The continuous dataset for each recording block was divided into 1s epochs (−100 to 900 ms post-stimulus onset), averaged for subjects and groups and low pass filtered at 10 Hz. Epochs were created for all sessions and stimulus conditions including single, superimposed, target and non-targets for flow and word stimuli. All stimuli preceded by correct response were included in the analyses. Grand averages were created for subjects and groups. These were low pass filtered at 10 Hz for display. N2 responses to target and non-target stimuli were identified as the first negative deflection 150–200 ms after stimulus onset.

Group and subject averages were peak detected in MATLAB by finding the time point where the first derivative of the voltage was approximately zero. Individual subject amplitudes were measured as the mean voltage in the 20 ms centered on the group peak latency. P1s were prominent in the ON and AD word responses, making P1N2 amplitudes the most consistent measure across all conditions and groups.

Latencies and amplitudes were derived for P1N2, N2b and P3s for each stimulus, task condition, and subject group and entered in to 3-way ANOVAs. The two stimulus frequencies (1.11, 1.57 Hz) did not effect P1N2, N2b or P3s (F3, 370 = 1.62, p = 0.184) but for shorter P3 latencies at the higher frequency (F3, 370 = 6.10, p< 0.001). Analyses of the two different stimulus frequency data sets yield nearly identical results for all reported measures. Thus, our analyses combined these data.

Spectral Analysis of EEG

Power spectra from Fourier transformation (EEGLAB) were estimated at a frequency resolution of 0.05 Hz. The resting, eyes-open condition was subtracted from the task-recorded spectra. Power at each stimulus fundamental frequency and their harmonics were measured peak to trough at OZ. Three YN subjects, two ON and one AD subject did not complete the two minute eyes-open session and were not included in the spectral analysis. The spectral peak amplitudes were entered into a 3-way analysis of variance to identify main effects of stimulus, task condition, and subject group. Tukey's Honestly Significantly Different (THSD) post-hoc tests (p<.05) were applied to ascertain the sources of significant effects.

Time-Frequency Coherence

The time-frequency analyses of inter-trial phase coherence was based-on the continuous data files from each stimulus and task condition [43]. These files were aligned on the onset of the target or non-target stimuli. Phase coherence (EEGLAB) was calculated over 4s windows across log-spaced frequencies from 0.5 to 40 Hz and increasing wavelet cycles from .5 to 1 cycle/Hz. Phase coherence measures the consistency in phase across time/ frequency points and trials and is scaled 0 to 1, where 1 represents identical phase coherence across trials. These measures were entered into 3-way ANOVAs to identify effects across stimuli, task condition, and subject group.

Results

Behavioral Task Performance

Despite the complexity of the behavioral tasks, all groups perform well with single and superimposed word and flow stimuli

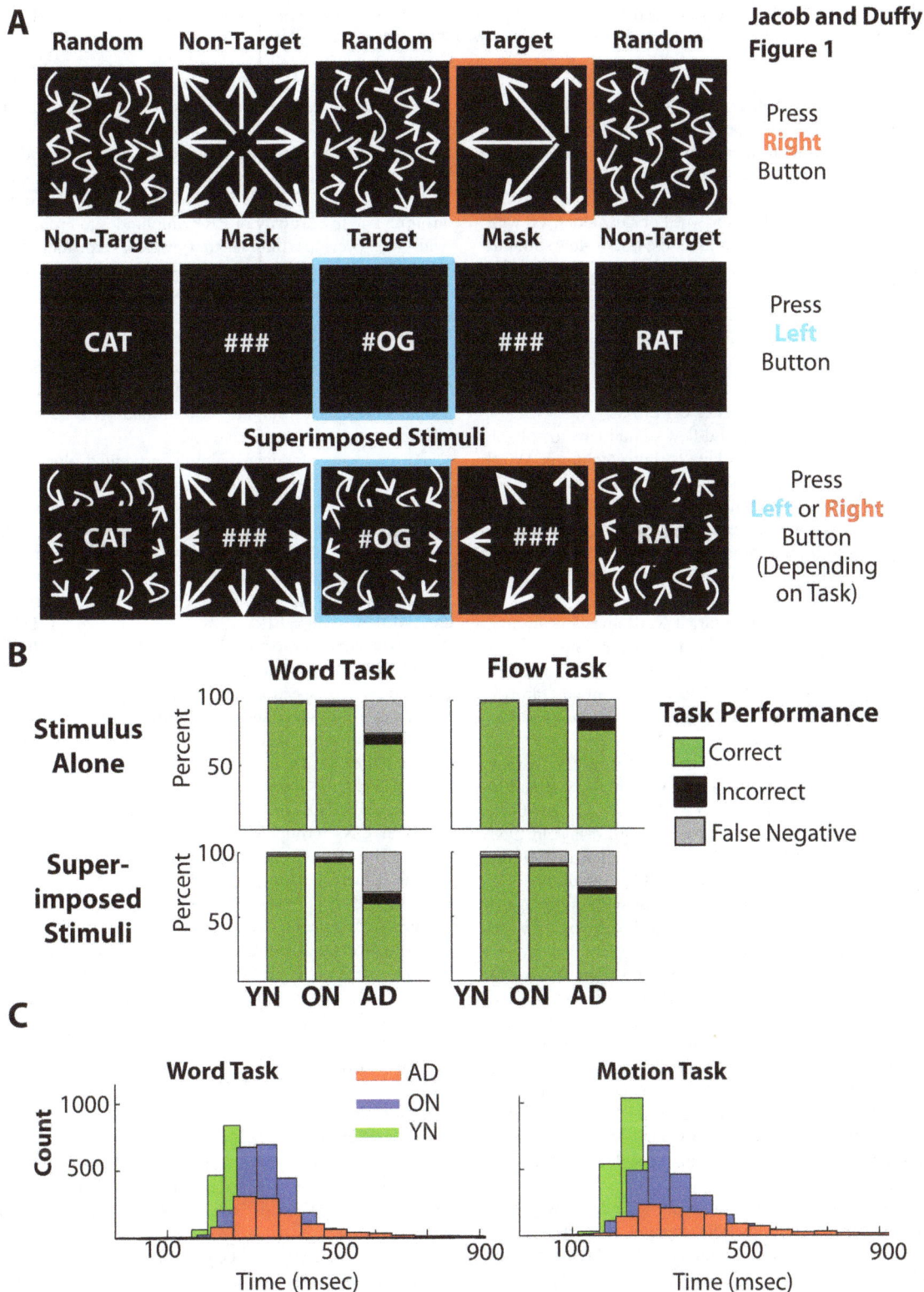

Figure 1. Behavioral paradigm and responses used in these studies. A. Schematic diagram of the visual stimuli and behavioral paradigm. Top: The optic flow stimulus stream consists of radial pattern motion alternating with random dot motion. The radial stimuli present a random series of non-targets with a centered focus of expansion (75%) and targets with a left or right side focus of expansion (25%). Middle: The word object stimulus stream consists of letters alternating with a dot grid. The letter stimuli present a random series of non-target three letter words (75%) and target letter pairs with a left or right side dot grid (25%). Bottom: Superimposed optic flow and word object stimulus streams including a word task left target (blue frame) and a flow task right target (red frame). B. Performance scored by button presses during the word task (left) and flow task (right) with stimuli presented alone at 1.11 Hz (top) or with superimposed stimuli (bottom). Bar graph of percent of total responses to target stimuli scored as correct (green), incorrect (black), and false negative (gray, no response to a target stimulus) for all subject groups (abscissa). ADs showed

lower accuracy than the other groups. C. Number of trials (ordinate) yielding the indicated push button response times (abscissa) for all conditions of the word and flow tasks in the three subject groups. ONs and AD showed longer response times then YNs.

(Figure 1) with differences attributable to group membership (Table S1). We assessed task performance in the alone and combined recording blocks, measuring accuracy, as percent correct push-button responses, and response time (RT). The only significant influence on these measures was subject group (MANOVA of accuracy and RT, for word or flow alone vs. with a 2nd stimulus, in the word or flow tasks, at the fast or slow stimulus frequencies, yields a group effect: F4, 328 = 38.5, p<.001; THSDs for accuracy: YNs = ONs > ADs; THSDs for RT: YNs < ONs < ADs). Thus, we considered task difficulty to be fairly well-balanced across the word and flow stimuli and tasks, with single and superimposed stimuli.

Stimulus, Task, and Group Effects on ERPs

Group averaged ERPs to word and flow stimuli have tri-phasic waveforms at occipital electrodes (Fig. 2, center column). Word P1N2s are largest at Oz, without significant lateralization (O1 vs. O2, Group-by-Electrode Interaction F1, 466 = 1.02, p = 0.313). Flow P1N2s were largest at Oz across groups, but equally so at Pz in YNs (Group-by-Electrode Interaction F1, 666 = 4.90 p<0.001). Peaks at Oz across stimuli and groups led us to focus on that site, but other active sites yield similar results.

We compared P1N2s evoked by target word and flow stimuli, for the three subject groups, recorded in three conditions: 1) word or flow presented alone, 2) word or flow presented with the other stimulus superimposed as a task-irrelevant 2nd stimulus, and 3) word or flow presented with the other stimulus superimposed as the task relevant stimulus.

P1N2 amplitudes are larger with task-irrelevant 2nd stimuli (condition F2, 421 = 6.87, p = .001), especially with flow added to word stimuli (condition-by-stimulus F2, 421 = 12.41, p<.001). Group effects are prominent in N2 latencies, with delays in ONs and ADs (group F2, 421 = 8.1, p<.001), especially to word stimuli (group-by-stimulus F2, 421 = 4.76, p = .009; condition F2, 421 = 14.49, p<.001, THSDs alone < combined; condition-by-stimulus F2, 421 = 7.11, p<.001, THSDs word with flow in word task > others). (Figures 2A and B).

Later response components (the negative and positive components following the N200 response, the N2b and P3) also showed significant effects of stimulus, condition, task, and subject group: N2b amplitudes are largest with flow in YNs (group-by-stimulus F2, 421 = 5.53, p = .004) and delayed in ONs and ADs, especially with words (stimulus-by-group F2, 421 = 3.99, p = .02, THSDs YN flow < others). P3s are also largest in YNs (group F2, 421 = 16.78, p<.001) and delayed in ONs and ADs, especially to flow (group-by-stimulus: F2, 421 = 17.67, p<.001, THSDs all others > YN).

P1N2 amplitudes evoked by non-target stimuli show larger responses to words, especially in YNs (stimulus F1, 416 = 39.52, p<.001, THSDs word > flow; group F2, 416 = 4.35, p = .014, THSDs YN > AD; stimulus-by-group F2, 416 = 6.95, p = .001, THSDs word > flow, YN = ON > AD; stimulus-by-condition F2, 416 = 12.2, p<.001, THSDs word combined > others). Non-target N2 latencies show group and condition effects, with the fastest peak in YNs (condition F2, 416 = 6.01, p = .003, THSDs combined with task > others; group F2, 416 = 4.02, p = .02, THSDs YN < AD). (Figure 2C and D).

Parallel analyses at Pz show a similar pattern of condition and group effects for word responses. At Pz, the flow responses are less distinct, but show the same pattern of relative response amplitudes

without statistical significance. Latency effects are the same across Oz and Pz.

Thus, stimulus and task conditions affect word and flow ERPs with unexpectedly larger responses with superimposed task-irrelevant 2nd stimuli, and delayed peaks in the older subject groups. The insensitivity of ERP amplitudes to group is consistent with our previous finding that rapidly repeating flow stimuli minimize group differences [34,44]. This prompted our use of spectral analyses that are suited to repetitive stimuli.

Spectral Power Analyses

The use of frequency tagged stimuli enables Fourier analysis of EEG data across the time period of each condition. These analyses reveal task effects, but not 2nd stimulus effects, on the power spectra at the stimulus frequency.

Power spectra for word stimuli, presented alone in the word task, show a peak at the stimulus frequency and at five harmonics with main effects of group but not of a 2nd stimulus (added flow) (MANOVA: group F12, 118 = 2.31, p = .011, THSD: ON > AD, condition p = 0.380, interaction p = 0.895). Power spectra for flow stimuli, presented alone, also show a clear peak at the stimulus frequency, with group effects but not 2nd stimulus effects (MANOVA group F12, 122 = 2.04, p = .026, THSD: ON > YN = AD; condition p = 0.577; interaction p = 0.992).

Mirroring our approach to the ERPs, we compared the amplitudes of spectral peaks at the stimulus fundamental frequencies for word and flow stimuli, across the three subject groups, and three stimulus conditions. A three-way ANOVA shows larger peaks to the task-linked stimulus (condition F2, 421 = 13.000, p<0.001; condition-by-stimulus F2, 421 = 33.01, p<0.001, THSDs task-relevant > irrelevant) with the largest peaks in ONs (group F2, 421 = 6.5, p = 0.002; THSDs ON > YN = AD). Task effects were also present in the higher harmonics of the word spectra (1st harmonic p<0.001; 2nd harmonic p = 0.005; 3rd harmonic p = 0.012) but not of the flow spectra. (Figure 3) Again, responses at Pz show the same main effects of task and group, as described above for the spectra recorded at Oz.

Thus, unlike the ERPs, the power spectra show similar task effects on both word and flow responses, but do not show effects of adding a 2nd task-irrelevant stimulus. The spectra also show robust group effects, with the surprising finding of spectral power increasing from YNs to ONs, but decreasing from ONs to ADs.

Phase Coherence Analyses

We considered that differences between the ERPs and the power spectra might reflect changes in the domain of response phase coherence. We focused our analyses on the frequency range of the stimuli with comparisons across stimuli, task conditions, and subject group.

Inter-trial coherence (ITC) in the 0–2 Hz range decreases across subject groups (group F2, 421 = 24.72, p<.001, THSDs YN > ON > AD). ITC is also affected by condition and stimulus, the strongest ITCs elicited with task-irrelevant 2nd stimuli, especially for flow (condition-by-stimulus F2, 421 = 88.49, p<.001). ITCs in the 2–7 Hz range of the spectral harmonics, only show group difference in YNs (F2, 421 = 21.24, p<.001, THSDs YN > ON = AD). These too are affected by condition and stimulus, especially with words in the word task (condition-by-stimulus F2, 421 = 88.49, p<001). These analyses show 2nd stimulus and task effects, with the largest responses to superimposed stimuli, and the

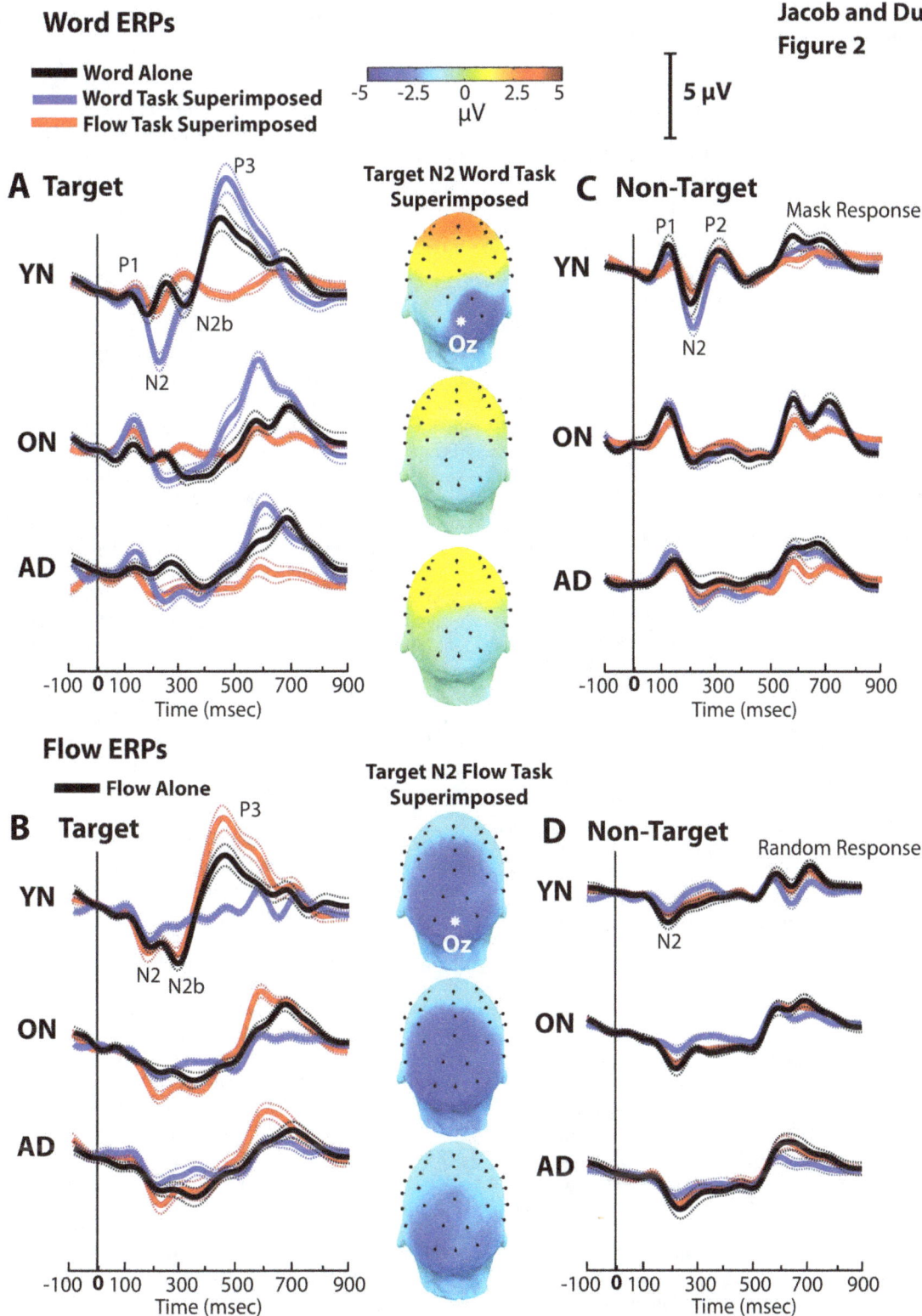

Figure 2. ERP traces and scalp maps of responses. Group average ERPs +/− sem envelope for YNs (top), ONs (middle), and ADs (bottom). A. Responses to target words presented alone (black), include P1, N2, N2b and P3 components. The amplitude of the N2 and P3 components increases with the addition of a task irrelevant flow stimulus superimposed on the word stimulus (blue). The N2 decreases, and the N2b and P3 are eliminated, when the superimposed flow and word stimuli are presented in the context of task change to the flow task (red). Voltage scalp maps (center) with prominent occipital/posterior activation of the N2 response to the word alone stimuli. B. ERPs target optic flow presented alone include N2, N2b and P3 (black) with the P3 increased by adding an irrelevant word stimulus (red). The N2b and P3 are eliminated when switching to the word task (blue). Voltage scalp maps (center) show prominent parietal/posterior activation of the optic flow N2. C. ERPs to non-target words presented alone (black) and the effect of adding an irrelevant motion stimulus (blue) or switching tasks (red). D. ERPs to non-target flow presented alone (black) and the

effect of adding an irrelevant word stimulus (red) or switching tasks (blue). The non-target responses after 700 ms illustrate subtler effects of the transition to the masking noise stimulus.

smallest responses to task-irrelevant stimuli, all most evident in YNs. (Figure 4A and B).

The ITCs evoked by non-target stimuli show the same stimulus, task, and group effects as the targets, but without effects of task-irrelevant 2nd stimuli. These effects are most prominent in YNs for word stimuli in the 0–2 Hz range (stimulus F1, 416 = 17.46, p< .001, THSDs word > flow stimuli; condition F2, 416 = 5.60, p = .004, THSDs word > flow tasks; group F2, 416 = 7.89, p< .001, THSDs YN > AD; condition-by-stimulus F2, 416 = 16.73, p<.001, THSDs word alone and combined > all others; group-by-stimulus F2, 416 = 10.15, p<.001, THSDs YN word > all others) with the same pattern of significant effects obtained for the 2–7 Hz range (all p<.001, THSDs as for the 0–2 Hz). (Figure 4C and D).

In sum, task-irrelevant 2nd stimuli greatly enhance target word and flow coherence with little effect on spectral power. In contrast, changing tasks greatly diminishes coherence, as well as decreasing power. Like task effects, aging and AD effect coherence and power, with successive decreases in coherence, but a paradoxical increase in power with aging, that is lost in AD.

Relating Neurophysiologic and Behavioral Measures

We explored relations between neurophysiological measures and task performance, focusing on ADs as the only group with substantial variability in performance. Multiple linear regression identified variables predicting percent correct responses in the word and flow selective attention conditions.

Word task accuracy (R^2 = 0.758, F3, 19 = 20.6, p<0.001) relates to phase coherence (β = 1.31), with small contributions from the word spectral fourth harmonic (β = 0.028) and P3 amplitudes (β = 0.002). Similarly, flow task accuracy relates (R^2 = 0.605, F3, 19 = 11.4, p<0.001) to phase coherence (β = 1.12), with small contributions from the third harmonic (β = 0.023), and P3 amplitudes (β = 0.0012). Thus, we find that phase coherence is, by far, the best predictor of selective attentional task performance in AD.

Discussion

Mechanisms of Selective Attention

ERPs to task-related words and flow are enhanced by superimposing a task-irrelevant 2nd stimulus, potentially related to increased phase coherence. Previously, task-irrelevant stimuli were seen to reduce responses to task-relevant stimuli. That distractor inhibition [45,46,47] is smaller with complex stimuli and larger with demanding tasks [48,49,50]. Our selective attention task reverses that effect, with the 2nd stimulus enhancing responses (Figure 2).

The attentional control of visual processing has been linked to fronto-posterior signals seen as late ERP components (N2b, N2pc, etc.) [51,52]. These late components are lost when distraction [45,53,54] blocks frontal stimulus selection [55,56]. Our 2nd stimuli do not distract our subjects, performance is not impaired, or block late ERPs. This may reflect the independence of ventral extrastriate word processing and dorsal extrastriate flow processing [57,58], controlled by parallel, reciprocal, fronto-posterior pathways.

The neural mechanisms of selective attention may be revealed by phase coherence increases when adding task-irrelevant 2nd stimuli, with increased coherence (Figure 4) potentially reflecting

phase locking on the task-relevant stimulus stream [59]. Phase locking could create fronto-posterior resonance, promoting the frontal propagation of task-relevant visual input [60,61,62]. In naturalistic circumstances, phase locking could be linked to intrinsic posterior cortical rhythms [63,64,65,66]. In our studies, phase locking is seen by synchronizing our analyses to the tagging frequency of the task-relevant stimulus.

Distinguishing Aging and AD

Aging is thought to be associated with a degradation of top-down fronto-posterior control mechanisms [12,13,67], with effects that may be compounded by cortico-cortical disconnection in AD [68,69,70]. In our studies, such effects are seen as successive declines in attention dependent phase coherence in aging and AD (Figure 4). Our cross-sectional data do not support inferences about disease progression in individual subjects. However, across our subjects and groups, phase incoherence is the best predictor of attentional dysfunction, which is consistent with the prominent group differences in executive function (Table S1).

Paradoxically, aging causes an increase in total spectral power, whereas AD causes a still greater decrease (Figure 3). Mechanistically the differential effect of aging and AD on total power and phase coherence may be linked. That is, in aging, the loss of signal coherence might trigger an enhancement of the net neural activity evoked by that signal to boost the reliability of signal transmission. Such an increase in net activity of engaged neuronal populations would cause more neurons, to be more active, more of the time. That would be the case whether individual neurons in a circumscribed area are responding more, or whether more neurons are responding in or across networked areas, or both.

Our study does not support definitive inferences about the underlying pathophysiologies of aging, AD, or their potential inter-relations. However, our finding that cortical hyper-responsiveness is task-dependent, may favor mechanisms operating at the level of network dynamics. One scenario for compensatory task-dependent hyper-responsiveness might link signal incoherence to the recruitment of functionally overlapping neuronal populations to maintain task performance. This is consistent with our finding that the neurophysiological changes seen in aging are associated with success in the behavioral tasks, and with reports suggesting that older adults show greater neural activity than younger subjects when achieving comparable levels of task performance [12,14,71]. Neuro-behavioral compensation could be actively engaged by greater effort in older adults, or by a passive feedback control process. In fact, subjective effortfulness could reflect such a process; effort as neural recruitment [72].

Aging related cortical hyperactivity may contribute to the pathophysiology of AD [2,3,6], potentially triggering the transition from aging to AD [7]. These views are consistent with likely molecular pathophysiologies of AD, with increased total power generation in aging causing hyper-metabolic changes [73] that promote excito-toxicity [5]. Excito-toxicity could promote changes in the generation and processing of endogenous proteins that compose the plaques and tangles of AD [74]. This might further exacerbate network incoherence [75] and critically impair spectral power generation [76]. Thus, aging and AD are neurophysiologically distinguishable, and their association may be causal.

Might Cortical Hyper-Responsiveness in Aging Contribute to Alzheimer's...

67

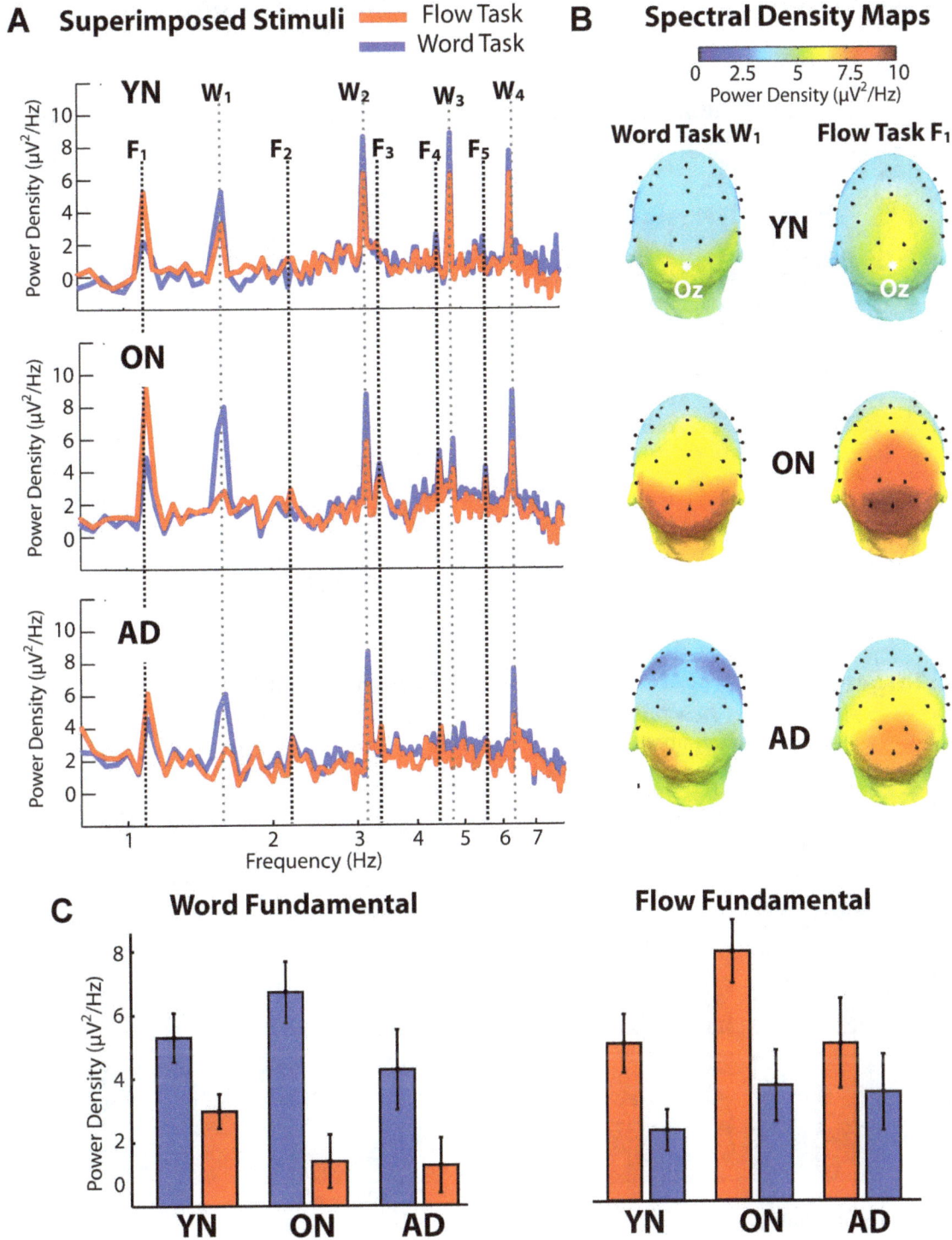

Figure 3. Frequency spectra of scalp recorded electrical activity. Stimulus specific frequency spectra of cortical responses to superimposed optic flow at 1.11 Hz and words at 1.57 Hz during the flow (red) or word (blue) button press tasks. A. Task effects are seen for all groups, with larger responses at the frequency of the task-relevant stimulus. B. Spectral density scalp maps with prominent occipital/posterior activation of the word (left) and flow (right) responses, substantially more evident in ONs than YNs or ADs. C. Bar graphs of spectral power (ordinate, mean +/− sem) show task effects for the word (left) and flow (right) stimuli at the fundamental frequencies, during the flow (red) and word (blue) push button tasks, for the three subject groups (abscissa).

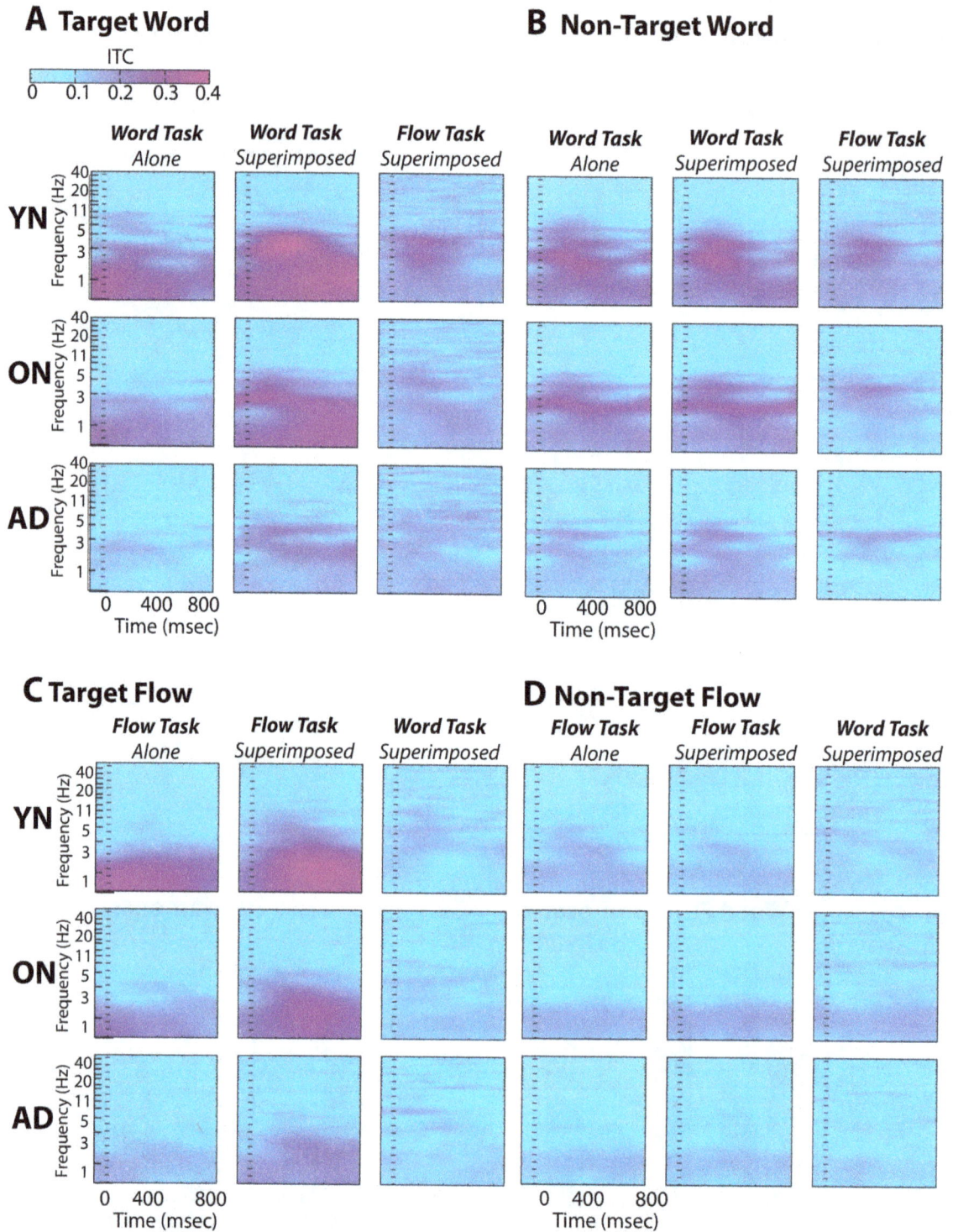

Figure 4. Inter-trial coherence (ITC) of recorded responses. Mean ITC of response phase (color) elicited across frequencies (ordinate) and the time-course of the 1.11 Hz stimulus cycle (abscissa). Phase coherence for target word (A) and flow (C) stimuli is most pronounced for superimposed stimuli during the word task (middle), relative to the word alone stimulus (left), or superimposed stimuli during the flow task (right). ITC for non-target word (B) and flow (D) stimuli show similar effects.

Might Cortical Hyper-Responsiveness in Aging Contribute to Alzheimer's...

69

Acknowledgments

We gratefully acknowledge the scientific and computer programming contributions of William Vaughn and the assistance of Dr. Anthony Monacelli, Teresa Steffenella, and Eva Perelstein in recording sessions. We appreciate the comments of Dr. William K. Page, William Vaughn, and Colin Lockwood on earlier drafts of the manuscript. This work was supported by NEI R01-EY022062, NEI P30-EY01319, R01-NIA AG17596, ONR N000141110525, and UofR CTSI RR024135.

Author Contributions

Conceived and designed the experiments: MSJ CJD. Performed the experiments: MSJ. Analyzed the data: MSJ CJD. Contributed reagents/materials/analysis tools: MSJ. Contributed to the writing of the manuscript: MSJ CJD.

References

1. Evans DA, Funkenstein HH, Albert MS, Scherr PA, Cook NR, et al. (1989) Prevalence of Alzheimer's disease in a community population of older persons. Higher than previously reported. JAMA: the journal of the American Medical Association 262: 2551–2556.

2. Jagust WJ, Mormino EC (2011) Lifespan brain activity, beta-amyloid, and Alzheimer's disease. Trends Cogn Sci 15: 520–526.

3. Sheline YI, Morris JC, Snyder AZ, Price JL, Yan Z, et al. (2010) APOE4 allele disrupts resting state fMRI connectivity in the absence of amyloid plaques or decreased CSF Abeta42. J Neurosci 30: 17035–17040.

4. Oh H, Mormino EC, Madison C, Hayenga A, Smiljic A, et al. (2011) beta-Amyloid affects frontal and posterior brain networks in normal aging. NeuroImage 54: 1887–1895.

5. Mamelak M (2007) Alzheimer' s disease, oxidative stress and gammahydroxybutyrate. NeurobiolAging 28: 1340–1360.

6. Dolev I, Fogel H, Milshtein H, Berdichevsky Y, Lipstein N, et al. (2013) Spike bursts increase amyloid-beta 40/42 ratio by inducing a presenilin-1 conformational change. Nat Neurosci 16: 587–595.

7. Suberbielle E, Sanchez PE, Kravitz AV, Wang X, Ho K, et al. (2013) Physiologic brain activity causes DNA double-strand breaks in neurons, with exacerbation by amyloid-beta. Nat Neurosci 16: 613–621.

8. Fernandez R, Kavcic V, Duffy CJ (2007) Neurophysiologic analyses of low- and high-level visual processing in Alzheimer disease. Neurology 68: 2066–2076.

9. Schmolesky MT, Wang Y, Pu M, Leventhal AG (2000) Degradation of stimulus selectivity of visual cortical cells in senescent rhesus monkeys. Nature Neuroscience 3: 384–390.

10. Fu Y, Yu S, Ma Y, Wang Y, Zhou Y (2013) Functional degradation of the primary visual cortex during early senescence in rhesus monkeys. Cerebral cortex 23: 2923–2931.

11. Hua T, Li X, He L, Zhou Y, Wang Y, et al. (2006) Functional degradation of visual cortical cells in old cats. NeurobiolAging 27: 155–162.

12. Prvulovic D, Van de Ven V, Sack AT, Maurer K, Linden DE (2005) Functional activation imaging in aging and dementia. Psychiatry Res 140: 97–113.

13. Tumeh PC, Alavi A, Houseni M, Greenfield A, Chryssikos T, et al. (2007) Structural and functional imaging correlates for age-related changes in the brain. Semin Nucl Med 37: 69–87.

14. Park DC, Reuter-Lorenz P (2009) The adaptive brain: aging and neurocognitive scaffolding. Annu Rev Psychol 60: 173–196.

15. Li L, Gratton C, Fabiani M, Knight RT (2013) Age-related frontoparietal changes during the control of bottom-up and top-down attention: an ERP study. Neurobiology of aging 34: 477–488.

16. Ungerleider LG, Mishkin M (1982) Two cortical visual systems. In: Ingle DJ, Goodale MA, Mansfield RJW, editors. Analysis of Visual Behavior. Cambridge: MIT Press. 549–586.

17. Goodale MA, Milner AD (1992) Separate visual pathways for perception and action. TINS: 20–25.

18. Hopfinger JB, Woldorff MG, Fletcher EM, Mangun GR (2001) Dissociating top-down attentional control from selective perception and action. Neuropsychologia 39: 1277–1291.

19. Gazzaley A, Rissman J, Cooney J, Rutman A, Seibert T, et al. (2007) Functional interactions between prefrontal and visual association cortex contribute to top-down modulation of visual processing. Cereb Cortex 17 Suppl 1: i125–135.

20. Siegel M, Donner TH, Engel AK (2012) Spectral fingerprints of large-scale neuronal interactions. Nat Rev Neurosci 13: 121–134.

21. Desimone R (1998) Visual attention mediated by biased competition in extrastriate visual cortex. Philosophical Transactions of the Royal Society of London - Series B: Biological Sciences 353: 1245–1255.

22. Cook EP, Maunsell JH (2002) Attentional modulation of behavioral performance and neuronal responses in middle temporal and ventral intraparietal areas of macaque monkey. Journal of Neuroscience 22: 1994–2004.

23. Reynolds JH, Heeger DJ (2009) The normalization model of attention. Neuron 61: 168–185.

24. Kishore S, Hornick N, Sato N, Page WK, Duffy CJ (2011) Driving Strategy Alters Neuronal Responses to Self-Movement: Cortical Mechanisms of Distracted Driving. Cereb Cortex 22: 201–208.

25. Mapstone M, Duffy CJ (2010) Approaching objects cause confusion in patients with Alzheimer's disease regarding their direction of self-movement. Brain 133: 2690–2701.

26. Morgan ST, Hansen JC, Hillyard SA (1996) Selective attention to stimulus location modulates the steady-state visual evoked potential. Proc Natl Acad Sci U S A 93: 4770–4774.

27. Hillyard SA, Vogel EK, Luck SJ (1998) Sensory gain control (amplification) as a mechanism of selective attention: electrophysiological and neuroimaging evidence. Philos Trans R Soc Lond B Biol Sci 353: 1257–1270.

28. Pei F, Pettet MW, Norcia AM (2002) Neural correlates of object-based attention. J Vis 2: 588–596.

29. Muller MM, Andersen S, Trujillo NJ, Valdes-Sosa P, Malinowski P, et al. (2006) Feature-selective attention enhances color signals in early visual areas of the human brain. Proc Natl Acad Sci U S A 103: 14250–14254.

30. Palomares M, Ales JM, Wade AR, Cottereau BR, Norcia AM (2012) Distinct effects of attention on the neural responses to form and motion processing: a SSVEP source-imaging study. J Vis 12: 15.

31. Kim YJ, Grabowecky M, Paller KA, Muthu K, Suzuki S (2007) Attention induces synchronization-based response gain in steady-state visual evoked potentials. Nat Neurosci 10: 117–125.

32. Gregoriou GG, Gotts SJ, Zhou H, Desimone R (2009) High-frequency, long-range coupling between prefrontal and visual cortex during attention. Science 324: 1207–1210.

33. Kavcic V, Duffy CJ (2003) Attentional dynamics and visual perception: Mechanisms of spatial disorientation in Alzheimer's disease. Brain 126: 1173–1181.

34. Fernandez R, Duffy CJ (2012) Early Alzheimer's disease blocks responses to accelerating self-movement. Neurobiol Aging 33: 2551–2560.

35. McKhann G, Drachman D, Folstein M, Katzman R, Price D, et al. (1984) Clinical diagnosis of Alzheimer's disease: report of the NINCDS- ADRDA Work Group under the auspices of Department of Health and Human Services Task Force on Alzheimer's Disease. Neurology 34: 939–944.

36. Folstein MF, Folstein SE, McHugh PR (1975) "Mini-mental state". A practical method for grading the cognitive state of patients for the clinician. Journal of Psychiatric Research 12: 189–198.

37. Wechsler D (1997) Wechsler memory scale-III Manual. San Antonio, TX: The Psychological Corp.

38. Money J, Alexander D, Walker HT (1965) A Standardized Road Map Test of Direction Sense. Baltimore, MD: Johns Hopkins Press.

39. Benton A, Hamsher K, Varney NR, Spreen O (1983) Contributions to neuropsychological assessment: a clinical manual. New York: Oxford University Press. 44–54 p.

40. Binetti G, Cappa SF, Magni E, Padovani A, Bianchetti A, et al. (1996) Disorders of visual and spatial perception in the early stage of Alzheimer's disease. Annals of the New York Academy of Sciences 777: 221–225.

41. Perry RJ, Hodges JR (1999) Attention and executive deficits in Alzheimer's disease. A critical review. Brain : a journal of neurology 122 (Pt 3): 383–404.

42. Terada S, Sato S, Nagao S, Ikeda C, Shindo A, et al. (2013) Trail making test B and brain perfusion imaging in mild cognitive impairment and mild Alzheimer's disease. Psychiatry research 213: 249–255.

43. Makeig S, Debener S, Onton J, Delorme A (2004) Mining event-related brain dynamics. Trends Cogn Sci 8: 204–210.

44. Fernandez R, Monacelli A, Duffy CJ (2013) Visual Motion Event Related Potentials Distinguish Aging and Alzheimer's Disease. J Alzheimers Dis.

45. Niedeggen M, Michael L, Hesselmann G (2012) Closing the gates to consciousness: distractors activate a central inhibition process. J Cogn Neurosci 24: 1294–1304.

46. Hesselmann G, Niedeggen M, Sahraie A, Milders M (2006) Specifying the distractor inhibition account of attention-induced motion blindness. Vision Res 46: 1048–1056.

47. Michael L, Hesselmann G, Kiefer M, Niedeggen M (2011) Distractor-induced blindness for orientation changes and coherent motion. Vision Res 51: 1781–1787.

48. Lavie N (2005) Distracted and confused?: selective attention under load. Trends Cogn Sci 9: 75–82.

49. Parks NA, Hilimire MR, Corballis PM (2011) Steady-state signatures of visual perceptual load, multimodal distractor filtering, and neural competition. J Cogn Neurosci 23: 1113–1124.

50. Hindi Attar C, Muller MM (2012) Selective attention to task-irrelevant emotional distractors is unaffected by the perceptual load associated with a foreground task. PLoS One 7: e37186.

51. Luck SJ, Hillyard SA (1994) Electrophysiological correlates of feature analysis during visual search. Psychophysiology 31: 291–308.

52. Eimer M (1996) ERP modulations indicate the selective processing of visual stimuli as a result of transient and sustained spatial attention. Psychophysiology 33: 13–21.

53. Zhao G, Liu Q, Zhang Y, Jiao J, Zhang Q, et al. (2011) The amplitude of N2pc reflects the physical disparity between target item and distracters. Neurosci Lett 491: 68–72.

54. Sawaki R, Geng JJ, Luck SJ (2012) A common neural mechanism for preventing and terminating the allocation of attention. J Neurosci 32: 10725–10736.

55. Cohen JY, Heitz RP, Schall JD, Woodman GF (2009) On the origin of event-related potentials indexing covert attentional selection during visual search. J Neurophysiol 102: 2375–2386.

56. Heitz RP, Cohen JY, Woodman GF, Schall JD (2010) Neural correlates of correct and errant attentional selection revealed through N2pc and frontal eye field activity. J Neurophysiol 104: 2433–2441.

57. Goodale MA, Meenan JP, Buxlthoff HH, Nicolle DA, Murphy KJ, et al. (1994) Separate neural pathways for the visual analysis of object shape in perception and prehension. Current Biology: 604–610.

58. Ungerleider LG, Haxby JV (1994) 'What' and 'where' in the human brain. Current Biology: 157–165.

59. Klimesch W, Sauseng P, Hanslmayr S, Gruber W, Freunberger R (2007) Event-related phase reorganization may explain evoked neural dynamics. Neurosci Biobehav Rev 31: 1003–1016.

60. Ullsperger P, Neumann U, Gille HG, Pietschmann M (1987) P300 and anticipated task difficulty. Int J Psychophysiol 5: 145–149.

61. Bledowski C, Prvulovic D, Goebel R, Zanella FE, Linden DE (2004) Attentional systems in target and distractor processing: a combined ERP and fMRI study. Neuroimage 22: 530–540.

62. Ng BS, Schroeder T, Kayser C (2012) A precluding but not ensuring role of entrained low-frequency oscillations for auditory perception. J Neurosci 32: 12268–12276.

63. Rousselet GA, Husk JS, Bennett PJ, Sekuler AB (2007) Single-trial EEG dynamics of object and face visual processing. Neuroimage 36: 843–862.

64. Kuba M, Kubova Z, Kremlacek J, Langrova J (2007) Motion-onset VEPs: characteristics, methods, and diagnostic use. Vision Res 47: 189–202.

65. Lakatos P, Karmos G, Mehta AD, Ulbert I, Schroeder CE (2008) Entrainment of neuronal oscillations as a mechanism of attentional selection. Science 320: 110–113.

66. Besle J, Schevon CA, Mehta AD, Lakatos P, Goodman RR, et al. (2011) Tuning of the human neocortex to the temporal dynamics of attended events. J Neurosci 31: 3176–3185.

67. Velasco ME, Smith MA, Siedlak SL, Nunomura A, Perry G (1998) Striation is the characteristic neuritic abnormality in Alzheimer disease. Brain Res 813: 329–333.

68. Morrison JH, Hof PR (2007) Life and death of neurons in the aging cerebral cortex. Int Rev Neurobiol 81: 41–57.

69. Andrews-Hanna JR, Snyder AZ, Vincent JL, Lustig C, Head D, et al. (2007) Disruption of large-scale brain systems in advanced aging. Neuron 56: 924–935.

70. Oh H, Jagust WJ (2013) Frontotemporal network connectivity during memory encoding is increased with aging and disrupted by beta-amyloid. The Journal of neuroscience : the official journal of the Society for Neuroscience 33: 18425–18437.

71. Buckner RL (2004) Memory and executive function in aging and AD: multiple factors that cause decline and reserve factors that compensate. Neuron 44: 195–208.

72. Henneman E, Somjen G, Carpenter DO (1965) Excitability and inhibitability of motoneurons of different sizes. Journal of neurophysiology 28: 599–620.

73. Scheef L, Spottke A, Daerr M, Joe A, Striepens N, et al. (2012) Glucose metabolism, gray matter structure, and memory decline in subjective memory impairment. Neurology 79: 1332–1339.

74. Jack CR Jr, Knopman DS, Jagust WJ, Petersen RC, Weiner MW, et al. (2013) Tracking pathophysiological processes in Alzheimer's disease: an updated hypothetical model of dynamic biomarkers. Lancet Neurol 12: 207–216.

75. Neufang S, Akhrif A, Riedl V, Forstl H, Kurz A, et al. (2011) Disconnection of frontal and parietal areas contributes to impaired attention in very early Alzheimer's disease. J Alzheimers Dis 25: 309–321.

76. Jardanhazy A, Jardanhazy T, Kalman J (2008) Sodium lactate differently alters relative EEG power and functional connectivity in Alzheimer's disease patients' brain regions. Eur J Neurol 15: 150–155.

8

Motor Imagery for Severely Motor-Impaired Patients: Evidence for Brain-Computer Interfacing as Superior Control Solution

Johannes Höhne[1]*, Elisa Holz[2], Pit Staiger-Sälzer[3], Klaus-Robert Müller[4,5,6]*, Andrea Kübler[2]*, Michael Tangermann[7]*

1 Neurotechnology group, Berlin Institute of Technology, Berlin, Germany, **2** Department of Psychology I, University of Würzburg, Würzburg, Germany, **3** Beratungsstelle für Unterstützte Kommunikation (BUK), Diakonie Bad Kreuznach, Bad Kreuznach, Germany, **4** Machine Learning Laboratory, Berlin Institute of Technology, Berlin, Germany, **5** Bernstein Center for Computational Neuroscience, Berlin, Germany, **6** Department of Brain and Cognitive Engineering, Korea University, Anam-dong, Seongbuk-gu, Seoul, Korea, **7** BrainLinks-BrainTools Excellence Cluster, University of Freiburg, Freiburg, Germany

Abstract

Brain-Computer Interfaces (BCIs) strive to decode brain signals into control commands for severely handicapped people with no means of muscular control. These potential users of noninvasive BCIs display a large range of physical and mental conditions. Prior studies have shown the general applicability of BCI with patients, with the conflict of either using many training sessions or studying only moderately restricted patients. We present a BCI system designed to establish external control for severely motor-impaired patients within a very short time. Within only six experimental sessions, three out of four patients were able to gain significant control over the BCI, which was based on motor imagery or attempted execution. For the most affected patient, we found evidence that the BCI could outperform the best assistive technology (AT) of the patient in terms of control accuracy, reaction time and information transfer rate. We credit this success to the applied user-centered design approach and to a highly flexible technical setup. State-of-the art machine learning methods allowed the exploitation and combination of multiple relevant features contained in the EEG, which rapidly enabled the patients to gain substantial BCI control. Thus, we could show the feasibility of a flexible and tailorable BCI application in severely disabled users. This can be considered a significant success for two reasons: Firstly, the results were obtained within a short period of time, matching the tight clinical requirements. Secondly, the participating patients showed, compared to most other studies, very severe communication deficits. They were dependent on everyday use of AT and two patients were in a locked-in state. For the most affected patient a reliable communication was rarely possible with existing AT.

Editor: Blake Johnson, ARC Centre of Excellence in Cognition and its Disorders (CCD), Australia

Funding: The authors are grateful for the financial support by several institutions: This work was partly supported by the European Information and Communication Technologies (ICT) Programme Project FP7-224631 and 216886, by the Deutsche Forschungsgemeinschaft (DFG) (grants MU 987/3-2, EXC 1086) and Bundesministerium fur Bildung und Forschung (BMBF) (FKZ 01IB001A, 01GQ0850) and by the FP7-ICT Programme of the European Community, under the PASCAL2 Network of Excellence, ICT-216886. This work was also supported by the World Class University Program through the National Research Foundation of Korea funded by the Ministry of Education, Science, and Technology, under Grant R31-10008. This publication only reflects the authors' views. Funding agencies are not liable for any use that may be made of the information contained herein.

Competing Interests: The authors have declared that no competing interests exist.

* Email: j.hoehne@tu-berlin.de (JH); klaus-robert.mueller@tu-berlin.de (KRM); Andrea.Kuebler@uni-wuerzburg.de (AK); michael.tangermann@blbt.uni-freiburg.de (MT)

Introduction

Aiming to develop communication pathways, which are independent of muscle activity, the research area of Brain-Computer Interfaces (BCIs, [1,2]) has significantly emerged over the last two decades. BCIs strive to decode brain signals into control commands, such that even severely handicapped people with no means of muscular control are enabled to communicate. Different types of brain signals can be used to control a BCI and a vast amount of studies have demonstrated the proof of concept, showing that healthy users are able to control noninvasive BCIs with a high accuracy and a communication rate of up to 100 bits/min [3]. Translating brain signals into digital control commands,

BCI systems can be applied for communication [4], interaction with external devices (e.g. steering a wheelchair) [5], rehabilitation [6] or mental state monitoring [7,8]. While recent studies also investigated the neuronal underpinnings of BCI control [9,10], the main objective of BCIs has always been to provide an alternative communication channel for patients that are in the locked-in state [11–13].

Brain signals suitable for BCI can be acquired with numerous acquisition technologies, such as electroencephalogram (EEG), magnetoencephalogram (MEG), functional magnetic resonance imaging (fMRI), functional near-infrared spectroscopy (fNIRS) or electrocorticogram (ECOG) in an invasive and non-invasive manner. While these different approaches are reviewed in

[1,2,14], we focus on non-invasive BCI systems which are based on EEG signals.

Based on experiments with healthy users, various improvements in the experimental design [15,16], and on the algorithmic side [17–21] have recently been presented. In particular, machine learning methods have been developed to improve feature extraction [18] and classification [22–26] of neuronal signals, enabling the field to set up an online BCI paradigm for naive healthy users within a single session. Until now, these improvements have mostly been tested on offline data from healthy subjects.

There are different types of BCI paradigms, which can generally be differentiated in (I) self-driven paradigms and (II) stimulus-driven paradigms. Stimulus-driven paradigms evaluate the neuronal response to multiple stimuli which are presented consecutively. The objective of the BCI is to detect to which stimulus the user is attending. Numerous stimulus-driven paradigms were introduced, with stimuli from the visual [3,27,28], auditory [29,30] or tactile [31] domain and they have proven successful in end-users with severe diseases leading to motor impairment [32,33]. Moreover, several types of neuronal responses (e.g. evoked potentials and steady-state potentials) enable to differentiate between the brain responses of attended and non-attended stimuli. As these paradigms are all relying on the user's perception of those stimuli, patients with sensory impairments may not be able to use such BCI systems [34].

Self-driven BCI paradigms are not relying on the perception of external stimuli, as these systems are based on brain signals which are intentionally produced by the user. Here, "Motor Imagery" (MI) is a widely used paradigm, in which the BCI detects changes of brain patterns (such as sensory motor rhythms), which are associated with the imagination of movements. In a common MI scenario, a computer can be controlled (e.g. moving a cursor on the screen) through either imagination of movements of the left hand/right hand/foot [35] or their attempted execution.

Although the proof-of-concept for noninvasive BCI technology has already been shown more than twenty years ago, patient studies are still very rare. Kübler (2013) [13] recently pointed out that "fewer than 10% of the papers published on brain-computer interfacing deal with individuals presenting motor restrictions, although many authors mention these as the purpose of their research". Moreover, within patient studies, those patients who were chosen to participate were rarely in need of a BCI, since their residual communication abilities with assisted technology (AT) were higher than the best state-of-the-art BCI could ever provide. Thus, there is a lack of studies with patients who are in a state that allows the BCI to become the best available communication channel. Some examples can be found in [4,11,34,36–44], also being reviewed in [12,45,46]. However, recent clinical studies have shown that it is even possible to set up BCI systems with patients in the complete locked-in condition. De Massari (2013) [47] introduced the idea of semantic conditioning as a potential alternative paradigm with completely paralyzed patients, and [48] applied a MI paradigm with patients diagnosed as being in the vegetative state. Moreover, patients with disorders of consciousness were trained to use BCI [49], however, no functional communication could be achieved. These studies reveal that it may be possible to obtain significant classification accuracies for those patients, but it has not yet been shown that patients in complete paralysis can "reliably" use a BCI system [50].

Our contribution describes the results of a MI-BCI study with four patients who showed severe brain damage. While all four patients had substantial difficulties with communication, two patients had a communication rate with their individually adapted

AT of less than 5 bits/min. This means that for these participants, a BCI has the chance to become their individually best available communication channel, with all the beneficial implications for the Quality-of-Life of these patients [51,52].

The objective of this study is to show that the application of state-of-the-art machine learning methods allows to set up a MI-BCI system for patients in need of communication solutions within a very small number of sessions. We addressed this issue within a BCI gaming paradigm, which was specifically adapted to the needs of each patient according to user-centered design principles [53]. Both, the BCI system and the feedback application were optimized in an iterative procedure in order to account for the users' individual preferences. For the first time, automatically adapting classifiers, as well as hybrid data processing and classification approaches were applied online with (locked-in) patients. Moreover, a thorough psychological evaluation was done [51].

More precisely, we demonstrate that by following the principle "let the machine learn," [54], patients gained significant BCI control within six sessions or less.

Materials and Methods

2.1 Patient Participants

The BCI system was tested with four severely disabled users in the information center of assistive technology, Bad Kreuznach, Germany. The patients were diagnosed with different diseases causing hemi- or tetraplegia. All patients were in a generally constant condition with no primary progress in their disease. No cognitive deficits were known. Table 1 summarizes disease- and demographic-related information. All patients had severe communication deficits and were using an AT solution on a daily basis. They had been continuously provided with individually optimized and cutting-edge AT (such as customized switches or eye-trackers) for more than five years. Only patient 3 had previously participated in BCI with MI training in a different study more than ten years ago - without gaining significant control (see patient KI in Kübler (2000) [55] and Kübler & Birbaumer (2008) [12]). It should be noted that the patient numbering was ordered with decreasing residual communication abilities. Two of the four patients (patients 3 and 4) were in the locked-in state. Patients in the locked-in state are restricted in their voluntary motor control to such an extent that they are not able to communicate. This definition however makes an exception for one remaining communication channel. For most patients in the locked-in state, eye movements are the last remaining form of muscular control. If no remaining form of voluntary muscular activity is available (including the control of eye gaze, blink or button press), patients are considered to be in the "complete locked-in state".

Since different disagreeing definitions of the (complete) locked-in state exist, Table 1 also provides the communication rate with AT (measured as Information Transfer Rate (ITR) in bits/min [56]) as an additional measure. Communication rates with AT were empirically estimated by quantifying the time that the users needed to answer yes/no questions or ratings on a visual analog scale (VAS) in the evaluation process of this study. In the following paragraphs, each individual patient and his current physical condition is described in further detail.

Patient 1. Amongst all patients enrolled in this study, patient 1 had the least impaired communication ability – being able to speak. Due to a stroke, his pronunciation is slurred, his language is considerably slowed down and needs to be amplified in volume. Although he has limited control over his left hand, he can reliably control his right hand to write, type or steer an electric wheelchair.

Table 1. Demographic and disease related data of all patients.

	Patient 1	Patient 2	Patient 3	Patient 4
Age	47	48	45	45
Diagnosis	Tetraparesis after pons infarct	Hemiplegia after cerebral bleeding	Infantile cerebral palsy	Tetraparesis after cerebral bleeding
Artificial Ventilation	No	No	No	No
Artificial Nutrition (PEG)	No	No	No	Yes
Wheelchair	Yes	Yes	Yes	Yes
Residual muscular control	Eye-movement Speech Residual movement of right hand	Eye-movement Residual movement of left arm, hand and head Mimic	Eye movement (unreliable) Mimic Residual movement of right hand/arm	Eye-movement (highly unreliable) Residual movement of left thumb (depending on physical state)
Computer input device	Keyboard PC	Keyboard PC	Joystick/switch with hand letterboard with eye movements	Button press with thumb (yes/no): yes: 1 button press no: 2 button presses
Use of ICT on a daily basis	Yes	Yes	Yes	Yes
Experience with AT since	2006	1982	1986	2000
ITR with AT ICT	>30 bits/min	>30 bits/min	1–5 bits/min	0–2 bits/min
Experience with MI -BCI	No	No	Yes	No

Patient 2. Although lacking the ability to speak, patient 2 has high residual communication abilities since he can voluntarily control the left hand, left arm and his facial muscles. Thus, he can gesture and also use a standard computer keyboard.

Patient 3. Patient 3 is communicating with trained caregivers (partner-scanning) by controlling his eye gaze. He has been trying to use numerous eye-tracking systems, without gaining sufficient control. However, he can control a computer with a slow, weak but reliable control of his right forearm through the press of a button. Being highly motivated to use BCI technology, he already participated in a BCI study more than ten years ago [55], which tested the control via slow cortical potentials (SCP) of the EEG. Unfortunately, he was not able to gain reliable control over the SCP-based BCI system in any session. Due to highly limited means of communication, a functioning BCI system would directly improve the quality of life of patient 3.

Patient 4. Having the goal to provide communication solutions for people who can hardly communicate with AT or otherwise, patient 4 represents the ultimate end-user target group for BCI technology. The one exclusively known voluntary muscular control is a rather unreliable movement of his right thumb. He thus uses his thumb to press a button (pinch grip), which reflects the only available communication channel.

When starting the study, he had been in this condition for more than nine years. His communication is very slow and unreliable to the extent, that he is sometimes completely unable to communicate at all for several hours. In principle, he uses the button press in order to communicate an answer upon a question. A single button press would represent a *yes*-answer/agreement, while disagreements are expressed by two consecutive button presses. He shows a high variation within and across days of his attentiveness (he spontaneously falls asleep), of his mood, and of his responsiveness. The median time for a single button press is estimated to be 12 s, but delays of tens of seconds appear frequently (approx. 40%). The variation of responsiveness is the biggest communication hurdle: whenever patient 4 wishes to

provide a negative response or disagreement, the second button press might be heavily delayed or not executed. Then the caregiver erroneously assumes an agreement. Given this communication quality and a communication rate at its best of 2 bits/min, patient 4 can be regarded to be close to the complete locked-in condition.

2.2 Study Protocol

The study protocol was approved by the Ethical Review Board of the Medical Faculty, University of Tübingen, Germany (case file 398/2011BO2). Written informed consent was obtained from each patient or their legally authorized representative. The study consisted of six EEG sessions per patient. There was not more than one EEG session per day and depending on the patient's condition, the session took 1–3 hours - including preparation time. Additionally, one introductory interview was conducted before the study and two interviews for evaluation were held after the last BCI session. Fig. 1A depicts details of the individual sessions. The psychological evaluation, with respect to the interview and questionnaires, is described in a separate article [51].

In the first EEG session, every patient was screened to explore individual brain patterns and to select the two MI classes (left-hand, right-hand and foot imagery) which resulted in highest and most robust class-discriminability. Moreover, standard auditory oddball ERP recordings and a labeled recording for eye-movements, blinking artifacts and eyes open/closed measurements were performed during this screening session. MI training with feedback was not performed during this first EEG session, but only during the following five BCI sessions.

Each feedback session (2–6) was split in two parts: patients first executed a copy task (CopyTask), afterwards they received full control of the application in the free game mode (FreeMode). Patients 3 and 4 attempted to perform a motor action, while patients 1 and 2 used motor imagery. In each trial, the task was

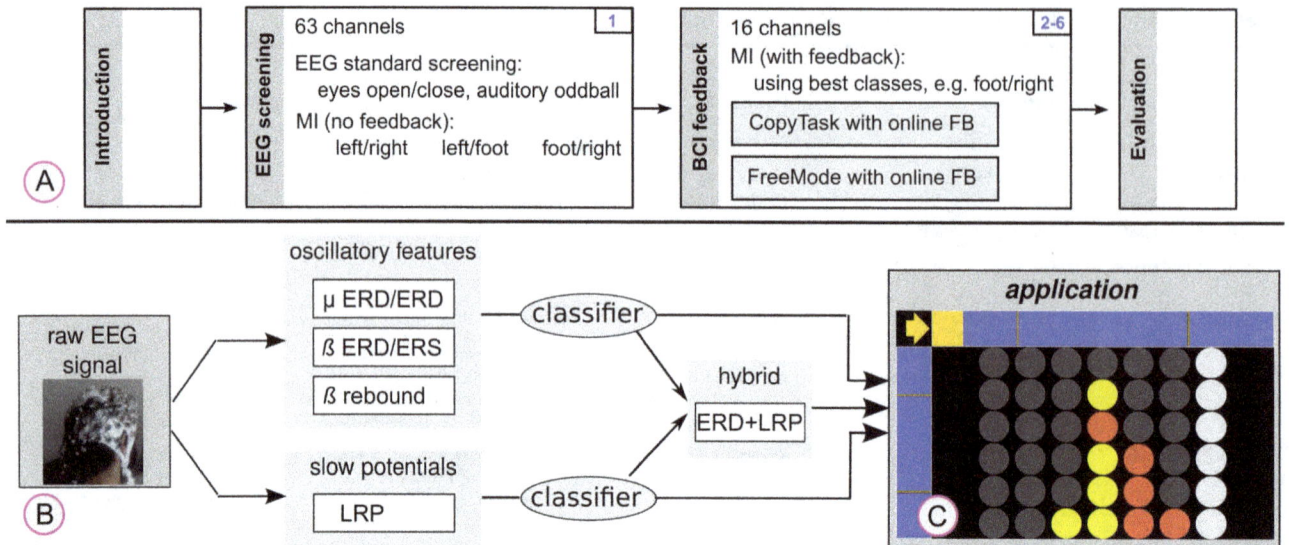

Figure 1. The experimental design is shown in plot (A). Plot (**B**) depicts the architecture of the flexible BCI system which simultaneously considers oscillatory features and slow potentials. Two classifiers are applied and the feedback application is receiving simultaneous output of both classifiers and their weighted combination. A screen shot of the "Connect-4" application in mode *FR* (foot vs. right hand) is plotted in (**C**). In the top-left corner, the cue is presented (an arrow pointing to the right) and based on the BCI output, the yellow bar is either extending rightwards or downwards. The rightmost column is currently selected and visually highlighted.

visually cued by an arrow, e.g. pointing rightwards or downwards (for right-hand or foot imagery), see Fig. 1B. During both the CopyTask and the FreeMode, patients received online feedback (see Fig. 1C) of their targeted brain activation. However, in the CopyTask the outcome of a trial did not initiate an action in the game. In the FreeMode, the directional cue was replaced by a question mark and the gaming application was fully controlled by the BCI with two available actions: "select next column" and "place coin". Each action was represented by one MI class. The FreeMode was only started if the patient had reached sufficient control ($\geq 70\%$) in the CopyTask (leading to less frequent and shorter FreeMode phases for early sessions).

In order to reduce the number of unintended actions in the FreeMode, an action (placement of a coin or selection of the next column) was only performed if a predefined threshold had been exceeded by the BCI classifier. This resulted in "noDecision" trials if the threshold was not exceeded. Consequently no action was elicited for these trials. Introducing "noDecision" trials lead to a decreased fraction of incorrect decisions, yet at the same time to a reduction of communication rate (here: actions per minute and ITR). The ITR values reported throughout this paper were calculated such that all pauses were taken into account [29].

Within the entire study, long durations of trials and inter-trial pauses led to an approximate speed of 4 trials/minute. Since one bit can be coded within one trial, the maximum achievable bit rate with this system was about 4 bits/min (with 100% correct trials). Although speeding up the communication rate by shortening the durations of trials and pauses would have been possible, we did not make use of this option in order to minimize the stress level and workload. Moreover, it should be noted that a reliable slow control might be preferable compared to a fast communication solution which is less reliable.

2.3 Application

Gaming applications represent a playful way to practice and improve the use of BCI systems, because they may provide long-

term and short-term motivation. Moreover, we considered the frustration of erroneous actions in a game to be lower than erroneous selections of letters in a spelling task. Therefore, a computer version of the game "Connect-4" was used within all sessions. "Connect-4" is a strategic game, in which two players take turns in filling a matrix of free slots with coins. The objective of the game is to connect four of one's own coins of the same color vertically, horizontally, or diagonally. The two players are alternately placing their coins in one of the seven columns. The gaming application can be controlled by a 2-class motor imagery BCI, since only two actions are needed to play the game: (1) select the next column, or (2) place the coin in the current column. The software was implemented as a standalone java-application. Fig. 1C shows a screen shot of the application.

2.4 EEG acquisition

Two different EEG systems were used within this study, both systems utilized passive gel electrodes. In the screening session, a 63-channel EEG system was used with most electrodes placed in motor-dense areas (cap: EasyCap, amplifier: BrainProducts, 2×32 channels, 1000 Hz sampling rate). One EOG channel was recorded additionally below the right eye. In sessions 2–6, a 16-channel EEG system was used (cap&amplifier: g.Tec, 1200 Hz sampling rate), while electrodes were placed symmetrically in areas close to the motor cortex. All EEG signals were referenced to the nose. Impedances were kept below 10 $k\Omega$, if possible. Data analysis and classification was performed with MATLAB (The MathWorks, Natick, MA, USA) using an inhouse BCI toolbox. For online processing and offline analysis, the EEG data was low-pass filtered to 45 Hz and down-sampled to 100 Hz.

2.5 BCI setup

This study focused on patients with severe brain injuries, thus the EEG signals and class-discriminative features were expected to be different to those known for healthy users. For this reason, the BCI was designed such that it could be driven by a wide range of features and their combinations. The incorporation of multiple features of the EEG or from other modalities into the BCI system is called a "hybridBCI" system, which is a rather recent line of research [57–59]. Fig. 1B shows the architecture of the BCI system used for this patient study. The BCI simultaneously delivered three control signals to the application. Spectral features (event related desynchronization (ERD) in μ, β, δ band or β rebound) as well as slower movement-related potentials (i.e. lateralized readiness potential, LRP) were processed and classified. The two classifier outputs and their individually weighted sum were received by the application. The experimenter could then choose (based on a prior offline analysis of the data), which of the three output signals should be used to control the application.

2.6 Feature extraction and classification

To extract oscillatory features, signals were band-pass filtered by a Butterworth filter of order 5 in the individually defined spectral band. After visual inspection of the channel-wise ERD, a discriminative time interval was defined to compute optimized spatial filters with the Common Spatial Patterns (CSP) method [60] and to train the classifier, a shrinkage-regularized linear discriminant analysis (LDA) [18]. In analogy to Blankertz and colleagues (2008) [60], offline classification accuracy was estimated using a (standard) cross-validation procedure, where the CSP filters and LDA weights were computed on the training set, and binary accuracy was assessed on the test set.

For the feature extraction of non-oscillatory slow potentials, raw EEG was band-pass filtered with a Butterworth filter (0.2–4 Hz) with a subsequent channel-wise baselining step (the interval of 300 ms duration before trial onset). In analogy to ERP classification [18], the mean amplitude in a manually selected (class-discriminative) time interval was taken from each channel in order to form the feature vector of a trial. A binary classifier (again LDA) was trained based on those features.

Both LDA classifiers were automatically adapted during the CopyTask phase. As described in [22], the pooled covariance matrix and the mean of the features was re-estimated after each trial, using the known labels (adaptation rate of 0.03). This also resulted in an implicit bias correction. In the FreeMode, no adaptation was performed. Besides the internal adaptation, the research team could recalibrate and fine-tune the classifiers between and within sessions. This was important in order to account for unstable features in the EEG data.

Results

3.1 Standard screening

The outcome of the standard screening (session 1) is depicted in Fig. 2. For patients 3 and 4 we found very atypical EEG signatures without any alpha or beta rhythms in the eyes-open and eyes-closed condition. It should be noted that these patients were unable to voluntarily open and close their eyes in response to an instruction/cue. Thus, eye-closure was supported by the caregiver who carefully moved the eyelids by hand.

3.2 ERD features and BCI performance

The BCI performance in this study was assessed for the two experimental conditions: during the CopyTask, the labels are known and the BCI performance can easily be evaluated using the fraction of correct trials (called "binary accuracy" in the following). A trial is correct, whenever the accumulated BCI output is pointing to the correct direction at the end of the trial, thus chance level is 50%.

For the FreeMode, labels are unknown, unless the patient is able to report his intention with AT in each trial. Moreover, the number of games which were won against a computer heuristic can also be assessed as a complex and very high-level performance measure for the FreeMode. Playing the game with random control was simulated with the finding that a random player won 10% of the games and 20% of the games ended with a draw. Thus, the computer heuristic would win 70% of the games when playing against a player with random control.

Offline analysis. One interesting question was whether or not class discriminant features are found consistently across sessions. Therefore, Fig. 3 shows the results of an offline analysis of the CopyTask data. For all patients except patient 3, we found at least one discriminative feature (e.g. β ERD) which was consistently present in all sessions. Patients 3 did not present any reliable feature with discriminative information. Notably, none of the patients featured a consistent ERD component in the α band. However, the spatial distribution of such features was observed to be variable for some patients. Fig. S2 visualizes the spatial distribution of class discriminative information for each patient across all sessions as scalp maps. This finding underlines the necessity of a flexible BCI system like it was used for this study. It should also be noted that the offline accuracy described in Fig. 3 cannot be directly translated into online BCI performance, as the cross-validation procedure was performed for each session separately. The resulting online BCI performance can be lower, if the features changed between sessions [61]. In a scenario of rather stable features across sessions, the online performance can also be higher, as the online classifier was trained with more data (from previous sessions).

Online BCI control. Fig. 4 and Fig. 5 show the online performance of the CopyTask for all four patients. All patients except patient 3 could gain significant control over the BCI. Excluding patient 3, we obtained 10/14 sessions with an online binary accuracy being significantly better than chance. Again, one should stress that this was done with a patient population and there were no more than six EEG sessions with each patient, and five of these with BCI feedback. Fig. S3 depicts the online accuracy in the FreeMode, which could only be assessed for patient 1 and 2.

In the following, EEG features and the resulting BCI performance for each of the four patients are discussed separately. Text S1 elaborates on the exact parameterization of the classifiers, which were used in the online study. After previously discussing offline results, we will only discuss online performances in the following.

Patient 1. Within the motor imagery study, a beta rebound as well as an LRP were found to be class-discriminant features for left-hand vs. right hand imagery, see Fig. 3. In the online framework, the beta-rebound was used to drive the system in session 4 and all following sessions. The LRP feature was not used, because it was more prone to (eye) artifacts and the patient featured involuntary eye-movements in the directions of the arrow. Although the beta-rebound was found quite consistently, the spatial distribution differed across sessions, see Fig. S2. Therefore, it was required to retrain CSP filters and to use LDA with adaptation. The user was then able to gain significant online control over the BCI, as shown in Fig. 4A. One can also observe that the BCI accuracy increased within sessions, resulting in the most reliable control towards the end of each session. The level of control was not perfect, but sufficient to drive the application in the FreeMode (cp. Fig. S3). Patient 1 played the game Connect-4 five times in total, and he could win three of those games.

Patient 2. A beta ERD as well as a LRP were found to be class-discriminant features for left-hand vs. foot imagery, see

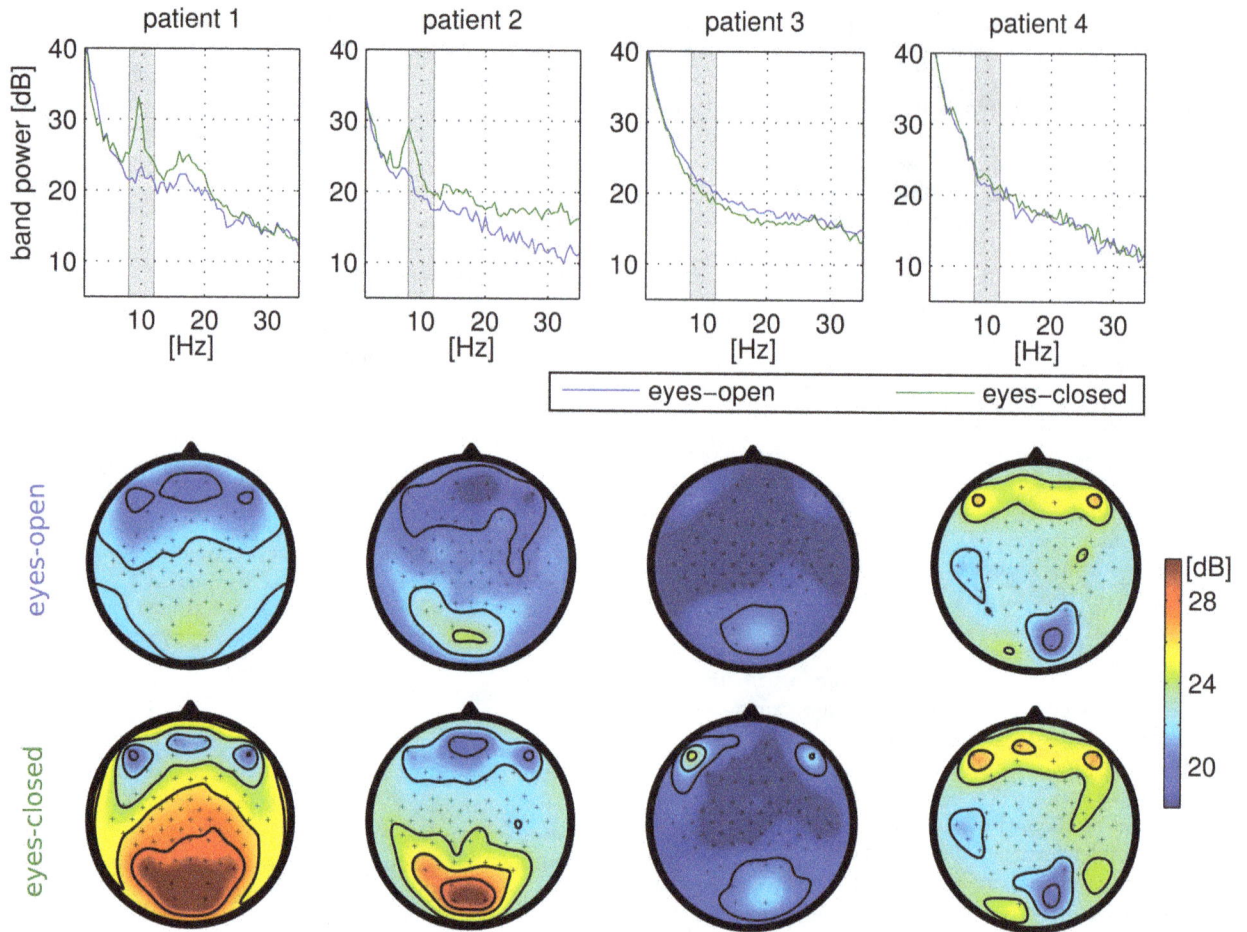

Figure 2. Standard physiological screening of the four patients. The top row shows the spectra at electrode '*Cz*' in the conditions eyes-open and eyes-closed. The spatial distribution of the channel-wise spectral power in the alpha-band [8–12 Hz] is depicted in the scalp maps of the lower row.

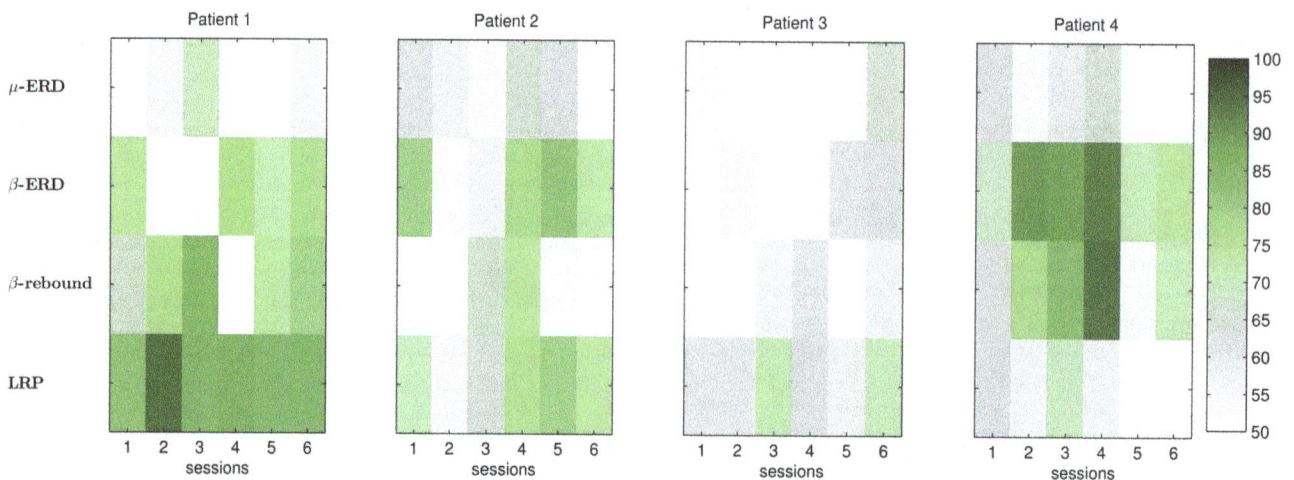

Figure 3. Discriminative power of each feature across sessions, obtained with offine reanalysis of the CopyTask data. Global parameters such as the frequency band and time interval were chosen individually for each patient after manually inspecting the data from all sessions. For each session, the same global parameters were taken – which might be suboptimal. The classification accuracy was then estimated with cross validation using the same parameters for each session. Note that the number of trails was varying across sessions with later sessions featuring less trials. Moreover, a β rebound was defined to as a discriminative feature in the β band, which was observed more than 500 ms after the end of a trial. As the β ERD of patient 4 was heavily delayed, it is also considered as β rebound in this analysis. Fig. S2 shows the corresponding spatial distribution of discriminative information as scalp maps.

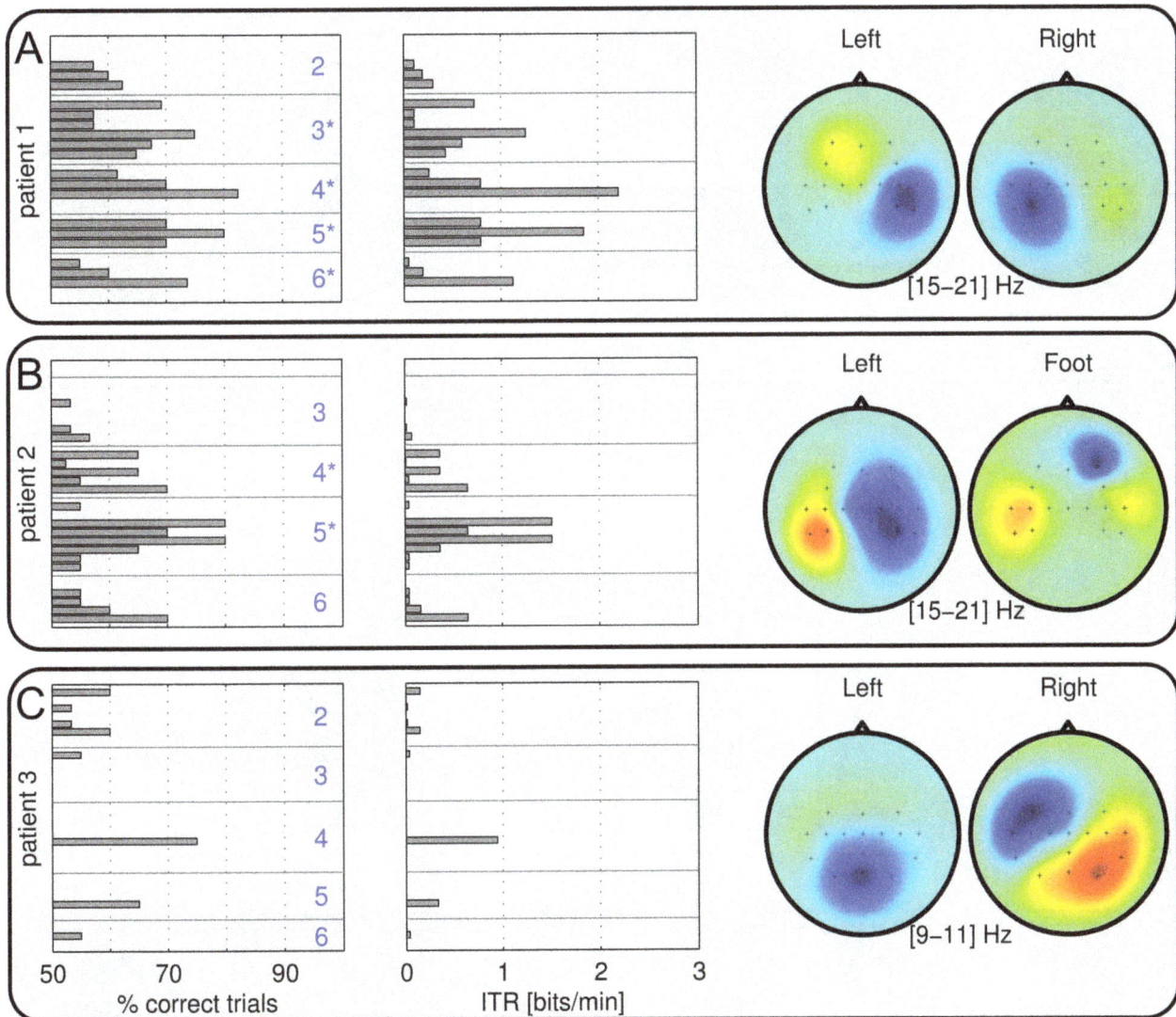

Figure 4. Binary online accuracies (left column) and estimated bit rates (middle column) in the CopyTask for patients 1–3. Each bar represents one block of at least 20 trials. Session numbers are specified in blue color (left column). Session numbers with a * mark sessions with significant online BCI control across all trials (χ^2 test with $p<0.05$). For patient 2, results for session 3 had to be disregarded due to technical problems. The right column depicts the scalp patterns of the most discriminant spectral features, based on data from all sessions. Results for Patient 4 are shown in Fig. 5.

Fig. 3. Since the beta ERD had a more consistent spatial pattern and was also less susceptible to artifacts, either the beta classifier or the meta classifier (beta + LRP) was used in the online BCI framework. However, although the ERD feature in the beta-band was found in almost every session, one could observe a high variation in class discrimination, spatial patterns as well as in BCI performance across and within sessions (see Fig. 4B and Fig. S2). Due to the adaptive methods mentioned above, patient 2 was nevertheless able to control the game in the FreeMode at the end of session 4 and all following sessions (Fig. S3). In total, he played four games in the FreeMode (winning two of them).

Patient 3. In analogy to a previous study [55], reliable class discriminant features could not be found in the EEG data of patient 3 (cp. Fig. 3). He was thus not able to control the BCI system, as shown in the CopyTask performance in Fig. 4C. For the online framework, either the meta classifier or the LRP classifier were applied. None of them performed reliably above chance level. Recall, that this user displayed very atypical EEG spectra at rest (Fig. 2): during the eyes-open and eyes-closed conditions, no alpha or beta peaks were present. Due to the lack of BCI control, patient 3 did not officially enter the FreeMode (see study protocol). However, although featuring insufficient BCI control, patient 3 insisted in attempting to play the BCI game in the FreeMode ("for the fun of it"). He could neither gain control, nor was the resulting data analyzed in the present evaluation.

Patient 4. A highly discriminative β ERD component was present during each session of patient 4 (cp. Fig. 3). His motor-related EEG patterns exhibited typical spatial distributions (see Fig. 5A). This finding is even more surprising, since patient 4 revealed very atypically EEG signatures in the resting state – stereotypical brain rhythms such as α and β were absent (cf. Fig. 2).

Despite his physical condition, patient 4 achieved the best BCI control amongst the four patients. Fig. 5A shows the online binary

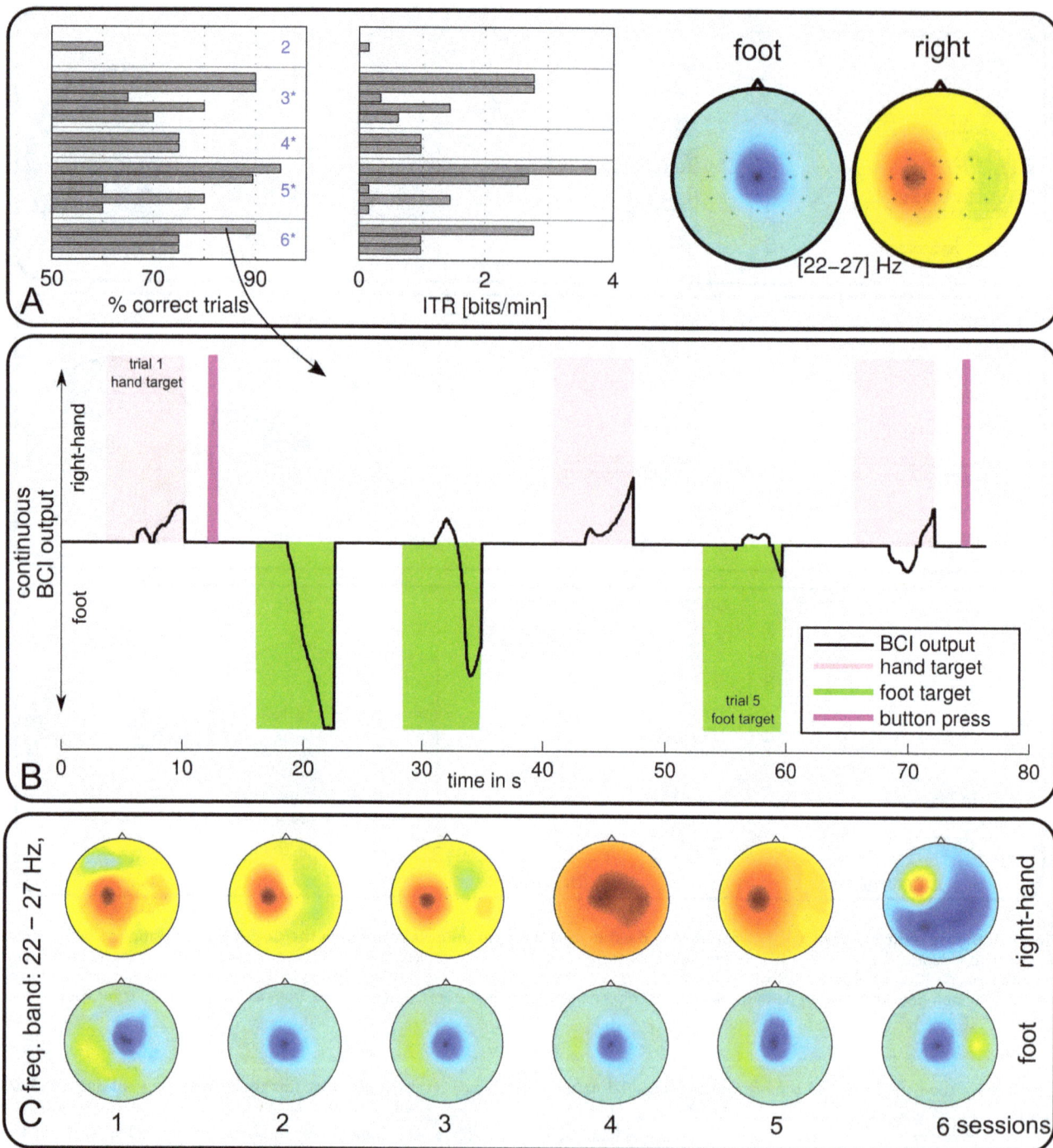

Figure 5. BCI performance and scalp patterns of patient 4. Online binary accuracies, estimated bit rates (left, middle) of the CopyTask, and CSP patterns (right) averaged across all sessions are depicted in the top row (**A**). Each bar represents one block of at least 20 consecutive trials. Middle row (**B**) relates the continuous online BCI output to the residual muscle control (button press) for a representative time segment. Colored areas mark trial periods where the patient was asked to initiate a motor action. The excerpt shown was extracted from session 6, revealing that the BCI can detect the users intention far before a muscle contraction can be initiated. The lower row (**C**) depicts the motor related patterns in the β band for each session individually.

performance, revealing that he gained highly accurate online control (up to 90% binary accuracy) over the BCI system within the third EEG session (which was the second session with BCI feedback), and all following sessions. Even when pooling across all six sessions, his BCI control was highly significant (χ^2 test with $p < 0.001$). He exhibited very typical EEG activity during the

right-hand and foot tasks of attempted motor execution, even though he had been unable to move his feet for more than nine years.

For this patient we could directly compare the communication rate of the BCI to his residual communication abilities with AT, by asking him to execute a button-press as soon as the corresponding cue appeared: we found, that the BCI-controlled feedback became discriminant after 1–3 seconds, while the button-press had a delay of 5–20 seconds — and sometimes the muscle contraction did not occur at all. As an example for this unbalanced communication behavior, a representative time window of 77 s was extracted for Fig. 5B. The interval contains six trials (three hand and three foot trials). The patient was requested to perform a button press in hand movement trial (marked in light magenta), but not during foot trials (marked in green). The BCI output and successful button presses are visualized. Patient 4 could only initiate a thumb muscle contraction successfully in two of the three trials. Moreover, any resulting button presses during this test were considerably delayed and occurred after the trial period of 7 s. The BCI, however, indicated the correct decisions at the end of each trial and even earlier in most cases. For the foot class, no motor action (i.e. muscle movement) was available; nevertheless the BCI could reliably detect the intention of a foot movement. Thus, to the best knowledge of the authors, this is the first quantitative report that shows that a BCI can uncover a patient's intention quicker and more reliable than the best available non-BCI AT.

Due to fatigue, temporal constraints and severe attention deficits, patient 4 entered the FreeMode only twice (sessions 4 and 6). In these two FreeMode sessions, he was not able to stay focused for more than 70 trials. As Table 1 reveals, he had the most severe deficits in communication. In practice, this means that he was mostly unable to communicate his intended action in the FreeMode. As a result, labels of the trials were not available and a data-driven evaluation of his BCI control in the FreeMode was impossible.

Discussion

Four end-users with severe motor restrictions, who heavily depended on AT for communication and interaction in their daily life, agreed to participate in this study. Two of them were impaired in their communication ability to an extent, that no available AT would enable a reliable and – given their physical state – high speed solution. For these two specific patients, a BCI-based solution for control and communication would indeed introduce a novel communication quality. The BCI could enable independent communication and thus represent an added value compared to the AT presently used.

During the course of six BCI sessions, we found that three out of the four subjects could gain significant BCI control using motor imagery. For the most severely impaired patient (patient 4), we found evidence that the BCI outperformed his existing communication solution with AT in terms of accuracy and information transfer – being discussed in a following section.

The chosen end-user environment posed severe limitations in terms of user availability, their concentration span and the communication quality with their standard AT. We responded to these challenges with a flexible BCI framework, enabling us to tailor three major components of the study to the individual needs of the patient: (1) details of the experimental MI paradigm, (2) the form of data processing and type of exploited brain signals, and (3) the software application, which the user interacted with. Many of the internal modules of the BCI system could flexibly be exchanged and such changes remained invisible to the patients. The result was an "out of the box" BCI system, which was adapting itself to the features and needs of each user. Thus, our BCI system was generic and adaptive to meet the extensive requirements of such a pragmatic patient study.

4.1 Reducing the number of sessions using machine learning

With our study we could show, that end-users are able to gain significant online BCI control within six sessions or less. Compared to other end-user studies [38] this is a very low number of sessions. Such a purposeful study design was enabled by the intense combined efforts of those users and the team, consisting of caregivers, psychologists, programmers and data analysts. We thereby followed the principles of user-centered design which implies an iterative process between developers and end-users of a product (see [53]). Thus, we used a setup which was flexible enough to adapt to the user's abilities and needs (e.g. choice of MI-classes, temporal constraints or the type of EEG feature such as ERD, β-rebound or LRP). Therefore, the system was designed to accommodate a wide variety of end users. Far from downplaying those individual contributions, the positive effect of advanced machine learning (ML) methods, such as hybrid classifiers with adaptation, should be mentioned. While motor-related BCI tasks are known to require a larger number of user training sessions compared to more salient ERP paradigms [38,44,62], we managed to apply our BCI system successfully within less than 6 sessions in three cases. While for one participant, no BCI control could be established, the remaining three participants gained sufficient online control to play the game relatively early on. (Patient 1: control from session three onwards, Patient 4: control from session four, and Patient 2: control from session five on.) The reduced time effort before BCI control was established represents a crucial step for bringing BCIs closer to clinical application for users in-need. In a comparable study with locked-in patients by Kübler et al. (2005) [38], machine learning methods were not applied. Reliable performance was achieved only after a substantial number of sessions.

4.2 Patient 4

The case of patient 4 deserves special attention. While displaying severely impaired communication abilities, his level of BCI control was en par with very good unimpaired BCI users performing motor imagery.

This is presumably the most exciting finding of the current study, given that practically the full spectrum of AT solutions had been tested for this patient over the past nine years by AT experts. It should be noted that also ERP based paradigms were tested with patient 4 after the presented MI study. Discriminant ERP components could neither be found for a visual multi-class paradigm (MatrixSpeller [63]) nor for an auditory ERP paradigm [64]. The only applicable AT solution (the pinch-grip button press) provided a limited one-class signal with low accuracy and high temporal variability. Nevertheless, the BCI-controlled signal was relatively robust (with up to ~90% accuracy) and available after 7 seconds at the latest.

Evaluating the speed and accuracy of his BCI control, we found evidence that the BCI could outperform his existing communication solution with AT in terms of accuracy and information transfer: during the online CopyTask, patient 4 accomplished commands which were presented visually through the software interface. Interestingly, he used *the same* (attempted) motor command for the right hand BCI class (i.e. the thumb movement) as for a real button press. Thus, a comparison of temporal dynamics and reliability of his BCI-responses with his button-press responses revealed interesting insights, as shown in Fig. 5B.

Contrary to the CopyTask mode, we could not show that patient 4 gained reliable control during the FreeMode. Even though the exact reason for this problem could not be clarified given the limited amount of data available for patient 4, the following – potentially accumulating – causes can be speculated: (1) identification problem, (2) attention problems and fatigue, (3) mental workload (4) self-initiation of actions. Text S2 discusses all mentioned aspects in further detail.

Conclusions

We could show that patients with severe motor impairments – even patients that are locked-in and almost completely locked-in – were able to gain significant control a noninvasive BCI by motor imagery. While applying state-of-the-art machine learning methods, this control was achieved within six or less sessions. The BCI was then used to operate a gaming application.

These findings are encouraging, since providing communication channels for patients in-need resembles the major goal of the interdisciplinary research field of BCI. Moreover, our study describes one patient (patient 4), whose communication abilities with existing AT were on the same performance level ($\leq$ 2 bits/min) than his BCI control. In a controlled CopyTask framework, we found evidence that the BCI could even outperform his existing AT solution in terms of accuracy, reaction times and information transfer. Thus, we showed for this patient that neuronal pattern detection of an attempted motor execution can indeed be faster than the muscular output. Future studies may evaluate the BCI control in follow-up sessions, also testing spelling applications. Moreover, broader patient groups will considered in order to further explore and evaluate the clinical usage of BCI.

Supporting Information

Figure S1   Description of the different classifiers used within for online BCI. Across and within sessions, the classifier was retrained on varying subsets of the data and different features. One classifier is described by the set of two neighboring lines (back and blue), a cross in magenta and the number in red. The black lines mark the chosen frequency band, the blue lines mark the time interval used to train and apply the classifier. The cross marks the accuracy of the classifier, estimated with cross-validation on training data. The number in red specifies the number of trails which were used to train the classifier. Note that beginning with the 6th session, the trial length for patient 1 was shortened to 3.5 seconds - resulting in a classification interval after the end of the trail (β rebound). For all other patients the trial length was 5–7 seconds.

References

1. Dornhege G, del R Millán J, Hinterberger T, McFarland D, Müller KR, editors (2007) Toward Brain-Computer Interfacing. Cambridge, MA: MIT Press.
2. Wolpaw JR, Wolpaw EW, editors (2012) Brain-computer interfaces: principles and practice. Oxford University press.
3. Bin G, Gao X, Wang Y, Li Y, Hong B, et al. (2011) A high-speed BCI based on code modulation VEP. J Neural Eng 8: 025015.
4. Sellers EW, Donchin E (2006) A P300-based brain-computer interface: initial tests by ALS patients. Clin Neurophysiol 117: 538–548.
5. Millan J, Galan F, Vanhooydonck D, Lew E, Philips J, et al. (2009) Asynchronous non-invasive brain-actuated control of an intelligent wheelchair. In: Conf Proc IEEE Eng Med Biol Soc. pp.3361–3364. doi:10.1109/IEMBS.2009.5332828.
6. Daly JJ, Wolpaw JR (2008) Brain-computer interfaces in neurological rehabilitation. Lancet Neurol 7: 1032–1043.
7. Blankertz B, Tangermann M, Vidaurre C, Fazli S, Sannelli C, et al. (2010) The Berlin Brain-Computer Interface: Non-medical uses of BCI technology. Front Neuroscience 4: 198.
8. Müller KR, Tangermann M, Dornhege G, Krauledat M, Curio G, et al. (2008) Machine learning for real-time single-trial EEG-analysis: From brain-computer interfacing to mental state monitoring. J Neurosci Methods 167: 82–90.
9. Halder S, Agorastos D, Veit R, Hammer EM, Lee S, et al. (2011) Neural

Figure S2   Class discriminant information for each patient across sessions. For each session, the spatial pattern of the most (left) and second-most (middle) discriminant CSP filter is depicted. Therefore, the same frequency band as well as the same time intervals were chosen for one subject and all sessions. The same parameters were used to generate Figure 3. The right scalpplot visualizes class discrimination of the LRP feature. The classification accuracy of the spectral (CSP-based) classifier and the LRP classifier is printed next the scalpplots. This classification accuracy is estimated with a 5 fold cross validation and gives a quantification of how separable the data was in the corresponding session. In the online scenario, a different classifier was used which was trained on more trails from preceding sessions. Note that the sign of the scalpmaps is arbitrary, thus red and blue (as well as their corresponding graduations) are exchangeable. Note that two colorbars (for CSP patterns and LRP discrimination) are given in the legend. The abbreviation "ssAUC" stands for a signed and scaled modification of the area under the curve (AUC).

Figure S3   BCI performance in the FreeMode. Patient 1 and patient 2 could communicate their intentions with AT. Their comments were used as labels for trials in the FreeMode. Note that the scaling of the bitrate is on the right axis. The patients did not enter the FreeMode in session 3 and session 4.

Text S1   Session to session transfer.

Text S2   Discussion of the performance of patient 4 in the FreeMode.

Acknowledgments

The authors would like to thank the patients and their families for participation and motivation. The authors gratefully acknowledge Benjamin Blankertz, Martijn Schreuder and Sven Dähne for fruitful discussions, Max Sagebaum for his programming efforts and Kathrin Veith for the support and advices when interacting with the patients.

Author Contributions

Conceived and designed the experiments: JH EH AK MT. Performed the experiments: JH EM PSS MT. Analyzed the data: JH KRM. Contributed reagents/materials/analysis tools: JH. Wrote the paper: JH AK KRM MT.

mechanisms of brain-computer interface control. Neuroimage 55: 1779–1790.
10. Grosse-Wentrup M, Scholkopf B, Hill J (2011) Causal influence of gamma oscillations on the sensorimotor rhythm. Neuroimage 56: 837–842.
11. Birbaumer N, Ghanayim N, Hinterberger T, Iversen I, Kotchoubey B, et al. (1999) A spelling device for the paralysed. Nature 398: 297–298.
12. Kübler A, Birbaumer N (2008) Brain-computer interfaces and communication in paralysis: extinction of goal directed thinking in completely paralysed patients? Clin Neurophysiol 119: 2658–2666.
13. Kübler A (2013) Brain-computer interfacing: science fiction has come true. Brain 136: 2001–2004.
14. Tangermann M, Müller KR, Aertsen A, Birbaumer N, Braun C, et al. (2012) Review of the BCI competition IV. Front Neuroscience 6.
15. Kaufmann T, Schulz S, Grünzinger C, Kübler A (2011) Flashing characters with famous faces improves ERP-based brain–computer interface performance. J Neural Eng 8: 056016.
16. Lotte F, Larrue F, Mühl C (2013) Flaws in current human training protocols for spontaneous brain-computer interfaces: lessons learned from instructional design. Front Hum Neurosci 7.
17. Dornhege G, Blankertz B, Curio G, Müller KR (2004) Boosting bit rates in non-invasive EEG single-trial classifications by feature combination and multi-class paradigms. IEEE Trans Biomed Eng 51: 993–1002.

18. Blankertz B, Lemm S, Treder MS, Haufe S, Müller KR (2011) Single-trial analysis and classification of ERP components – a tutorial. Neuroimage 56: 814–825.

19. Schreuder M, Höhne J, Blankertz B, Haufe S, Dickhaus T, et al. (2013) Optimizing ERP based BCI - a systematic evaluation of dynamic stopping methods. J Neural Eng 10: 036025.

20. Lemm S, Blankertz B, Dickhaus T, Müller KR (2011) Introduction to machine learning for brain imaging. Neuroimage 56: 387–399.

21. Kindermans PJ, Tangermann M, Müller KR, Schrauwen B (2014) Integrating dynamic stopping, transfer learning and language models in an adaptive zero-training erp speller. J Neural Eng 11: 035005.

22. Vidaurre C, Kawanabe M, von Bünau P, Blankertz B, Müller KR (2011) Toward unsupervised adaptation of lda for brain-computer interfaces. IEEE Trans Biomed Eng 58: 587–597.

23. Tomioka R, Müller KR (2010) A regularized discriminative framework for EEG analysis with application to brain-computer interface. Neuroimage 49: 415–432.

24. Lotte F, Congedo M, Lécuyer A, Lamarche F, Arnaldi B (2007) A review of classification algorithms for EEG-based brain-computer interfaces. J Neural Eng 4: R1–R13.

25. McFarland DJ, Sarnacki WA, Wolpaw JR (2011) Should the parameters of a bci translation algorithm be continually adapted? J Neurosci Methods 199: 103–107.

26. Höhne J, Blankertz B, Müller KR, Bartz D (2014) Mean shrinkage improves the classification of ERP signals by exploiting additional label information. In: Proceedings of the 2014 International Workshop on Pattern Recognition in Neuroimaging. IEEE Computer Society, pp.1–4.

27. Allison B, McFarland D, Schalk G, Zheng S, Jackson M, et al. (2008) Towards an independent brain-computer interface using steady state visual evoked potentials. Clin Neurophysiol 119: 399–408.

28. Riccio A, Mattia D, Simione L, Olivetti M, Cincotti F (2012) Eye gaze independent brain computer interfaces for communication. J Neural Eng 9: 045001.

29. Höhne J, Schreuder M, Blankertz B, Tangermann M (2011) A novel 9-class auditory ERP paradigm driving a predictive text entry system. Front Neuroscience 5: 99.

30. Höhne J, Tangermann M (2014) Towards user-friendly spelling with an auditory brain-computer interface: The charstreamer paradigm. PLoS ONE 9: e98322.

31. Brouwer AM, van Erp JBF (2010) A tactile P300 brain-computer interface. Front Neuroscience 4: 036003.

32. Kaufmann T, Schulz SM, Köblitz A, Renner G, Wessig C, et al. (2012) Face stimuli effectively prevent brain–computer interface inefficiency in patients with neurodegenerative disease. Clin Neurophysiol 124: 893–900.

33. Kaufmann T, Holz EM, Kübler A (2013) Comparison of tactile, auditory and visual modality for brain-computer interface use: A case study with a patient in the locked-in state. Front Neuroscience 7.

34. Murguialday AR, Hill J, Bensch M, Martens S, Halder S, et al. (2011) Transition from the locked in to the completely locked-in state: A physiological analysis. Clin Neurophysiol 122: 925–933.

35. Wolpaw JR, McFarland DJ (2004) Control of a two-dimensional movement signal by a noninvasive brain-computer interface in humans. Proc Natl Acad Sci U S A 101: 17849–17854.

36. Birbaumer N, Kübler A, Ghanayim N, Hinterberger T, Perelmouter J, et al. (2000) The thought translation device (TTD) for completely paralyzed patients. IEEE Trans Rehabil Eng 8: 190–193.

37. Kübler A, Kotchoubey B, Kaiser J, Wolpaw J, Birbaumer N (2001) Brain-computer communication: Unlocking the locked in. Psychol Bull 127: 358–375.

38. Kübler A, Nijboer F, Mellinger J, Vaughan TM, Pawelzik H, et al. (2005) Patients with ALS can use sensorimotor rhythms to operate a brain-computer interface. Neurology 64: 1775–1777.

39. Neuper C, Müller G, Kübler A, Birbaumer N, Pfurtscheller G (2003) Clinical application of an eeg-based brain-computer interface: A case study in a patient with severe motor impairment. Clin Neurophysiol 114: 399–409.

40. Birbaumer N, Murguialday AR, Cohen L (2008) Brain-computer interface in paralysis. Curr Opin Neurobiol 21: 634–638.

41. Neumann N, Kübler A (2003) Training locked-in patients: a challenge for the use of brain-computer interfaces. IEEE Trans Neural Syst Rehabil Eng 11: 169–172.

42. Birbaumer N (2006) Brain-computer-interface research: coming of age. Clin Neurophysiol 117: 479–483.

43. Hinterberger T, Birbaumer N, Flor H (2005) Assessment of cognitive function and communication ability in a completely locked-in patient. Neurology 64: 1307–1308.

44. Nijboer F, Sellers EW, Mellinger J, Jordan MA, Matuz T, et al. (2008) A P300-based brain-computer interface for people with amyotrophic lateral sclerosis. Clin Neurophysiol 119: 1909–1916.

45. Birbaumer N, Cohen L (2007) Brain-computer interfaces: communication and restoration of movement in paralysis. J Physiol 579: 621–636.

46. Mak JN, Wolpaw JR (2009) Clinical applications of brain-computer interfaces: current state and future prospects. Biomedical Engineering, IEEE Reviews in 2: 187–199.

47. De Massari D, Ruf CA, Furdea A, Matuz T, van der Heiden L, et al. (2013) Brain communication in the locked-in state. Brain 136: 1989–2000.

48. Cruse D, Chennu S, Chatelle C, Bekinschtein TA, Fernández-Espejo D, et al. (2011) Bedside detection of awareness in the vegetative state: a cohort study. Lancet 378: 2088–2094.

49. Lulé D, Noirhomme Q, Kleih SC, Chatelle C, Halder S, et al. (2013) Probing command following in patients with disorders of consciousness using a brain-computer interface. Clin Neurophysiol 124: 101–106.

50. Sellers EW (2013) New horizons in brain-computer interface research. Clin Neurophysiol 124: 2–4.

51. Holz EM, Höhne J, Staiger-Sälzer P, Tangermann M, Kübler A (2013) Brain-computer interface controlled gaming: Evaluation of usability by severely motor restricted end-users. Artificial Intelligence in Medicine 59: 111–120.

52. Lulé D, Häcker S, Ludolph A, Birbaumer N, Kübler A (2008) Depression and quality of life in patients with amyotrophic lateral sclerosis. Deutsches Ärzteblatt international 105: 397.

53. Zickler C, Riccio A, Leotta F, Hillian-Tress S, Halder S, et al. (2011) A brain-computer interface as input channel for a standard assistive technology software. Clinical EEG and Neuroscience 24: 222.

54. Blankertz B, Curio G, Müller KR (2002) Classifying single trial EEG: Towards brain computer interfacing. In: Diettrich TG, Becker S, Ghahramani Z, editors, Advances in Neural Inf. Proc. Systems (NIPS 01). volume 14, pp.157–164.

55. Kübler A (2000) Brain-computer communication - development of a brain-computer interface for locked-in patients on the basis of the psychophysiological self-regulation training of slow cortical potentials (SCP). Tübingen: Schwäbische Verlagsgesellschaft.

56. Wolpaw JR, Birbaumer N, McFarland DJ, Pfurtscheller G, Vaughan TM (2002) Brain-computer interfaces for communication and control. Clin Neurophysiol 113: 767–791.

57. Pfurtscheller G, Allison BZ, Bauernfeind G, Brunner C, Escalante TS, et al. (2010) The hybrid BCI. Front Neuroscience 4: 42.

58. del R Millán J, Rupp R, Müller-Putz G, Murray-Smith R, Giugliemma C, et al. (2010) Combining brain-computer interfaces and assistive technologies: State-of-the-art and challenges. Frontiers in Neuroprosthetics 4.

59. Fazli S, Mehnert J, Steinbrink J, Curio G, Villringer A, et al. (2012) Enhanced performance by a Hybrid NIRS-EEG Brain Computer Interface. Neuroimage 59: 519–529.

60. Blankertz B, Tomioka R, Lemm S, Kawanabe M, Müller KR (2008) Optimizing spatial filters for robust EEG single-trial analysis. IEEE Signal Process Mag 25: 41–56.

61. Samek W, Kawanabe M, Müller KR (2014) Divergence-based framework for common spatial patterns algorithms. IEEE Reviews in Biomedical Engineering 7: 50–72.

62. Sellers E, Kübler A, Donchin E (2006) Brain-computer interface research at the University of South Florida Cognitive Psychophysiology Laboratory: the P300 Speller. IEEE Trans Neural Syst Rehabil Eng 14: 221–224.

63. Farwell L, Donchin E (1988) Talking off the top of your head: toward a mental prosthesis utilizing event-related brain potentials. Electroencephalogr Clin Neurophysiol 70: 510–523.

64. Höhne J, Krenzlin K, Dähne S, Tangermann M (2012) Natural stimuli improve auditory BCIs with respect to ergonomics and performance. J Neural Eng 9: 045003.

9

Electroencephalographic Variation during End Maintenance and Emergence from Surgical Anesthesia

Divya Chander[1][*][9], **Paul S. García**[2][9], **Jono N. MacColl**[3], **Sam Illing**[3], **Jamie W. Sleigh**[3]

1 Department of Anesthesiology, Perioperative and Pain Medicine, Stanford University School of Medicine, Stanford, California, United States of America, **2** Department of Anesthesiology, Atlanta VA Medical Center/Emory University, Atlanta, Georgia, United States of America, **3** Department of Anaesthesia, Waikato Clinical School, University of Auckland, Hamilton, New Zealand

Abstract

The re-establishment of conscious awareness after discontinuing general anesthesia has often been assumed to be the inverse of loss of consciousness. This is despite the obvious asymmetry in the initiation and termination of natural sleep. In order to characterize the restoration of consciousness after surgery, we recorded frontal electroencephalograph (EEG) from 100 patients in the operating room during maintenance and emergence from general anesthesia. We have defined, for the first time, 4 steady-state patterns of anesthetic maintenance based on the relative EEG power in the slow-wave (<14 Hz) frequency bands that dominate sleep and anesthesia. Unlike single-drug experiments performed in healthy volunteers, we found that surgical patients exhibited greater electroencephalographic heterogeneity while re-establishing conscious awareness after drug discontinuation. Moreover, these emergence patterns could be broadly grouped according to the duration and rapidity of transitions amongst these slow-wave dominated brain states that precede awakening. Most patients progressed gradually from a pattern characterized by strong peaks of delta (0.5–4 Hz) and alpha/spindle (8–14 Hz) power ('Slow-Wave Anesthesia') to a state marked by low delta-spindle power ('Non Slow-Wave Anesthesia') before awakening. However, 31% of patients transitioned abruptly from Slow-Wave Anesthesia to waking; they were also more likely to express pain in the post-operative period. Our results, based on sleep-staging classification, provide the first systematized nomenclature for tracking brain states under general anesthesia from maintenance to emergence, and suggest that these transitions may correlate with post-operative outcomes such as pain.

Editor: Uwe Rudolph, McLean Hospital/Harvard Medical School, United States of America

Funding: This work was supported by a collaborative grant from the James S. McDonnell Foundation, and departmental resources of the authors. The funders had no role in study design, data collection and analysis, decision to publish, or preparation of the manuscript.

Competing Interests: The authors have declared that no competing interests exist.

* Email: dchander@stanford.edu

[9] These authors contributed equally to this work.

Introduction

Both sleep and anesthesia have been tracked in the human electroencephalogram (EEG) since the 1950s [1–3], but a staging nomenclature based on specific EEG features has only been well-developed for natural sleep [4,5]. While there are also stereotyped EEG features, such as a shift in the spectrum toward lower frequencies (<14 Hz), that correlate with anesthesia-induced unresponsiveness (the historical clinical marker of anesthetic adequacy) [6–11], a standardized nomenclature for anesthetic maintenance and emergence has never been universally accepted by clinicians. Recent focus has been placed on the spatial and temporal distribution of these frequency changes [12–15], and identifies an anteriorization of lower frequency power that correlates with the behavioral transition to loss of consciousness [8,9,16,17]. Studies in which volunteers have been exposed to slowly changing doses of propofol have described spectral power changes upon emergence that appear to be the inverse of induction, i.e. a decrease in power in these low frequency oscillations over the frontal EEG, followed by an increase in higher frequencies as the patient becomes behaviorally responsive to mild stimuli [8,9]. This is in contrast to the termination of natural sleep, which is typically preceded by cyclic transitions into progressively longer episodes of cortical activation [18]. Waking usually occurs from rapid eye movement (REM) sleep (reviewed in Steriade [19]).

Although sleep and anesthesia are not the same, significant overlap in neurotransmitters, circuitry and electrical patterns do exist [20,21], suggesting that anesthetics may achieve part of their hypnotic effect by acting on the normal sleep and arousal systems of the brain [22]. Pharmacologic enhancement of inhibitory signaling, mediated via the gamma aminobutyric acid type A (GABA$_A$) receptor, underlies the mechanisms of most commonly used anesthetic agents [23,24]. Similarly, a physiological GABAergic state also contributes to the thalamocortical oscillations characteristic of non-REM sleep [25], while pharmacologic inhibition of the GABA$_A$ receptor reverses sleepiness in hypersomnic patients [26]. It has been shown that sleep deprivation potentiates the efficacy of anesthetics [27], and these effects can be partially reversed by antagonists to adenosine, an endogenous ligand that accumulates during sleep pressure [28]. Furthermore, activation of subcortical endogenous arousal pathways (e.g. thalamus, basal forebrain, hypothalamus, brain stem) can reverse anesthesia in some animal models [29–36], significantly blurring the distinction between sleep and anesthesia. Perhaps most

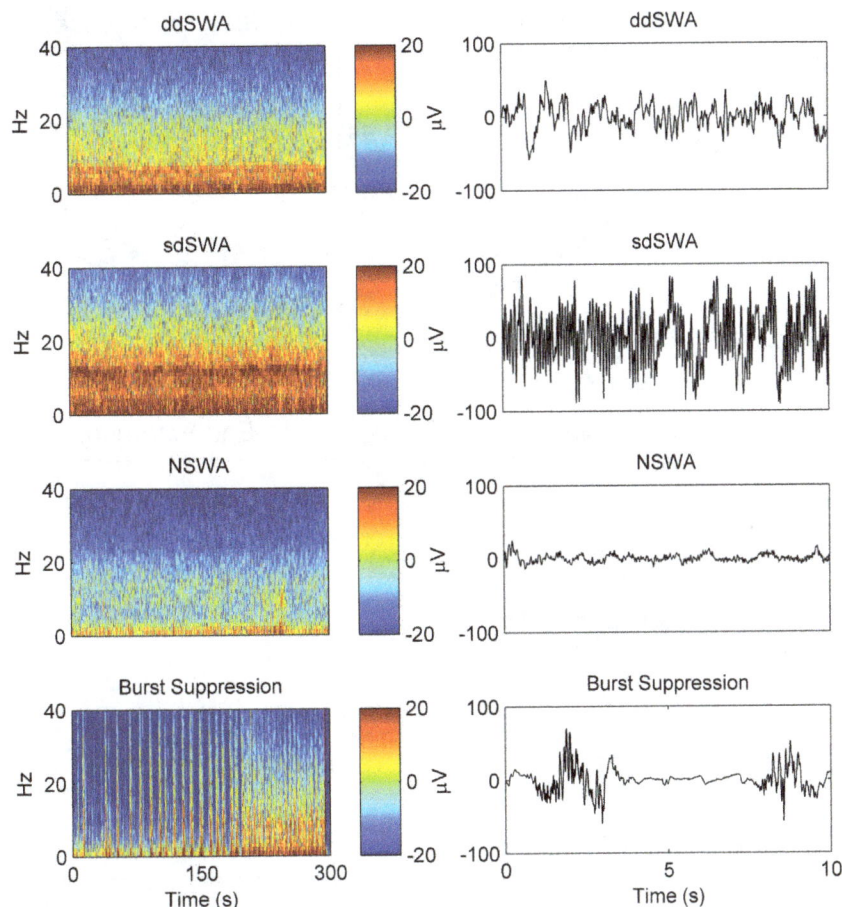

Figure 1. Spectral patterns at the end of maintenance under sevoflurane general anesthesia comprise 4 basic patterns. 'Slow-Wave Anesthesia' (SWA) is a spectral pattern in which there is both high delta and spindle power (>7 dB). Panel (A) shows the more common variant, or subclass, of the SWA spectrogram, calculated over 5 minutes prior to turning off the anesthetic, in which delta power is higher than spindle power (point #1 below the diagonal in Figure 2B) termed delta dominant SWA, or ddSWA. An example 10 second raw EEG tracing is take from this period and shown in the right column. Panel (B) is an SWA spectral variant/subclass in which spindle power is higher than delta power, termed spindle-dominant SWA, or sdSWA (point #2 above the diagonal in Figure 2B). Finally, a small subset of patients (5%) showed low amplitude power in both the spindle and delta frequency bands (C). We termed this pattern non Slow-Wave Anesthesia, or NSWA (point #3 in Figure 2B). For completeness, the spectrogram in panel (D) reflects a deeper anesthetic maintenance pattern, burst suppression, transitioning into a ddSWA pattern at approximately 1.5 minutes prior to End Maintenance. The representative 10 second EEG to its right is taken from the burst suppression period.

importantly, both non-REM (NREM) sleep and general anesthesia exhibit similar synchronization and slowing of the EEG [37,38]. Not surprisingly, the same range of lower frequency oscillations that indicate loss of consciousness are also used to separate natural sleep into specific stages [4,5,39,40]. Thalamocortical oscillations in the alpha band (8–14 Hz) are the electroencephalographic hallmark of the loss of perceptual awareness in synchronized sleep [41]. Generated by the reticular nucleus of the thalamus [42], these oscillations consist of waxing and waning of electrical potentials, and are often referred to as sleep spindles [43]. As sleep deepens, spindles are progressively reduced and replaced by slower oscillations (0.5–4 Hz) [44,45]. In contrast, REM sleep is characterized by profound inhibition of motor output, abolition of these low-frequency oscillations, and an EEG resembling the aroused brain [46]. Although the different sleep stages were arbitrarily and heuristically defined, based on EEG patterns described above [5,47], they have been successfully used by clinicians and researchers to relate sleep physiology to functional neuroanatomy [48], consolidation of memory [49–51], and sleep disorders [52,53].

We therefore designed a study with three objectives. The first was to catalogue and define a standardized nomenclature for the EEG during anesthetic maintenance, analogous to that used to describe natural sleep. The second was to characterize the evolution of the human EEG during emergence from general anesthesia during surgery, to determine if there was a single common path, or multiple pathways to re-establishing conscious awareness and interaction with the outside world. Our final goal was to determine if the path by which the patient emerged had any relationship to the quality of a patient's recovery.

We recorded the frontal EEG from 100 human subjects in the operating room, undergoing routine orthopedic surgery with general volatile anesthesia, prior to loss of consciousness, through the maintenance and recovery from anesthesia, until patients were able to be taken safely to the recovery room. Using spectral processing techniques, we propose a nomenclature of four basic EEG patterns, based on the relative dominance of low frequency oscillatory patterns seen during maintenance of general anesthesia (i.e. a degree of hypnosis considered to be commensurate with unconsciousness). We also identified four stereotypical trajectories

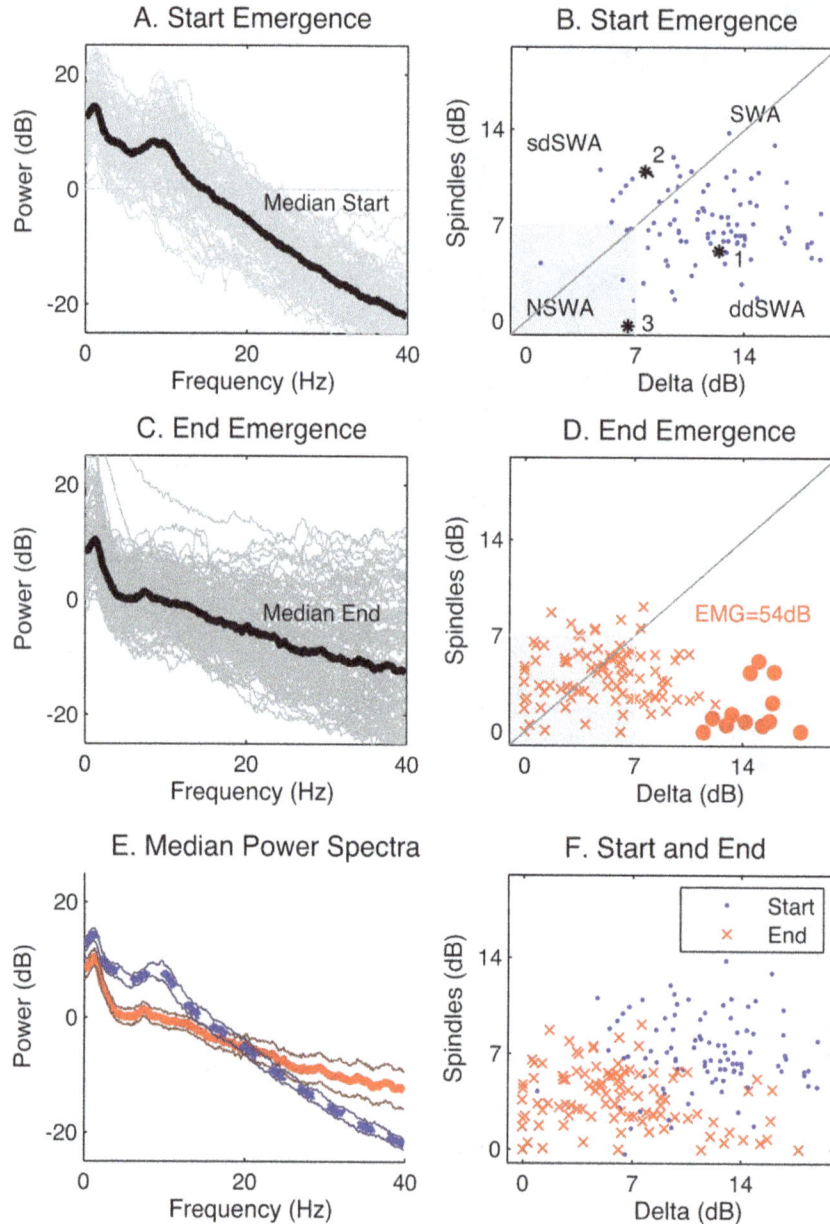

Figure 2. Emergence from general anesthesia is characterized by a loss in power in the slower spindle and delta frequency bands, and a recovery of power in the higher frequency bands. Power spectra and scatterplots of delta and spindle power (dB) for all patients, at the start (2A, 2B) and the end (2C, 2D) of emergence. The thick black lines are the median of the power spectra at each frequency for all patients. The median power spectra and 95% confidence intervals of the median, at the start and end, are shown in 2E. Patients were separated into two main spectral classes by thresholding spindle and delta power at 7 dB, whose boundary is marked by the gray box (see also Figure S1). Thus, the most common pattern, seen in 95% patients at Start Emergence, is characterized by high power (>7 dB) in both frequency bands, which we define as **'Slow-Wave Anesthesia (SWA)'**; the alternate pattern, defined as **'Non Slow-Wave Anesthesia (NSWA)'**, represents the 5% of patients that fall within the gray box. The fuzzy clusters in 2B are defined in the text: SWA = Slow-Wave Anesthesia, ddSWA = delta-dominant Slow-Wave Anesthesia, sdSWA = spindle-dominant Slow-Wave Anesthesia, NSWA = Non Slow-Wave Anesthesia (gray box). Red circles in 2D are those patients with a high delta power at End Emergence. All except one subject with high delta at End Emergence also had an EMG>40 dB. 2F is the same as 2B and 2D superimposed for ease of visual comparison.

that describe the progression toward conscious awareness during emergence. These emergence patterns do not consistently follow the averaged patterns of volunteers undergoing slow infusions of propofol described in prior studies [8,9], but in some instances do share similarities with sleep stages that precede awakening. Further, we noted that the trajectory taken to re-establish conscious awareness is not correlated to the brain state at the

cessation of the anesthetic (End Maintenance), but the path taken to re-establishing awareness does appear to have some correlation with a subject's subsequent level of sedation and post-operative pain. Our work suggests that the central nervous system may not always re-establish connectivity in a canonical sequence after unconsciousness produced by general anesthesia during surgery. We hypothesize that these less typical emergence sequences under

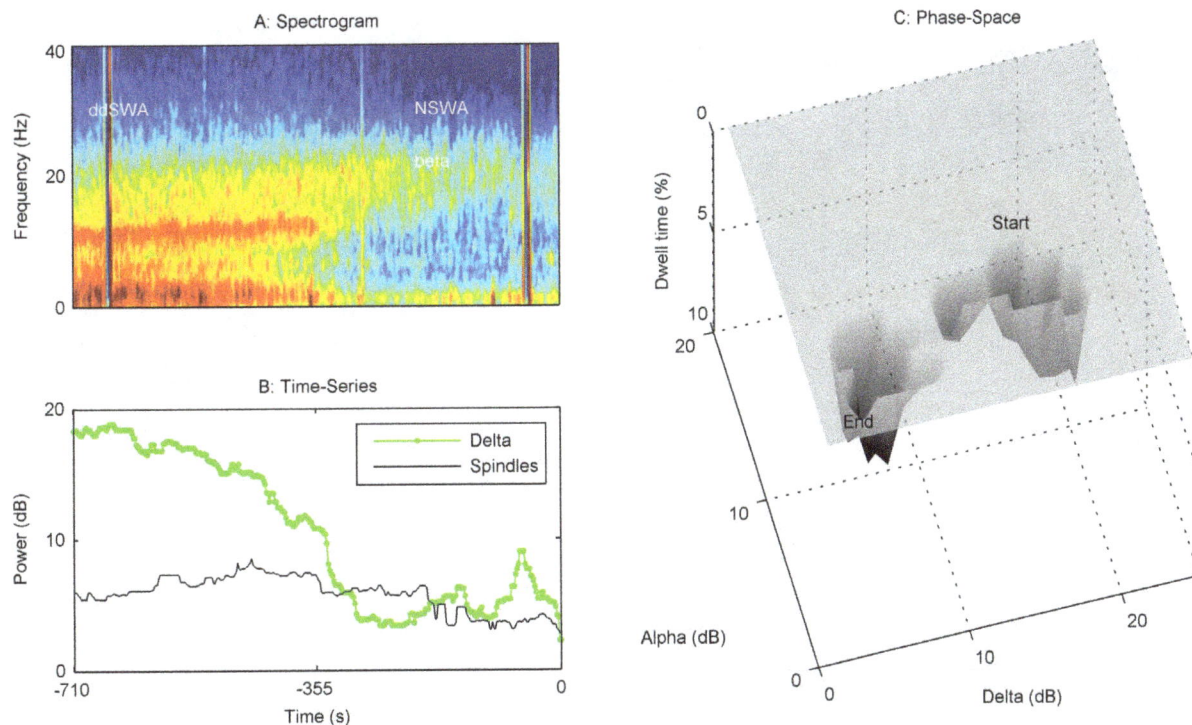

Figure 3. Emergence Trajectory 1, SWA → NSWA. The upper left panel (A) is the spectrogram from Start Emergence (measured in negative seconds) to End Emergence (time 0 seconds) for a representative patient (#81); this also corresponds to the time of anesthetic wash-out from the brain. Below it is a time series (B) that quantifies spindle and delta power (dB) over the same emergence period. To the right is a dwell time state-space plot (C). The evolution of spindle and delta power over the emergence trajectory from Start Emergence (upper right) to End Emergence (lower left) is shown where the depth of the contour (y-axis) reflects the time spent in each pixel of the state, as a percentage of the total emergence time. At the start of emergence, this patient remained for a signficant period in a slow-wave state (SWA) characterized by higher delta to spindle power ratio (ddSWA). There was a relatively abrupt transition period of approximately 60 seconds, to a second attractor characterized by lower delta and spindle power (NSWA) prior to waking-up. In our sample, 23% of patients had a similar trajectory.

anesthesia may predispose patients to undesirable wake-ups, in a similar way that parasomnias are exacerbated by disrupted sleep architecture [54].

Results

Patterns during maintenance in the human frontal electroencephalograph can be divided into four (4) basic spectral variants

In order to define a nomenclature for anesthetic maintenance, we analyzed the relative contribution amongst major oscillatory features found in the power spectra of the frontal electroencephalogram (EEG) of 100 patients undergoing routine orthopedic surgery under general anesthesia. The time at which the anesthetic was turned off was defined as the 'End Maintenance' or 'Start Emergence' point. A spectrogram of EEG data from a single frontal EEG electrode for 5 minutes prior to End Maintenance was computed for each individual patient. Visual inspection revealed clear peaks in the spectrogram within the delta and alpha bands of some patients, but these peaks showed considerable variation across the population (Figure 1A-D). The power spectra and a scatterplot of delta power against the oscillatory component of alpha power, computed over an 8 second EEG window (see Methods) for all 100 patients at Start Emergence, are shown in Figures 2A and 2B. The oscillatory component of alpha power was quantified by measuring the height of the alpha peak above the underlying broadband activity [55]. This has the advantage that it specifically targets the narrowband oscillatory component of

this peak, and is less influenced by the underlying broadband (1/f) components of the EEG, making the alpha oscillatory power more orthogonal to the delta power. In this study we have chosen to borrow the term 'spindles' from the sleep literature to describe the specific oscillatory component in the alpha range from the overall composite alpha power [5]. Although the scatterplot in Figure 2B does not readily segregate into discrete clusters, we followed statistical convention and separated the patients into two main spectral classes by thresholding spindle and delta power at 7 dB. Because the bi-variate data appears to follow a unimodal distribution, the 7dB theshold reflects the boundary below which only 5% of the Start Emergence data lay, and the region within which most of the End Emergence data lay (Figure S1). Thus, the most common pattern, seen in 95% patients at Start Emergence, is characterized by high power (>7 dB) in both frequency bands, which we define as '**Slow-Wave Anesthesia (SWA)**;' this includes patients above the 7 dB boundary marked by the gray box. Some patients have a relatively equal distribution of spindle and delta power during SWA, lying on or near the unity diagonal (Figure 2B). However, it was more common in this patient sample for delta power to be greater than spindle power during SWA. This is represented by the preponderance of points lying below the diagonal in Figure 2B. We therefore propose the term '**delta-dominant Slow-Wave Anesthesia**' (**ddSWA**, Figure 1A) to describe this sub-classification. Conversely when spindle power is greater than delta power (i.e. points above the diagonal, Figure 2B), we propose the term '**spindle-dominant Slow-Wave Anesthesia**' (**sdSWA**, Figure 1B). In this sample, we

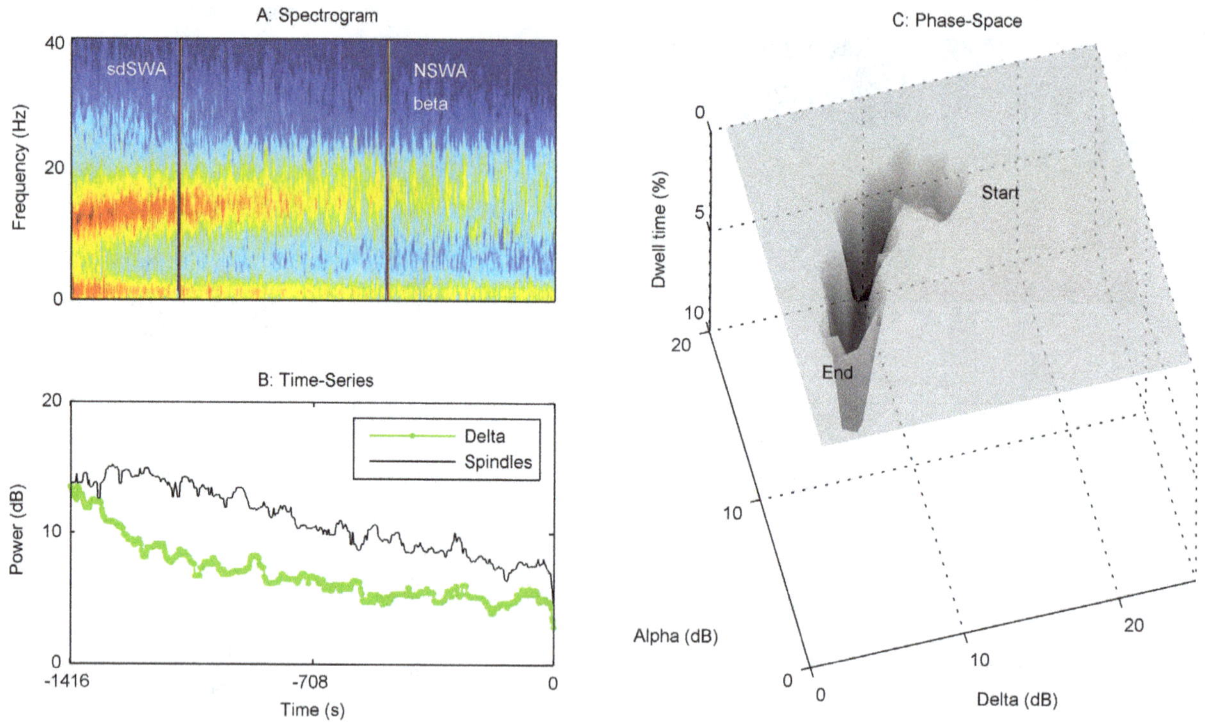

Figure 4. Emergence Trajectory 2, SWA→NSWA, continuous progression. The spectrogram (A) and time series (B) from Start Emergence to End Emergence for a representative patient (#36) are shown. To the right is dwell time state-space plot (C). This patient started in a slow-wave state (SWA). Over approximately 1.5 minutes, the patient transitioned into a state characterized by higher spindle power (sdSWA), and then showed a progressive decrease in delta and spindle power towards the NSWA region over about 20 minutes before waking. There was a converse increase in beta power as alpha/spindle power was diminished. No single deep attractor in state-space characterizes this patient's emergence path until reaching NSWA prior to wake-up. In our sample, 20% of patients had a similar trajectory.

noted a continuum of relative spindle and delta power between patients, and even within patients during the course of their anesthetic. Because of this we have purposely left the terms sdSWA and ddSWA somewhat loosely defined – they are convenient labels that indicate a patient (in SWA) has relatively stronger spindle or delta waves. These plots are generated over a short snap-shot in time; thus, a patient in a ddSWA pattern may gradually lose delta power and transition into an sdSWA pattern over the course of an anesthetic. Five percent (5%) of patients had Start Emergence EEGs with a very low spindle and delta power (<7 dB) – we termed these indeterminate patterns "**Non Slow-Wave Anesthesia**" (**NSWA**, Figure 1C). An example of another common maintenance pattern, that of burst suppression (transitioning into SWA) is shown in Figure 1D, for as complete a description as possible of spectral patterns encountered during surgical anesthesia. This pattern is more typically seen post-induction of general anesthesia (i.e. just after loss of consciousness is achieved with a bolus dose of propofol), but may be seen during the entire course of the maintenance phase of anesthesia.

Emergence from general anesthesia is characterized by a shift from a slow-wave pattern (SWA) to a more uniform distribution of power across all frequency bands

In order to characterize salient features of the EEG at the start (i.e. turning off anesthetic) and end of emergence (i.e. responsiveness to standard verbal stimulation), the power-spectral density (PSD) plots for individual patients were compared in each condition. The plots in the left column of Figure 2 show the power spectra for all patients (gray), derived from the 8 second

EEG segments at the start (Figure 2A) and end of emergence (Figure 2C). There is considerable variation in individual patient spectral power, encompassing a 30 dB range (equivalent to an approximately five-fold variation in raw voltage) at both Start and End Emergence, with greater spread in the higher frequency bands (>14 Hz) during End Emergence. The thick black line in both Figures 2A and 2C are the median power spectra for each condition. Distinct peaks are present at Start Emergence/End Maintenance in the delta and spindle frequency bands. At End Emergence, the spindle peak is lost, and the delta peak diminishes in amplitude. The scatterplots in Figures 2B and 2D, in which delta and spindle power are plotted against one another for each patient, clearly show the downward shift in power in both these frequency bands (from 2B to 2D). There is a small subset of patients (12%) at End Emergence that maintains high delta power (red dots in Figure 2D); this subset is also the group that showed high EMG at End Emergence (>40 dB) suggesting that the high delta power is actually broad-band contamination of the EEG with frontalis muscle activity rather than true frontal cortical activity. For ease of comparison, the shifts in median power spectra at Start (blue) and End Emergence (red) are shown in Figure 2E, while the downward shift in spindle-delta power at Start (blue) and End Emergence (red) is summarized in Figure 2F. As a whole, the median power spectra at End Emergence demonstrates a more uniform distribution of power in the 20–40 Hz range, consistent with recent studies in human volunteers receiving propofol infusions [8,9], but with more variability as evidenced by broader confidence intervals.

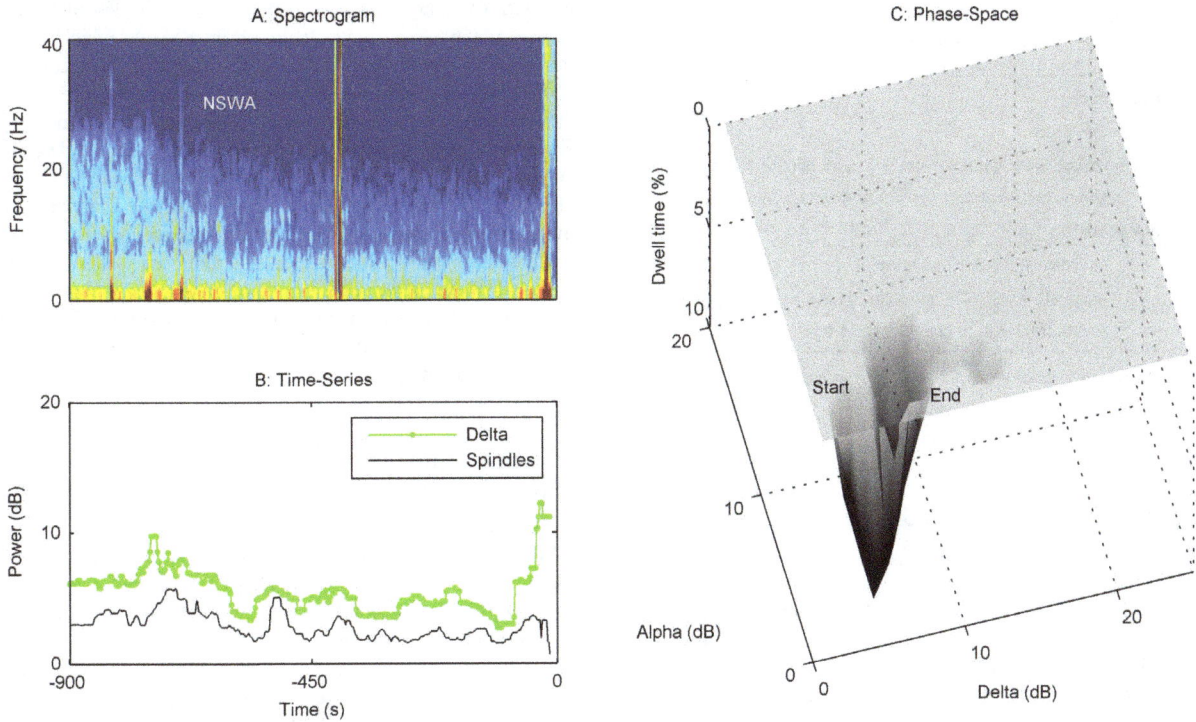

Figure 5. Emergence Trajectory 3, NSWA→Wakefulness. The spectrogram (A) and time series (B) from Start Emergence to End Emergence for a representative patient (#19) are shown. To the right is a dwell time state-space plot (C). This patient started and ended in a state characterized by a non slow-wave state (NSWA) attractor prior to waking up. The duration of emergence was long (15 minutes), and the attractor did not move significantly. In our sample, 16% of patients had a similar trajectory.

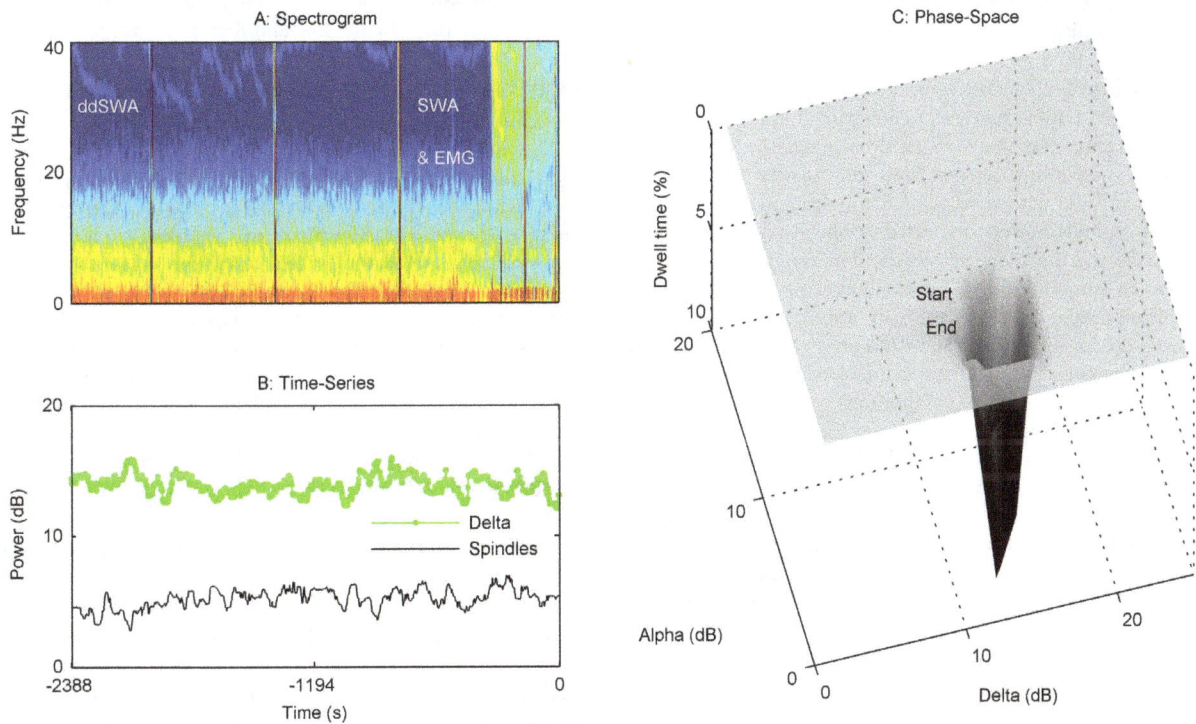

Figure 6. Emergence Trajectory 4, SWA→Wakefulness. The spectrogram (A) and time series (B) from Start Emergence to End Emergence for a representative patient (77) are shown. To the right is a dwell time state-space plot (C). This patient started and ended in a state characterized by a slow-wave state (SWA) attractor prior to waking up. Patients who woke up this abruptly from a slow-wave state of anesthesia were more likely to experience high pain in recovery. In our sample, 31% of patients had a similar trajectory.

Table 1. Level of Consciousness and Pain.

PACU-Cons Score	
0	Confused
1	Quickly alert (Ramsay score = 2 at 15 minutes)
2	Somnolent (Ramsay score = 3 or 4 at 15 minutes)
PACU-Pain Score	
0	Minimal (NRS = 0–3 and relaxed)
1	Moderate (NRS = 4–8 and relaxed or going back to sleep)
2	Severe (NRS = 8–10 or NRS>4 and signs of distress)

PACU = Post anesthesia care unit, Cons = consciousness, NRS = numerical rating scale

Evolution of trajectories from Start Emergence to End Emergence vary by patient

Figure 2 captures a static image of the state of the brain at the start and end of emergence. While a shift from one average state to another can be seen in Figure 2E, the variability of individual patient PSDs and spindle-delta power scatterplots suggests that the path from Start to End Emergence may not be identical or stereotyped. Clinically, this is often reflected in the length of time a patient takes to emerge from general anesthesia. We chose not to average patient trajectories, and instead looked for graphical methods to describe changes for individual patients. This involved construction of an 'emergence trajectory' for each patient. A spectrogram from Start to End Emergence was first calculated (Figure 3–6A), and a time series data of spindle and delta power extracted from the power spectrum (Figure 3–6B). Finally, we applied a dynamical systems approach to the data, creating a corresponding 3-D 'dwell time plot' for each patient's emergence trajectory (Figure 3–6C). These graphically depict how the relative spindle and delta power changes for each patient in response to the progressive decline in both anesthetic drug concentrations and the residuum of surgical nociception from the time the anesthetic is turned off until the patient responded to voice. In these 'phase-space' plots, spindle power is reflected on the y-axis, delta power on the x-axis, and the z-axis reflects the time spent in each 'pixel' of state-space as a percentage of the total emergence time ("dwell time"). From these surfaces, we can see that a continuous, progressive decrease in spindle and delta power was **not** the usual pattern of emergence. Instead the majority of patients tended to follow a more "punctated equilibrium" pattern, occupying restricted regions of the state-space for extended periods of time, before relatively rapidly moving to other areas of phase space, or to the waking state. At first approximation, these areas appear to functionally act as point attractors [56]. At Start Emergence, most (95%) of these point attractors can be classified as SWA, or a sub-classification (sdSWA or ddSWA), while at End Emergence, the majority (59%) are classified as NSWA. The path from Start Emergence to End Emergence took variable trajectories. These were roughly classified by the presence of one or two attractors, whether these attractors lay in the SWA or NSWA regions, and whether the transition to a new state was rapid or gradual through the phase-space. Figure 3 demonstrates a common emergence trajectory (23% of patients). It shows an initial attractor in the SWA region, which steps abruptly to a second attractor in NSWA space, followed by arousal. The second trajectory (20%) is similar to the first except it shows a more gradual transition between SWA

and NSWA state space (Figure 4). Figure 5 describes a third trajectory (16%), a single attractor in NSWA, which reflects a patient who spends nearly the entire duration of emergence in NSWA before responding to voice. The fourth trajectory (31%) is characterized by a patient who woke up directly from SWA (Figure 6). About 10% of patients fell into indeterminate categories. We would note that during emergence many patients who start emergence in the ddSWA go on to lose their delta power and gained spindle power during their emergence; this resulted in nearly half (49%) of patients spending more than 25% of their time in the sdSWA region. This transition pattern is analogous to that seen in the progression from deep to lighter natural NREM stage 2 sleep. At the other extreme, 27% patients spend no time in the sdSWA region at all, as if NREM stage 2 sleep was skipped during the process of waking.

Evolution of trajectories from Start Emergence to End Emergence are correlated to nociceptive state and level of consciousness upon waking

We next examined whether there was an association with, the relative time spent in SWA vs. NSWA, and the *quality of emergence*. Two post-anesthesia scores were used to quantify level of consciousness and post-operative pain (Table 1). Because sedation can interfere with reported pain, we measured pain heuristically by combining self-reported pain score with non-reported signs of distress. We found an association between lower pain scores and the relative amount of time spent in NSWA during emergence (Figure 7). Those who spent a long time in a non slow-wave state prior to wake-up were more likely to waken with minimal pain (PACU-Pain = 0) than those who woke directly from a slow-wave state ($p = 0.037$, Chi-squared test; $p = 0.0017$ for delta power distribution, $p = 0.05$ for alpha power distribution; Kolmogorov-Smirnov test). This is reflected in the averaged dwell-time contour map for the low and high pain groups (Figure 8).

Associations amongst patient variables with delta and spindle power

The delta power at the start of emergence was negatively correlated with age ($r = -0.44$, $p<0.0001$), and positively correlated with the C_eMAC ($r = 0.24$, $p = 0.015$). Combined in a multiple regression model, these two variables explained 21% of the variability in delta power. Addition of anesthetic agent, regional block and gender insignificantly increased this to 24%. Delta power was not correlated with $C_eOpioid$. The spindle power was also negatively correlated with age ($r = -0.34$, $p = 0.0003$) and with duration of operation ($r = -0.29$, $p = 0.002$). When combined with the C_eMAC, the model explained 23% of the variation in spindle power. However older patients were also more likely to have longer operations ($r = 0.25$, $p = 0.01$), and receive less volatile anesthetic drug ($r = -0.19$, $p = 0.05$).

Associations amongst patient variables, emergence time, and post-operative pain

Emergence time was positively correlated with the duration of operation ($r = 0.24$, $p = 0.014$), and weakly influenced by the C_eMAC ($r = 0.18$, $p = 0.07$). Consistent with prior studies [57–60], male patients were slower to emerge ($p = 0.02$) than females. In this study, we found that different volatile drugs had no significant influence on emergence time, but the number of patients receiving desflurane or isoflurane was small. The multivariate model of emergence time is given below (the presence of a regional block is coded as 1, the absence as 0; the difference between the genders was included as a categorical variable [1/0]).

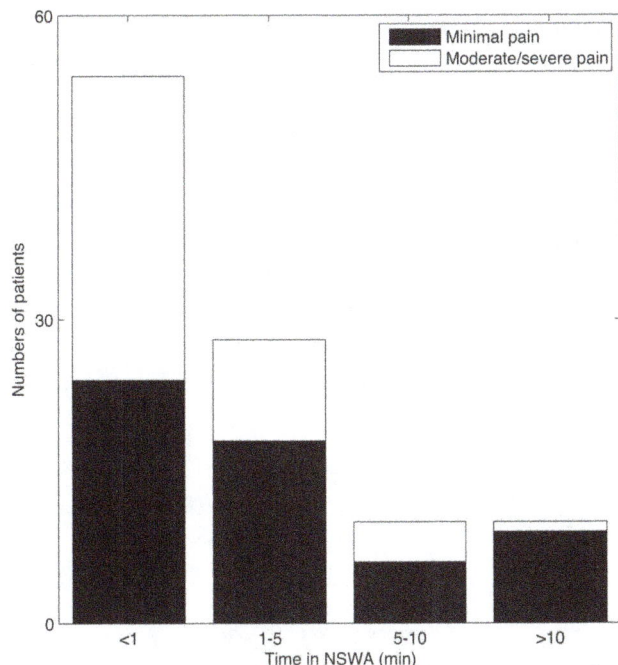

Figure 7. Increased time spent in a non slow-wave state (NSWA) during emergence is correlated with a lower nociceptive state. Patients had a variable duration of emergence from the time the anesthetic was turned off, ranging from 2 minutes to more than 10 minutes, as well as a variable dwell-time in the state of NSWA. When divided into 4 groups based on NSWA dwell-time, patients that spent more time in NSWA prior to emerging were more likely to have minimal pain (PACU-pain = 0, Table 1). Of the group that spent >10 minutes in NSWA prior to wake-up, 90% had minimal pain. Of the group that spent less than a minute in NSWA prior to wake-up, 44% had minimal pain ($p = 0.037$, Chi-squared test).

$$Log[Emergence\ Time(min)] = 0.75 + 0.004 \times [Rregional\ Block] +$$
$$0.20 \times [C_e MAC] + 0.036 \times [Delta\ Power] + 0.05 \times [gender\ Male - Female]\quad (1)$$
$$+ 0.001 \times [Operation\ Duration(min)]$$

Although the model is statistically significant, these explanatory variables are not a very good explanation of the variation in emergence time, as the r^2 value was only 0.16.

When combined in the logistic regression model, the effect site concentration of opioid at the start of emergence, expressed in fentanyl equivalents (C_eOpioid), duration of NSWA, and male gender were the most significant associations with postoperative pain. A higher opioid concentration was associated with more pain. We attribute this unusual observation to the fact that patients who were expected to have more painful operations would have been given more (but presumably not enough) opioids intraoperatively. This model had a modest predictive capability (area under ROC = 0.71), but again the strength of association was quite weak ($r^2 = 0.11$).

$$Probability[Severe\ pain/Mild\ pain] = -0.23 + 1.08 \times [C_e Opioid]$$
$$-0.004 \times [NSWA] - 0.61 \times [gender\ Male - Female]\quad (2)$$

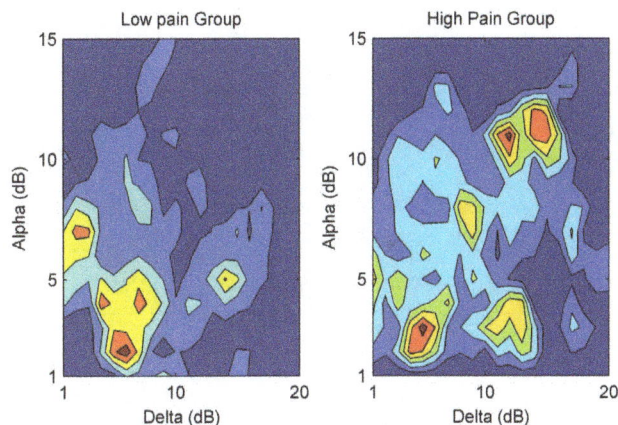

Figure 8. Patients with low pain scores (0) spend more time in a non slow-wave (NSWA) pattern during emergence while patients with higher pain scores (2) spend more time in a slow-wave pattern (SWA). This is reflected in the averaged trajectories through the spindle-delta state space for the low (left panel) and high pain (right panel) groups. The heat map from blue to red reflects least to most time.

Associations amongst patient variables and different EEG patterns of emergence

The heterogeneity in patterns of emergence seem to be largely determined by unknown intrinsic factors, and are not strongly related to the common clinical explanatory variables. We found no significant associations between the EEG emergence pattern group and simple clinical and demographic variables – namely postoperative pain, type of volatile anaesthetic drug, gender, the presence of a regional block, operation duration, or the C_eMAC. However those patients that started in SWA, but then spent a period of time in the NSWA attractor before transitioning to wakefulness tended to be younger (mean(SEM) 43(4) years vs. 58(3) years, $p = 0.015$) and have a higher C_eOpioid (0.80(0.09) vs. 0.44(0.08) ng/ml fentanyl equivalents, $p = 0.04$), than those who jumped directly from a SWA state to wakefulness. Thus the relationship between C_eOpioid, postoperative pain, and EEG emergence pattern, is complex and remains to be fully elucidated in larger studies.

EMG Activation During Emergence

The BIS EEG monitor attributes the power (dB) in the frequency range 70–110 Hz to the frontalis EMG signal, because it lies above the frequency band at which there is significant scalp EEG power. Typically the EMG power is low during general anaesthesia, and then rather abruptly increases in a stepwise fashion at various points during the emergence period. Often there are no overt clinical signs of an increase in muscle tone, or any gross motor movement. After examination of the EMG records, we chose the point at which the EMG power rose above 40 dB as a time point that reflected the activation of the EMG with reasonable face validity. The most striking feature was that the activation of the EMG often had quite a different time course to the EEG changes. The interval between EMG activation and End Emergence approximately followed an exponential probability distribution. For a quarter of the patients, their EMG became activated coincident with their waking (response to voice). Another one-half of patients woke within 74 seconds of EMG activation. However, a quarter of patients had a prolonged interval of at least 334 seconds between EMG activation and waking. The strongest

Emergence Hypnograms

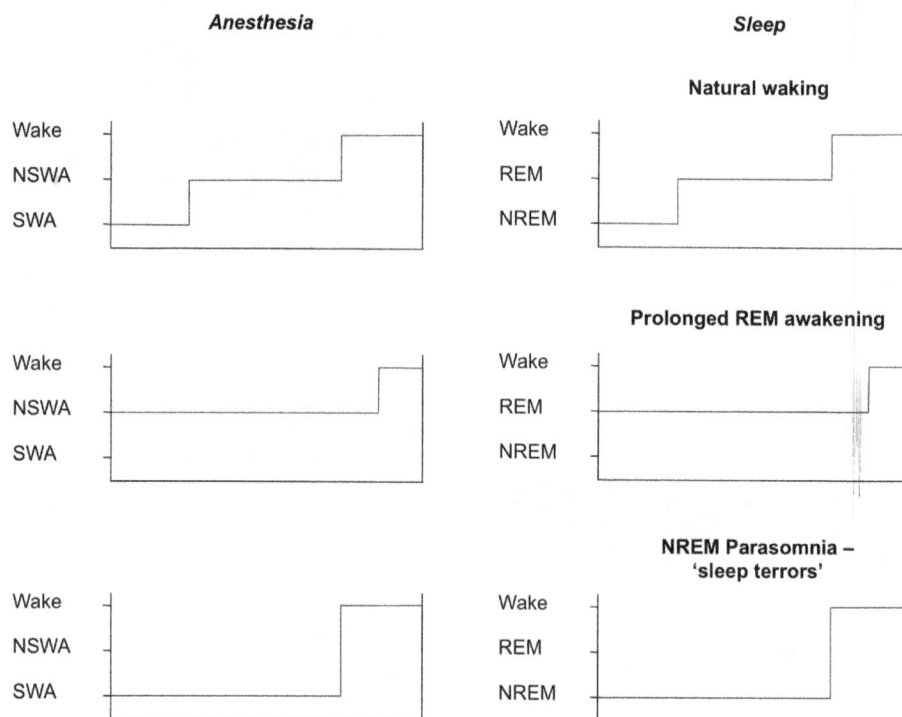

Figure 9. Hypnograms for emergence from general anesthesia and sleep. Temporal evolution of stages of arousal during emergence from general anesthesia (GA) are plotted in the left column, and from sleep in the right column. Each GA hypnogram on the left reflects an identified Emergence Trajectory as defined earlier in the text. These trajectories might be loosely correlated with arousal trajectories from various stages of sleep that are placed immediately to the right. SWA = Slow-Wave Anesthesia, NSWA = Non Slow-Wave Anesthesia; NREM = non-REM sleep, REM = REM sleep.

correlations were with duration of operation ($r = 0.23$, $p = 0.02$) and age ($r = 0.21$, $p = 0.03$).

Discussion

A Nomenclature for Distinguishing Between Anesthetic Maintenance States

In this study, we present a conceptual framework to discriminate four patterns of anesthetic maintenance comprised of two states, 'Slow-Wave Anesthesia' (SWA) and 'Non Slow-Wave Anesthesia' (NSWA), and two derivative sub-classes of the slow-wave state, 'delta-dominant' (ddSWA) and 'spindle-dominant' (sdSWA). These classes were defined by the relative contribution of delta (0.5–4 Hz) and spindle-alpha (8–14 Hz) power in their spectral signatures (Figure 2B). These sub-14 Hz oscillations that dominate the EEG during both NREM (slow-wave) sleep and general anesthesia have been shown to correspond to diminished responsiveness to mild stimuli in NREM sleep [41,61] and to more aversive stimuli during general anesthesia [9,62,63]. Because these oscillations can also be correlated with specific neural generators in a more generally hyperpolarized reticulothalamocortical circuit, they have been used for decades to classify stages of natural sleep. We were therefore able to capitalize on the methods by which sleep is staged and dynamically tracked over time (Figures 1, 9) to generate a new standardized taxonomy that could be used to describe the maintenace phase of general anesthesia. Although a pattern similar to the spindle-dominant slow-wave pattern (sdSWA) has been previously reported in studies in which

volunteers are exposed to slowly changing levels of propofol anesthesia [8,64], the greater diversity of patterns we observed may be due to the lack of spectral averaging in our subjects, the greater diversity of the typical surgical population (e.g. baseline neurological status and co-morbidities, pre-operative medication status, baseline pain sensitivity), and the highly variable surgical environment (e.g. intraoperative medication administration, surgical stimulation, nociception).

A Description of Emergence Trajectories

We examined the transition from unconsciousness back to conscious awareness (i.e. responsiveness) after general anesthesia was terminated at the conclusion of surgery, from End Maintenance/Start Emergence to End Emergence. We found a general shift from the slow-wave pattern (SWA) to a more uniform distribution of power across frequency bands (NSWA). This trend was immediately visible and highly significant when the grand average of EEG spectra across the entire patient population was performed at the beginning and end of emergence (Figure 2E, $p < 0.05$). However, just as with the maintenance patterns, individual patient emergence trajectories from unconsciousness to waking were more variable than averaged trajectories [8,9] (Figure 2F, Figures 3–6). We speculate that inactivation of endogenous sleep networks, activation of redundant arousal networks, and the nociceptive residuum experienced by the patient, contribute to this variability. In order to minimize non-surgical noxious stimuli, an LMA was used as the airway device, and auditory and tactile stimulation during emergence was limited (see Methods); we

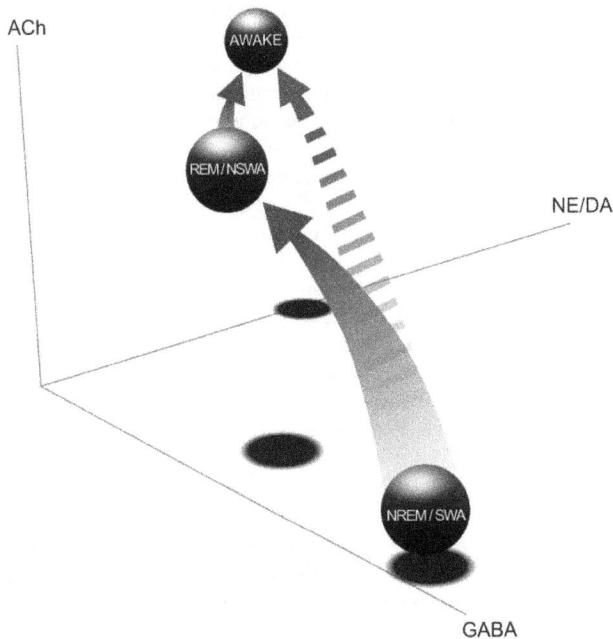

Figure 10. A putative (shared) 3-D neurotransmitter state space for emergence from sleep and general anesthesia. Based on spectral power and underlying neural generators, stages of anesthesia and stages of sleep may be analagous, especially on the path from thalamocortical hyperpolarization to waking. During natural NREM sleep, levels of GABA are high, while REM is characterized by high levels of both GABA and acetylcholine (ACh). As the brain passes from REM to waking, levels of GABA diminish, and monoamines such as norepinephrine and dopamine start to increase. The progression on the more typical anesthetic-emergence trajectory from SWA -> NSWA -> waking may reflect a similar shift in neurotransmitter balance as shown in this diagram (solid arrow). The "non-preferred" pathway of emergence that transitions directly from SWA -> waking (somewhat analogous to NREM -> waking) is represented by the broken arrow. NREM = non-REM sleep, REM = rapid eye movement sleep, SWA = Slow-Wave Anesthesia, NSWA = Non Slow-Wave Anesthesia, GABA = GABA-aminobutyric acid, ACh = acetylcholine, NE = norepinephrine, DA = dopamine.

therefore do not attribute this variability to tracheal or general environmental stimulation. More importantly, these diverse emergence patterns suggest that recovery from general anesthesia does not necessarily mirror the induction process, and may reflect a behavioral state barrier, which depends in part on the balance of activation in endogenous sleep and arousal pathways [31,65–67].

Using a dynamical systems approach, we grouped 100 observed emergence trajectories in state-space into categories based on the apparent number of attractors during emergence, the time each subject occupied that stable attractor state, and the time required to transition between attractor states (Figures 3–6). As with any empirical study, the exact dynamical system classification of the attractor topology is provisional. Although the attractors resembled simple point attractors, more detailed studies of the EEG dynamics might reveal some high dimensional chaotic or limit cycle structure within these attractors. With those provisos, almost half (43%) of patients exhibited a canonical sequence: loss of delta, followed by loss of spindles, and then a period of NSWA (characterized by the absence of low frequency oscillatory peaks in the EEG and behavioral unresponsiveness), before waking. In contrast, approximately one-third (31%) of subjects skip the NSWA stage and transition directly from SWA to wakefulness

(Trajectory 4), and 16% do not achieve SWA at any stage during end maintenance or emergence (Trajectory 3). We also observed a sharp increase in electromyographic power (EMG) that often precedes the return of consciousness, but is not a necessary prerequisite.

Connections between Emergence Trajectories and Post-operative Recovery

The time spent in NSWA prior to wake-up (defined on the dwell-time plots from Figures 3–6) was modestly predictive of subsequent pain (Figures 7–8). Patients who spent little of their emergence time in NSWA, were more likely to have high pain, and express a degree of agitation in recovery. (A similarly sudden transition from slow wave sleep directly to wakefulness is associated with some sleep pathologies such as night terrors [53,68], see also FIgure 9). These patients often had more frontal EMG activation during emergence, which in itself was weakly associated with a higher pain score in the PACU. Frontalis muscle activation (EMG) in patients can in itself confound the results. The EMG signature is broad-band and can potentially contaminate, distort or obscure the underlying EEG signal. Conversely EMG activation is a valuable indication of motor system activation as part of the emergence sequence from anesthesia, and we found it to be largely independent of the return of consciousness, as defined by recovery of responsiveness to voice. This observation is in accord with other work suggesting that components of motor systems are relatively resistant to the effects of anesthesia, and that recovery of motor tone is not captured by changing information in the EEG which tends to reflect the hypnotic axis [69]. Different central nervous subsystems may not always reconnect in a well-defined sequence after general anesthesia is discontinued; in some instances, alternate paths or sequences for bringing various brain arousal nuclei or networks on-line preceding the return of consciousness may predispose patients to undesirable wake-ups, in the same way that parasomnias are exacerbated by disrupted sleep architecture [54]. Our measurements also do not assess recovery along the axis of memory, another subsystem affected by anesthetics and sleep.

The evolution of trajectories from Start to End Emergence can be captured in an emergence hypnogram for general anesthesia

Figure 9 graphically depicts the evolution of each of the emergence trajectory patterns (Figures 3–6) and compares these patterns to arousal from specific stages of sleep. Carrying the analogy between waking from natural sleep and emergence from general anesthesia further, we propose using a hypnogram to capture the emergence trajectories from general anesthesia (left column) seen in Figures 3–6, where the length of the horizontal line at each stages reflects the relative dwell-time in the state-space plot (panel C of Figures 3–6). These can be compared to the sequences of emergence from natural sleep, seen in the right column, in the more classic version of the emergence hypnogram. A transition from SWA to NSWA before waking may correspond most closely to the waking from natural sleep. Waking from very prolonged NSWA may not have a correlate in normal sleep (prolonged REM awakening), but may instead reflect certain hypersomnia subtypes [70]. The emergence trajectory of an abrupt transition from SWA to wakefulness can be compared to arousal during NREM sleep, often associated with parasomnias or sleep disturbances resulting from fragmented sleep [53,54].

Table 2. Demographic Data.

Age (yrs)	48(19)
Gender (F/M)	48/52
Duration of surgery (min)	99(68)
Duration of emergence (min)	12.4 [8.4 to 18.9]
Sevo/Des/Isoflurane	81/8/11
$C_e MAC_s$	10.79 [0.66 to 0.98]
$C_e MAC_e$	0.06 [0.001 to 0.08]
$C_e fentanyl_e$ (ng/ml)	0.54 [0.31 to 0.78]
PACU-Cons (0/1/2)	17/42/41
PACU-Pain (0/1/2)	56/15/29

C_e denotes effect site concentration of the drug, and the subscripts 's' and 'e' denote the start and end of emergence. MAC indicates units of age adjusted Minimum Alveolar Concentration, PACU-Cons and PACU-Pain are defined in the text and in Table 1.

The Neurochemical Relationship Between Sleep Circuitry And General Anesthesia

The degree of thalamocortical hyperpolarization depends on the balance of activity in neurotransmitters systems [71,72]. While there are many regional and nuclear brain differences, NREM sleep tends to be dominated by high GABAergic and low cholinergic and monoaminergic tone, while REM sleep is dominated by both GABAergic and cholinergic tone, and low levels of monoamines [73,74]. We postulate that the presence of spindles and delta oscillations within the stage we define as SWA also reflects overwhelming GABAergic tone and low cholinergic tone, consistent with the mechanism of action of many of our volatile and intravenous anesthetics. The exact sequence of neuromodulator activation during emergence from anaesthesia is unknown, and is probably the main cause for the heterogeneity that we observed in the emergence trajectories. As anesthetic washes out of the brain, the residual GABAergic effects of the drug may be antagonized by depolarizing cholinergic (or aminergic) systems, pushing the brain into the NSWA state. The reason for transition from this point to waking is unclear, but probably involves a switch from high GABAergic tone to high monoaminergic and orexinergic tone, allowing the patient to fully emerge and reconnect with the external world. These pathways may be visualized in a 3-D neurotransmitter diagram for NREM/SWA, REM/NSWA, and waking states (Figure 10). The solid arrow signals a "preferred" wake-up sequence in which a patient moves from SWA to NSWA prior to waking, and experiences a higher degree of conscious awareness and a lower degree of pain and agitation in recovery (i.e. the classic cycle of NREM to REM to waking). The "non-preferred" sequence – in which the brain transitions directly from SWA to waking state – is reflected by the broken arrow, which if compared to sleep, would characterize a parasomnic or less desirable trajectory to re-establishing conscious awareness.

Underlying Neurobiology of EEG Signatures of Emergence and their Relationship to Sleep

Both sleep and general anesthesia share many similarities, including specific nuclei, circuitry, and neurotransmitter systems. Physiological recordings [75–76] and modeling [64,77] suggest that the oscillatory components of the alpha band (spindles between 8–14 Hz) in the frontal EEG during sleep and anesthesia

are generated by hyperpolarizing neurons of the reticular nucleus of the thalamus, in the permissive environment of depressed ascending cholinergic and monoaminergic brainstem activity [75], which switches them to a burst firing mode [78–80]. Spindles predominate in NREM stage 2 sleep, and are more commonly observed during general anesthesia when analgesics are administered to diminish noxious stimulation [63]. NREM stage 3 sleep reflects an even greater degree of thalamocortical hyperpolarization as spindle activity diminishes and slower delta oscillations (0.5–1 Hz) begin to dominate [40]. Because our data demonstrate a positive correlation between anesthetic dose and relative delta power [81] we suggest that NREM stage 3 sleep may be similar to a ddSWA pattern under anesthesia, and NREM stage 2 sleep to an sdSWA pattern. This notion is further supported by the observation that at the midpoint of emergence (with decreasing anesthetic dose) there is an increase in the number of subjects categorized as sdSWA.

A progressive depolarization within the corticothalamic system accompanies the ordered transition to waking from natural sleep. This state is termed REM and is typically the stage of sleep from which most individuals awaken. Similarly, most subjects emerging from general anesthesia appear to move progressively from SWA to NSWA. Can NSWA be likened to REM sleep? Approximately 25% of patients report dream mentation if queried immediately upon waking, and it was more common for the group who reported dreaming to be in NSWA (i.e. have low power in the < 14 Hz range) prior to waking [55]. Thus, SWA and NSWA may directly correspond to different levels of activation in the two distinct networks of conscious awareness (i.e. awareness of environment and awareness of self) described by others [82]. NSWA may reflect an unresponsive state in which some form of internally-directed consciousness has been established (e.g. fronto-parietal connectivity), but there is still insufficient brain function to connect externally. This is consistent with the concept of an unconnected (i.e. with the external world) or covert consciousness, which has been seen using carefully controlled propofol infusions in human volunteers with combined fMRI/EEG [9]. The thalamocortical network is rendered insensate to external inputs, yet activation to stimuli is still observed in cortical areas such as the precuneus. The role of the thalamus is less clear. It plays an important role in sleep, but its contribution to anesthesia has been questioned [83], and thalamic deactivation may not be the cause of unconsciousness but rather a consequence, via a functional thalamic de-afferentation from diminished cortical connectedness [84,85].

One significant limitation to this study is that we only used a frontal EEG electrode strip for our recordings. Our data is therefore constrained to data gathered from accessible frontal leads (corresponding approximatley to FPz, FP1/2 from a traditional 10–20 montage) without simultaneous recording from parietal, temporal or occipital regions. We therefore could not consider other markers of loss and return of consciousness such as global coherence [8,16] or the degree of connectedness and communication between different cortical regions [11,13–15,86]. However, EEG power is largely anteriorized upon loss of consciousness under general anesthesia [11,16,17,87], making the frontal leads reasonable markers for spectral changes that can be observed at the single electrode level. Use of commercially available EEG electrodes that can be easily placed on a patient's forehead intraoperatively as part of the placement of routine monitors also increases the likelihood that our methods for tracking and staging depth of consciousness could be used more routinely by clinicians making real-time decisions in the operating room. Our data indicate that a long period of NSWA before waking is associated with less pain than a direct transition from SWA to waking. Without further prospective randomized clinical studies, it is unclear whether it would actually be clinically useful to specifically titrate anesthetic (or analgesic) drugs to target any particular intraoperative spectral pattern. Apart from the effect of age on spectral power, we found relatively weak correlations between clinical variables and spectral pattern. This would suggest that the spectral pattern for each patient is largely determined by other unknown (possibly inherited) factors. Nevertheless we would hope that this study provides a methodological framework in which these questions could be answered.

Conclusions

The unconsciousness that accompanies general anesthesia during surgery is marked by several, distinct, oscillatory patterns in the EEG. Because these share features with those observed in natural sleep, it is possible that the underlying neural generators are conserved. Building upon a classification system used to stage sleep, we provide, for the first time, a standardized EEG-based nomenclature by which anesthetic maintenance can be staged and followed intraoperatively. We also applied a dynamical systems approach to characterize the return to consciousness after discontinuation of the anesthetic. We found that recovery of consciousness varies amongst individuals, and that deviations from a canonical sequence of SWA to NSWA occur. Further, the functional path by which the brain re-establishes conscious awareness is correlated with preferred wake-ups (e.g. diminished pain). We have created a descriptive means by which endogenous sleep rhythms and general anesthesia can be compared. Subsequent usage of this nomenclature should further our understanding of the overlapping neural mechanisms of sleep and anesthesia. As the homeostatic, learning and memory benefits of sleep are beginning to be characterized [88], future work may identify targets to improve post-operative cognitive health. The latter is of increasing concern as patients, researchers, and physicians become more apprehensive about the potential for anesthesia to cause or exacerbate adverse neurocognitive sequelae.

Methods

Ethics Statement

Studies were approved by the Northern Y Regional Ethics Committee of New Zealand (NTY/11/EXP/077), and written informed consent obtained from each patient. Free and public access to the de-identified data is available from the website: www.accesshq.org.

Patient Selection

We studied 100 adult patients presenting for routine orthopedic surgery under general anesthesia at Waikato Hospital, New Zealand, from November 2011 to January 2013. Data collection was restricted to patients eligible for laryngeal mask airway (LMA) management, considered less stimulating than an endotracheal tube [89], in order to minimize confounding effects of airway irritation, a strong non-surgical arousal stimulus, on the EEG. We specifically included patients who would be expected to have a wide range of post-surgical pain levels (some augmented with regional nerve blocks). We excluded patients with pre-existing psychiatric illness, chronic substance abuse, chronic pain, or obesity (BMI>35). Patient demographics are represented in Table 2.

Surgical Procedure and Data Collection

In order to determine the spread of emergence patterns at the conclusion of routine clinical anesthesia, we did not restrict the course of administration of the general anesthetic with the exception of limiting the airway device to an LMA, allowing it proceed according to the clinician's judgment. Patients were induced with a bolus dose of intravenous fentanyl (50–200 μg) followed by propofol (80–200 mg). Patients were maintained on a volatile general anesthetic (VA) of the clinician's choice - sevoflurane, desflurane, or isoflurane - delivered in a mixture of air and oxygen. No neuromuscular blocking drugs were used. Intraoperative analgesia was provided by intravenous morphine (0–25 mg); analgesic adjuncts of paracetamol (1 gm, n = 34), parecoxib (40 mg, n = 39), tramadol (100–200 mg, n = 22) or clonidine (60–120 μg, n = 18) were given as needed. 21 patients received a peripheral nerve block for post-operative analgesia; 14 of these were femoral blocks, done for reduction of postoperative muscle spasm for lower limb joint replacements. Because of the mutineuronal innervation of the knee and hip, most of these nerve blocks achieved incomplete analgesia. Of the others (mainly ankle blocks and brachial plexus blocks), 5 patients had pain scores of 0 on awakening – indicative of a completely successful block.

We used standard American Society of Anesthesiology [90] monitors (pulse oximeter, non-invasive blood pressure cuff, electrocardiogram, capnograph) to measure intraoperative oxygen saturation, hemodynamics, and end-tidal gas concentrations (O_2, CO_2, VA). In addition to these routine parameters, the times of surgery, tourniquet inflation and release, and drug administration were recorded.

A 2-lead EEG prefrontal electrode strip was placed on the patient's forehead, as per the manufacturer's recommendations (BIS, Covidien Vista). Frontal EEG data (sampling rate 128 Hz) was collected for the duration of the anesthetic, prior to induction through the end of emergence. The frontal EEG waveforms on the BIS sensor strip correlate approximately to the FPz and FP1/2 leads of standard 20 electrode EEG montage. Both electrodes are referenced by an additional electrode over the eyebrow. A separate lead over the temporalis muscle is used as an EMG electrode. Suitable electrode impedance (<5 kOhm) was confirmed using the manufacturer's automatic checking routine. To provide a mechanism to correlate external events with the patient's EEG, the times of surgical incision, cessation of the volatile anesthetic agent, and the exact moment of awakening were marked on the EEG record by tapping the electrodes 4 times in ~1.5 seconds to create a clear stimulus artifact. The patients were allowed to waken without excessive stimulation beyond the usual noise and activity of the operating room and post anesthesia care unit (PACU) environment (e.g. removal and replacement of monitors, background talking). Sustained awakening was confirmed by a positive response to verbal command ("Mrs. X, your operation is over, open your eyes."). 'Emergence' from general anesthesia was specifically defined as the time between the cessation of administration of the maintenance hypnotic drug (VA) and the point at which the patient became responsive to verbal command. Raw EEG and EMG data for each patient were downloaded post-operatively for further analysis.

Drug Effects

The decreasing effect-site concentrations (C_e) of the different volatile anesthetic drugs were estimated as a fraction of age adjusted MAC [91] at Start and End Emergence, and the estimated effect-site concentrations of the intraoperative opioids (fentanyl and morphine) were calculated using standard compartmental pharmacokinetic modeling [92,93]. In order to compare opioid effects across patients, and to take into account the fact that many patients had received both morphine and fentanyl intraoperatively, we expressed the morphine concentrations as fentanyl concentration equivalents (C_e fentanyl), assuming a conversion factor of 50. This data is also summarized in Table 2.

Evaluation of post-emergence level of consciousness and pain

It is common for patients to experience fluctuations in both level of consciousness and pain in the early postoperative period. These changes are hard to capture and analyze [94]. Accordingly we used simple, heuristically derived, descriptions of level of consciousness (PACU-Cons) and pain (PACU-Pain) as described in Table 1. We believe that these classifications have the advantage of capturing the clinically relevant, qualitative aspects of the recovery period. The PACU-Cons score is based on the change in the Ramsay Score over the first 15 minutes in the PACU [95]. The severity of the pain was quantified using a composite of the standard integer numerical verbal rating scale (NRS) – where 0 is no pain and 10 the worst imaginable pain. Because of the questionable validity of the fine gradations in these semi-quantitative scores, the PACU-Pain score bins the numerical rating scale into 'minimal', 'moderate' and 'severe' pain groups [96], which appear to have reasonable clinical validity. However, we also scored the degree of objective distress that the patient manifested, and used this added information to modify these scores as described in Table 1. The first pain score was obtained when the patient had achieved a level of consciousness at which they could maintain a brief conversation. These pain queries were then repeated every 15 minutes. If they were in pain, patients were treated with increments of 1–2 mg IV morphine, 25–50 µg of fentanyl, or 50–100 mg IV tramadol in the PACU, and then discharged to the ward according to institutional criteria based on the Aldrete score [97].

Spectral Processing, Statistical and Analytical Methods

All data was analyzed using custom scripts written in MATLAB (Mathworks, Natick, Massachusetts). The amplitude and frequency structure of the EEG signal was initially described by the mean power in the traditional frequency bands: delta (0.5–4 Hz), theta (5–7 Hz), alpha (8–14 Hz), and beta (15–25 Hz). The power in each band was then logarithmically transformed so that all spectral power was expressed in units of dB ($10\times$ logarithm base 10, referenced to 1 μV^2/Hz). These band-powers were then smoothed using a 30 second median smoothing filter. In addition we recorded the EMG output (dB) from the Vista monitor. We then extracted EEG features (the delta and alpha bands) that reflected the largest changes in spectral power seen in the prefrontal channels during emergence. Spindle power was specifically derived by measuring the height of the alpha peak above the underlying broadband activity to target the narrowband oscillatory component of this peak [55].

To follow these changes dynamically, we displayed the EEG using typical spectrograms and time series plots of salient features

(spindle, delta and EMG power). Spectrograms of the EEG data were made using the 'mtspecgramc.m' function and PSDs using the 'mtspectrumsegc.m' function of the Chronux toolbox (http://chronux.org) [98] on 8 second segments, with 6 second (75%) overlap and tapers of 13 and 8. This segment length was chosen to balance the time required to reliably estimate power in the delta band, while still being short enough to allow for changes in the detection of waveforms within a clinically relevant time frame. 95% confidence intervals for the median PSD for each condition (Start and End Emergence) were calculated using a jackknife estimation method. To create 3-D individualized dwell-time plots for each patient's emergence trajectory (Figures 3–6, panel C), spindle and delta power were plotted against one another in x-y plane, while depth on the z-axis reflected the total amount of time a patient remained in each x-y pixel of the spindle-delta state space as a fraction of total emergence time. This allowed us to capture the changing relationship between oscillations over time, and permitted comparisons across different patients with differing lengths of emergence.

Correlations between pairs of variables were quantified using Pearson's correlation co-efficient (r) if they followed a normal distribution (Kolmogorov-Smirnoff test), otherwise Spearman's rank correlation was used. The multivariate analysis of the interrelationships between all the variables in an observational study is subject to unknown confounding factors. Following conservative statistical practice, we limited the total number of explanatory variables for each model to 5, in order to have 20 data points to estimate the parameter for each variable with reasonable precision. We used multiple linear regression models, with stepwise forward selection, to discover which group of variables were most significantly associated with the continuous outcome variables: namely delta and alpha power at Start Emergence, and emergence time (which was logarithmically transformed to achieve a normal probability distribution). We used similar techniques, but using logistic regression, for binary outcome variables (pain group).

A patient's post-operative nociceptive status was loosely correlated with the emergence trajectory. In order to display those average trajectories, we combined the phase-space data (spindle vs. delta power) for all patients in the low (PACU-Pain =0) and high (PACU- Pain =2) groups (Figure 8). More stereotypical patterns were reflected in data points remaining tightly constrained in the 2-D phase space. More variable EEG emergence trajectories were reflected in points spread out over a large area of the 2-D phase space. Cumulative time spent in each area of the phase space was reflected in a color heat map from blue (little time) to red (large amount of time).

Author Contributions

Conceived and designed the experiments: DC PSG JWS. Performed the experiments: JWS JNM SI. Analyzed the data: JWS DC PSG. Contributed reagents/materials/analysis tools: JWS DC. Wrote the paper: DC PSG JWS.

References

1. Courtin RF, Bickford RG, Faulconer A Jr. (1950) The classification and significance of electro-encephalographic patterns produced by nitrous oxide-ether anesthesia during surgical operations. Proc Staff Meet Mayo Clin 25: 197–206.

2. Kiersey DK, Bickford RG, Faulconer A Jr. (1951) Electro-encephalographic patterns produced by thiopental sodium during surgical operations; description and classification. Br J Anaesth 23: 141–152.

3. Clark DL, Rosner BS (1973) Neurophysiologic effects of general anesthetics. I. The electroencephalogram and sensory evoked responses in man. Anesthesiology 38: 564–582.

4. Dement W, Kleitman N (1957) Cyclic variations in EEG during sleep and their relation to eye movements, body motility, and dreaming. Electroencephalogr Clin Neurophysiol 9: 673–690.

5. Rechtschaffen A, Kales A (1968) A manual of standardized terminology, techniques, and scoring system for sleep stages of human subjects. University of California, Los Angeles: Brain Information Service/Brain Research Institute.

6. Hudson RJ, Stanski DR, Saidman LJ, Meathe E (1983) A model for studying depth of anesthesia and acute tolerance to thiopental. Anesthesiology 59: 301–308.

7. Long CW, Shah NK, Loughlin C, Spydell J, Bedford RF (1989) A comparison of EEG determinants of near-awakening from isoflurane and fentanyl anesthesia. Spectral edge, median power frequency, and delta ratio. Anesth Analg 69: 169–173.

8. Purdon PL, Pierce ET, Mukamel EA, Prerau MJ, Walsh JL, et al. (2013) Electroencephalogram signatures of loss and recovery of consciousness from propofol. Proc Natl Acad Sci U S A 110: E1142–1151.

9. Ni Mhuircheartaigh R, Warnaby C, Rogers R, Jbabdi S, Tracey I (2013) Slow-wave activity saturation and thalamocortical isolation during propofol anesthesia in humans. Sci Transl Med 5: 208ra148.

10. Gugino LD, Chabot RJ, Prichep LS, John ER, Formanek V, et al. (2001) Quantitative EEG changes associated with loss and return of consciousness in healthy adult volunteers anaesthetized with propofol or sevoflurane. Br J Anaesth 87: 421–428.

11. John ER, Prichep LS, Kox W, Valdes-Sosa P, Bosch-Bayard J, et al. (2001) Invariant reversible QEEG effects of anesthetics. Conscious Cogn 10: 165–183.

12. Breshears JD, Roland JL, Sharma M, Gaona CM, Freudenburg ZV, et al. (2010) Stable and dynamic cortical electrophysiology of induction and emergence with propofol anesthesia. Proc Natl Acad Sci U S A 107: 21170–21175.

13. Lee U, Ku S, Noh G, Baek S, Choi B, et al. (2013) Disruption of frontal-parietal communication by ketamine, propofol, and sevoflurane. Anesthesiology 118: 1264–1275.

14. Ku SW, Lee U, Noh GJ, Jun IG, Mashour GA (2011) Preferential inhibition of frontal-to-parietal feedback connectivity is a neurophysiologic correlate of general anesthesia in surgical patients. PLoS One 6: e25155.

15. Boly M, Moran R, Murphy M, Boveroux P, Bruno MA, et al. (2012) Connectivity changes underlying spectral EEG changes during propofol-induced loss of consciousness. J Neurosci 32: 7082–7090.

16. Cimenser A, Purdon PL, Pierce ET, Walsh JL, Salazar-Gomez AF, et al. (2011) Tracking brain states under general anesthesia by using global coherence analysis. Proc Natl Acad Sci U S A 108: 8832–8837.

17. Vijayan S, Ching S, Purdon PL, Brown EN, Kopell NJ (2013) Thalamocortical mechanisms for the anteriorization of alpha rhythms during propofol-induced unconsciousness. J Neurosci 33: 11070–11075.

18. Steriade M, Timofeev I (2003) Neuronal plasticity in thalamocortical networks during sleep and waking oscillations. Neuron 37: 563–576.

19. Steriade M (2004) Acetylcholine systems and rhythmic activities during the waking—sleep cycle. Prog Brain Res 145: 179–196.

20. Zecharia AY, Nelson LE, Gent TC, Schumacher M, Jurd R, et al. (2009) The involvement of hypothalamic sleep pathways in general anesthesia: testing the hypothesis using the GABAA receptor beta3N265M knock-in mouse. J Neurosci 29: 2177–2187.

21. Nelson LE, Guo TZ, Lu J, Saper CB, Franks NP, et al. (2002) The sedative component of anesthesia is mediated by GABA(A) receptors in an endogenous sleep pathway. Nat Neurosci 5: 979–984.

22. Franks NP (2008) General anaesthesia: from molecular targets to neuronal pathways of sleep and arousal. Nat Rev Neurosci 9: 370–386.

23. Bonin RP, Orser BA (2008) GABA(A) receptor subtypes underlying general anesthesia. Pharmacol Biochem Behav 90: 105–112.

24. Garcia PS, Kolesky SE, Jenkins A (2010) General anesthetic actions on GABA(A) receptors. Curr Neuropharmacol 8: 2–9.

25. Huntsman MM, Porcello DM, Homanics GE, DeLorey TM, Huguenard JR (1999) Reciprocal inhibitory connections and network synchrony in the mammalian thalamus. Science 283: 541–543.

26. Rye DB, Bliwise DL, Parker K, Trotti LM, Saini P, et al. (2012) Modulation of Vigilance in the Primary Hypersomnias by Endogenous Enhancement of GABAA Receptors. Sci Transl Med 4: 161ra151.

27. Tung A, Szafran MJ, Bluhm B, Mendelson WB (2002) Sleep deprivation potentiates the onset and duration of loss of righting reflex induced by propofol and isoflurane. Anesthesiology 97: 906–911.

28. Tung A, Herrera S, Szafran MJ, Kasza K, Mendelson WB (2005) Effect of sleep deprivation on righting reflex in the rat is partially reversed by administration of adenosine A1 and A2 receptor antagonists. Anesthesiology 102: 1158–1164.

29. Berridge CW, Bolen SJ, Manley MS, Foote SL (1996) Modulation of forebrain electroencephalographic activity in halothane-anesthetized rat via actions of noradrenergic beta-receptors within the medial septal region. J Neurosci 16: 7010–7020.

30. Alkire MT, McReynolds JR, Hahn EL, Trivedi AN (2007) Thalamic microinjection of nicotine reverses sevoflurane-induced loss of righting reflex in the rat. Anesthesiology 107: 264–272.

31. Kelz MB, Sun Y, Chen J, Cheng Meng Q, Moore JT, et al. (2008) An essential role for orexins in emergence from general anesthesia. Proc Natl Acad Sci U S A 105: 1309–1314.

32. Solt K, Cotten JF, Cimenser A, Wong KF, Chemali JJ, et al. (2011) Methylphenidate actively induces emergence from general anesthesia. Anesthesiology 115: 791–803.

33. Chemali JJ, Van Dort CJ, Brown EN, Solt K (2012) Active emergence from propofol general anesthesia is induced by methylphenidate. Anesthesiology 116: 998–1005.

34. Taylor NE, Chemali JJ, Brown EN, Solt K (2013) Activation of D1 dopamine receptors induces emergence from isoflurane general anesthesia. Anesthesiology 118: 30–39.

35. Vazey EM, Aston-Jones G (2014) Designer receptor manipulations reveal a role of the locus coeruleus noradrenergic system in isoflurane general anesthesia. Proc Natl Acad Sci U S A 111: 3859–3864.

36. Solt K, Van Dort CJ, Chemali JJ, Taylor NE, Kenny JD, et al. (2014) Electrical Stimulation of the Ventral Tegmental Area Induces Reanimation from General Anesthesia. Anesthesiology.

37. Sleigh JW, Andrzejowski J, Steyn-Ross A, Steyn-Ross M (1999) The bispectral index: a measure of depth of sleep? Anesth Analg 88: 659–661.

38. Tung A, Lynch JP, Roizen MF (2002) Use of the BIS monitor to detect onset of naturally occurring sleep. J Clin Monit Comput 17: 37–42.

39. Walters AS, Lavigne G, Hening W, Picchietti DL, Allen RP, et al. (2007) The scoring of movements in sleep. J Clin Sleep Med 3: 155–167.

40. Silber MH, Ancoli-Israel S, Bonnet MH, Chokroverty S, Grigg-Damberger MM, et al. (2007) The visual scoring of sleep in adults. J Clin Sleep Med 3: 121–131.

41. Dang-Vu TT, Bonjean M, Schabus M, Boly M, Darsaud A, et al. (2011) Interplay between spontaneous and induced brain activity during human non-rapid eye movement sleep. Proc Natl Acad Sci U S A 108: 15438–15443.

42. Steriade M, Deschenes M, Domich L, Mulle C (1985) Abolition of spindle oscillations in thalamic neurons disconnected from nucleus reticularis thalami. J Neurophysiol 54: 1473–1497.

43. Steriade M, McCormick DA, Sejnowski TJ (1993) Thalamocortical oscillations in the sleeping and aroused brain. Science 262: 679–685.

44. McCormick DA, Pape HC (1990) Properties of a hyperpolarization-activated cation current and its role in rhythmic oscillation in thalamic relay neurones. J Physiol 431: 291–318.

45. Dossi RC, Nunez A, Steriade M (1992) Electrophysiology of a slow (0.5–4 Hz) intrinsic oscillation of cat thalamocortical neurones in vivo. J Physiol 447: 215–234.

46. Jones BE (1991) Paradoxical sleep and its chemical/structural substrates in the brain. Neuroscience 40: 637–656.

47. Moser D, Anderer P, Gruber G, Parapatics S, Loretz E, et al. (2009) Sleep classification according to AASM and Rechtschaffen & Kales: effects on sleep scoring parameters. Sleep 32: 139–149.

48. Dang-Vu TT, Schabus M, Desseilles M, Sterpenich V, Bonjean M, et al. (2010) Functional neuroimaging insights into the physiology of human sleep. Sleep 33: 1589–1603.

49. Gais S, Molle M, Helms K, Born J (2002) Learning-dependent increases in sleep spindle density. J Neurosci 22: 6830–6834.

50. Rasch B, Buchel C, Gais S, Born J (2007) Odor cues during slow-wave sleep prompt declarative memory consolidation. Science 315: 1426–1429.

51. Molle M, Eschenko O, Gais S, Sara SJ, Born J (2009) The influence of learning on sleep slow oscillations and associated spindles and ripples in humans and rats. Eur J Neurosci 29: 1071–1081.

52. Morgenthaler TI, Kapur VK, Brown T, Swick TJ, Alessi C, et al. (2007) Practice parameters for the treatment of narcolepsy and other hypersomnias of central origin. Sleep 30: 1705–1711.

53. Howell MJ (2012) Parasomnias: an updated review. Neurotherapeutics 9: 753–775.

54. Espa F, Ondze B, Deglise P, Billiard M, Besset A (2000) Sleep architecture, slow wave activity, and sleep spindles in adult patients with sleepwalking and sleep terrors. Clin Neurophysiol 111: 929–939.

55. Leslie K, Sleigh J, Paech MJ, Voss L, Lim CW, et al. (2009) Dreaming and electroencephalographic changes during anesthesia maintained with propofol or desflurane. Anesthesiology 111: 547–555.

56. Hilborn RC (2000) Chaos and nonlinear dynamics: an introduction for scientists and engineers. Oxford; New York: Oxford University Press.

57. Gan TJ, Glass PS, Sigl J, Sebel P, Payne F, et al. (1999) Women emerge from general anesthesia with propofol/alfentanil/nitrous oxide faster than men. Anesthesiology 90: 1283–1287.

58. Myles PS, McLeod AD, Hunt JO, Fletcher H (2001) Sex differences in speed of emergence and quality of recovery after anaesthesia: cohort study. BMJ 322: 710–711.

59. Hoymork SC, Raeder J (2005) Why do women wake up faster than men from propofol anaesthesia? Br J Anaesth 95: 627–633.

60. Bajaj P, Raiger LK, Jain SD, Kumar S (2007) Women emerge from general anesthesia faster than men. Middle East J Anesthesiol 19: 173–183.

61. Steriade M, Contreras D, Curro Dossi R, Nunez A (1993) The slow (<1 Hz) oscillation in reticular thalamic and thalamocortical neurons: scenario of sleep rhythm generation in interacting thalamic and neocortical networks. J Neurosci 13: 3284–3299.

62. Rampil IJ, Matteo RS (1987) Changes in EEG spectral edge frequency correlate with the hemodynamic response to laryngoscopy and intubation. Anesthesiology 67: 139–142.

63. MacKay EC, Sleigh JW, Voss LJ, Barnard JP (2010) Episodic waveforms in the electroencephalogram during general anaesthesia: a study of patterns of response to noxious stimuli. Anaesth Intensive Care 38: 102–112.

64. Ching S, Cimenser A, Purdon PL, Brown EN, Kopell NJ (2010) Thalamocortical model for a propofol-induced alpha-rhythm associated with loss of consciousness. Proc Natl Acad Sci U S A 107: 22665–22670.

65. Steyn-Ross ML, Steyn-Ross DA, Sleigh JW (2004) Modelling general anaesthesia as a first-order phase transition in the cortex. Prog Biophys Mol Biol 85: 369–385.

66. Friedman EB, Sun Y, Moore JT, Hung HT, Meng QC, et al. (2010) A conserved behavioral state barrier impedes transitions between anesthetic-induced unconsciousness and wakefulness: evidence for neural inertia. PLoS One 5: e11903.

67. Joiner WJ, Friedman EB, Hung HT, Koh K, Sowcik M, et al. (2013) Genetic and anatomical basis of the barrier separating wakefulness and anesthetic-induced unresponsiveness. PLoS Genet 9: e1003605.

68. Besset A, Espa F (2001) [Disorders of arousal]. Rev Neurol (Paris) 157: S107–111.

69. Illman H, Antila H, Olkkola KT (2010) Reversal of neuromuscular blockade by sugammadex does not affect EEG derived indices of depth of anesthesia. J Clin Monit Comput 24: 371–376.

70. (2005) International Classification of Sleep Disorders: Diagnostic and Coding Manual (ICSD-2). 2 ed. Westchester NY: American Academy of Sleep Medicine.

71. Basheer R, Sherin JE, Saper CB, Morgan JI, McCarley RW, et al. (1997) Effects of sleep on wake-induced c-fos expression. J Neurosci 17: 9746–9750.

72. Saper CB, Scammell TE, Lu J (2005) Hypothalamic regulation of sleep and circadian rhythms. Nature 437: 1257–1263.

73. Lydic R, Baghdoyan HA (2005) Sleep, anesthesiology, and the neurobiology of arousal state control. Anesthesiology 103: 1268–1295.

74. Van Dort CJ, Baghdoyan HA, Lydic R (2008) Neurochemical modulators of sleep and anesthetic states. Int Anesthesiol Clin 46: 75–104.

75. Keifer JC, Baghdoyan HA, Lydic R (1996) Pontine cholinergic mechanisms modulate the cortical electroencephalographic spindles of halothane anesthesia. Anesthesiology 84: 945–954.

76. Fuentealba P, Timofeev I, Steriade M (2004) Prolonged hyperpolarizing potentials precede spindle oscillations in the thalamic reticular nucleus. Proc Natl Acad Sci U S A 101: 9816–9821.

77. Gottschalk A, Haney P (2003) Computational aspects of anesthetic action in simple neural models. Anesthesiology 98: 548–564.

78. Contreras D, Curro Dossi R, Steriade M (1993) Electrophysiological properties of cat reticular thalamic neurones in vivo. J Physiol 470: 273–294.

79. Ferenets R, Lipping T, Suominen P, Turunen J, Puumala P, et al. (2006) Comparison of the properties of EEG spindles in sleep and propofol anesthesia. Conf Proc IEEE Eng Med Biol Soc 1: 6356–6359.

80. Kroeger D, Amzica F (2007) Hypersensitivity of the anesthesia-induced comatose brain. J Neurosci 27: 10597–10607.

81. Mulholland CV, Somogyi AA, Barratt DT, Coller JK, Hutchinson MK, et al. Association of innate immune single nucleotide polymorphisms with the electroencephalogram during desflurane general anaesthesia. Journal of Molecular Neuroscience: In press.

82. Vanhaudenhuyse A, Demertzi A, Schabus M, Noirhomme Q, Bredart S, et al. (2011) Two distinct neuronal networks mediate the awareness of environment and of self. J Cogn Neurosci 23: 570–578.

83. Alkire MT, Hudetz AG, Tononi G (2008) Consciousness and anesthesia. Science 322: 876–880.

84. Ferrarelli F, Massimini M, Sarasso S, Casali A, Riedner BA, et al. (2010) Breakdown in cortical effective connectivity during midazolam-induced loss of consciousness. Proc Natl Acad Sci U S A 107: 2681–2686.

85. Massimini M, Ferrarelli F, Sarasso S, Tononi G (2012) Cortical mechanisms of loss of consciousness: insight from TMS/EEG studies. Arch Ital Biol 150: 44–55.

86. Imas OA, Ropella KM, Ward BD, Wood JD, Hudetz AG (2005) Volatile anesthetics disrupt frontal-posterior recurrent information transfer at gamma frequencies in rat. Neurosci Lett 387: 145–150.

87. Tinker JH, Sharbrough FW, Michenfelder JD (1977) Anterior shift of the dominant EEG rhythm during anesthesia in the Java monkey: correlation with anesthetic potency. Anesthesiology 46: 252–259.

88. Tononi G, Cirelli C (2014) Sleep and the price of plasticity: from synaptic and cellular homeostasis to memory consolidation and integration. Neuron 81: 12–34.

89. Brimacombe J (1995) The advantages of the LMA over the tracheal tube or facemask: a meta-analysis. Can J Anaesth 42: 1017–1023.

90. (2010) American Society of Anesthesiologists Standards for Basic Anesthetic Monitoring. ASA House of Delegates (Standards and Practice Parameters Committee).

91. Whitlock EL, Villafranca AJ, Lin N, Palanca BJ, Jacobsohn E, et al. (2011) Relationship between bispectral index values and volatile anesthetic concentrations during the maintenance phase of anesthesia in the B-Unaware trial. Anesthesiology 115: 1209–1218.

92. Shafer SL, Varvel JR, Aziz N, Scott JC (1990) Pharmacokinetics of fentanyl administered by computer-controlled infusion pump. Anesthesiology 73: 1091–1102.

93. Villesen HH, Banning AM, Petersen RH, Weinelt S, Poulsen JB, et al. (2007) Pharmacokinetics of morphine and oxycodone following intravenous administration in elderly patients. Ther Clin Risk Manag 3: 961–967.

94. De Jonghe B, Cook D, Appere-De-Vecchi C, Guyatt G, Meade M, et al. (2000) Using and understanding sedation scoring systems: a systematic review. Intensive Care Med 26: 275–285.

95. Haenggi M, Ypparila H, Takala J, Korhonen I, Luginbuhl M, et al. (2004) Measuring depth of sedation with auditory evoked potentials during controlled infusion of propofol and remifentanil in healthy volunteers. Anesth Analg 99: 1728–1736.

96. Mei W, Seeling M, Franck M, Radtke F, Brantner B, et al. (2010) Independent risk factors for postoperative pain in need of intervention early after awakening from general anaesthesia. Eur J Pain 14: 149 e141–147.

97. Aldrete JA (1998) Modifications to the postanesthesia score for use in ambulatory surgery. J Perianesth Nurs 13: 148–155.

98. Mitra P, Bokil B (2008) Observed Brain Dynamics. New York: Oxford University Press.

10

Raised Middle-Finger: Electrocortical Correlates of Social Conditioning with Nonverbal Affective Gestures

Matthias J. Wieser[1]*, Tobias Flaisch[2], Paul Pauli[1]

1 Department of Psychology, University of Würzburg, Würzburg, Germany, **2** Department of Psychology, University of Konstanz, Konstanz, Germany

Abstract

Humans form impressions of others by associating persons (faces) with negative or positive social outcomes. This learning process has been referred to as social conditioning. In everyday life, affective nonverbal gestures may constitute important social signals cueing threat or safety, which therefore may support aforementioned learning processes. In conventional aversive conditioning, studies using electroencephalography to investigate visuocortical processing of visual stimuli paired with danger cues such as aversive noise have demonstrated facilitated processing and enhanced sensory gain in visual cortex. The present study aimed at extending this line of research to the field of social conditioning by pairing neutral face stimuli with affective nonverbal gestures. To this end, electro-cortical processing of faces serving as different conditioned stimuli was investigated in a differential social conditioning paradigm. Behavioral ratings and visually evoked steady-state potentials (ssVEP) were recorded in twenty healthy human participants, who underwent a differential conditioning procedure in which three neutral faces were paired with pictures of negative (raised middle finger), neutral (pointing), or positive (thumbs-up) gestures. As expected, faces associated with the aversive hand gesture (raised middle finger) elicited larger ssVEP amplitudes during conditioning. Moreover, theses faces were rated as to be more arousing and unpleasant. These results suggest that cortical engagement in response to faces aversively conditioned with nonverbal gestures is facilitated in order to establish persistent vigilance for social threat-related cues. This form of social conditioning allows to establish a predictive relationship between social stimuli and motivationally relevant outcomes.

Editor: Marina Pavlova, University of Tuebingen Medical School, Germany

Funding: Deutsche Forschungsgemeinschaft, FOR 605, Wi2714/3-2; Deutsche Forschungsgemeinschaft, SFB-TRR 58, project B05; This publication was funded by the German Research Foundation (DFG) and the University of Wuerzburg in the funding programme. The funders had no role in study design, data collection and analysis, decision to publish, or preparation of the manuscript.

Competing Interests: The authors have declared that no competing interests exist.

* Email: wieser@psychologie.uni-wuerzburg.de

Introduction

Traditionally, in classical aversive conditioning either highly aversive electric stimuli [1,2,3,4,5] or loud aversive bursts of (white) noise [6,7,8,9,10] have been used as aversive unconditioned stimulus (US), which have been proven to elicit strong fear reactions and enhanced amygdala activity in response to the conditioned stimulus (CS). Comparable effects were found for other types of US, such as odor stimuli [11] and negative emotional pictures [12]. From a social neuroscience perspective however, one has to note that affective and social learning processes outside the laboratory are rarely happening with these types of US stimuli. In contrast, one may consider these types of stimuli as ecologically less valid because humans seldom encounter such stimuli in everyday life. Admittedly, social stimuli (verbal or non-verbal) are much more likely to function as US in everyday social learning situations, and thus contribute to impression formation and social and affective learning. Particularly, the ability to identify individual faces based on the social consequences they have predicted in the past constitutes an essential form of associative learning in humans. This learning mechanism has been coined social conditioning, defined as process whereby an individual learns to identify other individuals that have predicted threats or rewards in the past [13].

Only recently researchers have started using social and hence ecologically more valid US such as verbal descriptions (sentences), affective prosody, and facial expressions [13,14,15,16] to investigate the effects and neural correlates of social conditioning. Using verbal feedback sentences as US (e.g., "He says you're stupid"), it was shown that faces associated with pleasant and unpleasant social outcomes elicited larger activations in the human amygdala compared to when subjects learned that a face predicted neutral social outcomes [13]. Consistent with these findings, pairing faces with aversive audiovisual US (negative faces combined with a male voice saying "Stupid") also led to efficient social aversive learning and concurrent amygdala activation to the fear-associated CS face [14]. These studies suggests that social US, although less intense than conventional US, are sufficient to cause conditioning and modulate amygdala responses to previously neutral stimuli. In a further study in which social conditioning was investigated in social anxiety disorder, participants underwent differential social conditioning incorporating socially stressful US such as critical facial expressions combined with derogatory verbal feedback [15]. Interestingly, only socially anxious subjects demonstrated fear conditioning, as a potentiated startle blink reflex to the CS face predictive of a negative compared to both CS predictive of a neutral or a positive social outcome indicated. The latter study points at the notion that socially relevant US may especially disseminate their anxiogenic effect in individuals with social anxiety disorder. This notion was also recently supported by findings of enhanced amygdala activity in socially anxious individuals in response to neutral faces which have been previously associated with videos of negative feedback [16].

The aim of the current study was to examine the electrocortical correlates of social conditioning, i.e. how the visual brain responds to socially conditioned faces. The conditioned stimuli consisted of three neutral faces which were paired with unpleasant, neutral, or pleasant hand gestures during the acquisition phase. Symbolic hand gestures carrying affective meaning appear well-suited as social US, as they have been shown to be preferentially processed by the brain [17,18,19]. Steady-state visually evoked potentials (ssVEPs) in response to faces were used to quantify the degree of visuocortical engagement to the different CS cues. The ssVEP is an oscillatory response of the visual cortex elicited by luminance- or contrast-modulated stimuli in which the frequency of the electrocortical response recorded from the scalp equals that of the driving [20,21]. Here, the frequency of the cortical response is precisely known and can therefore be reliably separated from noise and quantified in the frequency domain [22]. Moreover and of significant advantage in conditioning paradigms where the trial number is usually limited, ssVEPs possess excellent signal-to-noise ratios compared to traditional ERP components [23]. An amplitude enhancement of the ssVEP reflects heightened visuo-cortical activation in response to a stimulus, which has been demonstrated to be modulated both by bottom-up sources of signal salience [24] and top-down, task-related processes [25,26]. The neural sources of the ssVEP have been localized to the primary and extended visual cortex [27,28], with strong contributions from retinotopic areas, but also from cortices higher in the visual hierarchy [29]. In experiments on differential aversive conditioning, ssVEP and ssVEF responses (its magnetic relative measured by magnetencephalography) were found to be reliably enhanced for CS+ compared to CS- cues [9,10,30,31,32].

Based on the literature as reviewed above, we examined the hypothesis that affective CS cues elicit larger sensory responses compared to neutral CS cues, following differential social conditioning with pictures of affective and neutral gestures as US. Based on differential amygdala activity findings in social conditioning and larger motivational relevance of negative gestures of insult, we further explored whether visual cortex activity was also higher for CS cues paired with negative compared to CS cues paired with positive gestures.

Methods

Participants

Twenty undergraduate students (11 females, mean age $M = 20.8$, $SD = 2.6$ years) from the University of Würzburg with normal or corrected-to-normal vision participated in this study for course credits. All participants were screened for personal and family history of photic epilepsy. Nineteen participants were right-handed, one participant left handed. The institutional review board at the University of Würzburg approved all experimental procedures; all participants provided written informed consent.

Stimuli

The conditioned stimuli (CS) consisted of pictures of 3 male faces taken from the Radboud Faces database [33], which were converted to grey-scale, adjusted for brightness, luminance and

contrast, and presented using Presentation (Neurobehavioral Systems, Inc., Albany, CA, USA). Only male faces were used as it has been shown that male faces seem to be more efficient in fear conditioning and to elicit stronger responses in both men and women, for a review see [34]. The CS cues were delivered for 5000 ms in a flickering mode in front of a uniform gray background at a frequency of 12 Hz in order to elicit the ssVEP. The unconditioned stimuli (US) were pictures of unpleasant, neutral, and pleasant hand gestures [17,19], which were presented in the conditioning phase only, immediately at offset of the CS faces for 500 ms. Pictures used as CS and US are given in Figure 1.

Design and Procedure

The experiment contained three blocks (habituation, acquisition, extinction), each consisting of 60 trials (three faces, each presented 20 times) resulting in 180 total trials. In the habituation and extinction phase, faces were presented without any pairings with the US. In the acquisition phase, each face was paired with one of the three hand gestures such that the picture of the respective hand gesture immediately followed the 5000 ms presentation of the face stimulus. The combination of faces and hand gestures was counter-balanced across participants. The order of the stimuli within each block was pseudo-randomized such that no more than two of the same faces ever occurred consecutively during the different phases. After providing written informed consent and initial screening to rule out photic epilepsy/seizures, participants were seated in a sound-attenuated, dimly lit testing room where the electroencephalogram (EEG) sensor net was applied. Participants were instructed that they would view flickering faces of three different individuals, which would at some point during the experiment be combined with pictures of hand gestures. Participants were not informed of a specific relation between CSs and the US. Each picture was displayed centrally on a 19-inch computer monitor (resolution = 1280×1024 pixel) with a vertical refresh rate of 60 Hz, located approximately 80 cm in front of the participant, resulting in a picture presentation with a visual angle of $4.2°$ horizontally and $5.9°$ vertically. Each CS was presented on the screen for 5000 ms, with inter-trial intervals varying between 2000 and 3000 ms. Participants were asked to rate each CS stimulus for hedonic valence and arousal after each phase (Habituation, Acquisition, Extinction) using a computer-based version of the Self-Assessment Manikin Scale SAM [35]. The SAM is a language-free instrument for rating hedonic valence and consists of a graphic figure representing nine levels of pleasure/displeasure. Contingency awareness was also assessed using an online analogue scale, in which participants were to indicate the probability of the face to be paired with one of the three US. The purpose of the contingency rating was to determine whether participants successfully learned the CS-US pairing rule. The contingency ratings were obtained immediately after the conditioning phase. After the three experimental phases, participants were asked to rate the US stimuli for affective valence and arousal using the SAM scales.

EEG Data Recording

EEG was recorded continuously from 129 electrodes using an Electrical Geodesics (EGI) high-density EEG system and digitized at a rate of 250 Hz, using Cz as a recording reference. Impedances were kept below 50 kΩ, as recommended for the Electrical Geodesics high input-impedance amplifiers. All channels were filtered on-line with 0.1 and 100-Hz and 50 Hz notch filter.

CS

US

negative   neutral   positive

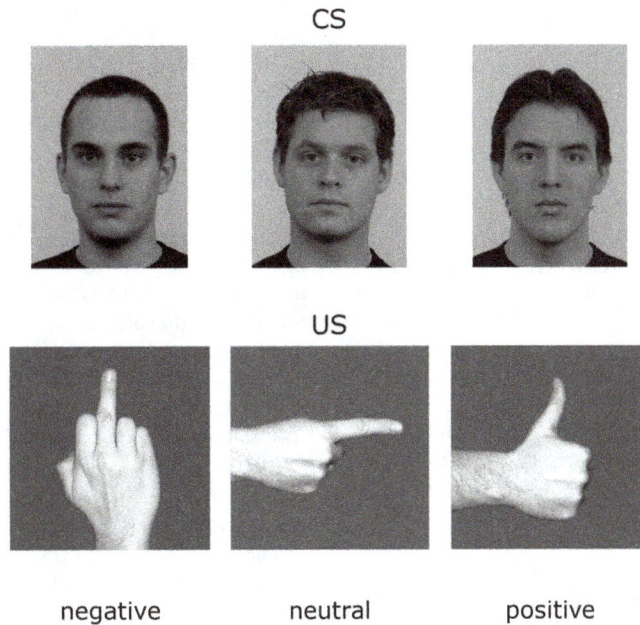

Figure 1. Three male neutral faces served as CS stimuli (upper panel). The affective hand gestures (middle finger, thumbs-up, point gesture) served as US for the differential conditioning procedure (lower panel).

EEG Data Reduction and Data Analysis

Offline EEG analyses were implemented using the Electro-MagnetoEncephalography toolbox for MATLAB [36]. Epochs of 600 ms pre-stimulus and 5600 ms post-stimulus onset were extracted offline. Data were filtered using a 40-Hz low-pass (45 dB/octave, 12th order Butterworth) filter. Artifact rejection was performed following the procedure proposed by Junghöfer, Elbert, Tucker, and Rockstroh [37]. This procedure creates distributions of statistical indices of data quality and allows to identify bad channels and trials, with the latter being discarded and the former being interpolated from the full channel set. In a subsequent step, data was re-referenced to average reference, and artifact-free trials were averaged for each subject according to experimental conditions. Trials were rejected when more than 20 channels out of 129 were outlying as per the statistical parameters used for artifact identification: the mean absolute (rectified) amplitude; the variability over time points; and the maximum first order derivate (gradient). Using this method, 74% of the trials were retained. A minimum number of 3 trials per condition were retained. The number of artifact-free trials did not differ between conditions per phase.

The artifact-free ssVEP epochs were averaged, and the time-varying amplitude of the ssVEP signal was then extracted by means of Hilbert transform on the time-domain averaged ssVEP data [9]. To this end, data were first bandpass-filtered with a 12th order Butterworth filter having a width of .5-Hz (48 dB/octave), around the target frequency of 12 Hz. To achieve high time resolution, instantaneous amplitudes of the band-pass filtered signal were computed using the Hilbert function implemented in MATLAB. The Hilbert transformation possesses high temporal resolution for indexing rapid changes in ssVEP amplitude. The absolute value of Hilbert transform corresponds to the envelope of the averaged waveform [38]. Figure 2 depicts the steady-state visually evoked potential (averaged across conditions and participants) in the time domain, demonstrating the onset of the oscillatory visuocortical response at the driving frequency (12 Hz) and its frequency spectrum as derived from FFT.

Statistical Analysis

As was seen in previous work with centrally presented stimuli [9,28,39,40,41,42], amplitudes of the ssVEPs were most pronounced at electrode locations near the medial occipital electrode Oz, over the occipital pole. Thus, to test conditioning-induced changes in visuo-cortical responses to the different CS, the ssVEP activity was averaged across 8 medial occipital sensors including Oz in the International 10/20 System (EGI sensors 70, 71, 72, 74, 75, 76, 82, 83; see Figure 3).

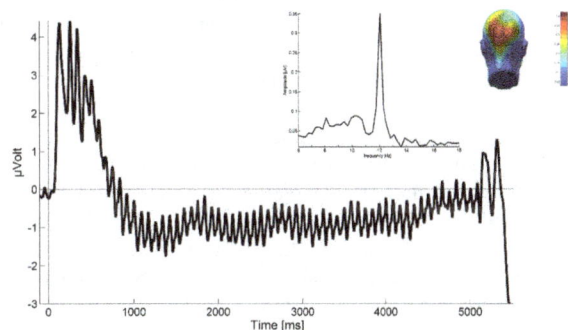

Figure 2. The grand mean steady-state visually evoked potential averaged across all participants and conditions, recorded from a medial occipital electrode (Oz) is presented. The ssVEP in the present study contains the driving frequency (12 Hz) of the face stimulus, as shown by the frequency domain representation (middle inlay) of the same signal (Fast Fourier Transformation of the ssVEP in a time segment between 200 and 5,000 ms. The right inlay shows the mean scalp topography of the very frequency over visual cortical areas.

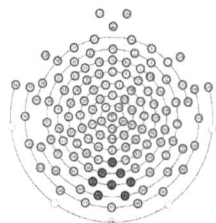

Figure 3. Layout of the dense electrode array. Locations of the electrodes grouped for regional means (used for statistical analysis) are in gray. Sensor #75 corresponds to Oz of the International 10–20 System.

Mean ssVEP amplitudes (100–4900 ms) were analyzed by means of repeated-measures analysis of variance (ANOVAs). The ANOVA contained the following within-subjects factors: Phase (Habituation, Acquisition, Extinction), and CS-Type (CS^{neg} vs. CS^{neu} vs. CS^{pos}). To investigate whether cortical activation differed across picture presentation time [9], an additional ANOVA analysis was carried out using two time windows of the ssVEP amplitudes (100–2500 ms and 2501–4900 ms), consequently including the factor time (early vs. late) as an additional within-subject factor. SAM ratings for valence and arousal were averaged for each stimulus and phase, and submitted to separate mixed-model ANOVAs, containing the within-subjects factors Phase and CS type. The Mauchly's test of sphericity was used to test for violations of this assumption and wherever relevant, the Greenhouse-Geisser corrected results are provided with uncorrected degrees of freedom, corrected F and p values [43].

Results

Electrocortical activity (ssVEPs)

The ANOVA on the mean amplitudes across the whole viewing time revealed a significant interaction of phase and CS type, $F(4,76) = 2.88$, GG-$\varepsilon = .63$, $p = .045$, $\eta_p^2 = .13$. (see Figure 4). Separate ANOVAs per phase revealed significant modulations of the ssVEP amplitude for the conditioning phase, only, $F(2,38) = 3.82$, $p = .031$, $\eta_p^2 = .17$. Planned contrasts showed that CS^{neg} faces evoked larger ssVEP amplitudes compared to CS^{neu} faces, $t(19) = 2.73$, $p = .013$ (Bonferroni-corrected $p = .017$), but CS^{pos} faces compared to CS^{neu} faces elicited only marginally larger amplitudes, $t(19) = 1.93$, $p = .069$ (Bonferroni-corrected $p = .017$). No differences emerged between CS^{neg} and CS^{pos} faces (Figure 5).

The analysis of the time course of the ssVEP amplitude including earlier and later time windows (100–2500 ms and 2501–4900 ms) did not find any interaction including the factor time, but a significant main effect of time, $F(1,19) = 8.91$, $p = .008$, $\eta_p^2 = .32$, with higher amplitudes in the first compared to the second time window. Additionally, the Phase x CS type interaction was significant, $F(4,76) = 2.88$, GG-$\varepsilon = .61$, $p = .045$, $\eta_p^2 = .13$.

Affective Ratings

As expected, arousal and valence ratings changed across the three phases of the experiment depending on the CS type, as the interaction of Phase X CS Type indicated, $F(4,76) = 3.35$, $p = .014$, $\eta_p^2 = .15$, and $F(4,76) = 2.81$, $p = .031$, $\eta_p^2 = .13$, respectively (see Figure 6).

For both ratings, also a significant main effect of CS type was observed: arousal ratings, $F(2,38) = 4.60$, GG-$\varepsilon = .77$, $p = .026$, $\eta_p^2 = .20$; valence ratings: $F(2,38) = 7.96$, $p = .001$, $\eta_p^2 = .30$. To

follow up on the interaction, separate ANOVAS per phase were run. For arousal ratings it turned out that differences were only significant in the conditioning phase, $F(2,38) = 7.60$, $p = .002$, $\eta_p^2 = .29$. This was due to CS^{neg} face cues were rated as to be more arousing compared to CS^{neu} faces, $t(19) = 4.09$, $p = .001$, whereas the comparison of CS^{pos} and CS^{neu} just missed significance, $t(19) = 2.24$, $p = .037$ (Bonferroni-corrected $p = .017$). For valence ratings, separate ANOVAS per phase revealed significant differences between CS types after the conditioning phase, $F(2,38) = 12.78$, $p<.001$, $\eta_p^2 = .40$, and the extinction phase, $F(2,38) = 6.32$, GG-$\varepsilon = .78$, $p = .009$, $\eta_p^2 = .25$. Post-hoc t-tests showed that after conditioning, CS^{neg} cues were rated as to be more unpleasant compared to CS^{neu} and CS^{pos}, $t(19) = 3.67$, $p = .002$, and $t(19) = 4.56$, $p<.001$ (Bonferroni-corrected $p = .017$). After extinction, only the difference between CS^{neg} and CS^{pos} cues was still significant, $t(19) = 4.76$, $p<.001$ (Bonferroni-corrected $p = .017$).

US ratings

The analysis of the US ratings revealed that the different gestures which served as US during conditioning were rated as differentially arousing as expected, $F(2,38) = 6.01$, $p = .005$, $\eta_p^2 = .24$. The middle finger gesture ($M = 5.80$, $SD = 1.74$) was rated as more arousing than the point gesture ($M = 4.15$, $SD = 1.76$), $t(19) = 3.38$, $p = .003$, whereas the arousal rating of the thumbs-up gesture ($M = 5.40$, $SD = 1.54$) was only marginally higher than the neutral point gesture, $t(19) = 5.93$, $p = .024$ (Bonferroni-corrected $p = .017$). No difference emerged between middle finger and thumbs-up gesture, $t(19) = 1.05$, $p = .31$. With regard to valence, ratings were also modulated by type of pictures, $F(2,38) = 85.21$, $p<.001$, $\eta_p^2 = .82$. As expected, the insult gesture ($M = 2.90$, $SD = 1.12$) was rated more unpleasant, whereas thumbs-up gesture was rated as more pleasant ($M = 7.30$,

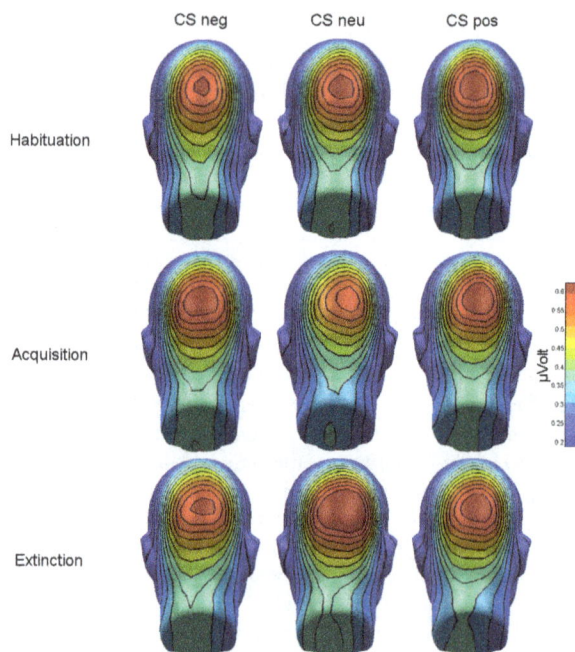

Figure 4. Mean scalp topographies of ssVEP amplitudes (100–4,900 ms) elicited by CS^{neg}, CS^{neu}, and CS^{pos} faces in during the three phases of the experiment (habituation, acquisition, extinction).

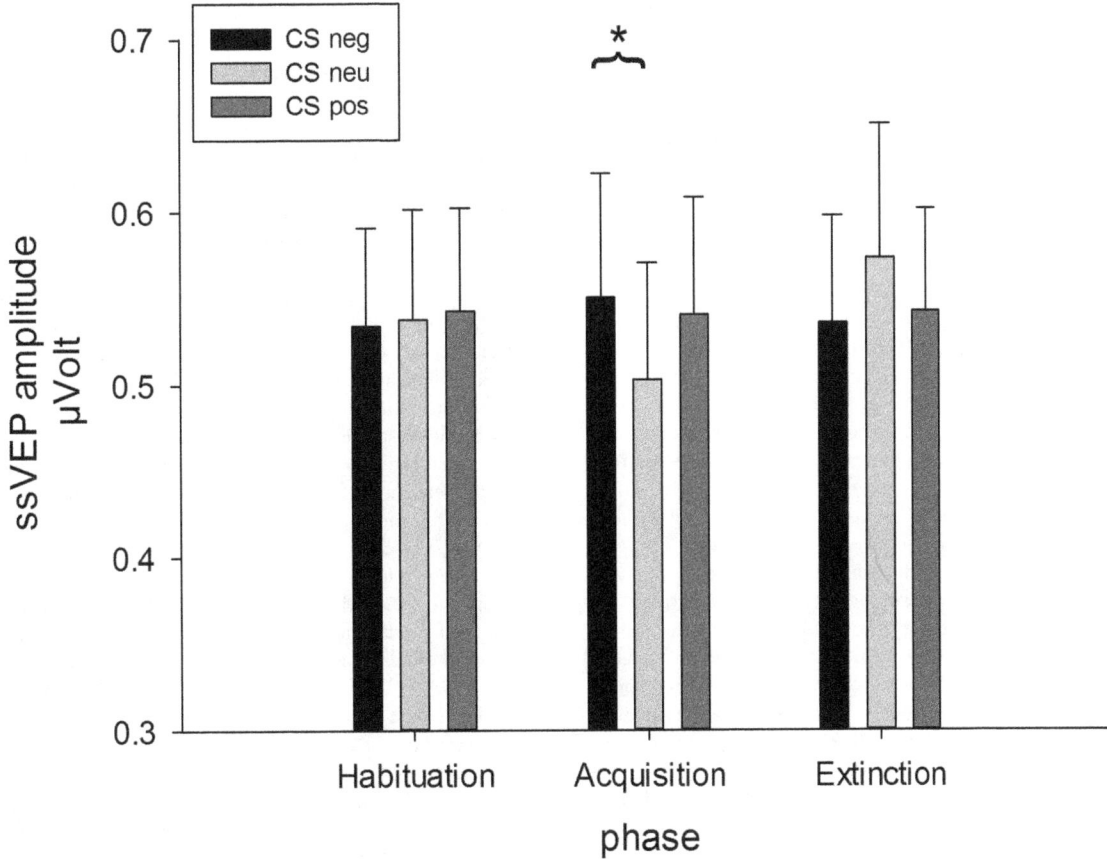

Figure 5. Mean ssVEP amplitudes (100–4,900 ms) +SEM evoked by CS^neg, CS^neu, and CS^pos faces in during the three phases of the experiment (habituation, acquisition, extinction). Amplitudes are averaged across a medial-occipital cluster comprising Oz and its 7 nearest neighbors.

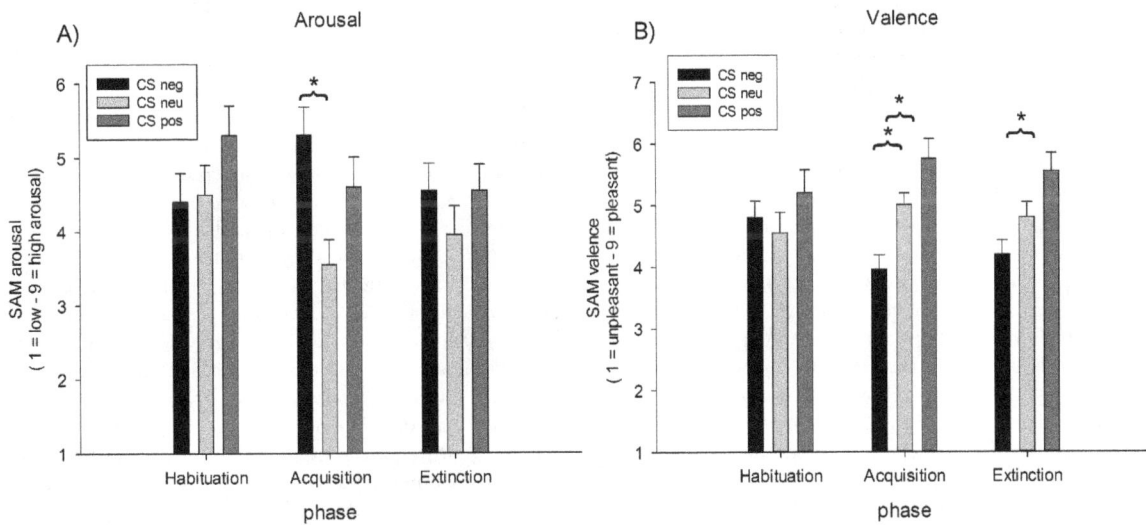

Figure 6. Mean SAM affective ratings collected after each phase. A) Mean arousal ratings (+SEM) of CS^neg, CS^neu, and CS^pos faces, B) mean valence ratings (+SEM) of CS^neg, CS^neu, and CS^pos faces.

$SD = 0.80$) than the neutral point gesture ($M = 4.55$, $SD = 0.95$), $t(19) = 4.44$, $p < .001$, and $t(19) = 9.23$, $p < .001$.

Contingency ratings

The analysis of correctly identified contingencies per category did not reveal any differences between CS types, $F(2,38) = 1.48$, $p = .241$, $\eta_p^2 = .07$. Faces were correctly identified as CS^{neg} in 97.5%, as CS^{neu} in 98.0%, and as CS^{pos} in 99.5% of cases.

Discussion

Faces associated with negative social cues (raised middle fingers) elicited stronger mass neuronal responses within the visual cortex compared to faces associated with neutral social signals. No differences were found between face-evoked cortical activity in response to faces that indicated negative compared to positive social consequences, however, the difference between neutrally and positively associated faces was only small. Affective ratings confirm these findings, but also demonstrate longer-lasting effects in explicit ratings, as differences were still observable after the extinction phase. Altogether, the findings suggest that response gain in local cortical population activity is modulated by the acquired social and motivational significance of the faces.

The enhanced electrocortical activation in response to faces predictive of negative social signals indicates that social conditioning alters visuocortical processing in a similar manner as more conventional aversive conditioning in which gratings were associated with aversive sounds or electrical shocks [9,10,30,31,32,41]. These adaptive changes in function of early visual cortices leads to augmented sensory gain and consequently enhanced processing of CS+ related features [44]. This change in sensory processing during social fear acquisition may be due to transient plasticity of sensory cortical networks [45]. Most likely, this short-term plasticity related to the individual learning history is due to re-entrant modulations of visual areas both by sub-cortical areas such as the amygdala as well as top-down influences of the fronto-parietal attention network. This corroborates findings which demonstrated that the amygdala shows elevated responses to socially conditioned stimuli [13,14,16]. Findings of conditioned responses in the lateral amygdala [46] and thalamus [47] preceding those that are observed in the primary sensory cortices support the notion that subcortical centers are necessary for the induction of sustained fear-related plasticity in the cortex. The amygdala can serve to enhance visual cortex activity given extensive bidirectional connectivity between amygdalar nuclei and multiple stages of visual hierarchy known to exist in the brains of human and non-human animals [48]. However, endogenous processes within sensory cortices may also underlie some transient forms of plasticity [49] in sensory cortical areas.

Notably, the amplification of sensory processing in response to socially conditioned faces bears striking similarities to the enhanced processing of visual cues which are inherently threatening such as aversive pictures or threatening faces [50,51]. Thus, sensory cortices seem to preferentially react to threatening information regardless of their threat values to be acquired by associated learning processes or inherent due to preparedness mechanisms of phylogenetic origin [52]. This observation is also in line with assumptions that sensory cortical networks are rather characterized as being highly adaptive and continuously shaped by the organism's learning history than just holding invariant representations of the external world [53,54]. Thus, features that are especially predictive of negative outcomes due to a learning history lead to enhanced sensory gain [41]. Future research may compare differences in the processing of inherent and acquired

threat cues directly to further shed light on the nature of the development of anxiety and anxiety disorders [55].

The nature of the US in the present study (affective symbolic gestures) points at the notion that nonverbal socio-communicative signals may serve as cues in social learning experience. Given the high emotional significance of particularly the aversive raised middle finger gesture [17,19], it seems plausible to regard the current paradigm as an excellent model for real-life situations in which subjects are exposed to social stress and form their impressions based on the social consequences they experienced with the very person. The result of the strongest learning effect with the negative gesture (raised middle finger) is in line with enhanced early cortical activity observed in the processing of this gesture of insult [19], which is most likely due to its immediate association with social threat and need of urgent action [17]. In line with other studies [13,14,16] using more ecologically valid US such as human voices, faces, verbal feedback, our results confirm that an emotional nonverbal gesture is sufficient to cause conditioning and modulate responses in the visual cortex. It has to be noted that this effect is observed although the US (picture) clearly is much less intense than conventional US such as electrical stimuli. Altogether, the present results make the paradigm of social conditioning with nonverbal gestures an interesting avenue for research on social learning and altered social conditioning in social anxiety, where enhanced sensitivity to social conditioning is assumed [15]. It has to be noted that the current paradigm is also a particular form of evaluative conditioning, in which pairings of positive or negative stimuli (US) with neutral stimuli (CS) induce the learning of evaluative reactions to the target stimuli [56]. Thus, originally neutral faces adopt the evaluative color of the US gestures with which they have been paired previously. Further research needs to clarify whether social conditioning is a different phenomenon such that social CS and US lead to stronger associative learning compared to evaluative conditioning by the easier association of two stimuli social in nature, i.e. a face and nonverbal gesture versus a face and aversive picture of a snake, for example. One may assume that social conditioning as presented here leads to stronger effects for implicit measures (such as visuocortical responses), which have been found to be rather weak in more conventional evaluative conditioning paradigms [57].

The present findings also add to the notion that the perception and evaluation of faces is critically dependent on the context in which faces appear [58,59]. For example, it has been shown in several studies where faces were combined with emotional bodies that a congruent affective value of the body helps the identification of the facial expression [60,61]. An important difference between these studies and the present study is that in our study the face gains affective value in a learning procedure through repeated association with affective gestures, whereas in the studies mentioned above the faces themselves were inherently affective (e.g., angry or happy facial expressions), but this recognition of this affective value was facilitated by congruent affective body postures. Nevertheless, both lines of research point to the notion that the affective value of a face is influenced by contextual factors such as concurrent affective body postures or learned associations between faces and affective gestures.

It also has to be noted that the faces paired with positive affective gestures also showed slightly higher electrocortical signal amplitudes compared to neutral faces, albeit non-significant. This effect which may have missed statistical significance due to statistical power, possibly indicates that the observed contextual modulation of face perception may not be entirely exclusive to negative USs, but that faces associated with positive outcomes may also attract more attention compared to neutrally associated faces.

In accordance with this notion, the positive hand gesture has consistently been shown to also receive priority processing which, however, is considerably reduced as compared to the higher arousing negative middle finger gesture [17,19].

Conclusion

The current study introduces a social conditioning paradigm incorporating socially relevant US of nonverbal affective gestures. The ssVEP in response to the CS faces as well as subjective ratings indicate that faces combined with aversive hand gestures (raised middle finger) are perceived as more negative and arousing, which is also accompanied by elevated visuocortical processing. Such results highlight the importance of using ecologically valid US in

conditioning when social learning processes in impression formation are the main area of interest. Moreover, the current paradigm offers a potential means for the study of social learning and its modulation in psychiatric disorders with deficits in social information processing such as in social anxiety disorder and autism.

Author Contributions

Conceived and designed the experiments: MW. Performed the experiments: MW. Analyzed the data: MW. Contributed reagents/materials/analysis tools: TF. Contributed to the writing of the manuscript: MW TF PP.

References

1. Alvarez RP, Chen G, Bodurka J, Kaplan R, Grillon C (2011) Phasic and sustained fear in humans elicits distinct patterns of brain activity. Neuroimage 55: 389–400
2. Andreatta M, Fendt M, Muhlberger A, Wieser MJ, Imobersteg S, et al. (2012) Onset and offset of aversive events establish distinct memories requiring fear and reward networks. Learn Mem 19: 518–526.
3. Kalisch R, Korenfeld E, Stephan KE, Weiskopf N, Seymour B, et al. (2006) Context-Dependent Human Extinction Memory is Mediated by a Ventromedial Prefrontal and Hippocampal Network. The Journal of Neuroscience 26: 9503–9511.
4. Knight DC, Cheng DT, Smith CN, Stein EA, Helmstetter FJ (2004) Neural Substrates Mediating Human Delay and Trace Fear Conditioning. The Journal of Neuroscience 24: 218–228.
5. Phelps EA, Delgado MR, Nearing KI, LeDoux JE (2004) Extinction learning in humans: role of the amygdala and vmPFC. Neuron 43: 897–905.
6. Büchel C, Dolan RJ (2000) Classical fear conditioning in functional neuroimaging. Current opinion in neurobiology 10: 219–223.
7. Büchel C, Dolan RJ, Armony JL, Friston KJ (1999) Amygdala-hippocampal involvement in human aversive trace conditioning revealed through event-related functional magnetic resonance imaging. The Journal of Neuroscience 19: 10869–10876.
8. Dunsmoor JE, Bandettini PA, Knight DC (2008) Neural correlates of unconditioned response diminution during Pavlovian conditioning. Neuroimage 40: 811–817.
9. Miskovic V, Keil A (2013) Visuocortical changes during delay and trace aversive conditioning: Evidence from steady-state visual evoked potentials. Emotion 13: 554.
10. Miskovic V, Keil A (2013) Perceiving Threat In the Face of Safety: Excitation and Inhibition of Conditioned Fear in Human Visual Cortex. The Journal of Neuroscience 33: 72–78.
11. Gottfried JA, Dolan RJ (2004) Human orbitofrontal cortex mediates extinction learning while accessing conditioned representations of value. Nature neuroscience 7: 1144–1152.
12. Nitschke JB, Sarinopoulos I, Mackiewicz KL, Schaefer HS, Davidson RJ (2006) Functional neuroanatomy of aversion and its anticipation. Neuroimage 29: 106–116.
13. Davis FC, Johnstone T, Mazzulla EC, Oler JA, Whalen PJ (2010) Regional response differences across the human amygdaloid complex during social conditioning. Cerebral Cortex 20: 612–621.
14. Iidaka T, Saito DN, Komeda H, Mano Y, Kanayama N, et al. (2010) Transient Neural Activation in Human Amygdala Involved in Aversive Conditioning of Face and Voice. Journal of Cognitive Neuroscience 22: 2074–2085.
15. Lissek S, Levenson J, Biggs AL, Johnson LL, Ameli R, et al. (2008) Elevated fear conditioning to socially relevant unconditioned stimuli in social anxiety disorder. American Journal of Psychiatry 165: 124.
16. Pejic T, Hermann A, Vaitl D, Stark R (2013) Social anxiety modulates amygdala activation during social conditioning. Social cognitive and affective neuroscience 8: 267–276.
17. Flaisch T, Hacker F, Renner B, Schupp HT (2011) Emotion and the processing of symbolic gestures: An event-related brain potential study. Social cognitive and affective neuroscience 6: 109–118.
18. Flaisch T, Schupp HT (2013) Tracing the time course of emotion perception: the impact of stimulus physics and semantics on gesture processing. Soc Cogn Affect Neurosci 8: 820–827.
19. Flaisch T, Schupp HT, Renner B, Junghofer M (2009) Neural systems of visual attention responding to emotional gestures. Neuroimage 45: 1339–1346.
20. Regan D (1989) Human Brain Electrophysiology: Evoked Potentials and Evoked Magnetic Fields in Science and Medicine. New York: Elsevier.
21. Vialatte F-B, Maurice M, Dauwels J, Cichocki A (2010) Steady-state visually evoked potentials: Focus on essential paradigms and future perspectives. Progress in Neurobiology In Press, Corrected Proof.
22. Wang J, Clementz BA, Keil A (2007) The neural correlates of feature-based selective attention when viewing spatially and temporally overlapping images. Neuropsychologia 45: 1393–1399.
23. Nunez PL, Srinivasan R (2006) Electric fields of the brain: The neurophysics of EEG. New York, NY: Oxford University Press.
24. Keil A, Gruber T, Müller MM, Moratti S, Stolarova M, et al. (2003) Early modulation of visual perception by emotional arousal: evidence from steady-state visual evoked brain potentials. Cognitive, Affective, & Behavioral Neuroscience 3: 195–206.
25. Andersen SK, Müller MM (2010) Behavioral performance follows the time course of neural facilitation and suppression during cued shifts of feature-selective attention. Proceedings of the National Academy of Sciences of the United States of America 107: 13878–13882.
26. Müller MM, Teder-Salejarvi W, Hillyard SA (1998) The time course of cortical facilitation during cued shifts of spatial attention. Nature Neuroscience 1: 631–634.
27. Müller MM, Teder W, Hillyard SA (1997) Magnetoencephalographic recording of steady-state visual evoked cortical activity. Brain Topography 9: 163–168.
28. Wieser MJ, Keil A (2011) Temporal Trade-Off Effects in Sustained Attention: Dynamics in Visual Cortex Predict the Target Detection Performance during Distraction. The Journal of Neuroscience 31: 7784.
29. Di Russo F, Pitzalis S, Aprile T, Spitoni G, Patria F, et al. (2007) Spatiotemporal analysis of the cortical sources of the steady-state visual evoked potential. Human Brain Mapping 28: 323–334.
30. Keil A, Miskovic V, Gray MJ, Martinovic J (2013) Luminance, but not chromatic visual pathways, mediate amplification of conditioned danger signals in human visual cortex. European Journal of Neuroscience 38: 3356–3362.
31. Moratti S, Keil A (2005) Cortical activation during Pavlovian fear conditioning depends on heart rate response patterns: an MEG study. Cognitive Brain Research 25: 459–471.
32. Moratti S, Keil A, Miller GA (2006) Fear but not awareness predicts enhanced sensory processing in fear conditioning. Psychophysiology 43: 216–226.
33. Langner O, Dotsch R, Bijlstra G, Wigboldus DHJ, Hawk ST, et al. (2010) Presentation and validation of the Radboud Faces Database. Cognition and Emotion 24: 1377–1388.
34. Kret ME, De Gelder B (2012) A review on sex differences in processing emotional signals. Neuropsychologia 50: 1211–1221.
35. Bradley MM, Lang PJ (1994) Measuring emotion: The Self-Assessment Manikin and the semantic differential. Journal of Behavior Therapy and Experimental Psychiatry 25: 49–59.
36. Peyk P, De Cesarei A, Junghöfer M (2011) Electro Magneto Encephalography Software: overview and integration with other EEG/MEG toolboxes. Computational Intelligence and Neuroscience 2011: Article ID 861705.
37. Junghöfer M, Elbert T, Tucker DM, Rockstroh B (2000) Statistical control of artifacts in dense array EEG/MEG studies. Psychophysiology 37: 523–532.
38. Kiebel SJ, Tallon-Baudry C, Friston KJ (2005) Parametric analysis of oscillatory activity as measured with EEG/MEG. Human Brain Mapping 26: 170–177.
39. Gruss LF, Wieser MJ, Schweinberger S, Keil A (2012) Face-evoked steady-state visual potentials: effects of presentation rate and face inversion. Frontiers in Human Neuroscience 6.
40. McTeague LM, Shumen JR, Wieser MJ, Lang PJ, Keil A (2011) Social vision: Sustained perceptual enhancement of affective facial cues in social anxiety. Neuroimage 54: 1615–1624.
41. Miskovic V, Keil A (2014) Escape from harm: Linking affective vision and motor responses during active avoidance. Social Cognitive and Affective Neuroscience: doi:10.1093/scan/nsu1013.
42. Wieser MJ, McTeague LM, Keil A (2012) Competition effects of threatening faces in social anxiety. Emotion 12: 1050–1060.
43. Picton TW, Bentin S, Berg P, Donchin E, Hillyard SA, et al. (2000) Guidelines for using human event-related potentials to study cognition: recording standards and publication criteria. Psychophysiology 37: 127–152.

44. Miskovic V, Keil A (2012) Acquired fears reflected in cortical sensory processing: A review of electrophysiological studies of human classical conditioning. Psychophysiology 49: 1230–1241.

45. Keil A, Stolarova M, Moratti S, Ray WJ (2007) Adaptation in human visual cortex as a mechanism for rapid discrimination of aversive stimuli. Neuroimage 36: 472–479.

46. Quirk GJ, Armony JL, LeDoux JE (1997) Fear conditioning enhances different temporal components of tone-evoked spike trains in auditory cortex and lateral amygdala. Neuron 19: 613–624.

47. Weinberger NM (2011) The medial geniculate, not the amygdala, as the root of auditory fear conditioning. Hear Res 274: 61–74.

48. Freese JL, Amaral DG (2009) Neuroanatomy of the primate amygdala. In: Whalen PJ, Phelps EA, editors. The human amygdala. New York, NY: Guilford Press. pp. 3–42.

49. Armony JL, Quirk GJ, LeDoux JE (1998) Differential effects of amygdala lesions on early and late plastic components of auditory cortex spike trains during fear conditioning. J Neurosci 18: 2592–2601.

50. Lang PJ, Bradley MM (2010) Emotion and the motivational brain. Biological psychology 84: 437–450.

51. Vuilleumier P (2005) How brains beware: neural mechanisms of emotional attention. Trends in Cognitive Sciences 9: 585–594.

52. Öhman A (2009) Of snakes and faces: An evolutionary perspective on the psychology of fear. Scandinavian journal of psychology 50: 543–552.

53. Engel AK, Fries P, Singer W (2001) Dynamic predictions: oscillations and synchrony in top–down processing. Nature Reviews Neuroscience 2: 704–716.

54. Gilbert CD, Sigman M (2007) Brain states: top-down influences in sensory processing. Neuron 54: 677–696.

55. Mineka S, Oehlberg K (2008) The relevance of recent developments in classical conditioning to understanding the etiology and maintenance of anxiety disorders. Acta psychologica 127: 567–580.

56. De Houwer J, Thomas S, Baeyens F (2001) Association learning of likes and dislikes: A review of 25 years of research on human evaluative conditioning. Psychological Bulletin 127: 853–869.

57. Hofmann W, De Houwer J, Perugini M, Baeyens F, Crombez G (2010) Evaluative conditioning in humans: a meta-analysis. Psychological bulletin 136: 390.

58. Hassin RR, Aviezer H, Bentin S (2013) Inherently ambiguous: Facial expressions of emotions, in context. Emotion Review 5: 60–65.

59. Wieser MJ, Brosch T (2012) Faces in context: A review and systematization of contextual influences on affective face processing. Frontiers in Psychology 3: 471.

60. Aviezer H, Trope Y, Todorov A (2012) Body cues, not facial expressions, discriminate between intense positive and negative emotions. Science 338: 1225–1229.

61. Kret ME, Stekelenburg JJ, Roelofs K, De Gelder B (2013) Perception of face and body expressions using electromyography, pupillometry and gaze measures. Frontiers in psychology 4.

11

Spatial Attention Effects of Disgusted and Fearful Faces

Dandan Zhang[1,2♥], Yunzhe Liu[2♥], Chenglin Zhou[3]*, Yuming Chen[1], Yuejia Luo[1]

1 Institute of Affective and Social Neuroscience, Shenzhen University, Shenzhen, China, **2** State Key Laboratory of Cognitive Neuroscience and Learning, Beijing Normal University, Beijing, China, **3** School of Kinesiology, Shanghai University of Sport, Shanghai, China

Abstract

Effective processing of threat-related stimuli is of significant evolutionary advantage. Given the intricate relationship between attention and the neural processing of threat-related emotions, this study manipulated attention allocation and emotional categories of threat-related stimuli as independent factors and investigated the time course of spatial-attention-modulated processing of disgusting and fearful stimuli. The participants were instructed to direct their attention either to the two vertical or to the two horizontal locations, where two faces and two houses would be presented. The task was to respond regarding the physical identity of the two stimuli at cued locations. Event-related potentials (ERP) evidences were found to support a two-stage model of attention-modulated processing of threat-related emotions. In the early processing stage, disgusted faces evoked larger P1 component at right occipital region despite the attention allocation while larger N170 component was elicited by fearful faces at right occipito-temporal region only when participants attended to houses. In the late processing stage, the amplitudes of the parietal P3 component enhanced for both disgusted and fearful facial expressions only when the attention was focused on faces. According to the results, we propose that the temporal dynamics of the emotion-by-attention interaction consist of two stages. The early stage is characterized by quick and specialized neural encoding of disgusting and fearful stimuli irrespective of voluntary attention allocation, indicating an automatic detection and perception of threat-related emotions. The late stage is represented by attention-gated separation between threat-related stimuli and neutral stimuli; the similar ERP pattern evoked by disgusted and fearful faces suggests a more generalized processing of threat-related emotions via top-down attentional modulation, based on which the defensive behavior in response to threat events is largely facilitated.

Editor: Cosimo Urgesi, University of Udine, Italy

Funding: This study was funded by the National Natural Science Foundation of China (31300867) and the National Basic Research Program of China (973 Program, 2014CB744600). The funders had no role in study design, data collection and analysis, decision to publish, or preparation of the manuscript.

Competing Interests: The authors have declared that no competing interests exist.

* Email: chenglin_600@126.com

♥ These authors contributed equally to this work.

Introduction

Rapid detection of impending danger is crucial for the interplay between humans and their environment. Our neural system has evolved to allow the expedient perception of potentially aversive stimuli [1]. In particular, humans always grant priority of attention allocation to threat-related stimuli; compared with non-threat events, humans disengage the fixation of attention more difficultly and less frequently from potentially dangerous events [2]. However, previous studies also suggested that the brain sometimes responses to threat automatically at the pre-attentive level [3,4]. Furthermore, attention may not be mandatory for the neural processing of all the threat-related information [1,5,6]. For example, both adults and young infants can response to threat involuntarily, without the focus of attention or even without the awareness of the stimulus occurrence [1,7,8].

Given the intricate relationship between emotion processing and attention, there is a need to manipulate attention allocation and emotional characteristics of stimuli (e.g., threat-related *vs.* non-threat-related; high-arousal *vs.* low-arousal) as independent factors and to investigate the interaction between them. However, most previous studies did not unambiguously discriminate between the focus of attention and emotion processing itself, thus failed to

demonstrate whether the privileged neural processing of threat-related information is independent of attention modulation [1,4,6–8]. Regarding the few studies that successfully distinguished the effects of attention and threat-related emotions, the results were inconsistent. For example, one functional magnetic resonance imaging (fMRI) study found that the blood-oxygen-level dependent (BOLD) signal of amygdala was larger in response to fearful faces as compared to neutral ones [9]. The authors also found that this emotion effect was not modulated by attention, suggesting that fearful stimuli may be detected pre-attentively [9]. Conversely, another fMRI study indicated that the attention influenced the amygdala function; compared with the unattended condition, the amygdala showed larger activity in the attend-to-fearful-face condition [10]. The discrepancy in these two studies may be due to the intrinsic limitation of fMRI technique: the BOLD signal varies slowly as compared to the rapidly-changed neuroelectrical activity, which may prevent the fMRI device from capturing the transient fluctuations of neural characteristics in these studies [11].

Meanwhile, although threatening events are typically associated with heightened neural responses [8,12], the model of threat-related processing is usually oversimplified with almost exclusive focus on the emotion of fear; other threat-related emotions have been overlooked in most of the previous literatures [13]. In the present study, we investigated and compared two subtypes of threat-related emotions, namely, fear and disgust. These two emotions represent different biological systems—the "self protection system" [14] and the "disease avoidance system" [15], respectively. Previous researches have demonstrated that fearful and disgusting emotions could induce divergent physiological responses and cognitive processes, i.e., disgust tends to activate parasympathetic system and suppresses action while fear stimulates sympathetic pathways and prompts fight or flight [16]; disgust provokes instant sensory rejection, whereas fear quickly orients attention so as to ensure sensory acquisition [17]. Vermeulen, Godefroid, & Mermillod employed an attentional blink task (with emotional faces as primes) and found that compared with the neutral faces, disgusted faces were associated with reduced attentional blinks [18]. One recent event-related potential (ERP) study asked participants to search the horizontal bar among seven vertical bars with fearful, disgusting or neutral affective pictures as visual background, which found a rapid discrimination between the two threat-related emotions as early as 96 ms after stimulus onset, represented by larger occipital P1 amplitudes in fearful condition and smaller P1 amplitudes in disgusting condition, compared with those in neutral condition [19]. However, while disgust is frequently considered as a warning signal for biological/psychological contamination and usually results in avoidant behavior [15], a few studies indicated that disgusting stimuli sometimes capture attention even faster than fearful stimuli [20]. For example, it is found in a masked presentation task that participants responded faster to disgusting words than to fearful or neutral words [21]. It is believed that the quick, early attention effects on different threat-related emotions could be further disclosed using the ERP technique, which has a high time resolution and could follow the neural dynamics timely.

Relevant studies have also suggested that after the early specialized processing, as described above, the threat-related emotions are further analyzed via a relatively general procedure with top-down modulation so as to facilitate subsequent defensive behavior; and that the attentional resources are necessary and essential at this stage. For example, one ERP study found that after an early P1 discrimination (peaked at 115 ms post-stimulus) between fearful and disgusting pictures, late ERP components within the time window of 388–425 ms converged between the two threat-related emotions [22]. In another ERP study, participants were presented with a rapid and continuous stream of high- and low-arousing affective pictures; the researchers found that high-arousing pictures evoked larger N2 amplitudes (~200 to 350 ms after stimulus onset) than low-arousing pictures both in attended and unattended conditions; in contrast, the P3 amplitudes (~400 to 600 ms) were markedly enhanced in high-arousing condition compared with low-arousing condition only when participants paid attention to the affective pictures [2]. Thus, unlike the early stage of the neural processing of threat-related emotions, the later stage may demand sufficient attention focused on target stimuli.

The present study employed ERPs to investigate whether the neural processing of fearful and disgusting stimuli is independent of attentional modulation. We manipulated spatial attention (i.e., stimuli appeared at attended or unattended locations) and emotional categories of presented stimuli as independent factors and examined the time course of the emotion-by-attention interaction. We hypothesized that fear and disgust may have distinct encoding patterns at early stage of attention-modulated processing, followed by a late, more generalized processing of threat-related information that may be strongly influenced by

attention. Previous ERP studies have indicated that two early ERP components, namely the occipital P1 and the occipito-temporal N170, are sensitive to both attention and emotion effects [1,23–25]. Besides P1 and N170, the N2pc has recently been proposed to be an effective biomarker of attention shift or selection [26]. For example, when the facial configuration contained both eyebrows and eyes, threatening angry targets showed a more pronounced occipital N2pc between 200 and 300 ms than friendly facial targets, which indicated that the advantage of rapid prioritized attention to facial threat is not driven by low-level visual features [27]. In addition, the centro-parietal P3 is typically found to reflect the neural process of selective spatial attention and serves as a measure of top-down modulation [28]. Therefore, it is expected that early ERP components such as P1 and N170 would show different patterns between emotion subtypes of fear and disgust, and that the amplitudes of later ERP components (e.g. P3) may be enhanced in both fearful and disgusting conditions, but only when participants paid attention to emotional stimuli.

Methods

Participants

Thirty-one healthy subjects (15 females; age range $= 21$ to 27 years) were recruited from Beijing Normal University in China as paid participants. All participants were right-handed and had normal or corrected-to-normal vision. They gave their written informed consent prior to the experiment. The individuals whose photographs are shown in this manuscript have given written informed consent (as outlined in PLOS consent form) to publish their photographs. The experimental protocol was approved by the local ethics committee (Beijing Normal University).

Stimuli

Faces were black and white photographs selected from the native Chinese Facial Affective Picture System (CFAPS) [29], with equal number of face pictures between males and females. A total of 60 faces (20 disgusted, 20 fearful, and 20 neutral faces) were used. Each picture had been assessed for its valence and arousal on a 9-point scale with a large sample of Chinese participants in a previous survey. The ANOVA performed on the average scores showed that the two categories of negative faces did not differ significantly in emotional valence ($F(2,38) = 172$, $p<.001$, $\eta_p^2 = .900$; mean $\pm$ standard deviation (SD): disgust $= 3.24\pm0.33$, fear $= 3.06\pm0.38$, neutral $= 4.81\pm0.24$; disgust $vs.$ fear: $p=.433$) or arousal ($F(2,38) = 1.54$, $p=.227$, $\eta_p^2 = .075$; disgust $= 5.69\pm0.45$, fear $= 5.78\pm0.52$, neutral $= 5.50\pm0.35$; disgust $vs.$ fear: $p=1.000$) while their valence ratings significantly differed from neutral faces (ps$<.001$). Of note, to prevent our results from being contaminated by the arousal across three emotional conditions, the 20 neutral faces were selected as with a relatively high arousal from a total of 422 neutral faces in the CFAPS (valence $= 4.29\pm0.52$; arousal $= 3.84\pm0.69$ of the 422 neutral faces). A total of 60 pictures of front-view houses were selected from internet. All stimuli were presented with the same contrast and brightness on the black background ($3.0°\times3.5°$ visual angle).

Procedure

The experimental procedure was similar to those employed in previous fMRI [9,30,31] and ERP studies [32]. Participants were seated in a dimly lit and sound-attenuated room. Stimuli were presented on a LCD monitor at a viewing distance of 100 cm. The experiment consisted of six blocks, each containing 64 trials.

Stimulus display and behavioral data acquisition were conducted using E-Prime 1.2 (Psychology Software Tools, Inc., Pittsburgh, PA). During the experiment, participants were required to always fix their eyes on the white cross in the center of the screen. As shown in Figure 1, each trial started with a 100-ms cue that consisted of two white rectangles ($3.0° \times 3.5°$ visual angle). The cue instructed subjects to direct their attention either to the two vertical or to the two horizontal locations; the stimulus pair at uncued locations should be ignored. After the cue, an interval was presented with the duration of 200 to 300 ms. Then two faces and two houses were presented for 300 ms. The two faces in each trial have the same emotion category and the same gender, which were selected randomly from one of the three facial expression categories and from one of the two genders. After the presentation of face/house stimulus array, subjects were required to respond as quickly and accurately as possible regarding the physical identity of the two stimuli at cued locations, with a "yes" key for an identical pair and a "no" key for a different pair. The response screen would not disappear until a button press or until 1500 ms elapsed. The inter-trial interval was 1000 ms. Participants were instructed to press the "F" and "J" buttons on the computer keyboard with their left and right index fingers. The assignment of keys to "yes" and "no" responses was counterbalanced across participants. In each block, the location (vertical *vs.* horizontal) of face and house pairs varied randomly across trials. The vertical and horizontal positions were equally likely cued or uncued.

EEG recording and ERP analysis

Brain electrical activity was recorded referentially against left mastoid and off-line re-referenced to the average of the left and right mastoids, by a 64-channel amplifier with a sampling frequency of 250 Hz (NeuroScan Inc., Herndon, USA). Besides electrooculogram electrodes, a 62-channel electroencephalography (EEG) data were collected with electrode impedances kept below 5 kΩ. Both vertical and horizontal ocular artifacts were removed from the EEG data using a regression procedure implemented in Neuroscan software (Scan 4.3). In particular, two electrooculogram templates (one for vertical and one for horizontal eye movements) were calculated from the EEG data. Then the software removed the ocular artifacts by performing two regression procedures.

The data analysis and result display in this study were performed using Matlab R2011a (MathWorks, Natick, USA). The recorded EEG data were filtered with a 0.01–30 Hz finite impulse response filter with zero phase distortion. Filtered data were segmented beginning 200 ms prior to the onset of face/house stimulus array and lasting for 1200 ms. All epochs were baseline-corrected with respect to the mean voltage over the 200 ms preceding the onset of the face/house stimulus array, followed by averaging in association with experimental conditions.

In the present study, we focused on the ERPs elicited by disgusted, fearful, and neutral facial expressions and in attend-to-face and attend-to-house conditions. The individual average ERPs of the 31 subjects were computed based on behaviorally correct trials, thus leading to 9.92 ± 5.84 trials (mean ± SD) being excluded from the data per condition per subject (the minimum number of accepted trials per condition in the individual average ERP was 39). The data were derived from all electrodes, but only the electrodes at which the components reached their peak values were entered into statistical analysis. We analyzed the potentials of occipital P1, occipito-temporal N170, and parietal P3 components across different sets of electrodes according to grand-mean ERP topographies. Time windows for mean amplitude calculation were centered at the peak latencies of ERP components in grand-mean waveforms, with a shorter window length for early components and a longer length for late component. The mean amplitudes of P1 were calculated at O1 and O2 within the time window of 100–130 ms [19,22]. The mean amplitudes of N170 were calculated at P7 and P8 within the time window of 170–200 ms [1,23]. The mean amplitudes of P3 were calculated at CPz and Pz within the time window of 520–680 ms [2,33].

Statistics

Statistical analyses were performed using SPSS Statistics 20.0 (IBM, Somers, USA). Descriptive data were presented as mean ± SD. The significance level was set at 0.05. Two-way repeated-measures ANOVAs were performed on measurements of accuracy rate (ACC), reaction time (RT), and the P3 amplitude, with emotion (disgust, fear, and neutral) and attention (attend to faces and attend to houses) as the two within-subject factors. Three-way repeated measures ANOVAs on the amplitudes of P1 and N170 components were conducted with emotion, attention, and hemisphere (left and right) as within-subject factors. Greenhouse-Geisser correction for ANOVA tests was used whenever appropriate. Post-hoc testing of significant main effects was conducted using Bonferroni method. Significant interactions were analyzed using simple effects model. Partial eta-squared (η_p^2) was reported to demonstrate the effect size in ANOVA tests, where 0.05 represents a small effect, 0.10 indicates a medium effect, and 0.20 represents a large effect. For the sake of brevity, effects that did not reach significance have been omitted.

Results

Behaviors

ACC. The main effect of emotion was significant ($F(2,60) = 25.1$; $p < .001$; $\eta_p^2 = .456$). The ACC in neutral condition (0.812 ± 0.107) was smaller than that in disgusting

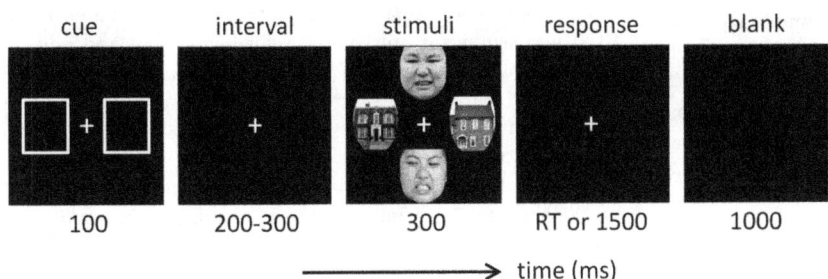

cue	interval	stimuli	response	blank
100	200–300	300	RT or 1500	1000

time (ms)

Figure 1. Illustration of one experimental trial in this study.

(0.862±0.081; $p<$.001) and fearful conditions (0.861±0.075; $p<$ .001).

The main effect of attention was significant ($F(1,30)=32.4$; $p<$ .001; $\eta_p^2 =.519$). The ACC in attend-to-face trials (0.812±0.102) was smaller than that in attend-to-house trials (0.878±0.065).

The interaction effect of emotion by attention was significant ($F(2,60)=27.5$; $p<$.001; $\eta_p^2 =.478$). Simple effect analysis showed that the emotion effect was significant in attend-to-face condition ($F(2,60)=47.7$; $p<$.001; disgust $=0.843\pm0.089$; fear $=0.847$ ±0.083; neutral $=0.747\pm0.101$) while there was no significant emotion effect in attend-to-house condition ($F(2,60)<1$; disgust $=0.880\pm0.069$; fear $=0.876\pm0.063$; neutral $=0.878\pm0.065$).

RT. The main effect of emotion was significant ($F(2,60)=6.07$; $p=.004$; $\eta_p^2 =.168$). The RT in neutral condition (773±89.7 ms) was longer than that in disgusting condition (741±87.2 ms; $p=.006$) while the neutral and fearful (761±91.9 ms) conditions showed no significant difference ($p=.123$).

The main effect of attention was significant ($F(1,30)=4.76$; $p=.037$; $\eta_p^2 =.137$). The RT in attend-to-face trials (765±96.5 ms) was larger than that in attend-to-house trials (752±83.2 ms).

The interaction effect of emotion by attention was significant ($F(2,60)=10.5$; $p<$.001; $\eta_p^2 =.259$). Simple effect analysis showed that the emotion effect was significant in attend-to-face condition ($F(2,60)=10.2$; $p<$.001; disgust $=741\pm91.7$ ms; fear $=764$ ±98.3 ms; neutral $=789\pm96.3$ ms) while there was no significant emotion effect in attend-to-house condition ($F(2,60)=2.07$; $p=.135$; disgust $=741\pm84.0$ ms; fear $=758\pm86.4$ ms; neutral $=757\pm80.8$ ms).

ERPs

P1. The main effect of emotion was significant ($F(2,60)=5.14$; $p=.009$; $\eta_p^2 =.146$). The P1 amplitude in response to disgusted faces (1.75±1.45 μV) was larger than that in response to fearful (1.40±1.79 μV; $p=.015$) and neutral faces (1.40±1.68 μV; $p=.017$).

The main effect of attention was significant ($F(1,30)=9.97$; $p=.004$; $\eta_p^2 =.249$). The P1 amplitude was larger when participants paid attention to faces (1.66±1.68 μV) than to houses (1.37±1.61 μV).

The interaction effect of emotion by hemisphere was significant ($F(2,60)=3.45$; $p=.038$; $\eta_p^2 =.103$) (Figure 2). Simple effect analysis indicated that the emotion effect on P1 was significant at the right hemisphere ($F(2,60)=9.11$; $p<$.001); the disgusted faces (1.94±1.23 μV) elicited larger P1 amplitudes than did fearful (1.29±1.56 μV) and neutral faces (1.27±1.49 μV). However, this emotion effect was not significant at the left hemisphere ($F(2,60)<$ 1).

N170. The main effect of attention was significant ($F(1,30)=44.8$; $p<$.001; $\eta_p^2 =.599$). The N170 amplitude was larger in attend-to-face condition (−6.27±4.39 μV) compared with that in attend-to-house condition (−4.66±3.62 μV).

The main effect of hemisphere was significant ($F(1,30)=19.5$; $p<$.001; $\eta_p^2 =.394$). The N170 amplitude in the left hemisphere was smaller (−3.70±2.94 μV) than that in the right hemisphere (−7.23±4.33 μV).

The interaction effect of emotion by hemisphere was significant ($F(2,60)=6.05$; $p=.004$; $\eta_p^2 =.168$). Simple effect analysis indicated that the emotion effect on N170 was significant at the right hemisphere ($F(2,60)=9.22$; $p<$.001); the N170 elicited by fearful faces (−7.72±4.43 μV) was larger than that elicited by

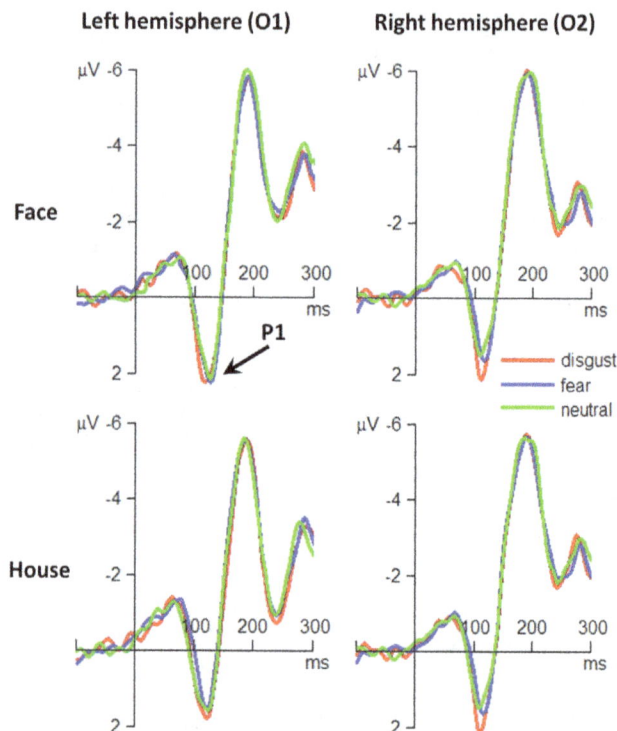

Figure 2. The grand-mean ERP waveforms at the occipital electrode sites of O1 and O2.

disgusted (−7.04±4.31 μV) and neutral faces (−6.93±4.28 μV). However, this emotion effect was not significant at the left hemisphere ($F(2,60)<1$).

The interaction effect of attention by hemisphere was significant ($F(1,30)=21.6$; $p<$.001; $\eta_p^2 =.419$). The attention effect was more significant at the right hemisphere ($F(1,30)=48.1$; $p<$.001) than at the left hemisphere ($F(1,30)=11.3$; $p=.002$). The N170 in attend-to-face condition (left $=-4.10\pm3.10$ μV; right $=$ -8.45 ± 4.42 μV) was larger than that in attend-to-house condition (left $=-3.31\pm2.73$ μV; right $=-6.01\pm3.90$ μV).

The interaction effect of emotion by attention was significant ($F(2,60)=4.08$; $p=.032$; $\eta_p^2 =.120$). The emotion effect was significant when participants attended to houses ($F(2,60)=5.61$; $p=.006$); the N170 elicited by fearful faces (−5.08±3.83 μV) was larger than that elicited by disgusted (−4.45±3.52 μV) and neutral faces (−4.44±3.52 μV). However, this emotion effect was not significant when participants attended to faces ($F(2,60)<1$).

The interaction effect of emotion by attention by hemisphere was significant ($F(2,60)=3.42$; $p=.043$; $\eta_p^2 =.102$) (Figure 3). Simple simple effect analysis indicated that the emotion effect on N170 was significant only at the right hemisphere and only in attend-to-house condition ($F(2,60)=18.4$; $p<$.001); the N170 elicited by fearful faces (−6.86±4.12 μV) was larger than that elicited by disgusted (−5.60±3.78 μV) and neutral faces (−5.57±3.75 μV).

P3. The main effect of emotion was significant ($F(2,60)=6.22$; $p=.004$; $\eta_p^2 =.172$) (Figure 4). The P3 amplitudes in response to disgusted (7.91±3.41 μV; $p=.025$) and fearful faces (7.69±4.06 μV; $p=.028$) were larger than those in response to neutral faces (6.63±4.16 μV).

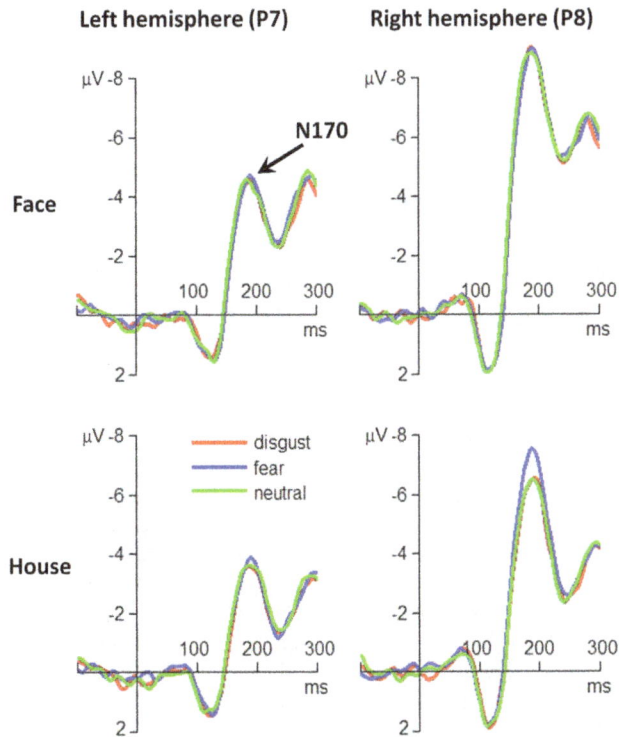

Figure 3. The grand-mean ERP waveforms at the occipito-temporal electrode sites of P7 and P8.

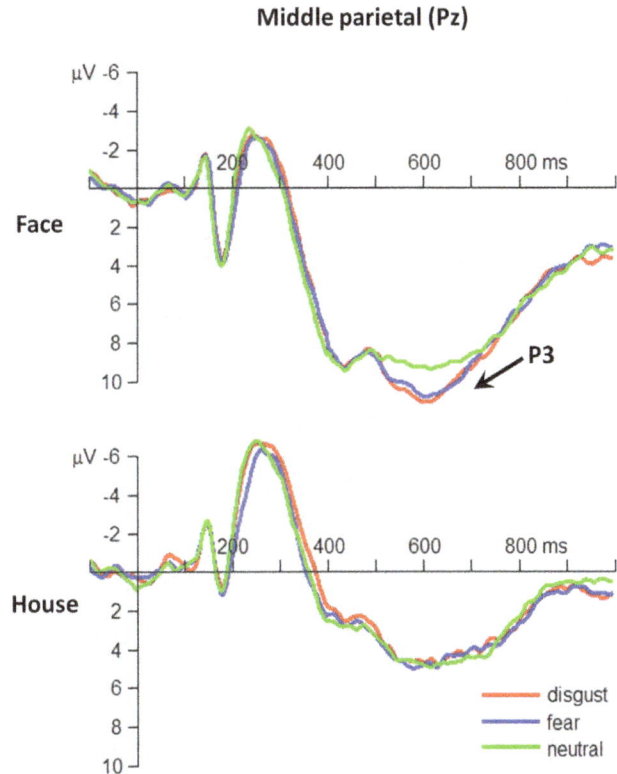

Figure 4. The grand-mean ERP waveforms at the middle parietal electrode site of Pz.

The main effect of attention was significant ($F(1,30) = 210$; $p < .001$; $\eta_p^2 = .875$). The P3 amplitude was larger when participants attended to faces (9.89 ± 3.32 μV) than to houses (4.92 ± 2.70 μV).

The grand-mean topographies of the ERP components of P1, N170, and P3 are shown in Figure 5.

Discussion

This study investigated the time course of the interaction effects between spatial attention and the two subtypes of threat-related emotions (fear vs. disgust). At the behavioral level, it was observed that fearful and disgusting stimuli resulted in higher ACC and shorter RT measures as compared to neutral stimuli, and that this phenomenon was only significant when participants attended to faces. At the electrophysiological level, we found neural evidences supporting a two-stage model of attention-modulated processing of threat-related emotions. The early stage was represented by the P1 and the N170 components that distinguished disgusting and fearful stimuli from neutral ones, respectively. In particular, the P1 component showed larger amplitudes in disgusting than in fearful and neutral conditions, irrespective of attention allocation. Meanwhile, the N170 component displayed larger amplitudes in fearful than in neutral and disgusting conditions when participants attended to houses. The late processing stage was represented by the P3 component, which was enhanced in response to both disgusted and fearful facial expressions when participants attended to faces.

The most novel finding of the present study is the neural evidence for early discrimination of disgusted faces, as evidenced by the larger P1 amplitude in disgusting condition compared with that in fearful and neutral conditions. The occipital P1 component has been proved to be sensitive to early emotional modulation in visual perception [24,25,34]. In this study, the enhanced P1

amplitude in response to disgusted faces was robust in both attended and unattended conditions, suggesting that disgusted faces can be detected without focus of attention at the early stage of emotion-related processing. Of note, the larger P1 evoked by disgusted faces is not necessarily contradictory to previous studies suggesting that disgusting stimuli suppress subsequent cognitive processing. For example, Krusemark and Li [19] observed in a visual searching task that the P1 amplitude following disgusting picture presentation was smaller than following fearful and neutral picture presentations. While Krusemark and Li [19] mainly investigated the influence of emotional stimuli on the subsequent cognitive processing (i.e., visual searching task), this study focused on the direct influence of the presented threat-related stimuli on the current task. Our finding of the early P1 separation between disgusting and neutral/fearful stimuli is consistent with previous behavioral evidences that suggested a neutral processing bias to disgusting information [20,21]. For example, people had more interference when responding to disgusting compared to fearful and neutral words in the Stroop color-naming task [20]; participants responded faster to disgusting words in the masked presentation task, compared with fearful and neutral conditions [21]. These converging behavioral and ERP evidences suggest a neutral bias to disgusting events/stimuli at early stage of emotion-related processing, which helps humans avoid potential contaminants timely and with a high success rate [21].

The early stage of attention-modulated emotion processing was also represented by larger occipito-temporal N170 amplitudes in fearful than in neutral and disgusting conditions. The N170 component is typically assumed to reflect structural encoding of faces and shows larger amplitudes for faces than other non-face objects [35,36]. More recent findings have suggested that the N170 is also modulated by emotional faces, with larger amplitudes

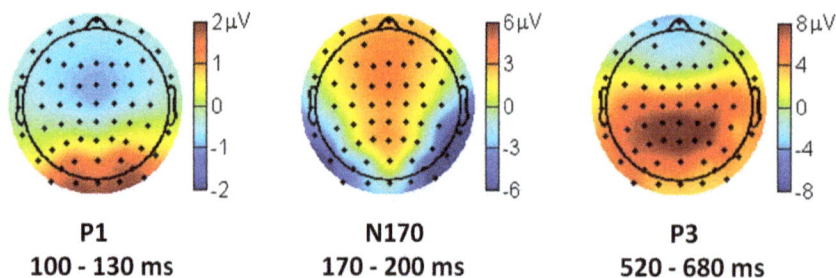

Figure 5. The grand-mean topographies of the P1, the N170, and the P3 components.

in response to fearful than neutral faces [9,12,23,25,37]. For example, employing a similar paradigm with in this study, Vuilleumier et al. [9] found that the right fusiform activity was influenced by emotional facial expressions, with a greater response to fearful than to neutral faces. However, the current finding seems to contradict the result obtained by Holmes et al. [5], who employed a very similar paradigm and found that the N170 component was unaffected by emotional facial expressions. The discrepancy between the present study and the Holmes' study may be due to the different tasks of participants (responses were required in a few *vs.* all trials in Holmes' and the present study, respectively) and/or different sets of electrode sites selected in the N170 analysis (T5 and T6 in Holmes' and P7 and P8 in this study). One of the most interesting results given by our data is the significant interaction between emotion and attention: the N170 showed larger amplitudes in fearful condition as compared to disgusting and neutral conditions only when participants attended to houses, i.e., when their attention was not focused on faces. It is known that fearful expressions are often associated with potential danger in the environment of which the source is usually undetermined [30]. It is of evolutionary advantage for fearful stimuli being processed rapidly, even when they occur in the periphery of the visual field [8,13,14]. Therefore, it is very likely that the attention capture effect of fearful faces is more prominent and easier to observe when participants pay their attention to emotion-irrelevant objects, such as the houses in this study [30]. In line with this interpretation, one previous fMRI research has found that amygdala showed larger activity in response to fearful faces, as compared to neutral and angry faces; and that this effect was only significant when the faces were out of attention [30].

The ERP data in the early processing stage of threat-related emotions indicated that the P1 component was able to separate disgust from fear and neutral in the attend-to-face condition. More importantly, we found that the discriminative index of disgusting stimuli (the P1) and fearful stimuli (the N170) were both valid in the unattended condition, suggesting that the early stage of threat-related processing may work automatically without specific attention allocation. In contrast, it was found that the later stage of emotion perception and interpretation was characterized as an attention-gated procedure, which was reflected by pronounced P3 amplitudes in fearful and disgusting conditions only when participants attended to faces. It has been proved that the amplitudes of the centro-parietal P3 component usually increase when the attention is allocated to target stimuli, as compared to unattended condition [38]. Therefore, it is believed that the P3 effect observed in this study indicated a voluntary attention modulation that occurred at the late stage of threat-related emotion processing [38,39]. In addition, previous studies have also found an arousal effect of the P3 component, i.e., the P3 shows larger amplitudes in response to high-arousal stimuli compared

with low-arousal or neutral stimuli [40,41]. By matching the arousal level of all the three categories of facial expressions (fear, disgust and neutral), the current finding of enhanced P3 amplitudes in disgusting and fearful conditions was highly unlikely to be attributed to the difference of arousal, but rather indicated the attention-modulation effect on threat-related emotion processing. Given the potential relationship between the P3 component and the top-down modulation [42–44], we further suggest that the late stage of threat-related processing may reflect a procedure of voluntary allocation of attention to biologically important events, with potential neural substrates located in the dorsal fronto-parietal pathways[40,45].

Some readers may note that the attend-to-face trials were associated with poorer performances (i.e., lower accuracy and longer reaction time) in this study. This result pattern may be due to the attention capture effect of facial expressions. It has been widely recognized that facial expressions are salient social signals, which tend to attract and hold attention more intensively as compared to other objects such as houses [46,47]. In the current study, when participants attended to faces, their attention was held by the emotion of faces, resulting in less attentional resources for the discrimination task. Therefore, attend-to-face condition had poorer behavioral performances as compared to attend-to-house condition. Furthermore, this attention capture effect of facial expressions may be more significant when the faces are threat-related [48,49]. Our finding is consistent with previous reports in the literature. For example, Vuilleumier et al. [9] found in a similar experiment that subjects made more errors in attend-to-face condition as compared to attend-to-house condition.

Conclusion

To sum up, the current study investigated the time course of spatial-attention-modulated processes of disgusting and fearful stimuli. It is proposed that the temporal dynamics of this procedure consist of two stages. The early stage is characterized by quick and specialized neural encoding of disgusting and fearful stimuli irrespective of voluntary attention allocation, indicating an automatic detection and perception of threat-related emotions. The late stage is represented by attention-gated separation between threat-related stimuli and neutral stimuli; the similar ERP pattern evoked by disgusted and fearful faces suggests a more general process of threat-related emotions via top-down attentional modulation, based on which the defensive behavior in response to threat events is largely facilitated. Altogether, the current study reveals a systematic progression of the relationship between spatial attention and threat-related emotion processing, highlighting the adaptability of the human defense system which always optimizes its function to deal with diverse dangers in the environment.

Author Contributions

Conceived and designed the experiments: DZ CZ YL. Performed the experiments: YL YC. Analyzed the data: DZ. Contributed reagents/materials/analysis tools: YL YC. Contributed to the writing of the manuscript: DZ YL.

References

1. Zhang D, Wang L, Luo Y, Luo Y (2012) Individual differences in detecting rapidly presented fearful faces. PloS one 7: e49517.
2. Schupp HT, Stockburger J, Codispoti M, Junghöfer M, Weike AI, et al. (2007) Selective visual attention to emotion. The Journal of Neuroscience 27: 1082–1089.
3. Anderson AK, Christoff K, Panitz D, De Rosa E, Gabrieli JD (2003) Neural correlates of the automatic processing of threat facial signals. The Journal of Neuroscience 23: 5627–5633.
4. Bishop SJ, Jenkins R, Lawrence AD (2007) Neural processing of fearful faces: effects of anxiety are gated by perceptual capacity limitations. Cerebral cortex 17: 1595–1603.
5. Holmes A, Vuilleumier P, Eimer M (2003) The processing of emotional facial expression is gated by spatial attention: evidence from event-related brain potentials. Cognitive Brain Research 16: 174–184.
6. Öhman A (2005) The role of the amygdala in human fear: automatic detection of threat. Psychoneuroendocrinology 30: 953–958.
7. Cheng Y, Lee S-Y, Chen H-Y, Wang P-Y, Decety J (2012) Voice and emotion processing in the human neonatal brain. Journal of cognitive neuroscience 24: 1411–1419.
8. Williams LM (2006) An integrative neuroscience model of "significance" processing. Journal of integrative neuroscience 5: 1–47.
9. Vuilleumier P, Armony JL, Driver J, Dolan RJ (2001) Effects of attention and emotion on face processing in the human brain: an event-related fMRI study. Neuron 30: 829–841.
10. Pessoa L, Padmala S, Morland T (2005) Fate of unattended fearful faces in the amygdala is determined by both attentional resources and cognitive modulation. Neuroimage 28: 249–255.
11. Devlin JT, Russell RP, Davis MH, Price CJ, Wilson J, et al. (2000) Susceptibility-induced loss of signal: comparing PET and fMRI on a semantic task. Neuroimage 11: 589–600.
12. Pourtois G, Dan ES, Grandjean D, Sander D, Vuilleumier P (2005) Enhanced extrastriate visual response to bandpass spatial frequency filtered fearful faces: Time course and topographic evoked-potentials mapping. Human brain mapping 26: 65–79.
13. Vaish A, Grossmann T, Woodward A (2008) Not all emotions are created equal: the negativity bias in social-emotional development. Psychological bulletin 134: 383–399.
14. Neuberg SL, Kenrick DT, Schaller M (2011) Human threat management systems: Self-protection and disease avoidance. Neuroscience & Biobehavioral Reviews 35: 1042–1051.
15. Oaten M, Stevenson RJ, Case TI (2009) Disgust as a disease-avoidance mechanism. Psychological bulletin 135: 303–323.
16. Ekman P, Levenson RW, Friesen WV (1983) Autonomic nervous system activity distinguishes among emotions. Science 221: 1208–1210.
17. Susskind JM, Lee DH, Cusi A, Feiman R, Grabski W, et al. (2008) Expressing fear enhances sensory acquisition. Nature neuroscience 11: 843–850.
18. Vermeulen N, Godefroid J, Mermillod M (2009) Emotional modulation of attention: fear increases but disgust reduces the attentional blink. PLoS One 4: e7924.
19. Krusemark EA, Li W (2011) Do all threats work the same way? Divergent effects of fear and disgust on sensory perception and attention. The Journal of Neuroscience 31: 3429–3434.
20. Charash M, McKay D (2002) Attention bias for disgust. Journal of anxiety disorders 16: 529–541.
21. Charash M, McKay D, Dipaolo N (2006) Implicit attention bias for disgust. Anxiety, stress, and coping 19: 353–364.
22. Krusemark EA, Li W (2013) From Early Sensory Specialization to Later Perceptual Generalization: Dynamic Temporal Progression in Perceiving Individual Threats. The Journal of Neuroscience 33: 587–594.
23. Smith ML (2012) Rapid processing of emotional expressions without conscious awareness. Cerebral Cortex 22: 1748–1760.
24. Vuilleumier P, Pourtois G (2007) Distributed and interactive brain mechanisms during emotion face perception: evidence from functional neuroimaging. Neuropsychologia 45: 174–194.
25. Zhang D, Gu R, Wu T, Broster LS, Luo Y, et al. (2013) An electrophysiological index of changes in risk decision-making strategies. Neuropsychologia 51: 1397–1407.
26. Galfano G, Sarlo M, Sassi F, Munafò M, Fuentes LJ, et al. (2011) Reorienting of spatial attention in gaze cuing is reflected in N2pc. Social neuroscience 6: 257–269.
27. Weymar M, Löw A, Öhman A, Hamm AO (2011) The face is more than its parts—Brain dynamics of enhanced spatial attention to schematic threat. Neuroimage 58: 946–954.
28. Cuthbert BN, Schupp HT, Bradley MM, Birbaumer N, Lang PJ (2000) Brain potentials in affective picture processing: covariation with autonomic arousal and affective report. Biological psychology 52: 95–111.
29. Gong X, Huang Y, Wang Y, Luo Y (2011) Revision of the Chinese facial affective picture system. Chinese Mental Health Journal 25: 40–46.
30. Ewbank MP, Lawrence AD, Passamonti L, Keane J, Peers PV, et al. (2009) Anxiety predicts a differential neural response to attended and unattended facial signals of anger and fear. Neuroimage 44: 1144–1151.
31. Wojciulik E, Kanwisher N, Driver J (1998) Covert visual attention modulates face-specific activity in the human fusiform gyrus: fMRI study. Journal of Neurophysiology 79: 1574–1578.
32. Eimer M, Holmes A, McGlone FP (2003) The role of spatial attention in the processing of rapid brain responses to six basic emotions. Cognitive, Affective, & Behavioral Neuroscience 3: 97–110.
33. Bledowski C, Prvulovic D, Hoechstetter K, Scherg M, Wibral M, et al. (2004) Localizing P300 generators in visual target and distractor processing: a combined event-related potential and functional magnetic resonance imaging study. The Journal of neuroscience 24: 9353–9360.
34. Eimer M, Holmes A (2007) Event-related brain potential correlates of emotional face processing. Neuropsychologia 45: 15–31.
35. Bentin S, Allison T, Puce A, Perez E, McCarthy G (1996) Electrophysiological studies of face perception in humans. Journal of cognitive neuroscience 8: 551–565.
36. Eimer M (2000) The face-specific N170 component reflects late stages in the structural encoding of faces. Neuroreport 11: 2319–2324.
37. Schyns PG, Petro LS, Smith ML (2007) Dynamics of visual information integration in the brain for categorizing facial expressions. Current Biology 17: 1580–1585.
38. Herrmann CS, Knight RT (2001) Mechanisms of human attention: event-related potentials and oscillations. Neuroscience & Biobehavioral Reviews 25: 465–476.
39. Hajcak G, Dunning JP, Foti D (2009) Motivated and controlled attention to emotion: time-course of the late positive potential. Clinical Neurophysiology 120: 505–510.
40. Capotosto P, Babiloni C, Romani GL, Corbetta M (2009) Frontoparietal cortex controls spatial attention through modulation of anticipatory alpha rhythms. The Journal of Neuroscience 29: 5863–5872.
41. Schupp HT, Markus J, Weike AI, Hamm AO (2003) Emotional facilitation of sensory processing in the visual cortex. Psychological science 14: 7–13.
42. Andersen SK, Fuchs S, Müller MM (2011) Effects of feature-selective and spatial attention at different stages of visual processing. Journal of Cognitive Neuroscience 23: 238–246.
43. Chong H, Riis JL, McGinnis SM, Williams DM, Holcomb PJ, et al. (2008) To ignore or explore: Top–down modulation of novelty processing. Journal of Cognitive Neuroscience 20: 120–134.
44. Zanto TP, Rubens MT, Bollinger J, Gazzaley A (2010) Top-down modulation of visual feature processing: the role of the inferior frontal junction. Neuroimage 53: 736–745.
45. Siegel M, Donner TH, Oostenveld R, Fries P, Engel AK (2008) Neuronal synchronization along the dorsal visual pathway reflects the focus of spatial attention. Neuron 60: 709–719.
46. Furey ML, Tanskanen T, Beauchamp MS, Avikainen S, Uutela K, et al. (2006) Dissociation of face-selective cortical responses by attention. Proceedings of the National Academy of Sciences of the United States of America 103: 1065–1070.
47. Langton SR, Law AS, Burton AM, Schweinberger SR (2008) Attention capture by faces. Cognition 107: 330–342.
48. Vuilleumier P, Schwartz S (2001) Emotional facial expressions capture attention. Neurology 56: 153–158.
49. Vuilleumier P (2002) Facial expression and selective attention. Current Opinion in Psychiatry 15: 291–300.

12

Nogo Receptor Inhibition Enhances Functional Recovery following Lysolecithin-Induced Demyelination in Mouse Optic Chiasm

Fereshteh Pourabdolhossein[1,2], **Sabah Mozafari**[1], **Ghislaine Morvan-Dubois**[2], **Javad Mirnajafi-Zadeh**[1], **Alejandra Lopez-Juarez**[2], **Jacqueline Pierre-Simons**[2], **Barbara A. Demeneix**[2], **Mohammad Javan**[1,3]*

1 Department of Physiology, Faculty of Medical Sciences, Tarbiat Modares University, Tehran, Iran, 2 UMR CNRS 7221, Evolution des Régulations Endocriniennes, Département Régulations, Développement et Diversité Moléculaire, Muséum National d'Histoire Naturelle, Paris, France, 3 Department of Stem Cells and Developmental Biology at Cell Science Research Center, Royan Institute for Stem Cell Biology and Technology, ACECR, Tehran, Iran

Abstract

Background: Inhibitory factors have been implicated in the failure of remyelination in demyelinating diseases. Myelin associated inhibitors act through a common receptor called Nogo receptor (NgR) that plays critical inhibitory roles in CNS plasticity. Here we investigated the effects of abrogating NgR inhibition in a non-immune model of focal demyelination in adult mouse optic chiasm.

Methodology/Principal Findings: A focal area of demyelination was induced in adult mouse optic chiasm by microinjection of lysolecithin. To knock down *NgR* levels, siRNAs against NgR were intracerebroventricularly administered via a permanent cannula over 14 days, Functional changes were monitored by electrophysiological recording of latency of visual evoked potentials (VEPs). Histological analysis was carried out 3, 7 and 14 days post demyelination lesion. To assess the effect of NgR inhibition on precursor cell repopulation, BrdU was administered to the animals prior to the demyelination induction. Inhibition of NgR significantly restored VEPs responses following optic chiasm demyelination. These findings were confirmed histologically by myelin specific staining. siNgR application resulted in a smaller lesion size compared to control. NgR inhibition significantly increased the numbers of BrdU+/Olig2+ progenitor cells in the lesioned area and in the neurogenic zone of the third ventricle. These progenitor cells (Olig2+ or GFAP+) migrated away from this area as a function of time.

Conclusions/Significance: Our results show that inhibition of NgR facilitate myelin repair in the demyelinated chiasm, with enhanced recruitment of proliferating cells to the lesion site. Thus, antagonizing NgR function could have therapeutic potential for demyelinating disorders such as Multiple Sclerosis.

Editor: Markus Reindl, Innsbruck Medical University, Austria

Funding: This study was supported by a grant from Tarbiat Modares University, Tehran, Iran. The work in B.A. Demeneix's lab, Paris France, was supported by the EU program (FP6, Crescendo), the AFM (Association Française contre les Myopathies) and grants from the CNRS and MNHN. The funders had no role in study design, data collection and analysis, decision to publish, or preparation of the manuscript.

Competing Interests: The authors have declared that no competing interests exist.

* Email: mjavan@modares.ac.ir

Introduction

Myelin associated inhibitory factors, including NogoA [1], myelin associated glycoprotein (MAG) [2] and oligodendrocyte myelin glycoprotein (OMgp) [3] are among the major factors known to inhibit regeneration in the CNS [4]. These factors bind to a common receptor called Nogo receptor 1 (NgR1) [5]. A large number of studies have shown that NgR is expressed by not only neurons [6] but also glial cells including oligodendrocyte progenitor cells (OPCs) [7,8], astrocytes [9], microglia [10], macrophages [11], dendritic cells [12] and neural precursor cells [13–15]. It has been reported that NgR exerts multiple inhibitory effects in neural pathological conditions [16–18], including inhibition of neural precursor migration during CNS development

[13]. While the focus of most of these studies has addressed the inhibitory roles of NgR or its ligands in axonal regeneration either in EAE demyelinating models [16,19,20] or non-demyelinating conditions [17,21,22], less is known about the roles of myelin inhibitory factors in demyelination condition in which the axons are intact or not targeted. Since it is well documented that myelin can protect axonal integrity and loss of myelin results in axonal loss and disability [23–26], it is important to better understand the role of myelin-derived inhibitory factors on myelin repair itself. This information is more pertinent given that NgR and its ligands are expressed in demyelinating lesions of MS tissues [9]. Chong et al. (2012) reported the role of NogoA in regulating oligodendrocyte myelination in vitro and in an in vivo focal model of demyelination

[27]. The roles of other myelin-bound ligands of NgR, also likely involved in myelin regeneration, remained to be studied.

Here we targeted the common receptor (NgR) of myelin inhibitory factors to analyze its effects on myelin repair in an in vivo context of demyelination. We previously developed a focal model of demyelination in the optic chiasm of adult rats [28] and mice [29] and showed that remyelination could be followed functionally by assessing visual evoked potentials and structurally, by assessing demyelination extension [28–30]. Furthermore, we observed that the caudal part of the optic chiasm displayed more remyelination than the rostral part [30], probably due to its vicinity to the third ventricle, which is a known neurogenic region both in development [31] and adulthood [32–34]. In this study, we used the same focal model, targeting the caudal part of optic chiasm to investigate the effects of NgR inhibition during demyelination. We also examined the response of the neurogenic niche around the third ventricle during this process and followed remyelination by histological examination. Recording visual evoked potentials (VEPs) allowed us to evaluate the functional recovery of the optic chiasm. Our results demonstrate that siRNA directed against NgR significantly enhanced the remyelination process and functional recovery of optic chiasm. Further, NgR inhibition significantly increased the number of Olig2+ cells recruited in the lesion site and enhanced the numbers of third ventricle progenitor cells produced following chiasm demyelination.

Material and Methods

Animals

All animal studies were conducted according to the principles and procedures described in Guidelines for care and use of experimental animals and were approved by Tarbiat Modares University-Ethics Committee for Research on Animals. Eight week-old (25–30 gr) male C57BL/6 mice were purchased from Razi institute (Karaj, Iran) and JANVIER (Le Genest St Isle, France). Animals (five per cage) were kept under 12 h light/dark cycles with controlled temperature (22±20°C). Food and water were available ad libitum.

Demyelination procedure

Animals were deeply anesthetized with intraperitoneal injection of Ketamine (100 mg/kg wt; Imalgen from Merial) and Xylazine (10 mgkg wt; Rompun from Bayer) diluted in 0.9% sterile saline. Meloxicam (Metacam from Boehringer Ingelheim) was used for analgesia throughout all operations.

Demyelination was induced by stereotaxic injection of 1 µl of 1% lysolecithin (LPC; sigma, St. Louis, USA) dissolved in 0.9% NaCl [28]. Mice were positioned in a stereotaxic device (Stoelting, USA) in a skull flat situation. The LPC was injected into the optic chiasm over 2 min, using the coordinates of 3.9 mm anterior to the Lambda, 5.75 mm deep from Dura surface and zero laterality [35]. The needle was kept in place for an additional 5 min to equilibrate tissue and inject solution, to avoid the possible reflux through the needle tract. Control animals were injected with equal volume of sterile saline.

Interventions

For intracerebroventricular administration of siRNAs, animals were cannulated unilaterally in the right lateral ventricle (3.6 mm anterior to lambda, 1.1 mm lateral, and 2.2 mm deep from the Dura surface) [35]. siNgR was injected from cannula, 24 pmol (2 µl)/animal/days. Control groups received same volume of saline.

Formulation of siRNA complexes

siRNA against pGL2 (for control group) and NgR1 (Rtn4r, 4 different sequences, Cat no: SI02722888, SI02699186, SI02748333, SI02678249) were purchased from Qiagen (validated siRNA). siRNA (24 pmol per animal) was diluted in glucose (5%) and mixed with monocationic lipid (IC10, Polyplus-transfection) at a ratio of 15 monocationic lipid nitrogens per RNA phosphate as described before [36,37]. Complexes prepared at room temperature are stable for two hours after preparation. Unilateral injection of siRNA (2 µl) was performed every day from permanent cannula stereotaxically placed into right lateral ventricle. Details of siRNA sequences are presented in Table S1.

Real time PCR

The rim of third ventricle of adult mice was dissected under a binocular microscope, snap-frozen in liquid nitrogen and stored at −80°C until processed. Total RNA was extracted based on the protocol provided with the RNAble reagent (Eurobio, Les Ulis, France). Concentration of total RNA was measured, and RNAs were stored in Tris 10 mM/EDTA 0.1 mM (pH 7.4) at −80°C. To quantify mRNAs 1 µg of total RNA was reverse-transcribed using High capacity cDNA Reverse Transcription kit (Applied Biosystems, Courtaboeuf, France). Control reactions without reverse transcriptase were done in parallel. Primers for the detection of NgR (Taqman gene expression assays, references: Mm00710554_m1) and control assay GAPDH (Mm99999915_g1) were purchased from Applied Biosystems. Direct detection of the PCR product was monitored by measuring the increase in fluorescence generated by the TaqMan probe (NgR, GAPDH) as described previously by Decherf et al. (2010) [38].

Visual evoked potential (VEP)

Visual evoked potentials (VEPs) are evoked electrophysiological potential that can be extracted, using signal averaging, from the electroencephalographic activity recorded at the scalp. The VEPs can provide important diagnostic information about the functional integrity of the visual system. The surgical process is similar to the method described previously [28,39,40]. The animals were anesthetized and fixed to stereotaxic apparatus. To facilitate VEP recordings, a monopolar electrode was implanted into the occipital cortex (A: 0.0, L: ±3.0 mm, Lambda) and the anterior end of the skull served as the reference electrode. The electrodes were connected to a miniature receptacle, which was embedded in the skull with dental cement. For VEP recording, mice were immobilized in a box and allowed to adapt to darkness for 10 minutes. The cylinder was placed in a sound-attenuating dark and electrically shielded box (60 cm×60 cm ×60 cm). Flash light stimulation was delivered by a general evoked response stimulator (SMP-3100, Nihon Kohden, Tokyo, Japan) 300 times with a frequency of 0.5 Hz. The illumination of the reflecting surface was approximately 40 lx. Responses were amplified with high and low filter settings of 30 and 0.08 Hz, respectively, using a biophysical amplifier (AVB-10, Nihon Kohden), and displayed on a memory oscilloscope (VC-11, Nihon Kohden). Amplified waveforms were afterwards averaged (DAT-1100, Nihon Kohden). For each VEP recording, we studied the latency between the flashlight and the first negative or positive peaks.

Cell tracing

Bromodeoxyuridine (5-bromo-2-deoxyuridine, (BrdU)) incorporates into DNA during S phase of the cell cycle; therefore it is appropriate for labeling of newly divided cells used for tracing of these cells while they are migrating. Mice received seven injections of Brdu (sigma, USA) at intervals of 2 hours (70 mg/kg each, i.p.) 24 hours prior to induction of demyelination. Using this tracing protocol, labeled cells is restricted to the germinative area of the CNS like lateral and third ventricles rims in controls. Afterward, detection of labeled cells in structures other than these areas implies that they originated from ventricular zone [41–44].

Tissue processing

Mice were deeply anesthetized with Pentobarbital (130 mg/kg from Sanofi) on 3, 7, 14 days post lesion and perfused with a fresh phosphate buffered saline 0.1 M (PBS) and followed by 4% paraformaldehyde solution (PFA, pH 7.4). Brains were excised and post-fixed 2 hours in same fixative solution at room temperature and cryoprotected by 20% sucrose/PBS overnight then embedded in optimum cutting temperature compound, frozen and stored at −80°C. Coronal sections (12 μm) were obtained using a Cryostat (Leica, Rueil-mal maison, France) and collected on superfrost plus slides (Thermo Scientific). Coronal serial sections with 120 μm intervals (+20-880 μm) were analyzed. Therefore we were able to determine the migration pattern of third ventricle proliferative cells towards optic chiasm.

Immunohistochemistry

Cryosections were rehydrated in 0.1 M PBS three times for 5 min (for myelin staining sections incubated in ethanol 95% for 10 min at RT washed two times with PBS) and incubated 1 h with blocking solution containing 10% normal goat serum (Vector Laboratories, France 501000) and BSA 2 mg/ml (Vector Laboratories- sp50-50) and 0.3% Triton ×100 (Sigma, France) in PBS. Slides were incubated overnight at 4°C with primary antibodies (Table S2) diluted in blocking solution and cover slipped. After slides were rinsed three times for10 min with PBS and incubated with secondary antibody (Table S3) for 1 h at RT. For double labeling with BrdU, sections were washed three times in PBS for 10 min and incubated in HCl 2N for 30 min at 37°C, after two washes 5 min in borate buffer (pH: 8.4) and PBS, sections were incubated with the same blocking solution and incubated overnight at 4°C with the anti Brdu antibody diluted in blocking solution. After washing, sections were incubated with secondary antibody for 1 h at RT. After several washes with PBS, brain sections were mounted in antifade reagent with DAPI (P3693, Invitrogen) and analyzed under fluorescent microscopy on an Olympus AX70 microscope and camera Olympus DP50.

For cell counting in the third ventricle and optic chiasm 12 μm sections were used. The number of total BrdU+ cells and Brdu+/Olig2+, Brdu+/GFAP+ or Brdu+/PSA-NCAM+ positive cells were averaged from three different levels 120 μm apart and three consecutive sections per level. For each brain (nine sections), data were expressed in number of cells per mm^2 and are deduced from three mice per experimental group.

The extent of demyelination, as the ratio of lesion size per total area, was determined using Image J software [45]. Data obtained from individual animals in each group was averaged from 9 sections (n = 3 animals per treatment time point). The number of Iba-1+ cells in the lesion site were averaged from four sections per brain and data were expressed in number of cells per mm^2 using a total of three mice per experimental group.

Statistical Analysis

The result are expressed as mean± SEM. Data were analyzed by two way analysis of variance (ANOVA) followed by Bonferroni post-tests with Graph pad PRISM software (Graph pad software, Inc, San Diego. CA). Data were determined to be significant when p<0.05.

Results

siNgR successfully mediated knock-down of Nogo receptor in vivo

The putative role of NgR in myelin repair and NPCs migration was studied by a loss of function strategy based on RNA interference. Remaud (et al. 2013), showed that siRNA/IC10 is the first generation of lipid based siRNA vectors to provide efficient, spatially and temporally defined knockdown in the adult brain [37]. The observed distribution of labled siRNA indicated that IC10 vectorizes siRNA in to cells expressing markers characteristic of NSC and transient amplifying progenitor cells (TAPs) in the adult SVZ [37]. To knock down NgR, a validated siRNA targeting NgR1 complexed with IC10 was injected stereotaxically into the lateral ventricle of adult mice brain. The areas lining the third ventricle of brain injected with either NgR (siNgR) or Control (siControl) were carefully sampled under dissecting microscope 24, 48 and 72 hrs after siRNA injection. RNA was extracted for qPCR analysis. A significant (p<0.001) decrease (0.40 fold change) in NgR mRNA expression was observed 24 hrs after the injection, in the group injected with NgR-siRNA when compared to control-siRNA (Fig. 1). No significant differences were observed between siNgR and siControl groups for later time points. This result indicates that siRNA-mediated knockdown of NgR was efficient and transient. To knockdown NgR during the process of the LPC demyelination/remyelination (2 weeks), 24 pmol siNgR/IC10 were daily injected in the ventricle of stereotaxically cannulated adult mice.

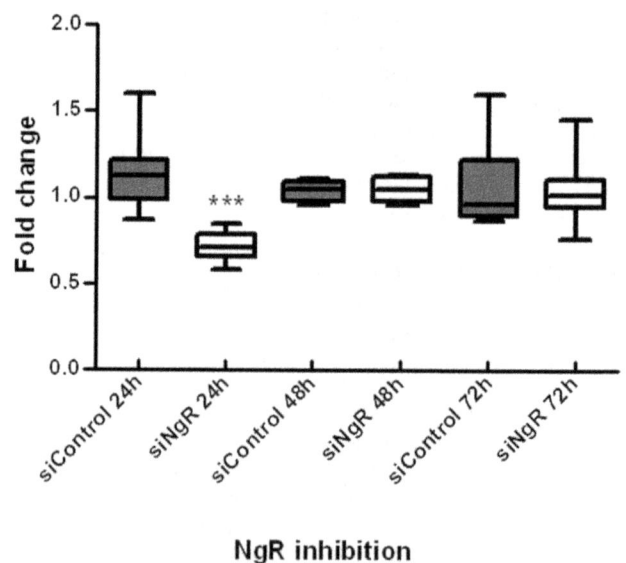

NgR inhibition

Figure 1. siRNA-mediated knockdown of NgR. qPCR of third ventricle samples show levels of NgR expression at 24, 48 and 72 hrs after single siRNA injection. Gene expression was normalized with Gapdh. Data are pooled from three independent experiments providing similar results (total number of mice for each data point =6). Graph shows fold changes in NgR mRNA using qPCR analysis. Boxes represent the fifth to ninety-fifth percentiles around the median with whiskers for minimum and maximum values. Statistical analysis used two-way ANOVA and Bonferroni's post -test. Treatment had significant effects on the level of NgR gene expression. NgR gene expression was decreased significantly 24 h after siNgR injection compared to siControl, the asterisk indicates that the difference between the pairs denoted are significant at the confidence levels ***p<0.001.

Functional recovery in demyelinated optic chiasm of mice following NgR inhibition

To investigate the role of NgR in a demyelinating context, we induced a focal lesion in the optic chiasm using LPC injection. We confirmed the physiological pertinence of the model by immunostaining against the myelin specific marker MOG (Fig. 2A) and LFB staining (data not shown). We observed that, at all time points axons were not affected by LPC injection when tissues were stained for axonal neurofilament (Fig. 2C–H). No demyelination was detected in the optic chiasm of saline-treated controls (Fig. 2B). Demyelination was observed as early as 3 days post injection. Demyelination extent was assessed as percentage of total area of optic chiasm. The demyelination extent was maximal at 7 dpi compared to controls (p<0.001, Figs. 2C, D). In LPC treated animals after 14 days the extent of demyelination was reduced compared to LPC 7 dpi (Fig. 2E). In siNgR treated animals the demyelination area was not different at 3 dpi compared to LPC but was considerably reduced at day 7 and 14 post injection (p<0.001 for all comparisons, Figs. 2F–H).

Since NgR is expressed also by microglia and macrophages [10,12]; and these cells are involved in LPC-mediated lesions and/or remyelination [46,47], we carried out immunocytochemistry on sections to label Iba-1+ cells at the lesion site and counted the number of Iba-1+ cells in LPC and LPC+siNgR treated animals at 3 and 14 dpi and compared it to saline treated chiasm evaluated at dpi 3. The number of Iba-1+ cells significantly increased in LPC and LPC+siNgR treated groups at all time points compared to control (p<0.001, Fig. 3 A–F). In LPC+siNgR groups the number of Iba-1+ cells was slightly higher than LPC but these changes were non-statistically significant (Fig. 3D).

To functionally investigate the effect of NgR knockdown in demyelinated optic chiasm, Visual Evoked Potentials (VEPs) were recorded from the occipital cortex of the control and treated mice. VEPs consist of specific P1–N1, N1–P2 and P2–N2 components (Fig. 4A). P1-N1 component represented the more stable wave and was therefore used for measuring timing of the response to the light stimulus [28,48]. P1 latency was calculated from VEP profiles as shown in (Fig. 4A). The reference is given by the mean P1 latency observed in the saline group (58 ms) (Fig. 4B). LPC treatment significantly increased the P1 latency observed at 3, 7 and 14 dpi (n=6, p<0.001). However, the P1 wave latency was reduced at 14 dpi compared to 7 dpi in LPC group (Figs. 4C–E). Treatment with siNgR reduced the P1 latency at 7 and 14 dpi compared to LPC 7 and 14 dpi (p<0.001, Figs. 4C–I). These electrophysiological results were consistent with our histological data (Figs. 2C–E) showing the reduction of extent of demyelination at 14 dpi. Demyelination was observed in all treatment groups but siNgR treated mice presented reduced demyelination. This difference was particularly remarkable at 7 and 14 dpi (Fig. 2, 4). The reduction in the P1 latency and demyelination extent demonstrated that knockdown of NgR potentiates repair process of demyelinated optic chiasm by inducing a functional recovery. Next, to assess the cellular basis of this functional recovery we tracked the production and migration of progenitor cells to the demyelinated chiasm following NgR inhibition.

Characterization of BrdU+ cells in demyelinated optic chiasm

To study the effect of siNgR on cell repopulation within the lesioned area, cells were labeled with BrdU before demyelination induction and were analyzed at 3, 7 and 14 dpi. The analysis showed that in saline treated animals few BrdU+ cells were present (Fig. 5H, 6G). However, the total number of BrdU+ cells increased progressively in LPC treated animals and at 14 dpi this increase was significant compared to controls (p<0.001, Table 1). In siNgR treated animals the number of total BrdU+ cells showed an almost 2 fold increase compared to LPC groups (p<0.001, Table 1). To characterize the BrdU+ labeled cells, tissues were stained for Olig2, GFAP, PSA-NCAM. The number of BrdU+/Olig2+ cells in the optic chiasm of LPC group did not change significantly over the time, however, the number these cells increased markedly in optic chiasm of siNgR-treated animals from 7 to 14 dpi as compared to controls (p<0.01, p<0.001, Fig. 5B-H). This increase was also significant between LPC 7, 14 dpi and siNgR 7 and 14 dpi (p<0.05, p<0.001, Fig. 5 I). Numbers of BrdU+/GFAP+ cells were significantly increased in LPC 7 and 14 dpi compared to control (p<0.05, Fig. 6 A–C). However, in siNgR treated LPC-groups the numbers of these cells significantly increased at 7 and 14 dpi compared to controls and LPC 14 dpi respectively (p<0.001, Fig. 6 A–H). BrdU+ cells in the optic chiasm were principally co-labeled with Olig2 and GFAP, but none, in any experimental group, expressed PSA-NCAM.

Third ventricle progenitor cells activation to demyelinated optic chiasm is increased in response to NgR knockdown

We previously showed that LPC-induced demyelination in adult rat optic chiasm activated proliferation in the subventricular zone (SVZ) around the third ventricle [30]. In this study we observed that inhibition of NgR resulted in a greater response from third ventricle following LPC lesion in the mouse optic chiasm. The analysis showed that progenitor cells residing in third ventricle wall were not mitotically active in saline treated animals (Fig. S1A). Third ventricle SVZ was reactivated in response to LPC induced lesion in optic chiasm. We observed that total number of BrdU+ cells increased at day 3 and 7 dpi in LPC treated mice. However in siNgR+LPC treated animals the number of total BrdU+ cells showed a two-fold increase compared to LPC groups at 3 and 7 dpi. The total number of BrdU+ cells at 14 dpi decreased significantly compared to siNgR 7 dpi (p<0.001, Table 1).

To identify proliferating cell types in third ventricle, BrdU+ cells were co-labeled with the antibodies against Olig2, PSA-NCAM and GFAP. Numbers of BrdU+/GFAP+ cells were not significantly modified in LPC treated animals compared to controls, whereas in siNgR treated animals BrdU+/GFAP+ cells significantly increased in the third ventricle SVZ at 3, 7 and 14 dpi compared to controls (p<0.05, p<0.001, p<0.01, Fig. 7A–F, M) respectively. Numbers of BrdU+/Olig2+ cells in LPC groups increased at 3 and 7 dpi compared to control (p<0.05, p<0.001 respectively), then decreased slightly at 14 dpi, (Fig. S1A–D, N). In siNgR-treated animals, BrdU+/Olig2+ cell numbers increased at 3, 7 and 14 dpi compared to controls (p<0.01, p<0.001, p<0.001, respectively) with an almost two fold increase in siNgR 7 dpi compared to LPC 7 dpi (P<0.001, Fig. 7 G–I, N). The number of these cells then decreased at siNgR14 dpi compared to siNgR 7 dpi (Fig. 7 H–I, N).

In LPC alone and siNgR-treated animals, some third ventricle BrdU+ cells expressed PSA-NCAM; and the number of BrdU+/PSA-NCAM+ cells in these groups was significantly higher than control group, however, these changes were not statistically significant when LPC and LPC+siNgR groups were compared (Fig. 7 J–L, O; Fig S2C, G–I).

Taken together, our results suggest that dividing cells are mobilized toward the lesion area in demyelinated optic chiasm. These cells mainly expressed Olig2 and GFAP, indicating a glia fate for progenitor cells at this neurogenic region.

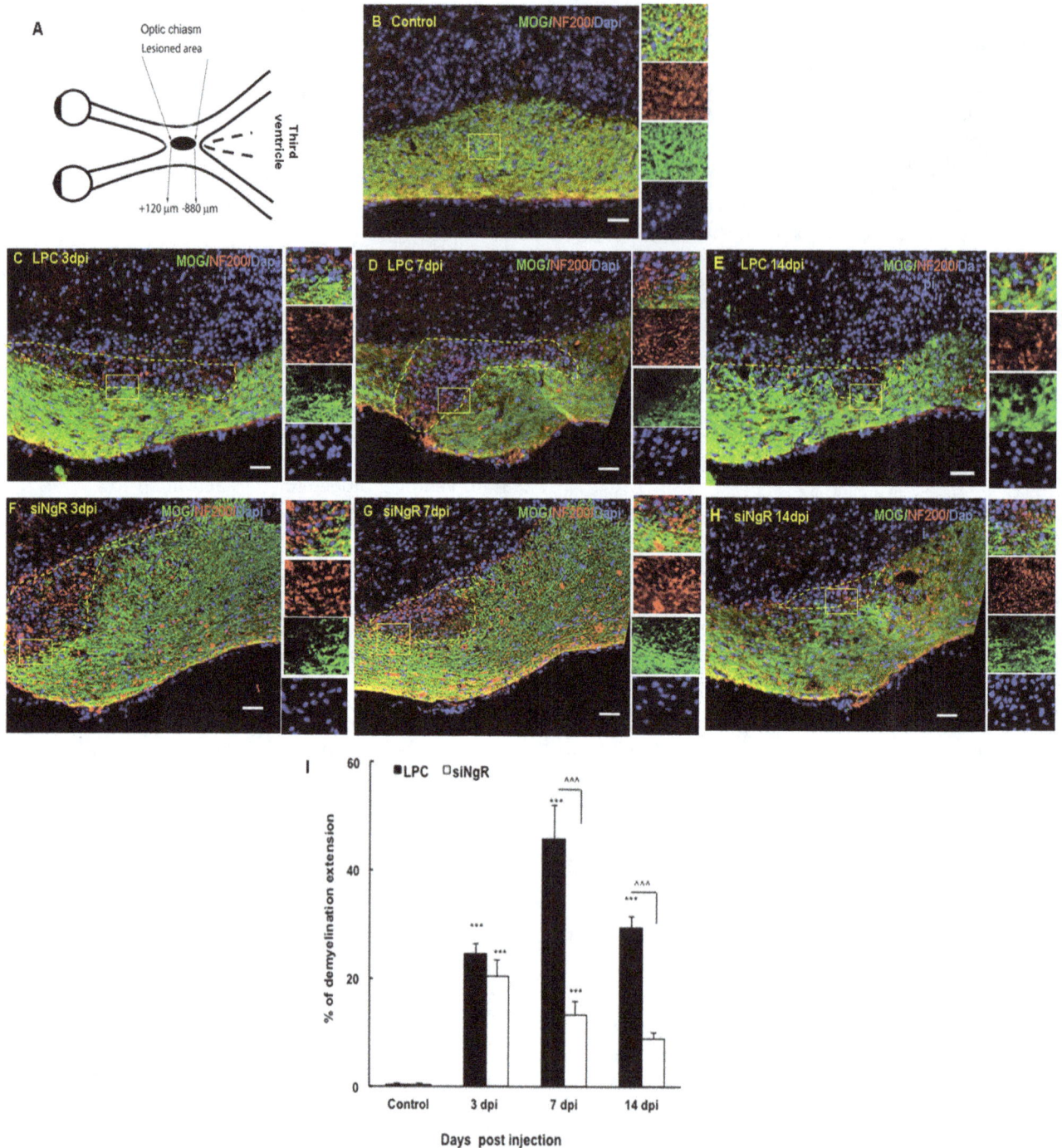

Figure 2. Extent of demyelination is decreased following NgR knock down. Coronal sections of adult mouse brains (12 μm) treated with saline, LPC and LPC+siNgR were double stained with MOG (green) and NF200 (red) and nuclei are labeled with DAPI (blue). (A) Schematic picture of injection site and demyelination area. (B) Saline-treated chiasm at 7 days post injection (dpi), no detectable demyelination is seen 7 days after a single injection of saline (Control). (C–E) Demyelination at optic chiasm of LPC-treated animals at 3, 7 and 14 dpi, respectively. (F–H) Demyelination at optic chiasm of LPC+siNgR treated animals at 3, 7 and 14 dpi, respectively. (I) The extent of demyelination in different groups are quantitatively analyzed and presented as percent of total area. Control group represents demyelination level in animals treated with saline at dpi 7. Statistical analysis used two-way ANOVA and Bonferroni's post -test. Treatment and time had a significant effect on the remyelination process. In LPC treated-animals significant demyelination is seen at 3, 7 and 14 dpi compared to saline (***$P<0.001$). At 14 dpi, demyelination was partially reduced compared to 7 dpi. Between groups, there was a significant reduction of demyelination in LPC+siNgR 7 dpi compared to LPC 7 dpi (^^^$P<0.001$) and in LPC+siNgR 14 dpi compared to LPC 14 dpi (^^^$P<0.001$). Each data point shows data obtained from experiments carried out on three mice (n = 3), and represents Mean ± SEMs, Bars: 50 μm, Dashed line indicates lesion area.

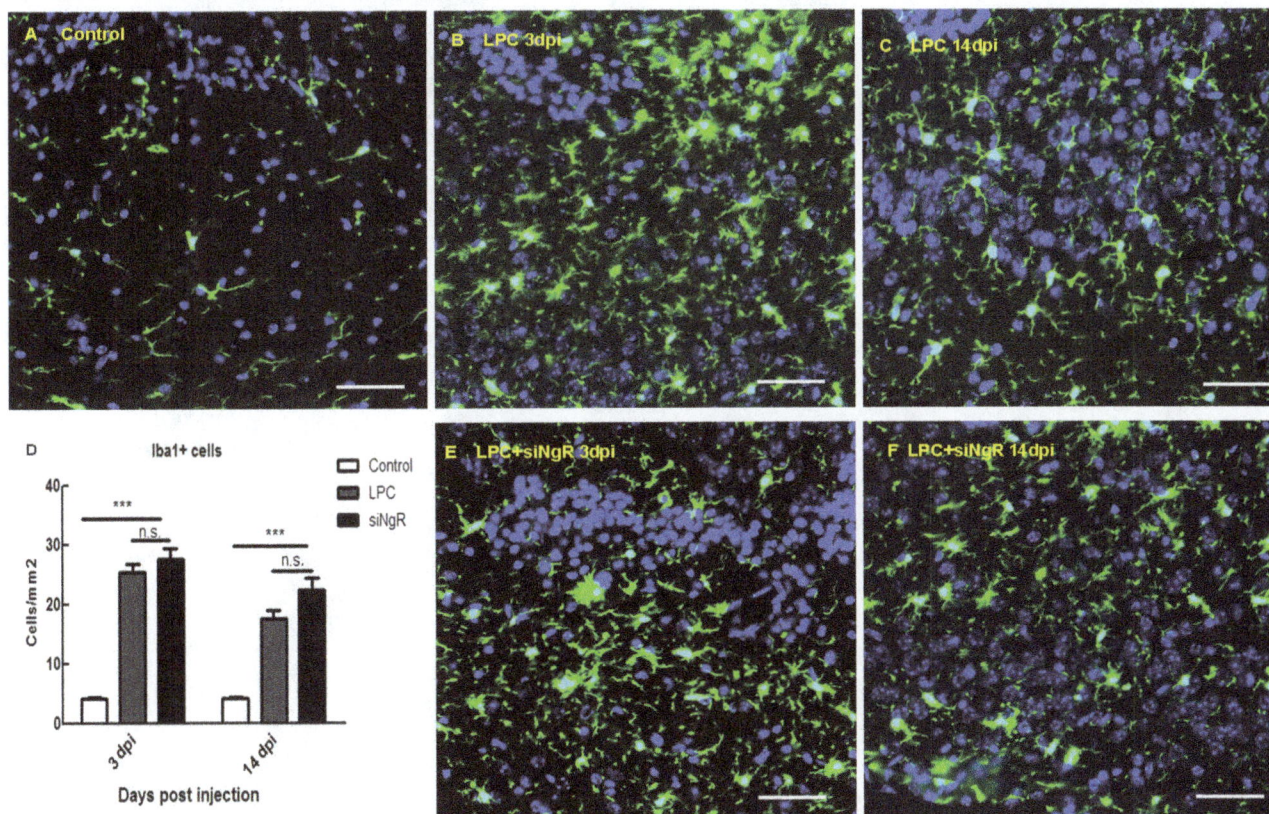

Figure 3. Macrophages and microglia response to LPC-induced demyelination. Sections from lesion sites were stained for Iba-1 (green) and DAPI (blue) at 3 and 14 dpi in both LPC and LPC+siNgR treated groups. (A) The number of Iba-1+ cells in saline treated animals (Control) was low at 3 dpi. (B–C) Increased number of microglia and macrophages in the lesion site following LPC induced demyelination at 3 (B) and 14 dpi (C). (E–F) In siNgR treated mice in LPC induced lesion also the number of Iba-1+ cells was increased at 3 (E) and 14 dpi (F). (D) Iba1+ cells per area/mm^2 are averaged from the counts of four sections of each chiasm (n = 3). Statistical analysis used two-way ANOVA with Bonferroni's post-test. The effects of treatment and time were significant. Further analysis using post-test showed significant difference between Control and LPC treated mice (p<0.001), and between Control and LPC+siNgR treated mice (p<0.001) at 3 and 14 dpi. The difference between the LPC and LPC+siNgR treated groups was non-significant (n.s.). Data are expressed as Mean ±SEMs, Bars: 50 µm.

Discussion

It has been reported that NgR is expressed not only by neurons [6] but also by other neural cells including neural stem cells [13–15], oligodendrocyte precursor cells [7,8], astrocytes [9], Schwann cells [12], microglia [10] or even non-neural cells [49]. This suggests a widespread role for NgR in many biological systems. NgR and its ligands have shown to hamper plasticity following neural damage or in CNS diseases [16–20]. Interacting with NgR, myelin derived inhibitory factors are the major candidates affecting axon outgrowth in the adult CNS [5]. Numerous experimental approaches have been used to assess the role of these inhibitory factors or their common receptor on axonal repair, including molecular blocking strategies, transgenic mice and models of CNS damage from spinal cord injury [17,18], stroke [22] to immune-mediated models of demyelination [16,19,20,50]. It is well documented that inhibition of NgR can functionally enhance axonal repair, but divergent neurobiological outcomes have been observed following NgR inhibition in EAE models. Since OPCs, NPCs and also immune cells express NgR, the effect of NgR inhibition in non-immune models of demyelination has not been fully investigated.

Here, by partially blocking NgR, we provide functional evidence from an inhibitory role of NgR on progenitor cell repopulation and myelin repair following optic chiasm demyelination. Recording visual evoked potentials following NgR knocking down enabled us to assess the myelin repair process electrophysiologically.

To locally inhibit NgR, we injected siRNA against NgR into lateral ventricle of adult mouse and evaluated the efficiency of NgR blockade by real time PCR for NgR mRNA in the tissue isolated from third ventricle surroundings which is anatomically close to the optic chiasm. Real time PCR quantification showed that the siRNA inhibits NgR gene expression by up to 40% 24 hours after in vivo injection. We thus applied siRNAs against NgR (siNgR) on a daily basis through permanent cannula. Our previous study [37] showed that with this technique the in vivo viability of siRNA is about 24 hours. This short term knock-down efficiency actually ensures that such RNAs interference method exerts transient and hence reversible effects [37].

This siNgR was applied following LPC-induced demyelination localized in the optic chiasm. Our results show that in animals treated with LPC alone, lesions were maximal at 7 dpi. In contrast, in groups receiving siNgR over 14 days LPC-induced demyelination was maximal at 3 dpi and progressively and significantly

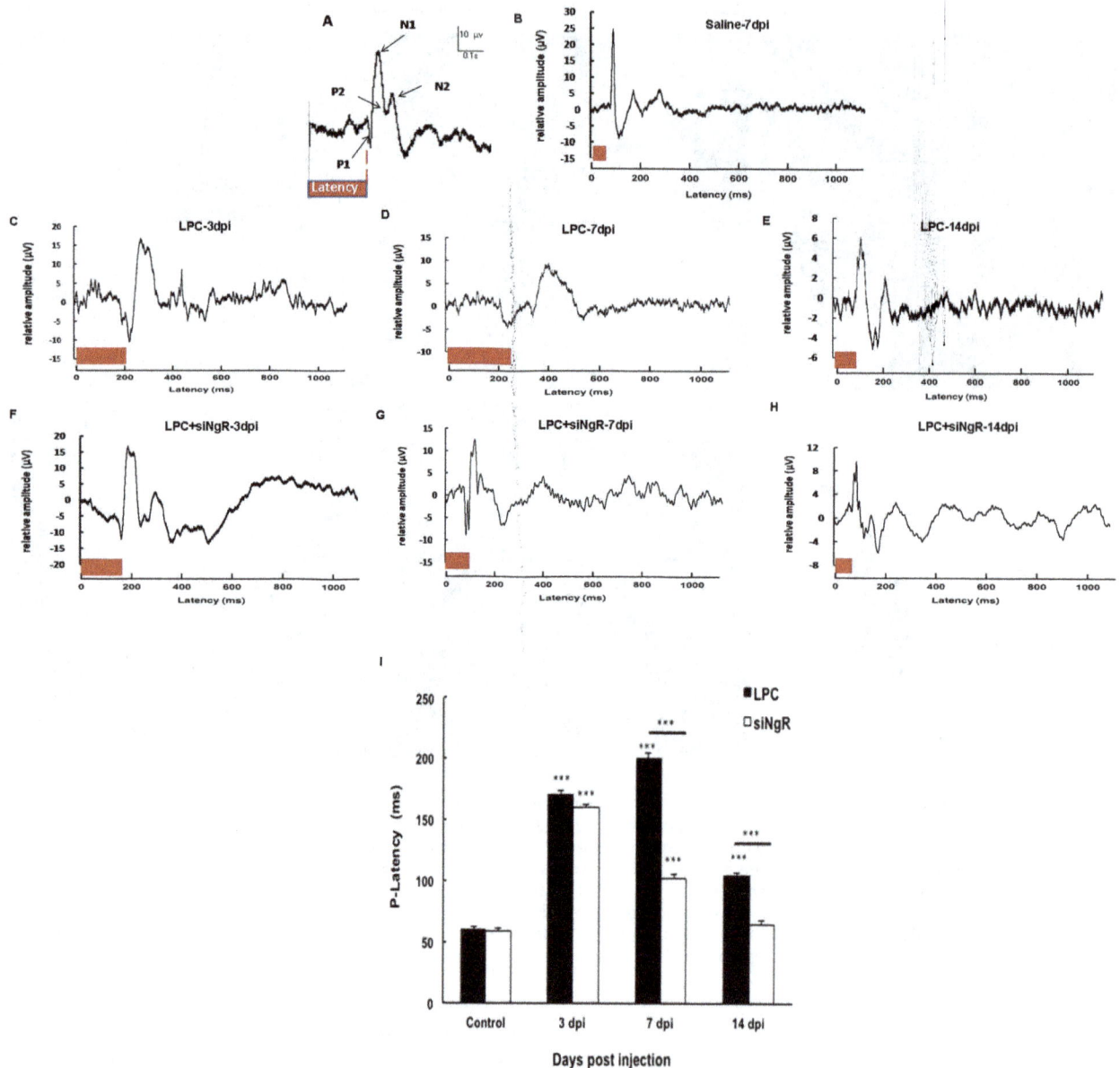

Figure 4. Functional recovery is induced by NgR inhibition in demyelinated optic chiasm. (A) Visual evoked potential (VEP) sample recordings from electroencephalographic activity and its components. The trace represented is the average of 300 sweeps of 300 ms duration with 1 Hz frequency. P1 latency (red bar) was measured by Biochart software. (B) VEP sample from animals treated with saline inside the chiasm (control) recorded at 7 dpi. (C–E) Changes in the P1 wave latency at 3, 7 and 14 dpi in the LPC treated animals. (F–H) VEP sample recordings from LPC+siNgR treated animals at 3, 7 and 14 dpi. (I) Quantitative analysis of changes in P1 latency in different groups. Statistical analysis used two-way ANOVA with Bonferroni's post-test. Treatment and time had a significant effect in this study. In LPC treated animals P1- latency was increased at 3, 7 and 14 dpi compared to control (all, [***]p<0.001) but was partially diminished at 14 dpi (E). In LPC+siNgR group, there was a significant increase in p-latency at 3 and 7 dpi compared to control (both, [***]P<0.001). NgR inhibition induces functional recovery at 7 and 14 dpi compared to LPC 7 and LPC 14, respectively (both, P<0.001) and there was no significant change in p-latency between LPC+siNgR and Control at14 dpi. Data was pooled from three independent experiments on mice (n=6), Bars: Mean ± SEMs.

reduced over the following 10 days (7 to 14 dpi). Our histological findings were functionally substantiated with VEPs recording. We used P1-latency delay, which closely reflects the degree of demyelination in the visual pathway. Recent studies show that latency prolongation of VEPs corresponds to size of the lesion area in the visual pathway in optic nerve demyelination or neuritis [28,48,51]. Here we show that LPC injection into the optic chiasm leads to increased P1-latency at 3 and 7 dpi, followed by significant reduction in the latency at 14 dpi. However, P1-latency was

recovered as early as 7 days post lesion in siNgR treated groups. Thus, inhibition of NgR facilitates functional recovery of visual pathways. This data fits with that of Chong et al. [27] who showed that mice lacking NogoA (NogoA-/-) have increased myelinogenic potential of oligodendrocytes, enabling enhanced remyelination after LPC-induced demyelination in the adult spinal cord [52]. The inhibitory effect of NogoA on OPCs differentiation in vitro has been also show by Syed and others (2008) [15]. However, Wang and others reported that exposure of neural stem cells with

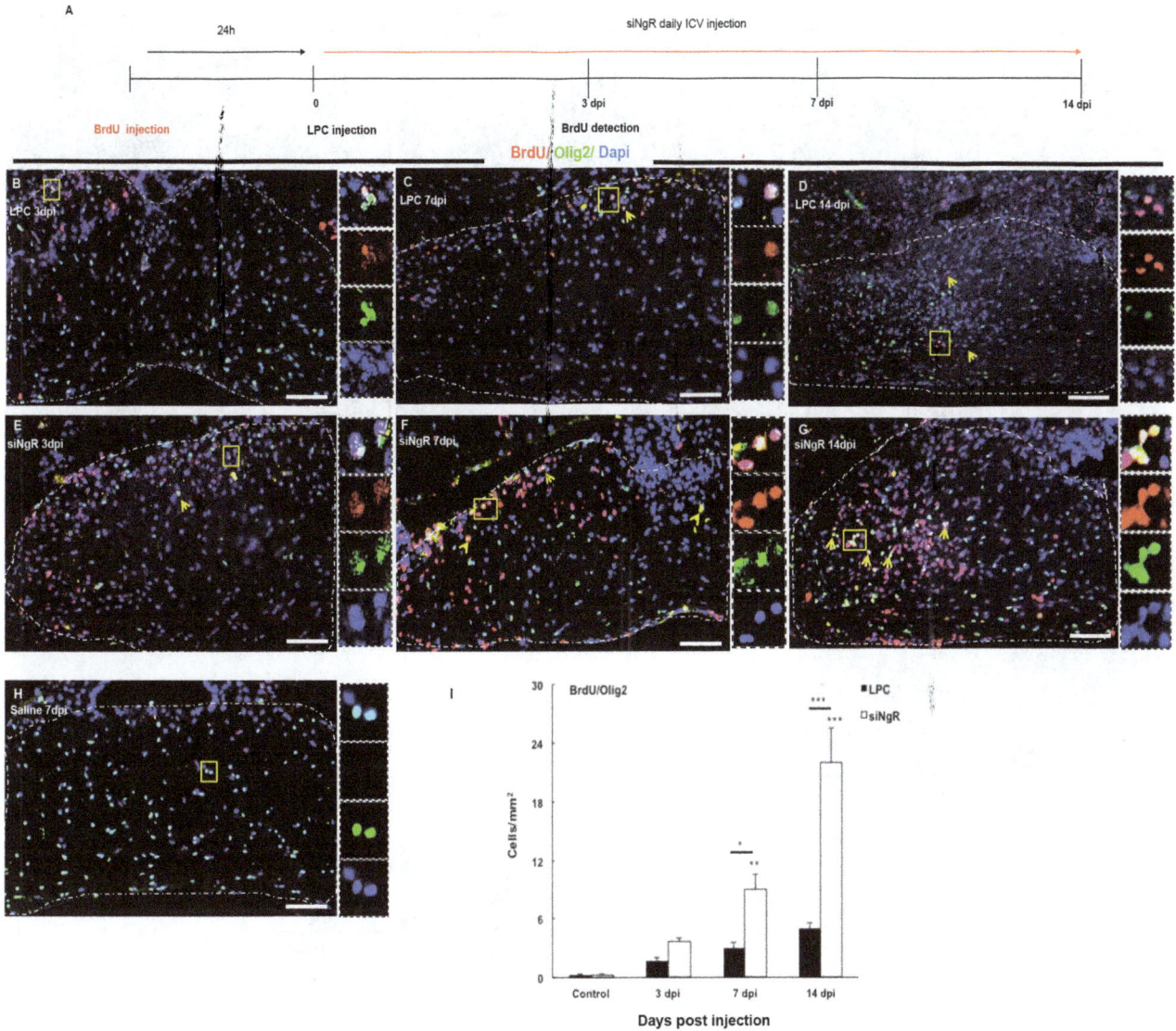

Figure 5. Increased BrdU+/Olig2+ cell numbers in demyelinated optic chiasm following NgR inhibition. Double immunohistochemistry (IHC) of BrdU (red) and Olig2 (green)-labeled cells was done on coronal section of optic chiasm in different groups. (A) Time line of BrdU injection and sampling in different groups. Mice received seven injections of Brdu at intervals of 2 hrs, 24 hrs prior to demyelination, and were sacrificed 3, 7 or 14 days after LPC injection. (B–D) BrdU+/Olig2+ cells in optic chiasm of LPC-treated animals at 3 (B), 7 (C) and 14 (D) dpi. (E–G) Optic chiasm of LPC+ siNgR treated animals at 3 (E), 7 (F) and 14 (G) dpi. (H) Low number of BrdU+/Olig2+ cells in optic chiasm of saline-treated animals at 7 dpi (Control). Arrows indicate double-labeled cells and Square shows the cells magnified in inset. Dashed line indicates optic chiasm border. (I) BrdU+/Olig2+ cells per area/mm^2 are averaged from the counts of nine sections of each chiasm. Statistical analysis used two-way ANOVA with Bonferroni's post-test. The effects of treatment and time were significant (p<0.001). In LPC treated groups the number of BrdU+/Olig2+cells was increased over the time but changes were not significant compared to Control. In LPC+siNgR treated animals, the number of BrdU+/Olig2+cells at 7 and 14 dpi in the lesion site was increased compared to control ([**]p<0.01, [***]p<0.001; respectively). Between groups significant changes exist at 7 dpi ([*]p<0.05) and 14 dpi ([***]p<0.001). Data are expressed as Mean±SEMs, n = 3, Bars: 100 µm.

nogo-66 promotes glial but inhibits neuronal differentiation in vitro [16].

Furthermore, the time course of repair with siNgR in our data fits with the recent report by Petratos and others [16] in which they showed a reduction in clinical score, inflammatory cell infiltrates, demyelination and axonal degeneration in EAE-induced *NgR-/-* mice. More specifically, their data shows that myelin repair in EAE-induced *NgR-/-* mice occur between 12-18 dpi [19,53]. Further, vaccination against Nogo A [20], or its systemic silencing using intravenously injected siRNA for NogoA suppresses EAE [50]. However, Steinbach and others reported

that complete depletion of NgR did not promote functional recovery in another EAE model [10,49]. These different observations in EAE models are most likely due to the expression of NgR by immune cells as well as neural cells which exert inhibitory roles on their migration [11]. We used immunocyto-chemistry with an Iba-1 antibody on sections and observed that the number of Iba-1+ cells in LPC and LPC+siNgR groups were significantly increased at 3 and 14 dpi. The number of Iba-1+ cells was slightly increased in the lesion site when NgR was partially inhibited; however, the result was not statistically significant compared to LPC-treated animals. So, we suggest that partial

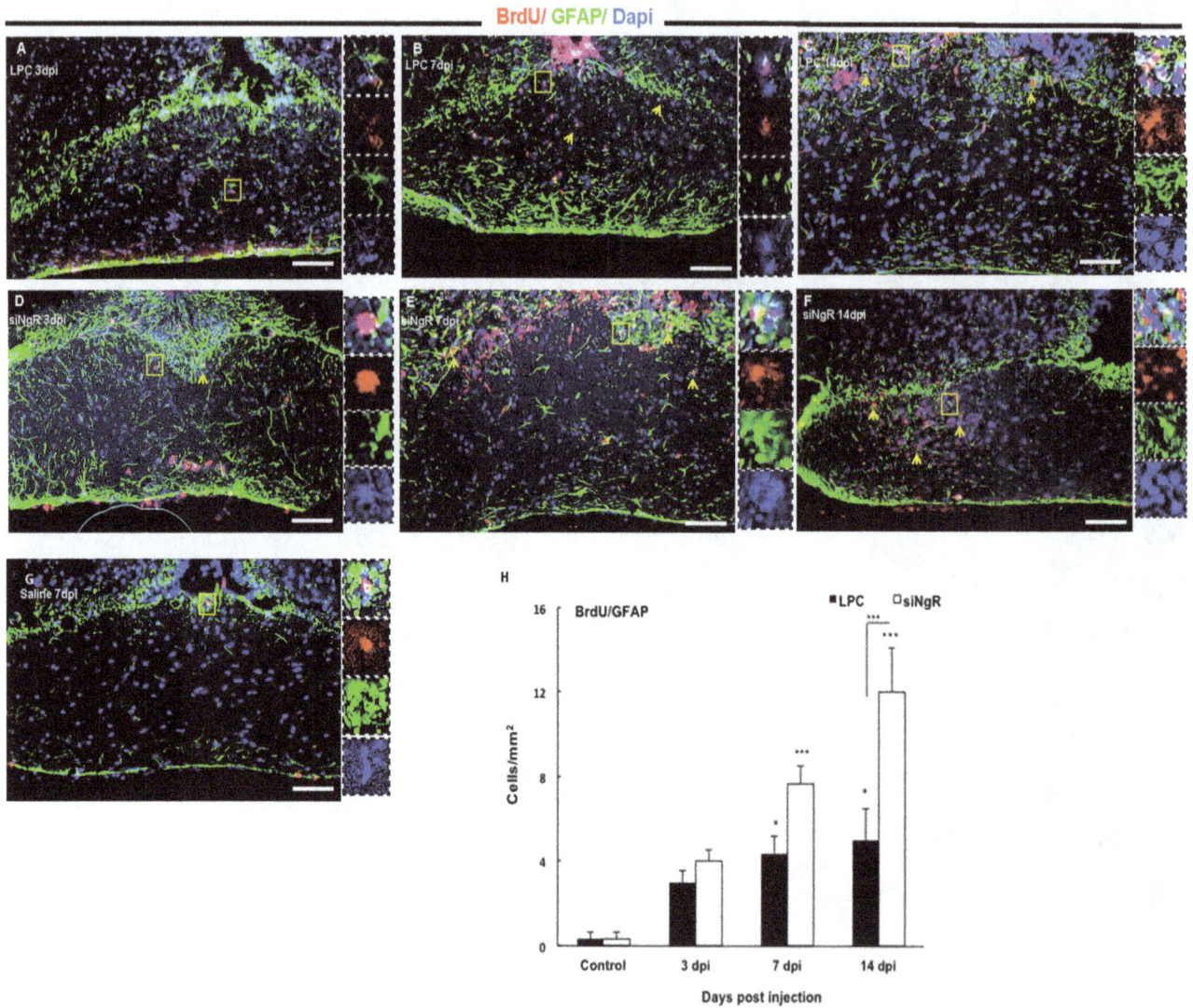

Figure 6. Increased numbers of BrdU+/GFAP+ cells within the lesion site following NgR inhibition. (A–C) Immunofluorescent images of Optic chiasm in LPC-treated animals at 3, 7 and 14 dpi. The number of BrdU+/GFAP+ cells at LPC 3 dpi (A), LPC 7 dpi (B) and 14 dpi (C) was increased. (D–F) Optic chiasm images of LPC+siNgR treated animals at 3 (D), 7 (E) and 14 dpi (F). The number of BrdU+/GFAP+ cells at 7 and 14 dpi in the lesion site was increased. (G) The number of BrdU+/GFAP+ cells in optic chiasm of saline-treated animals (Control) at 7 dpi was low. Arrows indicate double-labeled cells and Square shows the cells magnified in inset. (H) BrdU+/GFAP+ cells per area/mm^2 are quantified and averaged from the counts of nine sections of each chiasm. Statistical analysis of the differences between numbers of BrdU+/GFAP+ cells in the optic chiasm of all groups was done by two-way ANOVA followed by Bonferroni's post-test. Differences between groups were significant ($p < 0.001$). Post-test showed that the number of BrdU+/GFAP+ cells in LPC treated animals at 7 dpi and 14 dpi was increased significantly compared to Control (both, $p < 0.05$). In LPC+siNgR treated animals the number of BrdU+/GFAP+ cells at 7 and 14 dpi in the lesion site was increased significantly compared to Control (both, ***$p < 0.001$). NgR inhibition enhance the number of BrdU+/GFAP+ cells in optic chiasm compered to LPC groups and this change was significant between siNgR 14 dpi and LPC 14 dpi (***$p < 0.001$). Data are expressed as Mean ± SEMs, N = 3, Bars: 100 μm.

Table 1. Total number of BrdU+ cells in third ventricle and optic chiasm in different groups.

Total number of BrdU+ cells	Saline 7 dpi	LPC 3 dpi	LPC 7 dpi	LPC 14 dpi	siNgR 3 dpi	siNgR 7 dpi	siNgR 14 dpi
Third ventricle	0.3±0.12	7.3±1.97	9.1±1.5*	6±1.16	21.3±2.5***	16±2.49**	7±1.55^^
Optic chiasm	3.66±0.88	10±1.73	15±1.82	25.3±3.6***	14.67±2.6	32±2.25***	50.6±3.7

Data in all groups evaluated by one way ANOVA and *$p < 0.05$, **$p < 0.01$ and ***$p < 0.001$ show significance changes compared to saline and ^^$p < 0.01$ compared to siNgR 7 dpi.

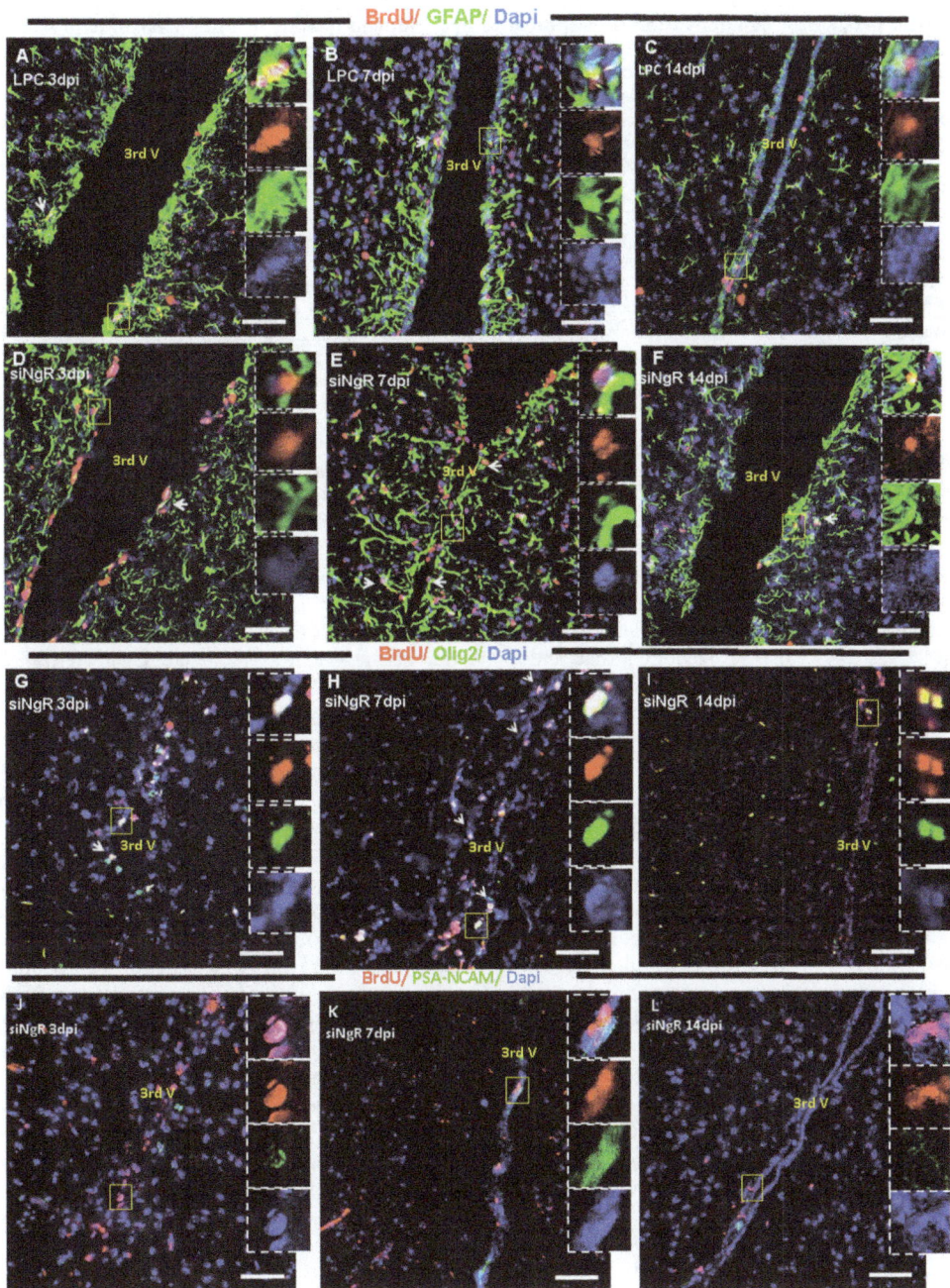

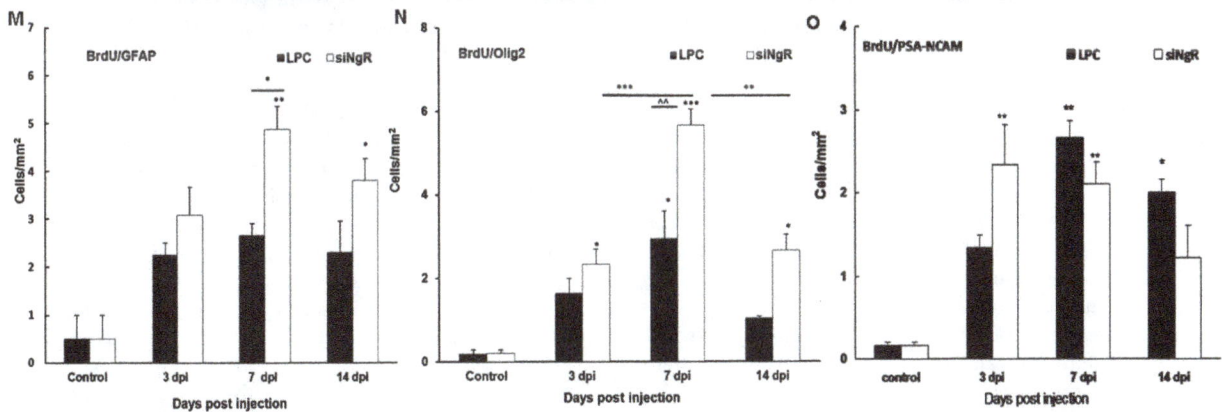

Figure 7. Third ventricle progenitor cell activation in response to LPC-induced lesions in optic chiasm is greater following NgR inhibition. Double labeling of BrdU (red) with Olig2, GFAP or PSA-NCAM (green) was done in coronal sections of third ventricle area in different groups. (A–C) BrdU+/GFAP+ cells in the rims of third ventricle of LPC group at 3 (A), 7 (B) and 14 dpi (C). (D–F) BrdU+/GFAP+ cells in the rims of third ventricle of LPC+siNgR treated animals at 3 (D), 7 (E) and 14 dpi (F). (G–I) BrdU/Olig2 double staining in third ventricle of LPC+siNgR treated animals at 3 (G), 7 (H) and 14 (I) dpi (see fig. S1D–F for BrdU+/Olig2+ cells in LPC group). (J–L) BrdU/PSA-NCAM positive cells in the third ventricle of LPC+siNgR treated animals at 3 (J), 7 (K) and 14 dpi (L) (see fig. S1G-I for BrdU+/PSA-NCAM+ cells in LPC group). Square shows the cells magnified in inset. Arrows show double marker positive cells. (M–O) Histograms show quantification of double marker positive cells, BrdU+/GAFP+ (M), BrdU+/Olig2+ (N) and BrdU+/PSA-NCAM+ (O) in different groups. Double marker positive cells per area/mm^2 are averaged from the counts of nine sections of each brain, n = 3. Statistical analysis used two-way ANOVA with Bonferroni's post-test. Differences between groups were significant (p<0.001). The number of BrdU+/GFAP+ cells in third ventricle of LPC 3, 7 and 14 dpi was increased but changes were not significant compared to Control 7dpi (mice received saline inside chiasm), but this type of cells in LPC+siNgR treated animals at 3, 7 and 14 dpi were considerably increased compared to Control (*p< 0.05, ***p<0.001, **p<0.01, respectively) (M). The number of BrdU+/Olig2+ cells was considerably increased in siNgR-LPC group at 3, 7 and 14 dpi compared to Control (**p<0.01, ***p<0.001; respectively) (N). Additionally in these animals, at 7 dpi the number of BrdU+/Olig2+ was considerably increased compared to LPC 7 dpi (∿∿p<0.001) (N). The number of BrdU/PSA-NCAM positive cells in the third ventricle of LPC+siNgR treated animals was significantly increased at 3 and 7 dpi (both, p<0.01), while it was significantly increases in LPC treated animals at 7 and 14 dpi (p<0.05, p<0.01; respectively). Data are expressed as Mean ±SEM, Bars: 50 µm.

blockade of NgR in our study might not favor the myelination through inflammatory cells mediated mechanisms. Although it has been reported that NgR expression by dendritic cells [10], microglia [12] and macrophages [46] helps repulsion of these cells from myelin debris or the lesion site, Kotter et al. (2001) showed that depletion of these cells in LPC-induced demyelination by inhibiting inflammatory responses impairs remyelination [47]. Furthermore, Miron et al. (2013) recently reported that anti-inflammatory microglia and macrophages drive oligodendrocyte differentiation during CNS remyelination [7]. So, we suggest that partial blockade of NgR in our study might not favor the repair through inflammatory cells mediated mechanisms.

It has been reported that myelin associated inhibitory factors inhibit OPCs migration [13] and depletion of NogoA increases progenitor cell migration during cortical development [28,30]. To investigate the effect of NgR inhibition on precursor cell recruitment in vivo, we pre-labeled the proliferating cells by BrdU before induction of LPC lesion in adult mouse optic chiasm. Our previous data showed that BrdU+ cells were recruited to the demyelinated rat optic chiasm over time and this was concurrent with recovery in myelin repair and VEP features [54]. In the current study we adjusted this model in mice to assess the effect of NgR inhibition on precursor cell repopulation. Interestingly our results reveal that total number of BrdU+ cells was significantly increased in demyelinated mice treated with siNgR over time when compared to LPC-induced control mice. Furthermore, we observed that these recruited cells expressed Olig2 but also GFAP markers of glial cells. Our observations show that NgR inhibition functionally increases myelin repair, as evidenced by an enhancement in progenitor cell migration to the lesion site. The mechanisms by which NgR inhibition favors cell recruitment need to be addressed. However, since there is evidence that OPC migration is governed by PDGF-AA and FGF-2 [55], and as FGF-2 has been suggested to interact with NgR1, which antagonizes FGF-2 signaling [13], it is plausible that NgR expressed on oligodendroglial lineage cells may play a role in their migration. Also NgR blockade in vitro increases the total covered distance and the maximum speed of migration of precursors in neurospheres [56]. Nogo A could also enhance the adhesion and inhibit the migration of OECs via NgR regulation of RhoA [10,12]. Roles for NgR on immune cell migration [57] or human glioma cells [32,34] have been also reported.

In adult human and rodents, the optic chiasm is anatomically proximal to the third ventricle. Several studies showed that third ventricle neurogenic zone contains multipotent cells that can give rise into neurons, oligodendrocytes and astrocytes in vitro [30]. Xu and others (2005) reported that cells located in ependymal layer of the third ventricle were able to migrate into hypothalamic

parenchymal regions and differentiate into functional neurons. Our previous study [41] also showed that progenitor cells in the third ventricle surroundings could be reactivated by adjacent chiasm demyelination. Ernest and others (2005) also showed that in response to brain damage, there was a significant increase in numbers of BrdU+ cells in third ventricle. We also observed that numbers of BrdU+ cells were significantly greater than control at 7 dpi when NgR was inhibited. Characterization of cell types revealed that NgR inhibition plus chiasm demyelination increases BrdU+/Olig2+ or BrdU+/GFAP+ populations in comparison with control animals.

The number of Olig2+ precursor cells significantly decreased in third ventricle in NgR treated mice at 14 dpi. The reduction of BrdU+/Olig2+ cells in the third ventricle at days 7 to 14 was correlated with the appearance of increased numbers of these cells within the chiasm as early as 7 dpi. These increases at 14 dpi suggest that progenitor cells located in third ventricle were mobilized and migrated in response to the LPC-induced demyelination in the optic chiasm. These mobilization and migration process were more marked when NgR was blocked. Mobilization of proliferating cells from SVZ of lateral ventricle in response to periventricular demyelination has been also reported [30]. We also observed that the number of BrdU+/GFAP+ cells increased in the area around the third ventricles in siNgR treated animals. GFAP reactivation may be an immediate astrocytic response to damage as in other brain areas. GFAP gene expression increases in response to demyelination in optic chiasm [58] indicating astrocyte reactivity in the lesion site. Although astrocyte activation has positive and negative effects on survival, migration and differentiation of OPCs, the data from GFAP-/- mice suggest that astrocytes are required for the long-term maintenance of CNS remyelination [59] and OPC remyelination fails in their absence [31,60,61]. Our results suggest that inhibition of NgR facilitated third ventricle progenitor activation and cell mobilization in response to demyelinated optic chiasm. It is also well documented that developmental origin of myelinating cells in the optic chiasm is an area in third ventricle neurogenic zone [62].

It has been also reported that inhibition of LINGO-1, a NgR co-receptor enhances oligodendrocyte differentiation and myelination in LINGO-/- [63] and in EAE model in LINGO-/- mice [64]. The authors of these reports, however, did not study expression of NgR in oligodendrocyte lineage cells, but did highlight the expression and role of LINGO-1 on neurons and mature oligodendrocytes. They showed that expression of LINGO-1, similar to its co-receptor NgR on neurons, can inhibit axonal regeneration by activation of RhoA signaling pathway; though LINGO-1 function on oligodendrocyte was not mediated through binding to NgR [65–67]. Huang et al. (2012); however, suggested that antagonizing NgR *in vitro* increased the number of PDGFRα+ OPCs and prolonged their processes but hampered their differentiation. They suggested that the effect of myelin inhibitory factors on OPC differentiation and process extending via NgR expressed by OPCs were mainly mediated via Erk1/2 and PI3/Akt signaling pathways and also involved various cell proliferation and differentiation effects [68,69], including oligodendrocyte differentiation [17].

In the present study, we observed a reduced demyelination area at 7 dpi in the optic chiasm of siNgR treated groups. Two major conclusions can be drawn from our observations. First, inhibition of NgR could induce a neuroprotective effect against demyelination. Second, NgR signaling exerts a negative role on progenitor cell migration and myelin repair. Yu and coworkers suggested that in addition to stimulating axon regeneration, NgR inhibition might also be neuroprotective, contributing to the overall functional recovery after spinal cord injury, which can be attributed to neuroprotective effect of NgR inhibition. However, the mechanism underlying such possible effects remains to be investigated.

To our knowledge, the current data are the first to show that the therapeutic effect of NgR inhibition on functional myelin recovery in a non-immune model of demyelination. Further studies need to be carried out to elucidate the molecular mechanisms by which NgR exerts its inhibitory effects on plasticity *in vivo*. Such information about the nature of the changes in the endogenous cell niche in response to demyelination will clarify to what extent the potential of self-repair in adult CNS can be enhanced following damage. Such research would contribute to therapeutic perspectives for successful repair in demyelinating disorders including Multiple Sclerosis.

Supporting Information

Figure S1 Third ventricle response to LPC-induced demyelination. (A–C) Double immunostaining of BrdU (red) and Olig2, GFAP and PSA-NCAM (green)-labeled cells in coronal section of third ventricle in saline treated animals showed that progenitor cells residing in third ventricle wall were not mitotically active. (D–F) Brdu (red)/Olig2 (green) double staining in third ventricle of LPC treated animals at 3, 7 and 14 dpi respectively. The number of BrdU+/Olig2+ cells increased at 7 dpi (E) compared to control. (G–I) The number of BrdU (red) and PSA-NCAM (green) positive cells in the third ventricle of LPC treated animals at 3(G), 7 (H) and 14 dpi (I) respectively. There were no remarkable changes between these groups. (PDF)

Table S1 Four different sequences of siRNA against NgR were combined in the same tube for injection.

Table S2 Primary antibodies used in this study.

Table S3 Secondary antibodies used in this study.

Raw Data S1 Raw data are presented as an attached Excel file.

Acknowledgments

We thank Dr. Anne Baron Van-Evercooren for critically reviewing this manuscript and giving many interesting and provocative comments and Miss Samaneh Dehghan for her technical assistance. We also thank Dr. Sarah Moyon from Dr. Catherine Lubetzki team for their collaborations. First author thanks Multiple Sclerosis International Federation (www.msif.org) for sabbatical support to complete this project. Work in B. Demeneix' laboratory is supported by the Association Française contre les Myopathies (AFM). The project also received support from Tarbiat Modares University as a PhD dissertation.

Author Contributions

Conceived and designed the experiments: MJ BAD. Performed the experiments: FP SM GMD. Analyzed the data: FP SM GMD JMZ ALJ JPS BAD MJ. Contributed reagents/materials/analysis tools: JMZ BAD MJ. Contributed to the writing of the manuscript: FP SM GMD BAD MJ.

References

1. GrandPre T, Nakamura F, Vartanian T, Strittmatter SM (2000) Identification of the Nogo inhibitor of axon regeneration as a Reticulon protein. Nature 403: 439–444.
2. McKerracher L, David S, Jackson DL, Kottis V, Dunn RJ, et al. (1994) Identification of myelin-associated glycoprotein as a major myelin-derived inhibitor of neurite growth. Neuron 13: 805–811.
3. Wang KC, Kim JA, Sivasankaran R, Segal R, He Z (2002) P75 interacts with the Nogo receptor as a co-receptor for Nogo, MAG and OMgp. Nature 420: 74–78.
4. Schwab ME (2010) Functions of Nogo proteins and their receptors in the nervous system. Nature reviews Neuroscience 11: 799–811.
5. Fournier AE, GrandPre T, Strittmatter SM (2001) Identification of a receptor mediating Nogo-66 inhibition of axonal regeneration. Nature 409: 341–346.
6. Hunt D, Mason MR, Campbell G, Coffin R, Anderson PN (2002) Nogo receptor mRNA expression in intact and regenerating CNS neurons. Molecular and cellular neurosciences 20: 537–552.
7. Lee JY, Petratos S (2013) Multiple sclerosis: does Nogo play a role? The Neuroscientist: a review journal bringing neurobiology, neurology and psychiatry 19: 394–408.
8. Huang JY, Wang YX, Gu WL, Fu SL, Li Y, et al. (2012) Expression and function of myelin-associated proteins and their common receptor NgR on oligodendrocyte progenitor cells. Brain research 1437: 1–15.
9. Satoh J, Onoue H, Arima K, Yamamura T (2005) Nogo-A and nogo receptor expression in demyelinating lesions of multiple sclerosis. Journal of neuropathology and experimental neurology 64: 129–138.
10. Yan J, Zhou X, Guo JJ, Mao L, Wang YJ, et al. (2012) Nogo-66 inhibits adhesion and migration of microglia via GTPase Rho pathway in vitro. Journal of neurochemistry 120: 721–731.
11. McDonald CL, Steinbach K, Kern F, Schweigreiter R, Martin R, et al. (2011) Nogo receptor is involved in the adhesion of dendritic cells to myelin. Journal of neuroinflammation 8: 113.
12. Fry EJ, Ho C, David S (2007) A role for Nogo receptor in macrophage clearance from injured peripheral nerve. Neuron 53: 649–662.
13. Mathis C, Schroter A, Thallmair M, Schwab ME (2010) Nogo-a regulates neural precursor migration in the embryonic mouse cortex. Cerebral cortex 20: 2380–2390.
14. Wang F, Zhu Y (2008) The interaction of Nogo-66 receptor with Nogo-p4 inhibits the neuronal differentiation of neural stem cells. Neuroscience 151: 74–81.
15. Wang B, Xiao Z, Chen B, Han J, Gao Y, et al. (2008) Nogo-66 promotes the differentiation of neural progenitors into astroglial lineage cells through mTOR-STAT3 pathway. PloS one 3: e1856.
16. Petratos S, Ozturk E, Azari MF, Kenny R, Lee JY, et al. (2012) Limiting multiple sclerosis related axonopathy by blocking Nogo receptor and CRMP-2 phosphorylation. Brain: a journal of neurology 135: 1794–1818.
17. Yu P, Huang L, Zou J, Yu Z, Wang Y, et al. (2008) Immunization with recombinant Nogo-66 receptor (NgR) promotes axonal regeneration and recovery of function after spinal cord injury in rats. Neurobiology of disease 32: 535–542.
18. Harvey PA, Lee DH, Qian F, Weinreb PH, Frank E (2009) Blockade of Nogo receptor ligands promotes functional regeneration of sensory axons after dorsal root crush. The Journal of neuroscience: the official journal of the Society for Neuroscience 29: 6285–6295.
19. Karnezis T, Mandemakers W, McQualter JL, Zheng B, Ho PP, et al. (2004) The neurite outgrowth inhibitor Nogo A is involved in autoimmune-mediated demyelination. Nature neuroscience 7: 736–744.
20. Yang Y, Liu Y, Wei P, Peng H, Winger R, et al. (2010) Silencing Nogo-A promotes functional recovery in demyelinating disease. Annals of neurology 67: 498–507.
21. Jiang W, Xia F, Han J, Wang J (2009) Patterns of Nogo-A, NgR, and RhoA expression in the brain tissues of rats with focal cerebral infarction. Translational research: the journal of laboratory and clinical medicine 154: 40–48.

22. Wang T, Wang J, Yin C, Liu R, Zhang JH, et al. (2010) Down-regulation of Nogo receptor promotes functional recovery by enhancing axonal connectivity after experimental stroke in rats. Brain research 1360: 147–158.

23. Edgar JM, Garbern J (2004) The myelinated axon is dependent on the myelinating cell for support and maintenance: molecules involved. Journal of neuroscience research 76: 593–598.

24. Griffiths I, Klugmann M, Anderson T, Yool D, Thomson C, et al. (1998) Axonal swellings and degeneration in mice lacking the major proteolipid of myelin. Science 280: 1610–1613.

25. Irvine KA, Blakemore WF (2008) Remyelination protects axons from demyelination-associated axon degeneration. Brain: a journal of neurology 131: 1464–1477.

26. Lappe-Siefke C, Goebbels S, Gravel M, Nicksch E, Lee J, et al. (2003) Disruption of Cnp1 uncouples oligodendroglial functions in axonal support and myelination. Nature genetics 33: 366–374.

27. Chong SY, Rosenberg SS, Fancy SP, Zhao C, Shen YA, et al. (2012) Neurite outgrowth inhibitor Nogo-A establishes spatial segregation and extent of oligodendrocyte myelination. Proceedings of the National Academy of Sciences of the United States of America 109: 1299–1304.

28. Mozafari S, Sherafat MA, Javan M, Mirnajafi-Zadeh J, Tiraihi T (2010) Visual evoked potentials and MBP gene expression imply endogenous myelin repair in adult rat optic nerve and chiasm following local lysolecithin induced demyelination. Brain research 1351: 50–56.

29. Dehghan S, Javan M, Pourabdolhossein F, Mirnajafi-Zadeh J, Baharvand H (2012) Basic fibroblast growth factor potentiates myelin repair following induction of experimental demyelination in adult mouse optic chiasm and nerves. Journal of molecular neuroscience: MN 48: 77–85.

30. Mozafari S, Javan M, Sherafat MA, Mirnajafi-Zadeh J, Heibatollahi M, et al. (2011) Analysis of structural and molecular events associated with adult rat optic chiasm and nerves demyelination and remyelination: possible role for 3rd ventricle proliferating cells. Neuromolecular medicine 13: 138–150.

31. Ono K, Yasui Y, Rutishauser U, Miller RH (1997) Focal ventricular origin and migration of oligodendrocyte precursors into the chick optic nerve. Neuron 19: 283–292.

32. Xu Y, Tamamaki N, Noda T, Kimura K, Itokazu Y, et al. (2005) Neurogenesis in the ependymal layer of the adult rat 3rd ventricle. Experimental neurology 192: 251–264.

33. Ernst C, Christie BR (2005) Nestin-expressing cells and their relationship to mitotically active cells in the subventricular zones of the adult rat. The European journal of neuroscience 22: 3059–3066.

34. Dahiya S, Lee da Y, Gutmann DH (2011) Comparative characterization of the human and mouse third ventricle germinal zones. Journal of neuropathology and experimental neurology 70: 622–633.

35. Paxinos GF, Franklin KBJ (2004) The mouse brain in stereotaxic coordinates. San Diego, California: Academic Press.

36. Lopez-Juarez A, Remaud S, Hassani Z, Jolivet P, Pierre Simons J, et al. (2012) Thyroid hormone signaling acts as a neurogenic switch by repressing Sox2 in the adult neural stem cell niche. Cell stem cell 10: 531–543.

37. Remaud S, Lopez-Juarez SA, Bolcato-Bellemin AL, Neuberg P, Stock F, et al. (2013) Inhibition of Sox2 Expression in the Adult Neural Stem Cell Niche In Vivo by Monocationic-based siRNA Delivery. Molecular therapy Nucleic acids 2: e89.

38. Decherf S, Seugnet I, Kouidhi S, Lopez-Juarez A, Clerget-Froidevaux MS, et al. (2010) Thyroid hormone exerts negative feedback on hypothalamic type 4 melanocortin receptor expression. Proceedings of the National Academy of Sciences of the United States of America 107: 4471–4476.

39. Ishikawa T, Fujiwara A, Takechi K, Ago J, Matsumoto N, et al. (2008) Changes of visual evoked potential induced by lateral geniculate nucleus kindling in rats. Epilepsy research 79: 146–150.

40. Kuroda K, Fujiwara A, Takeda Y, Kamei C (2009) Effects of narcotics, including morphine, on visual evoked potential in rats. European journal of pharmacology 602: 294–297.

41. Picard-Riera N, Decker L, Delarasse C, Goude K, Nait-Oumesmar B, et al. (2002) Experimental autoimmune encephalomyelitis mobilizes neural progenitors from the subventricular zone to undergo oligodendrogenesis in adult mice. Proceedings of the National Academy of Sciences of the United States of America 99: 13211–13216.

42. Decker L, Picard-Riera N, Lachapelle F, Baron-Van Evercooren A (2002) Growth factor treatment promotes mobilization of young but not aged adult subventricular zone precursors in response to demyelination. Journal of neuroscience research 69: 763–771.

43. Nait-Oumesmar B, Decker L, Lachapelle F, Avellana-Adalid V, Bachelin C, et al. (1999) Progenitor cells of the adult mouse subventricular zone proliferate, migrate and differentiate into oligodendrocytes after demyelination. The European journal of neuroscience 11: 4357–4366.

44. Lois C, Alvarez-Buylla A (1994) Long-distance neuronal migration in the adult mammalian brain. Science 264: 1145–1148.

45. Chitnis T, Imitola J, Wang Y, Elyaman W, Chawla P, et al. (2007) Elevated neuronal expression of CD200 protects Wlds mice from inflammation-mediated neurodegeneration. The American journal of pathology 170: 1695–1712.

46. Kotter MR, Setzu A, Sim FJ, Van Rooijen N, Franklin RJ (2001) Macrophage depletion impairs oligodendrocyte remyelination following lysolecithin-induced demyelination. Glia 35: 204–212.

47. Miron VE, Boyd A, Zhao JW, Yuen TJ, Ruckh JM, et al. (2013) M2 microglia and macrophages drive oligodendrocyte differentiation during CNS remyelination. Nature neuroscience 16: 1211–1218.

48. You Y, Klistorner A, Thie J, Graham SL (2011) Latency delay of visual evoked potential is a real measurement of demyelination in a rat model of optic neuritis. Investigative ophthalmology & visual science 52: 6911–6918.

49. Satarian L, Javan M, Kiani S, Hajikaram M, Mirnajafi-Zadeh J, et al. (2013) Engrafted human induced pluripotent stem cell-derived anterior specified neural progenitors protect the rat crushed optic nerve. PloS one 8: e71855.

50. Steinbach K, McDonald CL, Reindl M, Schweigreiter R, Bandtlow C, et al. (2011) Nogo-receptors NgR1 and NgR2 do not mediate regulation of CD4 T helper responses and CNS repair in experimental autoimmune encephalomyelitis. PloS one 6: e26341.

51. Klistorner A, Graham S, Fraser C, Garrick R, Nguyen T, et al. (2007) Electrophysiological evidence for heterogeneity of lesions in optic neuritis. Investigative ophthalmology & visual science 48: 4549–4556.

52. Syed YA, Baer AS, Lubec G, Hoeger H, Widhalm G, et al. (2008) Inhibition of oligodendrocyte precursor cell differentiation by myelin-associated proteins. Neurosurgical focus 24: E5.

53. Fontoura P, Ho PP, DeVoss J, Zheng B, Lee BJ, et al. (2004) Immunity to the extracellular domain of Nogo-A modulates experimental autoimmune encephalomyelitis. Journal of immunology 173: 6981–6992.

54. de Castro F, Bribian A (2005) The molecular orchestra of the migration of oligodendrocyte precursors during development. Brain research Brain research reviews 49: 227–241.

55. Lee H, Raiker SJ, Venkatesh K, Geary R, Robak LA, et al. (2008) Synaptic function for the Nogo-66 receptor NgR1: regulation of dendritic spine morphology and activity-dependent synaptic strength. The Journal of neuroscience: the official journal of the Society for Neuroscience 28: 2753–2765.

56. Su Z, Cao L, Zhu Y, Liu X, Huang Z, et al. (2007) Nogo enhances the adhesion of olfactory ensheathing cells and inhibits their migration. Journal of cell science 120: 1877–1887.

57. Liao H, Duka T, Teng FY, Sun L, Bu WY, et al. (2004) Nogo-66 and myelin-associated glycoprotein (MAG) inhibit the adhesion and migration of Nogo-66 receptor expressing human glioma cells. Journal of neurochemistry 90: 1156–1162.

58. Liedtke W, Edelmann W, Chiu FC, Kucherlapati R, Raine CS (1998) Experimental autoimmune encephalomyelitis in mice lacking glial fibrillary acidic protein is characterized by a more severe clinical course and an infiltrative central nervous system lesion. The American journal of pathology 152: 251–259.

59. Talbott JF, Loy DN, Liu Y, Qiu MS, Bunge MB, et al. (2005) Endogenous Nkx2.2+/Olig2+ oligodendrocyte precursor cells fail to remyelinate the demyelinated adult rat spinal cord in the absence of astrocytes. Experimental neurology 192: 11–24.

60. Colello RJ, Devey LR, Imperato E, Pott U (1995) The chronology of oligodendrocyte differentiation in the rat optic nerve: evidence for a signaling step initiating myelination in the CNS. The Journal of neuroscience: the official journal of the Society for Neuroscience 15: 7665–7672.

61. Gao L, Miller RH (2006) Specification of optic nerve oligodendrocyte precursors by retinal ganglion cell axons. The Journal of neuroscience: the official journal of the Society for Neuroscience 26: 7619–7628.

62. Mi S, Miller RH, Lee X, Scott ML, Shulag-Morskaya S, et al. (2005) LINGO-1 negatively regulates myelination by oligodendrocytes. Nature neuroscience 8: 745–751.

63. Mi S, Hu B, Hahm K, Luo Y, Kam Hui ES, et al. (2007) LINGO-1 antagonist promotes spinal cord remyelination and axonal integrity in MOG-induced experimental autoimmune encephalomyelitis. Nature medicine 13: 1228–1233.

64. Jepson S, Vought B, Gross CH, Gan L, Austen D, et al. (2012) LINGO-1, a transmembrane signaling protein, inhibits oligodendrocyte differentiation and myelination through intercellular self-interactions. The Journal of biological chemistry 287: 22184–22195.

65. Cantley LC (2002) The phosphoinositide 3-kinase pathway. Science 296: 1655–1657.

66. Chen Z, Gibson TB, Robinson F, Silvestro L, Pearson G, et al. (2001) MAP kinases. Chemical reviews 101: 2449–2476.

67. Kandel ES, Hay N (1999) The regulation and activities of the multifunctional serine/threonine kinase Akt/PKB. Experimental cell research 253: 210–229.

68. Bibollet-Bahena O, Cui QL, Almazan G (2009) The insulin-like growth factor-1 axis and its potential as a therapeutic target in central nervous system (CNS) disorders. Central nervous system agents in medicinal chemistry 9: 95–109.

69. Hu JG, Fu SL, Wang YX, Li Y, Jiang XY, et al. (2008) Platelet-derived growth factor-AA mediates oligodendrocyte lineage differentiation through activation of extracellular signal-regulated kinase signaling pathway. Neuroscience 151: 138–147.

13

Arousal vs. Relaxation: A Comparison of the Neurophysiological and Cognitive Correlates of Vajrayana and Theravada Meditative Practices

Ido Amihai[1], Maria Kozhevnikov[1,2]*

1 National University of Singapore, Psychology Department, Singapore, Singapore, **2** Martinos Center for Biomedical Imaging, MGH & Harvard Medical School, Charlestown, Massachusetts, United States of America

Abstract

Based on evidence of parasympathetic activation, early studies defined meditation as a relaxation response. Later research attempted to categorize meditation as either involving focused or distributed attentional systems. Neither of these hypotheses received strong empirical support, and most of the studies investigated Theravada style meditative practices. In this study, we compared neurophysiological (EEG, EKG) and cognitive correlates of meditative practices that are thought to utilize either focused or distributed attention, from both Theravada and Vajrayana traditions. The results of Study 1 show that both focused (Shamatha) and distributed (Vipassana) attention meditations of the Theravada tradition produced enhanced parasympathetic activation indicative of a relaxation response. In contrast, both focused (Deity) and distributed (Rig-pa) meditations of the Vajrayana tradition produced sympathetic activation, indicative of arousal. Additionally, the results of Study 2 demonstrated an immediate dramatic increase in performance on cognitive tasks following only Vajrayana styles of meditation, indicating enhanced phasic alertness due to arousal. Furthermore, our EEG results showed qualitatively different patterns of activation between Theravada and Vajrayana meditations, albeit highly similar activity between meditations within the same tradition. In conclusion, consistent with Tibetan scriptures that described Shamatha and Vipassana techniques as those that calm and relax the mind, and Vajrayana techniques as those that require 'an awake quality' of the mind, we show that Theravada and Vajrayana meditations are based on different neurophysiological mechanisms, which give rise to either a relaxation or arousal response. Hence, it may be more appropriate to categorize meditations in terms of relaxation vs. arousal, whereas classification methods that rely on the focused vs. distributed attention dichotomy may need to be reexamined.

Editor: J. David Creswell, Carnegie Mellon University, United States of America

Funding: This research is funded by the National University of Singapore. The funders had no role in study design, data collection and analysis, decision to publish, or preparation of the manuscript.

Competing Interests: The authors have declare that no competing interests exist.

* Email: psymaria@nus.edu.sg

Introduction

In spite of the increasing interest in meditation, evidenced by its global popularity and output of scientific papers, the failure to accurately define or categorize different types of meditations has been consistently mentioned in the scientific literature [1]. One of the reasons for these difficulties stems from an insufficient understanding of the theoretical and cultural differences between different meditative traditions, which has led to inconsistent findings in the scientific literature about the nature of meditation and its neurophysiological correlates [1]. The first major attempt to provide an operational definition of meditation was proposed by Benson [2] who reported that meditation activated the parasympathetic nervous system, and described the effect of meditation as a "relaxation response". The relaxation response refers to a physical state of deep rest, physiologically defined as a decrease in sympathetic activity (decreased heart and respiratory rate, blood pressure, oxygen consumption and reduction in cortisol and noradrenaline). Based on Benson's approach, an evolutionary theory was proposed, where meditation was viewed as a wakeful metabolic state of parasympathetic dominance – a state of deep

bodily rest – similar to hibernation, where the potential of acute mental ability nevertheless remains [3].

Furthermore, a number of early studies, consistent with Benson's approach, showed that other relaxation techniques, such as self-hypnosis and progressive relaxation, produce the same reduction effect as meditation on heart and respiration rates, as well as systolic and diastolic blood pressure [4–8]. However, most previous studies on the physiological, electrophysiological, and neural correlates of meditation, including research that demonstrated a relaxation response, have been conducted on *Theravada* or *Mahayana* Buddhist styles of meditation. On the other hand, studies on meditative practices of the *Vajrayana* tradition (also referred to as *Tantric Buddhism*), which is central to Tibetan Buddhism (see Supporting Information S1), have been relatively limited in scope. Indeed, previous research focused primarily on Theravada meditation styles such as Shamatha or Vipassana [6,9], both of which emphasize avoiding discursive thought by letting the practitioner concentrate on the object of meditation or his/her own mental activity, respectively [10]. In addition to Shamatha and Vipassana, which are the main meditative techniques of Theravada Buddhist schools, "compassion meditation" received much attention in recent scientific studies [11–13]. This type of meditation, however, pertains to all the Buddhist traditions, and it is not unique to Theravada or Vajrayana [14,15].

While meditative techniques of all Buddhist teachings stress liberation from all conceptual delusions, the means of achieving it are quite different. Specifically, Buddhist texts emphasize that Theravada styles of meditation, such as Shamatha or Vipassana, are techniques that emphasize "internally steadying" or stabilizing the "unstable mind", and cultivating the state of quiescence and tranquility, through which the nature of the mind could be seen without obstruction [16,17]. Vajrayana, in contrast, emphasizes the training "which is not exactly the same as keeping the mind still and quiet" [18], but rather aims at the realization of 'self-existing wakefulness' or 'an awake quality' of the mind, free from dualistic thoughts, which is "like a radiant flame of a candle which exists all by itself" [19]. Furthermore, Vajrayana teaching emphasizes that the preoccupation with "being too calm" blocks "the recognition of self-existing wakefulness", and that in a Vajrayana context, "it is sometimes said that stillness is not absolutely necessary..." [20]. Thus, from a Vajrayana perspective, the conceptualization of meditation as a relaxation response seems to be incongruent with Tibetan views of Vajrayana Tantric practices, which do not presuppose relaxation [21]. Indeed, Vajrayana "generation stage" practices, such as "visualization of self-generation-as-Deity", which are to precede the "completion stage" practices pertaining to realization of emptiness (Rig-pa) are aimed at achieving a wakeful state of enhanced cognition and emotions through the use of visual imagery and the emotional arousal associated with it, when the practitioner is required to imagine his/her mind, emotions, and feelings as the ones of a specific Deity [14,22].

Indeed, Benson [23] himself reported a contradictory and "unclear" phenomenon, that two of the three g-tummo practitioners from the Vajrayana tradition who participated in his research exhibited an activation of the sympathetic system as evidenced by increased metabolism and oxygen consumption, which is consistent with arousal but not with a relaxation response. Similarly, Corby and colleagues [24] showed that Hindu Tantric practices, which share some commonalities with Vajrayana Tantric practices, generated neural activity that promotes increased Alpha power in Electroencephalographic (EEG) recordings, as well as a small heart rate increase during meditation, suggesting the possibility of arousal rather than a relaxation response.

Based on the above review, we suggest that Vajrayana meditative practices could be described more accurately as generating arousal rather than a relaxation response. In contrast to relaxation, arousal is a physiological and psychological state of being awake or reactive to stimuli. It is characterized by an increase in the activity of the sympathetic system, which is followed by the release of epinephrine and norepinephrine from the endocrine system [25–27], and results in the state of *phasic alertness*, a significant temporary boost in the capacity to respond to stimuli [28–30]. This is in contrast to *tonic alertness*, which indicates a state of optimal vigilance where attention is sustained for a prolonged period of time. While tonic alertness can happen concurrently with relaxation, and indeed has been reported to occur during Theravada styles of meditation [31], phasic alertness is a result of the activity of the sympathetic system, and is elicited by different neurophysiological and cognitive mechanisms than tonic alertness, which are inconsistent with the state of relaxation. Thus, the first goal of this research was to examine whether Vajrayana meditative practices indeed lead to arousal, as reflected by sympathetic activation and behavioral markers of phasic

alertness, such as an immediate boost in performance on cognitive tasks, instead of a relaxation response that would characterize meditative practices of the Theravada tradition.

One of the more recent approaches to characterize meditation has been to define a type of meditation in terms of the attentional mechanisms that are engaged during its practice. Several researchers [11,32] have proposed two broad categories of meditative practices. The first category, termed Focused Attention (FA) meditation, includes meditative practices that require prolonged focused attention on a certain object, process, or state of mind. Specifically, Shamatha (Theravada style), where a special emphasis is given to an object of meditation and Deity-yoga practice (Vajrayana style) which involves holding the focus of attention on an internally generated image of a Deity, have been classified by a number of researchers as FA type of meditation [9,33]. The second category, Open Monitoring (OM) meditation techniques, do not require sustained attention on a particular object, process, or mental state, but rather that the practitioner would view his or her cognitive states from a disengaged point of view, developing a detached awareness of his or her feelings and thoughts [11]. Examples of OM include Vipassana meditation (Theravada), which was classified by previous researchers as belonging to this category because, as stated in [34], it emphasizes "open, nonjudgmental awareness of the sensory and cognitive fields and include a meta-awareness or observation of the ongoing contents of thought" (see also [9,11,35]), as well as Open Presence (Vajrayana style) meditation, in which the meditator is instructed to evenly distribute attention and to not direct his or her attention toward any particular object or experience [33].

In spite of the extensive use of the above classification, the empirical support for the focused attention vs. distributed attention categorization method has been inconclusive. In one study, Manna and colleagues [36] recorded fMRI signals during Shamatha (FA), Vipassana (OM), and during rest. They reported enhanced activity in the frontal cortex and reduced activity in the prefrontal cortex in Shamatha meditation relative to rest, and enhanced activity in the prefrontal cortex during Vipassana meditation relative to rest. In contrast, another fMRI study [13] reported that FA (Shamatha) was associated with enhanced and not reduced activity in the prefrontal cortex. Moreover, in an EEG study conducted by Dunn et al. [32], the authors reported decreased Theta power over the entire scalp during both Shamatha and Vipassana relative to rest, while Cahn, Delorme and Polich [37] observed a frontal Theta increase during Vipassana. Hence, there is no unequivocal evidence that supports the fact that FA and OM differ in terms of their neurophysiological substrates. The inconsistencies in the empirical studies may be attributed to that fact that not only from a Buddhist perspective, but also from a scientific standpoint, the classification of meditations into FA and OM seems to be an oversimplification of the different processes that are involved in meditative practices. Many meditation practices are complex, and require both focused and distributed attention. For instance, Deity-yoga meditation, although classified as FA due to the emphasis on focusing on a single object of meditation [33], also requires that during the meditative practice, the meditator would be continuously mindful of the symbolic meaning of the Deity's entourage, the ornaments and environment around Deity, as well as the cognitive, physical, and emotional states of the Deity [38]. Similarly, during Vipassana meditation, the practitioner does attend to individual objects and states of mind arising in his/her awareness using focused attention. Thus, the second goal of this study was to reexamine the validity of the FA-OM classification that distinguishes between different types of meditation based on the attentional systems that they involve, versus the classification that distinguishes between meditative practices from different traditions (Theravada or Vajrayana) resulting in arousal vs. relaxation responses.

In the present paper, four different types of meditative practices were compared: two types of Vajrayna practices: Visualization of self-generation-as-Deity (FA) and Rig-pa (OM) and two types of Theravada practices: Shamatha (FA) and Vipassana (OM). We collected Electrocardiographic (EKG) and Electroencephalographic (EEG) responses (Study 1) and measured behavioral performance on cognitive tasks (Study 2) using a participant pool of experienced Theravada practitioners from Thailand (Yannawa Temple, Bangkok) and Nepal (the International Buddhist Meditation Center and Amarapura Buddhist Nunnery, New Baneshwor) and Vajrayana practitioners from Nepal (Shechen monastery, Kathmandu). In order to measure the physiological correlates of arousal and relaxation responses, in Study 1 we used EKG measures, which have been shown to be reliably related to the activity of autonomic system [25,39–42]. Since relaxation type responses are expected to increase parasympathetic activity, meditations that produce relaxation should elicit the following EKG markers indicative of parasympathetic activation: 1) an increase in high-frequency power (HF), 2) a lower ratio between low and high frequencies (LF/HF) [25]. We did not use other conventional physiological measures of the output of the autonomic system, such as skin conductance resistance (GSR) or respiration rates, as the validity of these measures could not have been established in the present research. Respiration rates are highly influenced by certain types of meditations, which intentionally utilize breathing in order to alter the levels of relaxation and arousal, and could therefore present a mediating factor to EKG changes rather than an independent measure of the state of arousal or relaxation. GSR is highly influenced by humidity and temperature and could not be reliably measured in the present experimental conditions [43,44]. To complement EKG measures of autonomic system activity used in Study 1, in Study 2 we measured changes in performance on cognitive tasks following Vajrayana and Theravada styles of meditation as a behavioral marker of phasic alertness, which occurs during increased arousal. We expected to find an immediate significant increase in cognitive performance following Vajrayana but not Theravada styles of meditation.

Furthermore, to examine the validity of the FA-OM classification that distinguishes between different types of meditations based on the attentional systems they involve, versus the classification that distinguishes between meditative traditions (Vajrayana-Theravada), we compared EEG data recorded during each type of meditation. We expected that the neurophysiological correlates of the four types of meditations examined in this study would differ significantly across traditions but not across the FA-OM classification.

Methods

Study 1

Since Vajrayana and Theravada practitioners are not trained in the same meditative practices, a within-subjects design was not feasible. As a consequence, we used a mixed design, with the data from the Theravada style practitioners recorded at Yannawa Temple (Bangkok, Thailand), and the data from the Tibetan Vajrayana style practitioners recorded at the Shechen Monastery (Kathmandu, Nepal).

Participants. Ten long-term Theravada style practitioners who practice meditation at Yannawa Temple in Thailand, Bangkok (mean age = 41.4, 2 females), with an average of 8 years of meditation experience participated in the study. In addition, nine long-term Vajrayana practitioners (mean age = 47.5, 1 female), with an average of 7.4 years of meditation experience from Shechen monastery in Nepal participated in the study. All of the participants reported having no cardiovascular conditions, and were free of medication for the duration of the study. The subjects provided written, informed, consent for their participation in the study. The study was approved by the National University of Singapore's review board, which implements commonly used procedures for data deposition.

Theravada practices. In Buddhist scriptures, Shamatha practice relates to training in the concentration of attention. During the practice of Shamatha, the practitioners are instructed to place undistracted attention on the object of meditation, while withdrawing their focus from other objects [45]. Vipassana refers to insight into the true nature of reality, entailing an understanding of the impermanence of everything that exists, which is coupled with pacification (serenity) of the mind [17]. In meditation research, Vipassana practice typically begins with Shamatha (with a focus on the breath), but when awareness wanders away from the meditator's breathing, he or she is instructed to recognize that the mind has wandered, as well as the content that is currently occupying his or her mind [9].

For the purpose of this research, we used Kasina meditation as a particular type of Shamatha practice. Kasina meditation refers to objects of meditation that possess certain characteristics described in the Pali Tipitaka [46]. Kasina objects of meditation are typically colored disks, which differ from each other in terms of their color, size, object composition and other properties, depending on the type of Kasina used. The Pali Tipitaka [46] describes the following most commonly used Kasinas: earth, water, fire, air, blue, yellow, red, and white (see **Figure 1**). In the current study, Kasina was used in place of the more popular Shamatha practice where a meditator focuses on the breath for a long period of time [9] to dissociate it more easily from Vipassana, which implements focusing on the breath.

Vajrayana practices. Visualization of self-generation-as-Deity practice (Tibetan "Kyerim"; hereafter referred to as Deity meditation) originated in Hindu and Buddhist Tantric traditions in India and was later adopted by Tibetan Buddhism [47]. The practice involves holding the focus of attention on an internally generated image of a Deity surrounded by his or her entourage (see **Figure 2**). The content of Deity meditation is rich and multimodal, requiring the generation of colorful three-dimensional images (e.g., the Deity's body, ornaments, and environment), as well as representations of sensorimotor body schema, feelings, and emotions of the Deity. The image temporarily replaces one's sense of self and internal perception of the real world [38]. In Vajrayana, visualization of oneself as a Deity is related to the *generation or development stage*, which is the first stage of the meditation practice [48].

During Rig-pa meditation, which follows the final stages of Deity meditation, and represents the *completion stages* of the meditative practice [14], a meditator visualizes the dissolution of the Deity and its entourage into emptiness, and aspires to achieve awareness devoid of conceptualization. While performing Rig-pa, the meditator attempts to evenly distribute his or her attention so that it is not directed toward any object or experience. Although various aspects of experience may arise (e.g. thoughts, feelings, images, etc.), the meditator is instructed to let them subside on their own, without dwelling on them or examining them [49,50]. The important distinction between Vipassana and Rig-pa is that Rig-pa is considered to be a meditative practice with no object of meditation; it does not require noticing or watching the content of

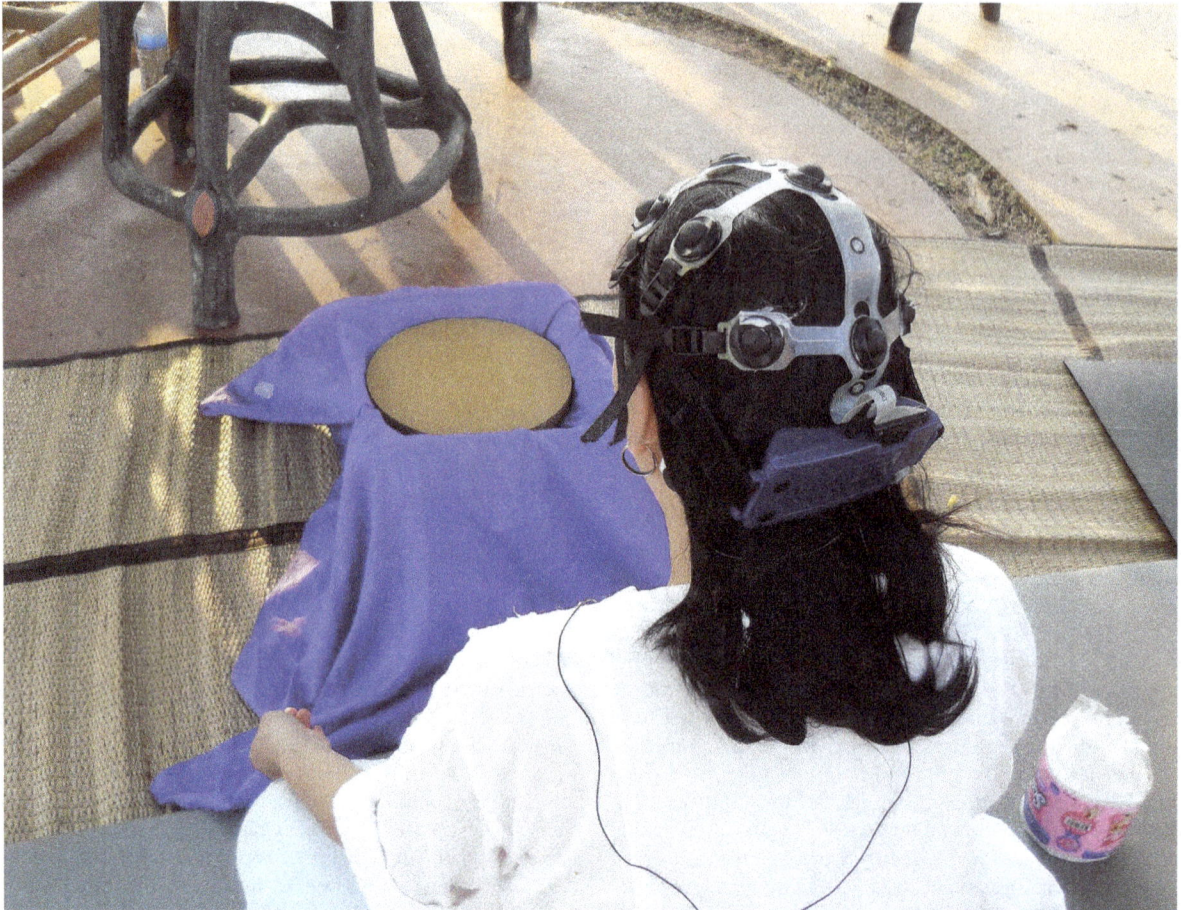

Figure 1. Participant meditating on earth Kasina while her EEG and EKG recordings are taken.

attention, the activity that is associated with a dualistic mind, but only to be fully aware of it [14].

Procedure. The data from the Theravada style practitioners were recorded in a meditation hall at the Yannawa Temple (Bangkok, Thailand), and the data from the Tibetan Vajrayana style practitioners was recorded at the Shechen Monastery library (Kathmandu, Nepal). EEG and EKG were continuously recorded throughout the study. At the beginning of the session, each participant performed a 10 minute Rest condition, during which they were explicitly instructed not to meditate but to remain seated with their eyes closed, and to simply relax. Following a 5 minute break, the Theravada practitioners were asked to perform 15 minutes of Shamatha meditation followed by 15 minutes of Vipassana. Tibetan Vajrayana practitioners were asked to perform 15 minutes of Deity meditation after the Rest condition, followed by 15 minutes of Rig-pa meditation. The orders of meditation were chosen per request of the participants who found that it is more natural first to meditate in Shamatha followed by Vipassana. Similarly, since Rig-pa (completion stages) follow the end of Deity practice (generation stage), Vajrayana practitioners performed Deity first followed by Rig-pa. For participants who did not speak English, interpreters translated all the instructions into their native language.

In contrast to Theravada styles of meditation, which are performed with closed eyes, Vajrayana practices are often performed with open eyes. However, to make the experimental conditions as similar as possible, we instructed all the practitioners to meditate with closed eyes. Importantly, we ensured that all our Vajrayana practitioners were comfortable with such a request, and they all confirmed that this would not affect their meditation.

EEG and EKG Recordings and Protocol. EEG was continuously recorded at the POz,Pz,Fz,C3,C4,F3,F4,P3 and P4 scalp regions, positioned according to the standard 10/20 system [51] using a B-Alert portable EEG cap (Advanced Brain Monitoring, Inc.), as well as from 2 additional electrodes placed on the right and left mastoids. EKG was recorded via two electrodes placed over on the right collar bone and below the left rib cage. EEG and EKG were sampled at 256 Hz, and referenced to the average between the two mastoid electrodes. Signals showing ocular and muscular artifacts were manually excluded from the study, and a high-band pass filter of 0.1 Hz was applied to the EEG data. Moreover, a digital notch filter was applied to the data at 50 Hz to remove artifacts caused by nearby electrical devices.

Heart rate variability analysis. Prior to the mid-1980s, heart rate variability (HRV) was typically analyzed through time domain methods but not frequency domain methods [25,41,42]. It has since been established that the reliability of time domain methods is highly dependent on the length of the EKG recordings, and that they are ideal for analyzing recordings that are typically longer than 18 hours [25]. On the other hand, during short term recordings, such as the ones conducted during meditation studies, frequency domain methods can be used reliably [25]. Specifically, the frequencies used in the analysis of autonomic system activity

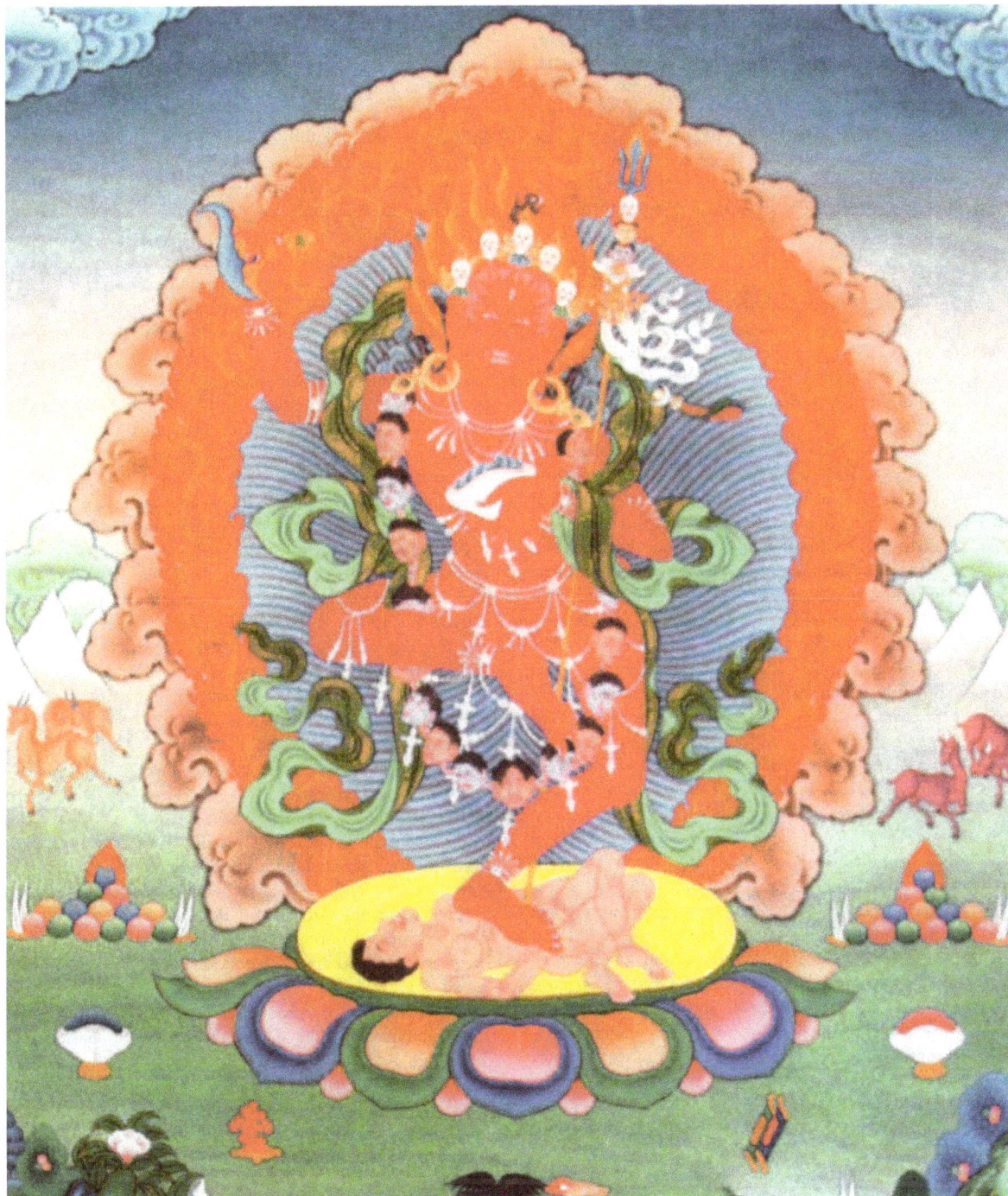

Figure 2. An example of a meditation Deity (Vajrayyogini) used by the participants in the practice of Deity Visualization.

are EKG high frequencies (HF), and the ratio of low to high frequencies (LH/HF) [25]. While some researchers [52–55] proposed that LF is a marker of sympathetic modulation, others attribute its activity to both sympathetic and parasympathetic influences [56,57]. In contrast, increases in HF could be reliably attributed to the activity of the parasympathetic system [41,52,56]. Under normal circumstances, HF decreases indicate decreased parasympathetic and increased sympathetic activation [58,59], although in some extreme cases (e.g. stress or physical exercise),

increases in HF could accompany an increase in sympathetic response [58–60].

A cubic spline interpolation with a 500 Hz sampling rate was performed on the EKG data, in order to improve the accuracy of the heart rate variability estimations [61,62]. Subsequently, HF and LF/HF were computed using Welch's periodogram method (FFT spectrum), and were measured in absolute power (milliseconds squared). Since a 2 minute recording period is needed to accurately assess LF/HF [25], we analyzed EKG from an additional minute preceding the 3 minute period that was used for EEG analysis. Hence, EKG sampled at 256 Hz was extracted from a 4 minute period, and interpolated to produce a 2 minute period sampled at 500 Hz. The HF frequencies were 0.15–0.4 Hz and LF frequencies were 0.04–0.15 Hz, which are the frequency ranges that are most commonly used in EKG analysis [58,63–66]. HF and LF/HF were then analyzed as dependent variables in separate repeated measures ANOVAs. Since the Theravada and Vajrayana meditations were performed by separate groups of subjects, we first compared each of them to the control Rest condition using within subject ANOVAs, with Condition (Meditation, Rest) as an independent factor. Subsequently, significant effects were contrasted using a mixed design ANOVA (2×2), with Tradition (Theravada-Vajrayana) as the between-subject factor, and Attention (FA-OM) as the within-subject factor.

Spectral Analysis. For each electrode and 1 second epoch, the power spectral distribution (PSD) was calculated using Welch's method [67], where power values are averaged and a 512 millisecond time window is applied. Subsequently, the mean power at the Delta (1–4 Hz), Theta (4.5–7.5 Hz), Alpha (8.5–12.5 Hz), Beta (13–25 Hz), and Gamma (35–44.5 Hz, 60–95.5 Hz, 110–128 Hz) frequencies were used as the dependent variables in the analyses. Importantly, we analyzed only a 3 minute epoch at the end of the meditation period, during which the meditators were most likely to be in a deep meditative state.

Theravada and Vajrayana meditations were first analyzed using within subject ANOVAs, for which the independent factors were Condition (Meditation, Rest) and Location. In order to test for potential effects of hemisphere (laterality), which are often observed [68], we divided the scalp into 3 regions, each of which consisted of the average of 3 electrodes that were selected according to their location: Left – C3,F3,P3; Right – C4,F4,P4; Center – Cz,Fz,POz. Subsequently, significant effects were contrasted using a mixed design ANOVA (2×2×3). The between-groups factor was Tradition (Theravada-Vajrayana), and the within-subject factors were Attention (FA-OM) and Location (Left, Right or Center).

Coherence Analysis. The mean squared coherence was measured between electrodes F3 and F4 (Frontal), the average between F3 and F4 and the average between electrodes C3 and C4 (Fronto-Central), P3 and P4 (Posterior), and the average between P3 and P4 and the average between F3 and F4 (Fronto-Posterior), separately for Alpha, Beta, and Gamma power. Subsequently, each one of the 12 frequency-coherence combinations (Alpha: Frontal, Fronto-Central, Posterior, Fronto-Posterior; Beta: Frontal, Fronto-Central, Posterior, Fronto-Posterior; Gamma: Frontal, Fronto-Central, Posterior, Fronto-Posterior) was separately analyzed as the dependent variable in a repeated measures ANOVA, with Condition (meditation vs. rest) as the independent factor. Furthermore, significant results were analyzed in a mixed ANOVA (2×2) using Attention (FA vs OM) as the within-subject factor, and Tradition (Vajrayana vs Theravada) as the between groups factor.

Study 2

In Study 2 we investigated whether the practice of Vajrayana or Theravada types of meditation will elicit an immediate significant enhancement in cognitive tasks as a result of an increase in phasic alertness, associated with arousal [28–30]. Indeed, previous research demonstrated a positive correlation between arousal and cognitive performance [69–71], so that the amount of pre-stimulus arousal predicted the probability of success on a number of visual tasks, including attention and memory guided delay tasks. Furthermore, a dramatic temporary enhancement (of about 15–20 minutes duration) on visual tasks such as dynamic spatial

transformations and the maintenance of a static image in visual working memory, was previously demonstrated to occur in experienced Vajrayana practitioners immediately following 20 minutes of Deity meditation practice [33].

Similarly to [33], we used a between-subject design, in which meditators were administered two computerized tasks assessing different aspects of visual processing (mental rotation and visual memory tasks) before and immediately after a 20 minute meditation session. Since we were interested in the effect of each type of meditation on cognitive performance, in contrast to Study 1, where EEG and EKG measures were taken from Vajrayana practitioners who performed Rig-pa meditation immediately after Deity, and from Theravada practitioners who performed Vipassana right after Kasina, in Study 2 each participant performed only one type of meditation practice (Kasina, Vipassana, or Rig-pa. As explained below, data from Deity practitioners was taken from a previously published study [33]). We hypothesized that Vajrayana types of meditation would lead to an immediate improvement in these tasks following meditation practice, due to an increase in phasic alertness associated with arousal. On the other hand, Theravada meditators should not significantly differ in their performance on these tests before and after meditation.

Participants. As in Study 1, all participants reported having no cardiovascular conditions, and were free of medication for the duration of Study 2. The first (Kasina) group of participants consisted of 12 long-term Theravada practitioners from Yannawa Temple, Bangkok (mean age = 43.2, 2 female) with an average of 10 years of meditation experience (10 practitioners from this group participated in Study 1). This group of participants performed Kasina meditation. The data of this group were collected at the Yannawa Temple (Bangkok, Thailand).

The second (Vipassana) group consisted of 14 Theravada practitioners who were asked to perform Vipassana meditation (mean age = 43.2, 4 female) with an average of 12.3 years of meditation experience. The ten male practitioners were recruited from the International Buddhist Meditation Center (Sankhamul, New Baneshwor, Nepal), and the four female practitioners were recruited from the Amarapura Buddhist Nunnery in Nepal. The data of this group of participants were collected at the International Buddhist Meditation Center (New Baneshwor, Nepal).

The third (Rig-pa) group consisted of the same 9 long-term Vajrayana practitioners from the Shechen monastery in Nepal (mean age = 47.5, 1 female) who participated in Study 1, and have an average of 7.4 years of meditation experience. The data from this group of participants were collected at the Shechen monastery library and they were asked to perform Rig-pa meditation. Although Rig-pa is usually practiced right after Deity meditation in one session, our experimental design required that each participant would perform only one type of meditation. All participants acknowledged that they were comfortable in performing Rig-pa meditation not preceded by Deity.

The behavioral data from two visual tasks administered before and after a meditation session in the above three groups were compared with the data from the same tasks performed before and after Deity meditation, which were previously published in Kozhevnikov et al.'s study [33] that incorporated the same experimental procedure. The group of Deity meditators [33] consisted of 15 Vajrayana long-term practitioners (mean age = 42, 5 female) with an average meditation experience of 13 years. (It should be noted that Kozhevnikov et al. [33], in addition to Deity meditators, investigated a group of practitioners who performed "Open Presence" practices, which although in some respects were similar to Rig-pa practice, included a mixture of OM meditations from different schools of Tibetan Buddhism, not necessarily Tantric).

Mental Rotation Test (MRT). On each trial of the MRT, participants viewed a pair of three dimensional pictures, which were rotated relative to each other around the x, y, or z-axis. Across trials, the amount of rotation ranged from 40° to 180°, in 20° increments. Participants were required to judge whether the two pictures were of the same form, or whether the forms were mirror-reversed. The test consisted of 36 trials, 18 in which the forms were the same, and 18 in which they were mirror-reversed.

Visual Memory Test (VMT). The VMT [72] consisted of two parts. In the first part, participants performed 6 trials during which a single image first appeared for 5 seconds and was subsequently replaced by an array of six images. The array consisted of the original image along with 5 distractors, and the participants were asked to determine which image in the array was the first image (**see Figure 3**). The second part of the VMT consisted of 18 trials, during which participants first viewed an array of seven images that appeared for 8 seconds. This array was subsequently replaced by another array of seven images, 6 which appeared in the previous array and one novel image. Participants were asked to determine which image in the second array did not appear in the first.

Procedure. The procedure for Study 2 was similar to the procedure reported in [33]. All the participants were tested individually in a testing session that lasted from 1.5–2 hours. First, the participants completed the MRT and VMT pre-tests, the order of which was counterbalanced. Similarly to Study 1, for those who did not speak English, interpreters translated all the instructions into the native language of the participants before each test began. After completing the pre-test, the Theravada (Thai) participants from the Kasina group were asked to perform Kasina meditation. The Theravada (Nepalese) participants were asked to perform Vipassana, and Vajrayana practitioners were asked to perform Rig-pa. Similarly to [33], all the groups meditated for 20 minutes.

Although different groups of meditators were tested in different locations, we tried to make the testing conditions as similar as possible. In particular, during all the tests, we used a quiet room in the monasteries with moderate temperature; the same laptop computers were used during all the procedures, and the same training session and instructions (apart from the meditation instructions) were given to all the participants. Importantly, the Vipassana meditators in this study were from the International Buddhist Center in Nepal, enabling us to compare Theravada and Vajrayana (Rig-pa) meditations in a similar environment. As Kasina is not practiced in Nepal, this data was collected in Thailand.

Results

Study 1

Heart Rate Variability. The Heart Rate Variability results are summarized in Table S1. For Theravada meditation, we observed a marginally significant main effect of Condition (Rest, Kasina, Vipassana): $F(2,18) = 3.2$, $p = 0.06$. As we hypothesized that HF would increase during Theravada meditations, we performed planned pairwise comparisons between Vipassana and Rest, and Kasina and Rest. These comparisons showed that the difference between Vipassana and Rest was significant ($p < 0.05$), whereas the difference between Kasina and Rest was not significant ($p > 0.4$), see **Figure 4**. Furthermore, we observed a significant main effect of Condition on LF/HF, $F(2,18) = 3.67$, $p < 0.05$. Since we hypothesized that LF/HF would decrease during

Theravada meditations, we performed planned pairwise comparisons between Vipassana and Rest, and Kasina and Rest, which showed that the differences between Kasina and Rest ($p < 0.05$), and Vipassana and Rest ($p < 0.05$), were both significant. Moreover, the post-hoc comparison between Kasina and Vipassana was not significant ($p > 0.8$). This suggests that both Kasina and Vipassana induced an increase in parasympathetic activity, corresponding to a relaxation response, with a clearer pattern of parasympathetic increase for Vipassana than Kasina, as evidenced by both an increase in HF and a decrease in LF/HF.

For Vajrayana meditation, the analysis demonstrated a marginally significant Condition (Rest, Deity, Rig-p) effect for HF, $F(2,16) = 3.19$, $p = 0.07$. As we hypothesized that HF would decrease during Vajrayana meditations, we performed planned pairwise comparisons between Deity and Rest, and Rig-pa and Rest. HF was significantly decreased in Deity relative to Rest ($p < 0.05$) and in Rig-pa relative to Rest ($p < 0.05$). The post-hoc comparison between Deity and Rig-pa was not significant ($p > 0.8$), see **Figure 4**. The effect of Condition on LF/HF was also not significant, $F(2,16) = 1.3$, $p > 0.2$. Overall, the HRV analysis showed that although there were no significant changes in LF/HF, there was a significant decrease in HF, which is primary marker of increase in sympathetic activity, suggesting that during both Vajrayana practices, the practitioners exhibited an arousal response.

Furthermore, the between traditions comparison showed a significant Tradition (Theravada, Vajrayana) effect on HF, $F(1,17) = 7.02$, $p < 0.05$, so that HF was significantly decreased during Vajrayana in comparison to Theravada, see **Figure 4**. However, the main effect of Attention (FA, OM) on HF was not significant ($F < 1$) as well as Attention X Tradition interaction ($F < 1$). The between-tradition analysis of LF/HF showed non-significant main effects of Tradition: $F(1,17) = 1.34$, $p > 0.2$ and Attention: $F(1,17) = 2.13$, $p > 0.1$, as well as a non-significant Attention X Tradition interaction: $F(1,17) = 1.77$, $p > 0.2$.

Overall, the results suggest that Theravada and Vajrayana meditative practices lead to very different patterns of HRV responses, exhibiting patterns that are consistent with a relaxation response for Theravada practices and arousal responses for Vajrayana practices.

Spectral analysis. The statistical results for all the frequencies are summarized in Table S2, and are described here in ascending order (Delta, Theta, Alpha, Beta, Gamma).

Delta. For Theravada style of meditation, the analysis showed a significant main effect of Condition: $F(2,18) = 8.37$, $p < 0.01$, so that Delta power was reduced during meditation in comparison to Rest. However, posthoc comparisons using Bonferroni adjusted α levels of 0.017 per test ($\alpha = 0.05/3 = 0.017$) did not reveal significant differences between Rest, Kasina, and Vipassana. The main effect of Location was significant: $F(2,18) = 7.19$, $p < 0.01$, suggesting that Delta power was greater at the Center (see **Figure 5**). The Condition X Location interaction was not significant: $F(4,36) = 1.41$, $p > 0.2$.

We also found a significant main effect of Condition for Vajrayana meditation: $F(2,16) = 5.11$, $p < 0.05$, indicating that Delta power was reduced during Vajrayana in comparison to Rest (see **Figure 5**). Using a Bonferroni correction ($\alpha = 0.05/3 = 0.017$), we found a significant difference between Deity and Rest ($p < 0.001$), but the difference between Rig-pa and Rest was not significant ($p > 0.1$). There was no significant difference between Deity and Rig-pa ($p > 0.3$). The main effect of Location was not significant: $F(2,16) = 2.36$, $p > 0.1$, as well as the Condition X Location interaction: $F(4,32) = 1.08$, $p > 0.3$.

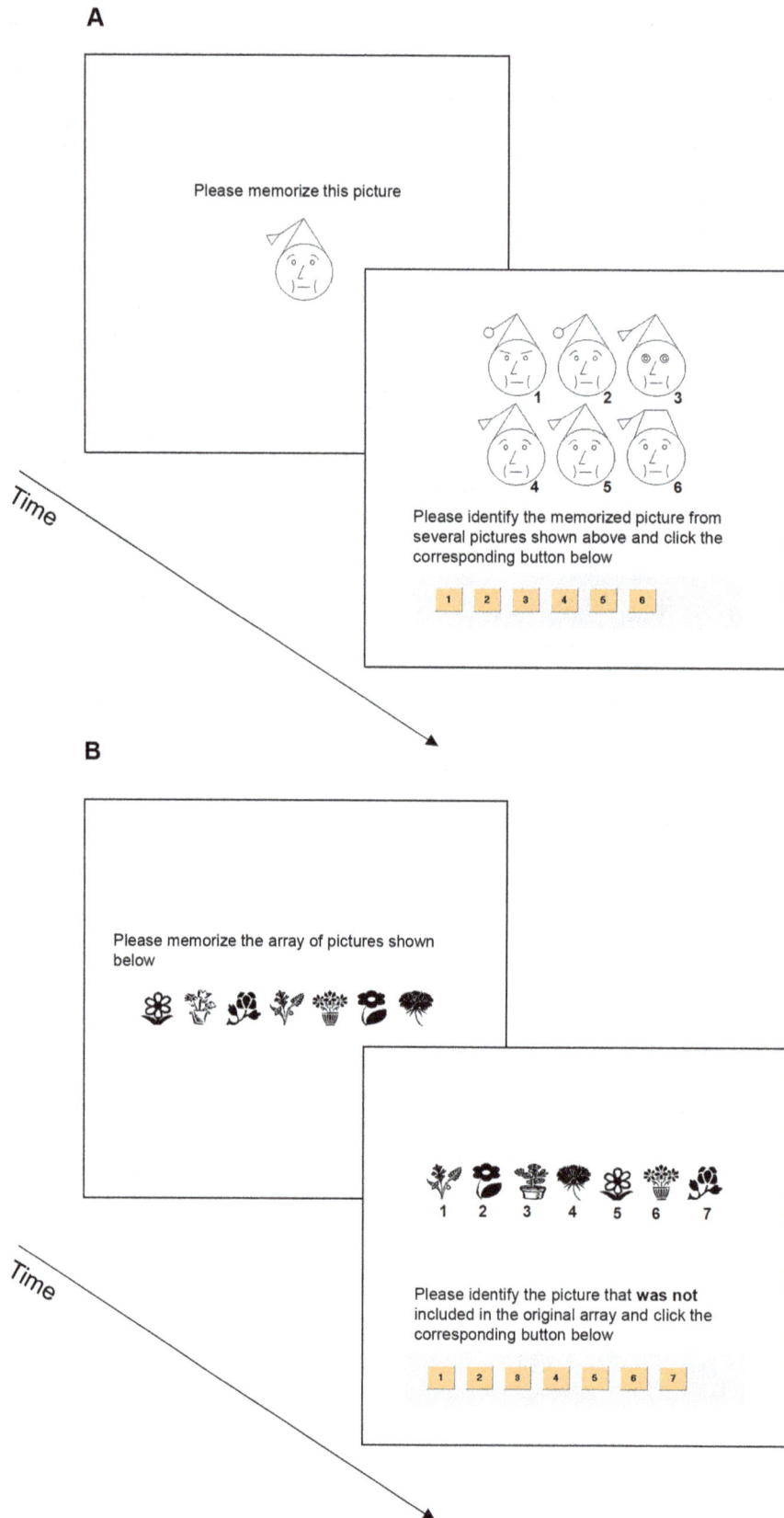

Figure 3. Examples of items from the Visual Memory Test.

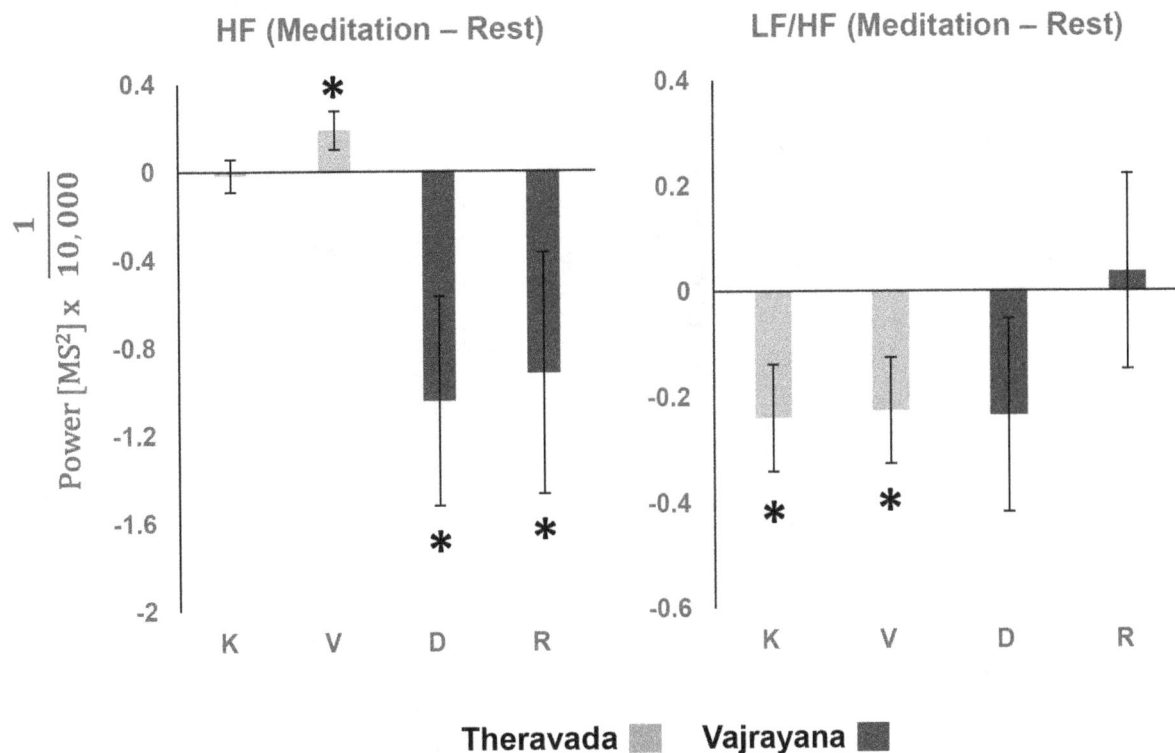

Figure 4. EKG differences between Meditation and Rest (K – Kasina, V – Vipassana, D – Deity, and R – Rig-pa).

The comparison between traditions showed that the main effects of Attention, $F<1$, and Tradition, $F_{(1,17)}=1.97$, $p>0.1$, were not significant, as well as the Attention X Tradition interaction, $F_{(1,17)}=1.48$, $p>0.2$.

Theta. The effect of Condition was not significant for either Theravada, $F_{(2,18)}=1.11$, $p>0.3$ or Vajrayana styles of meditation, $F_{(2,16)}=2.5$, $p>0.1$, as was the Condition X Location interaction – Theravada style: $F_{(4,36)}=1.9$, $p>0.1$; Vajrayana style: $F<1$. We found a significant main effect of Location that was unrelated to meditation – Theravada style: $F_{(2,18)}=20.16$, $p<0.001$; Vajrayana style: $F_{(2,16)}=3.5$, $p=0.055$ – suggesting that Theta power was higher at central scalp regions for both meditation and Rest.

Alpha. Although meditative states were often reported to produce an increase in Alpha power [32,73,74], when adequate control conditions were applied to account for general relaxation, then either decreased Alpha power, or no differences between meditation and rest were demonstrated [34,37,75,76]. Indeed, other neuroscience research also showed that decreased Alpha power is associated with deep relaxation, while increases in Alpha are associated with wakefulness, attention, and task load [77,78]. Therefore, we expected to find reductions in Alpha power for Theravada meditations, and increases in Alpha power for Vajrayana practices.

For Theravada styles of meditation, the analysis revealed a significant main effect of Condition, $F_{(2,18)}=6.84$, $p<0.01$, indicating that Alpha power was reduced during meditation relative to Rest (see **Figure 5**). The main effect of Location was also significant: $F_{(2,18)}=13.49$, $p<0.001$, as was the Condition X Location interaction: $F_{(2,18)}=6.84$, $p<0.01$. Hence, follow up ANOVAs were performed at each Location. The effect of Condition was significant at all Locations [Left: $F_{(2,18)}=6.49$, $p<0.01$; Right: $F_{(2,18)}=8.19$, $p<0.01$; Center: $F_{(2,18)}=5.72$, $p<$

0.05]. Moreover, the planned pairwise comparisons between Kasina and Rest were significant at all Locations [Left: $p<0.05$, Right: $p<0.01$, Center: $p<0.05$]. The difference between Vipassana and Rest was significant at the Left, $p<0.05$, and Right Location, $p=0.051$, but not at the Center, $p>0.1$. Using a Bonferroni correction ($\alpha=0.017$), we did not find significant differences between Kasina and Vipassana at any Location.

For Vajrayana types of meditation, in contrast to our predictions, there were no significant differences in Alpha power between Deity, Rig-pa, and Rest ($p>0.8$ for all main effects and interactions).

The comparison between traditions showed that the main effects of Attention: $F_{(1,17)}=2.68$, $p>0.1$, and Tradition: $F_{(1,17)}=1.86$, $p>0.1$, were not significant, as well as the Attention X Tradition interaction ($F<1$). The main effect of Location was not significant ($F<1$), nor were there any significant interactions between Location and other factors ($p>0.3$ for all comparisons).

Beta. For Theravada styles of meditation, ANOVA showed a significant effect of Condition: $F_{(2,18)}=3.68$, $p<0.05$, demonstrating that Beta power was reduced during meditation (see **Figure 5**). The effect of Location was not significant ($F<1$), however the Condition X Location interaction was significant, $F_{(4,36)}=3.77$, $p<0.05$, suggesting that the difference between the Conditions was most prominent at the Right, followed by the Center Location (see **Figure 5**). Using a Bonferroni correction ($\alpha=0.017$), we did not find any significant difference between Kasina and Rest ($p>0.03$), Vipassana and Rest ($p>0.15$) and Vipassana and Kasina ($p>0.05$) at any Location.

For Vajrayana style, there was also a significant main effect of Condition: $F_{(2,16)}=8.42$, $p<0.01$, demonstrating that Beta power was reduced during meditation relative to Rest (see **Figure 5**). Using a Bonferroni correction ($\alpha=0.017$), we observed significant differences between Deity and Rest ($p<0.01$), and Rig-pa and Rest

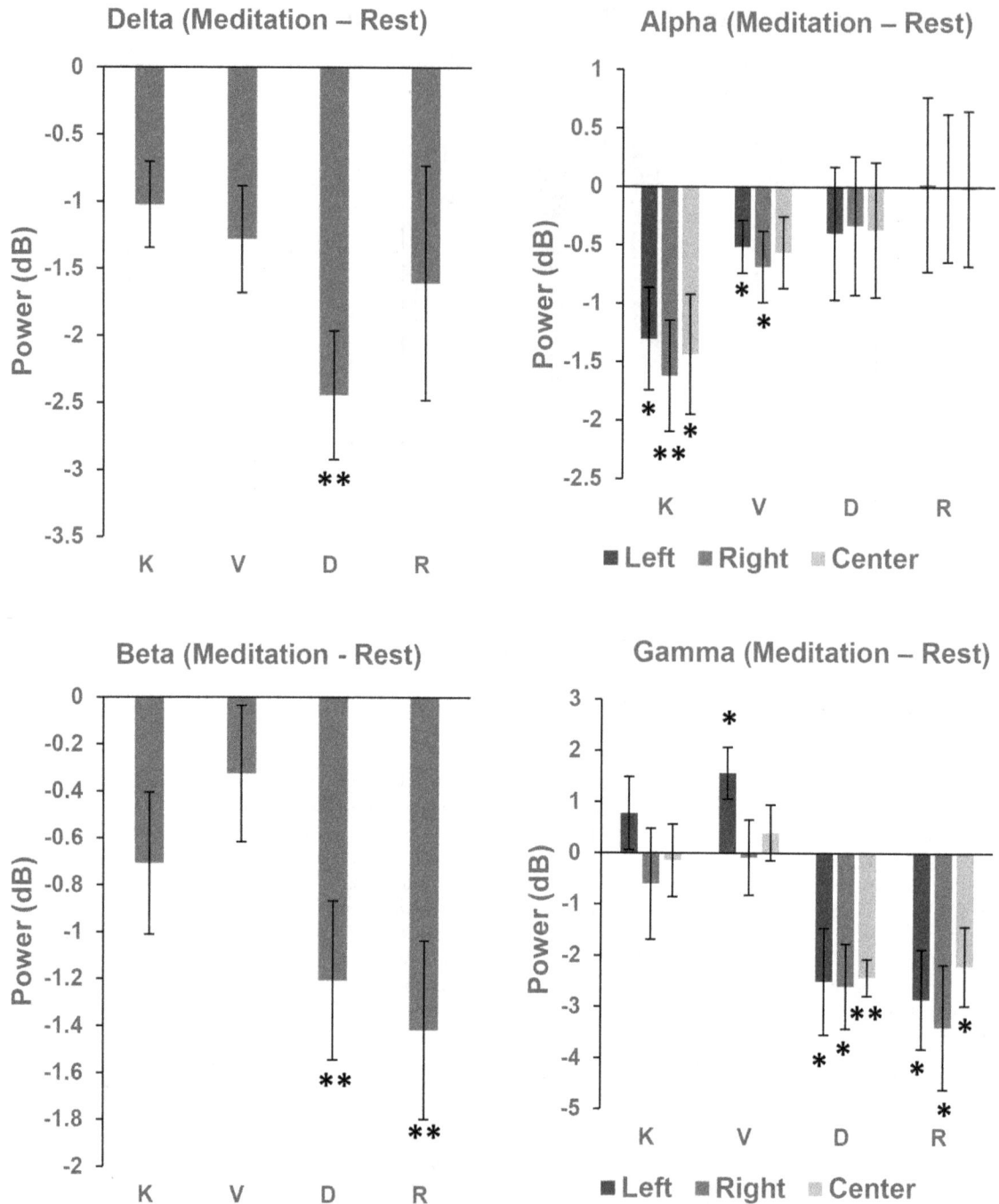

Figure 5. Differences in EEG frequency power between Meditation and Rest (K – Kasina, V – Vipassana, D – Deity, and R – Rig-pa).

(p<0.01). However the comparison between Deity and Rig-pa was not significant (p>0.6). A marginal effect of Location was obtained: F(2,16) = 3.43, p = 0.058, suggesting that Beta power was higher over the left hemisphere for both Meditation and Rest (see **Figure 5**), and we did not find an interaction between Condition and Location: F(2,16) = 1.01, p>0.4.

The between traditions analysis demonstrated a marginally significant main effect of Tradition, F(1,17) = 3.69, p = 0.07, which suggests that Beta power was more decreased during Vajrayana than Theravada (see **Figure 5**). No other main effects or

interactions were observed between traditions (p>0.1 for all comparisons).

Gamma. For meditations belonging to the Theravada tradition, although the main effects of Condition (F<1), and Location: F(2,18) = 1.48, p>0.2 were not significant, we found a significant Condition X Location interaction: F(4,36) = 3.09, p< 0.05, and separate ANOVAs at each level of the Location factor showed a significant trend at the Left Location: F(2,18) = 2.76, p = 0.09, but not the at the Right or Center (F<1 for both comparisons). Since previous studies found increases in Gamma during Theravada meditation [37], we performed planned pairwise comparisons between both Theravada meditations and Rest at each Location. These comparisons revealed that Gamma power was increased for Vipassana relative to Rest at the Left Location (p<0.05), but not at the Right or Center (p>0.2). The planned pairwise comparisons between Kasina and Rest were not significant (p>0.3 at all Locations), as were the comparisons between Vipassana and Kasina (p>0.2 at all Locations).

As for Vajrayana, there was a significant main effect of Condition: $F(2,16) = 6.16$, p<0.01, demonstrating a significant reduction in Gamma power during Deity and Rig-pa relative to Rest (see **Figure 5**). Moreover, using a Bonferroni correction ($\alpha = 0.017$) we observed significant differences between Deity and Rest (p<0.01), and Rig-pa and Rest (p = 0.012), but there was no difference between Deity and Rig-pa (p>0.7). We also observed a main effect of Location, $F(2,16) = 6.33$, p<0.01, indicative of lower Gamma power at the Center (see **Figure 5**). However this effect was not influenced by meditation, as the Condition X Location interaction was not significant (F<1).

The differences in Gamma power between Theravada and Vajrayana were significant, as demonstrated by a significant Tradition main effect: $F(1,17) = 12.27$, p<0.01. No other main effects or interactions were found in the between traditions analysis (p>0.1 for all comparisons).

Overall, the results show large EEG differences between Theravada and Vajrayana traditions. In particular, we observed a reduction in Alpha power for Theravada (both Kasina and Vipassana), but not Vajrayana practices. Furthermore, Gamma power was increased during Vipassana, but decreased during Vajrayana (both Deity and Rig-pa) practices. Interestingly, decreases in Beta power were observed in both Theravada and Vajrayana meditation, but they were more prominent during Vajrayana. On the other hand, we did not find any significant differences in EEG frequency power within traditions that could be explained through the FA-OM framework.

Coherence Analysis. The statistical results are shown in Table S3. For Theravada styles, the analysis showed a marginally significant Condition effect for Alpha Frontal Coherence: $F(2,18) = 2.74$, p = 0.09, suggesting that Alpha Frontal Coherence may be reduced in meditation relative to Rest (see **Figure 6**). No other significant effects were found (p>0.15 for all other comparisons of Alpha, Beta, or Gamma Coherence).

For Vajrayana style of meditation, Alpha Frontal Coherence also showed a marginally significant effect of Condition, $F(2,17) = 3.16$, p = 0.07, suggesting that it is reduced during Vajrayana as well. In addition, for Vajrayana meditation, the analysis of Beta Fronto-Central Coherence revealed a marginally significant effect of Condition: $F(2,16) = 3.34$, p = 0.06, suggesting that it was increased during Vajrayana meditation relative to Rest (see **Figure 6**). No other significant effects were obtained (p>0.1 for all comparisons of Alpha, Beta, or Gamma Coherence).

The comparison between traditions showed that for Alpha Frontal Coherence, although the main effects of Attention, p>0.2, and Tradition, F<1, were not significant, a significant Attention X Tradition interaction was observed: $F(1,17) = 4.98$, p<0.05. This interaction shows that, whereas Alpha Frontal Coherence was greater for Rig-pa (OM) than Deity (FA) of the Vajrayana tradition, the opposite trend was observed for Theravada, so that more coherence was observed for Kasina (FA) than Vipassana (OM) (see **Figure 6**). No other effects of Alpha Frontal Coherence were observed (p>0.2 for all main effects and interactions). Moreover, the Beta Fronto-Central Coherence analysis revealed a marginally significant main effect of Tradition, $F(1,17) = 4.15$, p = 0.057, suggesting that it was increased during Vajrayana relative to Theravada (see **Figure 6**). No other effects of Beta

Coherence were observed between traditions (F<1 for all comparisons).

In summary, the results of the coherence analysis support a tradition-based classification of meditations, but not the attention-based classification. While we found an increase in Beta Fronto-Central Coherence for Vajrayana practices relative to Rest, no such effect was found for Theravada meditative practices. Furthermore, we observed an increase of Alpha Frontal Coherence for Rig-pa (OM) relative to Deity (FA) in Vajrayana, but a decrease for Vipassana (OM) relative to Kasina (FA) during Theravada meditation, which is incompatible with the attention-based classification.

Study 2

The results of the study are summarized in Table S4. Outlier response times (RTs±2.5 SD from a participant's mean) were deleted, which accounted to less than 3% of responses in every condition.

As in [33], to avoid issues of speed-accuracy trade-off that are often observed during visual tasks [79], we calculated the visual processing efficiency for each participant for the MRT and VMT tasks by dividing each participant's proportion of correct responses by their logarithmically transformed average reaction time (lnRT).

MRT. The MRT results were analyzed through a 2 (Time: pretest vs. post-test) X 4 (Condition: Kasina/Vipassana/Deity/Rig-pa) ANOVA, which indicated a significant main effect of Time, $F(1,47) = 14.73$, p<0.001. The effect of Condition was not significant, F<1. However, there was a significant interaction between Time and Condition, $F(3,47) = 9.52$, p<0.001. Follow-up ANOVAs revealed a Time effect for Deity, $F(1,14) = 19.36$, p< 0.001, and Rig-pa, $t(9) = 7.68$, p<0.05, but not Kasina, F<1, and Vipassana, F<1 (see **Figure 7**).

VMT. Similarly to the MRT results, VMT were analyzed through a 2 (Time: pretest vs. post-test) X 4 (Condition: Kasina/Vipassana/Deity/Rig-pa) ANOVA, which showed a significant main effect of Time, $F(1,45) = 20.73$, p<0.001 (df = 45 as two Vipassana meditators did not perform the VMT). Again, the main effect of Condition was not significant, p>0.16, albeit a significant Time X Condition interaction was found, $F(3,45) = 8.57$, p< 0.001. Follow-up ANOVAs revealed a significant efficiency increase for Deity, $F(1,14) = 26.41$, P<0.001, and Rig-pa, $F(1,9) = 19.46$, p<0.01, but not Kasina, F<1, or Vipassana, F< 1, see **Figure 7**.

Overall, the results of Study 2 demonstrated a significant improvement in cognitive performance on two visual tasks, MRT and VMT, immediately after both Deity and Rig-pa Vajrayana styles of meditation, but not Theravada styles of meditation. Such dramatic improvements in cognitive performance in comparison with the baseline suggest enhanced phasic alertness takes place during Vajrayana meditation. The results are consistent with previous research on meditation [33] which demonstrated that, although the improvements are not long-lasting and return to baseline in about 20 min, certain types of meditation (e.g., Deity) can dramatically boost performance on visual tasks.

Discussion

Whereas previous research mostly emphasized the power of Theravada styles of meditation to induce a relaxation response, even after short practices (e.g. 20 minutes) [2,4–6,80] as well as to promote tonic alertness [31], the findings of our research show that Vajrayana styles of meditation induce an arousal response during a comparable time interval, characterized by an increase in sympathetic activation, and promote enhanced phasic alertness.

Alpha Frontal Coherence
(Meditation – Rest)

Beta Fronto-Central
Coherence (Meditation – Rest)

Theravada ░ **Vajrayana** ■

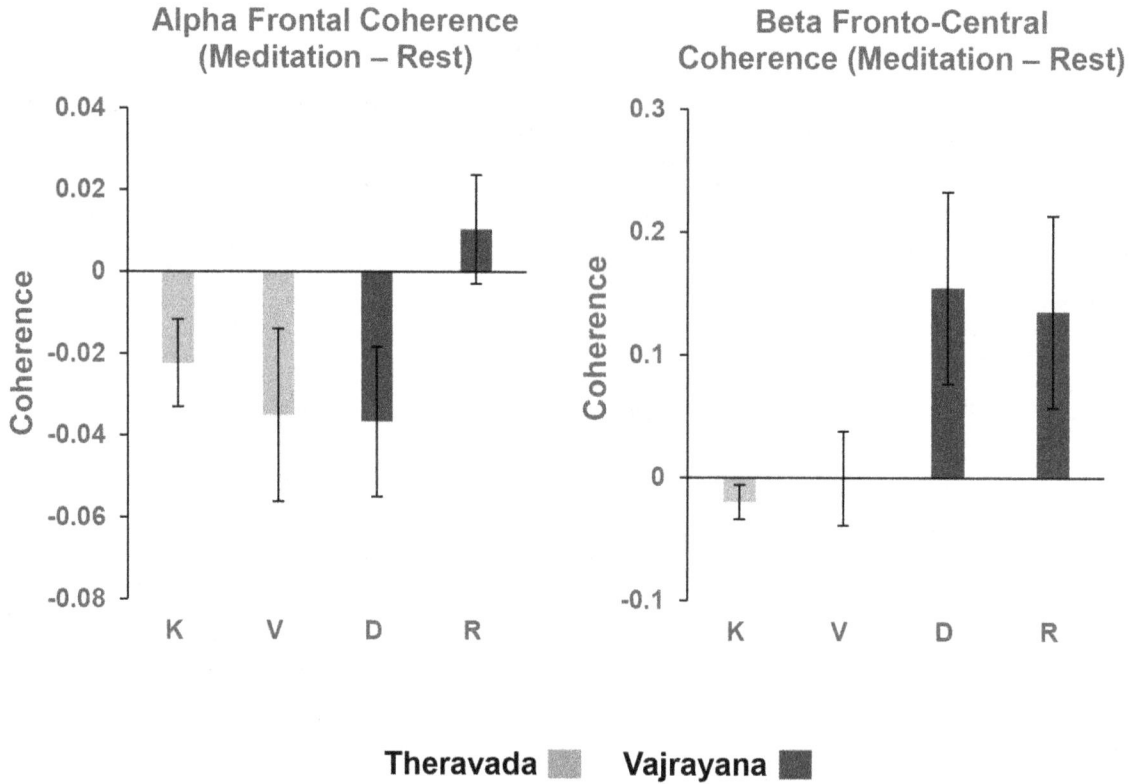

Figure 6. Differences in Coherence between Meditation and Rest (K – Kasina, V – Vipassana, D – Deity, and R – Rig-pa).

Specifically, Study 1 demonstrated that the meditators were more relaxed during Vipassana (Theravada) meditation practices than during rest, as manifested by increased HF for Vipassana meditation and decreased LF/HF and Alpha power. As for Kasina (Theravada), although we did not observe an HF increase, a decrease in LF/HF, decrease in Alpha power, and the overall similarity to the responses obtained for Vipassana also suggest a relaxation response. The opposite pattern of responses was observed for both Vajrayana practices. A decrease in HF power during Deity and Rig-pa meditations indicated that the meditators showed more arousal while engaging in Vajrayana meditation relative to rest. Additionally, only Vajrayana meditators demonstrated significantly enhanced performance on the MRT and VMT tasks following Vajrayana styles of meditation in Study 2.

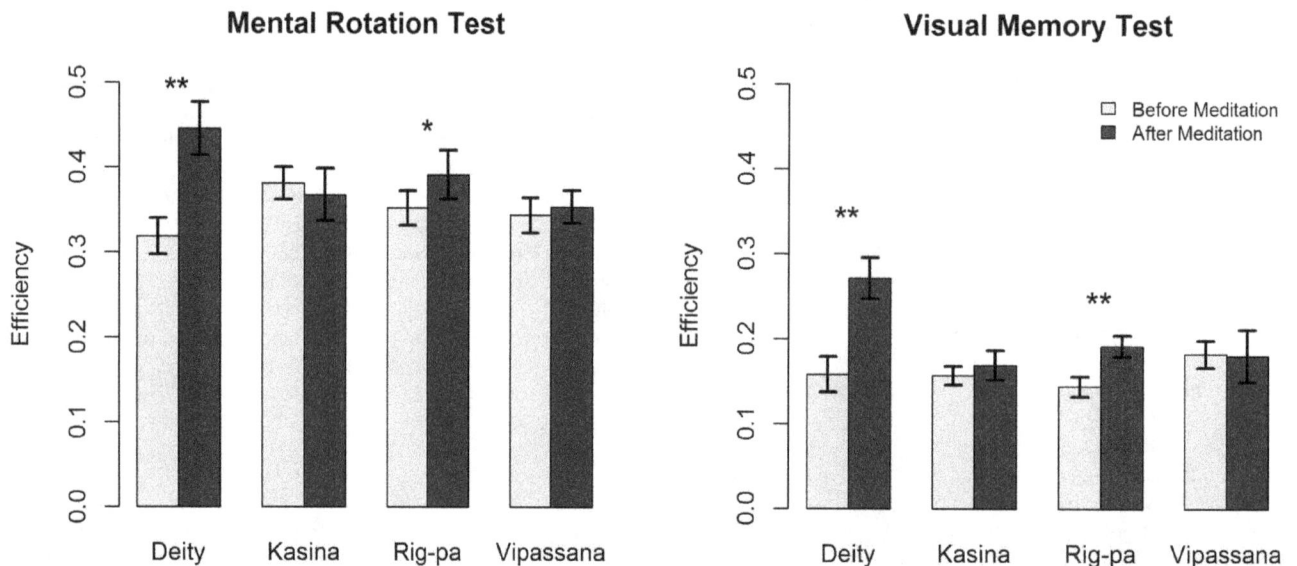

Mental Rotation Test

Visual Memory Test

Figure 7. Efficiency scores before and after Meditation for the MRT (left panel) and VMT (right panel) tasks.

Such immediate dramatic improvements on cognitive task performance could only be attributed to enhanced phasic alertness due to arousal, which reflects rapid mobilization of resources to process stimuli and prepare the system for response [29,71]. Moreover, our findings are consistent with those of a recent study that showed that the practice of g-Tummo Vajrayana meditation can lead to increases not only in peripheral but also in core body temperature [81], which is, to a large extent, mediated by increased sympathetic activation [82]. It is not likely that the enhanced performance we observed in our research is due to the fact that Vajrayana practice involves visualization, and thus results in more efficient metabolic processes necessary to successfully perform the visual imagery tasks administered to the practitioners. The practice of Rig-pa meditation, which is not a visualization type of meditation, produced improvements on the cognitive tasks, while the practice of Kasina meditation, which is a visualization type of meditation, did not lead to any improvements. Nevertheless, further studies are still needed in order to assess whether the performance enhancements which were observed in the current research are modality specific (effecting only visual performance). This should be examined in future studies through the administration of non-visual tests, such as verbal working memory or auditory attention tasks, before and after Vajrayana meditation.

It should be noted that although arousal and "fight-or-flight" or stress responses are related, since both result from the activation of the sympathetic system, they are not the same. Whereas arousal is "an energizing function" responsible for harnessing the body's resources for intense activity, fight-or-flight or the acute stress response (also called *hyperarousal*) is a physiological reaction that occurs in response to a perceived harmful event, attack, or threat to survival [83]. It is important to mention that while Vajrayana meditation activated the sympathetic system, it did not lead to a stress response, which according to recent studies [84–86] would be characterized by increases in Beta power. Our results showed not only that Vajrayana meditative practices led to significant decreases in Beta power, but also that these decreases were even larger than those that occurred to Theravada practitioners. Similarly, the relaxation response produced by Theravada or Vajrayana meditation cannot be reduced to a state of drowsiness or sleep, typically associated with increased Delta power [87], since meditators from both traditions exhibited Delta power decrease during their meditation. This suggests that both Theravada and Vajrayana styles of meditation are neither associated with drowsiness nor with stress, but rather that the meditators were in an alert and non-drowsy state. Furthermore, while it was shown in previous studies that Theravada styles of meditation can induce tonic alertness [31], the results of Study 2 demonstrated that Vajrayana styles of meditation induced phasic alertness as reflected by significant improvements on cognitive tasks immediately after Deity and Rig-pa practices.

An additional goal of our research was to re-examine the validity of the FA-OM classification vs. the classification based on arousal vs. relaxation responses that distinguishes between different meditative traditions. Our EEG results showed qualitatively different patterns of activation between Theravada and Vajrayana meditations, albeit highly similar activity between Kasina and Vipassana, and between Deity and Rig-pa. First, whereas both Theravada practices led to decreases in Alpha power, Vajrayana practices did not, consistent with recent studies that have established that relaxation is correlated with decreased Alpha power [77,78]. Second, while we found a significant decrease in Beta power for both Theravada and Vajrayana meditations, it was significantly larger for Vajrayana. While increases in Beta power have been shown to occur during the

active maintenance of current cognitive and sensorimotor states, decreases in Beta power have been attributed to the processing of upcoming stimuli [88], which is important for both Theravada and Vajrayana (e.g. noticing the content of one's mental activity). The more significant attenuation of Beta power in Vajrayana could be attributed to enhanced readiness to respond to stimuli during increased phasic alertness states, which occur during Vajrayana practices.

Third, whereas Vajrayana meditations showed a decrease in Gamma power relative to Rest, Vipassana meditation showed a Gamma power increase, consistent with a recent study that also demonstrated increased Gamma power during Vipassana [37]. Several other studies also reported increased Gamma power during meditations other than Vipassana. For instance, [12] found increased Gamma synchronization during loving-kindness meditation, which they interpreted to mean that neurons become more synchronized when meditators engage in this type of meditation (see also [89]). Although one must be careful when interpreting Gamma power in EEG, as some researchers believe it to be an artifact generated by miniature eye movements [90], there is nevertheless research that suggests that Gamma power might be linked to object representation and feature binding [91–94], as well as changes in awareness during meditation [37], and the current results might reflect the fact that Theravada and Vajrayana meditations produce states of awareness that are qualitatively different.

Fourth, while we observed only a marginally significant decrease in Alpha Coherence for both Theravada and Vajrayana meditations, we found a significant interaction between the attention and tradition classification of meditations. In particular, the increase in Alpha Coherence was larger for FA (Kasina) than OM (Vipassana) meditation for Theravada, but the opposite effect was observed for Vajrayana, where Alpha Coherence was larger for OM (Rig-pa) but not FA (Deity), inconsistently with the FA-OM classification. Considering that decrease in Alpha Coherence is associated with a more relaxed state [95], it is possible that Kasina requires more effort than Vipassana, while Rig-pa requires more effort than Deity.

Lastly, the difference in Beta Fronto-Central Coherence between Theravada and Vajrayana practices, manifested by an increase only during Vajrayana meditations, may be indicative of enhanced emotion evaluation and affective value choices [96]. This might be related to the emphasis on transformations of emotional states during Vajrayana versus the emphasis on nonattachment from emotions in Theravada practices [14,97].

Thus, based on our findings, we suggest that the categorization of meditations as either "focused attention" or "open monitoring" cannot fully accommodate the range of behaviors and neural processes that are involved during meditation. Indeed, the utilization of focused or distributed attention is not clear cut for the majority of, if not all, meditation techniques, and both attentional systems are probably active at some level in most types of meditations. On the other hand, the distinction between relaxation and arousal is dichotomous: something either induces relaxation or arousal (or neither), but cannot induce both. Our data demonstrate reliable and consistent differences between meditative techniques across traditions, and that meditative practices can be appropriately classified on the basis of whether they produce relaxation or arousal. Importantly, neither relaxation nor arousal are simple by-products of the meditative practice, but play an essential role in the process of attaining insight, and the possibility that the insight obtained would differ depending on whether a relaxation or arousal approach is chosen ought to be investigated in future studies. Whereas the elicitation of an arousal or relaxation response cannot provide a complete description of any type of meditation, the results of the current research provide evidence that it is possible to reliably categorize different types of meditation in this manner.

The implications of our findings are important in several ways. First of all, the present research showed Vajrayana practices can lead to dramatic enhancement in cognitive performance, suggesting that Vajrayana practices can be useful in tasks where optimal performance is required. However, it is important to note that we did not assess long term (i.e. trait) effects of meditations in this research. While the improvements on cognitive tasks following Vajrayana meditation are immediate and dramatic, it is still to be investigated in further research whether they lead to long-term changes. At the same time, while such improvement were not observed after Theravada practices, there is evidence that Theravada meditations might lead to long-term improvement on attentional tasks [31,98,99].

Moreover, our results show that Theravada meditations produce relaxation responses, while Vajrayana types of meditation produce arousal, suggesting that Theravada meditations could be more appropriate for stress reduction than Vajrayana, while Vajrayana meditation could be more problematic in people with higher stress levels. However, it should be noted that our research was conducted on a sample of long-term practitioners. While previous research has shown that stress reduction can be achieved through Theravada types of meditation (i.e. Mindfulness Based Stress Reduction [100,101]), even after just 4–5 weeks of training [102,103], no studies have yet addressed how training in Vajrayana meditation affects stress levels. Thus, investigating how Vajrayana practitioners learn to respond to stressful situations as they gain additional meditation experience, especially practitioners with pre-existing stress or anxiety, is an important direction for future research. It is possible that during long-term practice, Vajrayana meditators develop unique strategies that can be utilized to cope with stressful situations, for instance by transforming their negative emotions into the positive emotional states of the visualized deity.

Limitations affecting the generalizability of our findings is the small sample size due to the difficulties in accessing experienced Vajrayana practitioners, as well as that meditators from different traditions did not have the same cultural background. Additionally, although our findings demonstrate that there are qualitative differences in the manner in which different types of meditation traditions influence the autonomic system, the degree to which Vajrayana and Theravada meditations activate the sympathetic and parasympathetic nervous systems, respectively, still requires further investigation. This could be done, for example, by assessing the level of epinephrine and nor-epinephrine that would be

directly measured through blood samples taken before and after meditation. Furthermore, it would be an interesting research direction to explore whether the nature of the particular Deity that is meditated upon (e.g. peaceful, wrathful, etc.) would influence the level of arousal generated during Deity meditation. It is possible that wrathful Tantric Deities might generate higher levels of arousal in comparison to more peaceful Deities. In addition, since certain meditations utilize breathing specifically to alter the level of relaxation and arousal, it would be valuable for future studies to obtain concurrent respiration and EKG measures.

Despite the limitations, we were able for the first time to show that Vajrayana and Theravada styles of meditation are correlated with different neurophysiological substrates. More generally, the current findings undermine the prevalent view that all meditation practices bring about the same results, of enhancing cognitive performance and reducing stress levels. Indeed, it shows that the physiological and cognitive influences that meditations induce can vary greatly between traditions. Even though the benefits that can follow from different types of meditations of different traditions are often similarly described, leading to the widespread belief that they are in fact highly similar and that the choice to practice one meditation over another would not greatly influence the outcome of the practice, the current research shows not only that this is a misconception, but also that it has greatly hindered the progress of the scientific study of meditation. Our research shows that the large body of research on Theravada meditation is not generalizable to Vajrayana meditation, and thus Vajrayana practices should receive a greater emphasis in future research. Indeed, we show that the term "meditation" is in many ways too general, and have taken a step toward establishing a terminology that can appropriately distinguish the various practices from different traditions.

Acknowledgments

The experiments were conducted by Maria Kozhevnikov at the Shechen Monastery in Nepal and Yannawa Temple in Thailand. We thank Wandrak Gebhack Rinpoche, Elizabeth McDouglas, and George Samuel for providing guidance on Buddhist concepts and theories, and Matthew Ricard for help with the recruitment of subjects. We also thank Charlotte Davis and Konchog Lladripa for help in running experiments and the recruitment of subjects in Nepal and Charoon Wonnakasinanont and Pawana Fongcharoen for arranging the experiments in Thailand. Lastly, we thank Gaelle Desbordes for advising us to use HRV recordings to measure arousal levels in Study 1.

Author Contributions

Conceived and designed the experiments: MK. Performed the experiments: MK IA. Analyzed the data: IA MK. Wrote the paper: IA MK.

References

1. Awasthi B (2013) Issues and perspectives in meditation research: in search for a definition. Front Psychol 3: 1–9.
2. Benson H (1975) The relaxation response. New York, U.S.A.: HarperCollins. 240 p.
3. Young J, Taylor E (1998) Meditation as a voluntary hypometabolic state of biological estivation. News Physiol Sci: 149–153.
4. Boswell PC, Murray GJ (1979) Effects of meditation on psychological and physiological measures of anxiety. J Consult Clin Psychol 47: 606–607.
5. Cauthen N, Prymak C (1977) Meditation versus relaxation. J Consult Clin Psychol 45: 496–497.
6. Morse DR, Martin S, Furst ML, Dubin LL (1977) A physiological and subjective evaluation of meditation, hypnosis, and relaxation. Psychosom Med 39: 304–324.

7. Walrath I, Hamilton D (1975) Autonomic correlates of meditation and hypnosis. Am J Clin Hypn 17: 190–197.

8. Travis T, Kondo C, Knott J (1976) Heart-rate, muscle tension, and alpha production of transcendental meditators and relaxation controls. Biofeedback Self Regul 1: 387–394.

9. Lutz A (2006) Meditation and the neuroscience of consciousness: an introduction. In: P. D . Zelazo and E . Thompson, editors. The Cambridge Handbook of Consciousness. New York, U.S.A.: Cambridge University Press. pp. 499–551.

10. Powers J (1995) Wisdom of Buddha: The Saṃdhinirmocana Sūtra. Berkeley: Dharma Publishing. pp. 153.

11. Lutz A, Slagter HA, Dunne JD, Davidson RJ (2008) Attention regulation and monitoring in meditation. Trends Cogn Sci 12: 163–169.

12. Lutz A, Greischar LL, Rawlings NB, Ricard M, Davidson RJ (2004) Long-term meditators self-induce high-amplitude gamma synchrony during mental practice. Proc Natl Acad Sci U S A 101: 16369–16373.

13. Brefcynski-Lewis JA, Lutz A, Schaefer HS, Levinson DB, Davidson RJ (2007) Neural correlates of attentional expertise in long-term meditation practitioners. Proc Natl Acad Sci USA 104: 11483–11488.

14. Tulku Urgyen Rinpoche (1999) As it is. Hong Kong: Ranjung Yeshe Publications. 224 p.

15. Buddhaghosa B (2010) Visuddhimagga: the path of purification. Kandy, Sri Lanka: Buddhist Publication Society. 794 p.

16. Walshe M (1995) The long discourses of the Buddha: a translation of the Digha Nikaya (teachings of the Buddha). Boston, U.S.A.: Wisdom Publications. pp. 152–153 (I.165), 335 (II.290).

17. Bodhi B (2012) The numerical discourses of the Buddha: a translation of the Anguttara Nikaya. Boston, U.S.A.: Wisdom Publications. pp. 1287–1288 (IV.1410).

18. Tulku Urgyen Rinpoche (1999) As it is. Hong Kong: Ranjung Yeshe Publications. pp. 118.

19. Tulku Urgyen Rinpoche (1999) As it is. Hong Kong: Ranjung Yeshe Publications. pp. 88.

20. Tulku Urgyen Rinpoche (1999) As it is. Hong Kong: Ranjung Yeshe Publications. pp. 85–86.

21. Stutchbury E (1998) Tibetan meditation, yoga, and healing practices: mind-body interactions. In: M. M . DelMonte and Y . Haruki, editors. The Embodiment of Mind: Eastern Western Perpsectives. Delft, Netherlands: Eburon Publishers. pp. 103–127.

22. Beyer S (1978) The Cult of Tara. Berkeley, U.S.A.: University of California Press.

23. Benson H, Malhotra MS, Goldman RF, Jacobs GD, Hopkins PJ (1990) Three case reports of the metabolic and electroencephalographic changes during advanced Buddhist meditation techniques. Behav Med 16: 90–95.

24. Corby JC, Roth WT, Zarcone VP, Jr., Kopell BS (1978) Psychophysiological correlates of the practice of trantric yoga meditation. Arch Gen Psychiatry 35: 571–577.

25. Camm AJ, Malik M, Bigger JT, Breithardt G, Cerutti S, et al. (1996) Heart rate variability - standards of measurement, physiological interpretation, and clinical use. Circulation 93: 1043–1065.

26. Chess GF, Tam RMK, Calaresu FR (1975) Influence of cardiac neural inputs on rhythmic variations of heart period in the cat. Am J Physiol 228: 775–780.

27. Levy MN (1971) Sympathetic-parasympathetic interacitons in the heart. Circul Res 29: 437–445.

28. Weinbach N, Henik A (2011) Phasic alertness can modulate executive control by enhancing global processing of visual stimuli. Cognition 121: 454–458.

29. Sturm W, Simone A, Krause B, Specht K, Hesselmann V, et al. (1999) Functional anatomy of intrinsic alertness: Evidence for a fronto-parietal-thalamic-brainstem network in the right hemisphere. Neuropsychologia 37: 797–805.

30. Petersen SE, Posner MI (2012) The attention system of the human brain: 20 years after. Annual Reviews Neuroscience 21: 73–89.

31. Britton WB, Lindahl JR, Cahn BR, Davis JH, Goldman RE (2013) Awakening is not a metaphor: the effects of Buddhist meditation practices on basic wakefulness. Ann N Y Acad Sci 1307: 64–81.

32. Dunn BR, Hartigan JA, Mikulas WL (1999) Concentration and mindfulness meditations: Unique forms of consciousness? Appl Psychophysiol Biofeedback 24: 147–165.

33. Kozhevnikov M, Louchakova O, Josipovic Z, Motes MA (2009) The enhancement of visuospatial processing efficiency through Buddhist Deity Meditation. Psychol Sci 20: 645–653.

34. Cahn BR, Polich J (2006) Meditation states and traits: EEG, ERP, and neuroimaging studies. Psychol Bull 132: 180–211.

35. Valentine ER, Sweet PLG (1999) Meditation and attention: a comparison of the effects of concentrative and mindfulness meditation on sustained attention. Mental Health, Religion and Culture 2: 59–70.

36. Manna A, Raffone A, Perrucci MG, Nardo D, Ferretti A, et al. (2010) Neural correlates of focused attention and cognitive monitoring in meditation. Brain Res Bull 82: 46–56.

37. Cahn BR, Delorme A, Polich J (2010) Occipital gamma activation during Vipassana Meditation. Cogn Process 11: 39–56.

38. Gyatrul R (1996) Generating the deity. Ithaca, New York, U.S.A.: Snow Lion. 100 p.

39. van de Borne P, Nguyen H, Biston P, Linkowski P, Degaute JP (1994) Effects of wake and sleep stages on the 24-h automatic control of blood pressure and heart rate in recumbend men. Am J Physiol 266: H548–H554.

40. van Dijk AE, van Lien R, van Eijsden M, Gemke RJ, Vrijkotte TG, et al. (2013) Measuring cardiac autonomic nervous system (ANS) activity in children. Journal of Visualized Experiments 74: e50073.

41. Pomeranz M, Macaulay RJB, Caudill MA, Kutz I, Adam D, et al. (1985) Assessment of autonomic function in humans by heart rate spectral analysis. Am J Physiol 248: H151–H153.

42. Pagani M, Lombardi F, Guzzetti S, Rimoldi O, Furlan R, et al. (1986) Power spectral analysis of heart rate and arterial pressure variabilities as a marker of sympathovagal interactin in man and conscious dog. Circul Res 59: 178–193.

43. Schulte-Mecklenbeck M, Kuhberger A, Ranyard R (2011) A handbook of process tracing methods for decision research: a critical review and user's guide. UK: Psychology Press: Taylor and Francis Group. pp. 272.

44. Boucsein W (1992) Electrodermal activity. New York: Plenum Press. 624 p.

45. Wallace A (2006) The attention revolution: unlocking the power of the focused mind. Somerville MA, U.S.A.: Wisdom Publications. 224 p.

46. (2005) Tipitaka: The Pali Canon. Access to Insight. Available: http://www.accesstoinsight.org/tipitaka/. Accessed 30 November 2013.

47. Snellgrove D (2003) Indo-Tibetan Buddhism: Indian Buddhists and their Tibetan successors. Boston, U.S.A.: Shambala. 666 p.

48. Sogyal Rinpoche (1990) Dzogchen and Padmasambhava. California, U.S.A.: Rigpa Fellowship. 95 p.

49. Wangyal T (1993) Wonders of the natural mind: the essence of Dzogchen in the Native Bon tradition. Ithaca, New York, U.S.A.: Snow Lion. 224 p.

50. Goleman D (1996) The meditative mind: the varieties of meditative experience. New York, U.S.A.: G.P. Putnam's Sons. 214 p.

51. American Electroencephalographic Society (1994) Guidelines for standard electrode position nomenclature. J Clin Neurophysiol 11: 111–113.

52. Malliani A, Pagani M, Lombardi F, Cerutti S (1991) Cardiovascular neural regulation explored in the frequency domain. Circulation 84: 1482–1492.

53. Kamath MV, Falen EL (1993) Power spectral analysis of heart rate variability: a noninvasive signature of cardiac autonomic function. Crit Rev Biomed Eng 21: 245–311.

54. Rimoldi O, Pierini S, Ferrari A, Cerutti S, Pagani M, et al. (1990) Analysis of short-term oscillations of R-R and arterial pressure in conscious dogs. Am J Physiol 258: H967–H976.

55. Montano N, Ruscone TG, Porta A, Lombardi F, Pagani M, et al. (1994) Power spectrum analysis of heart rate variability to assess the changes in sympathovagal balance during graded orthostatic tilt. Circulation 90: 1826–1831.

56. Akselrod S, Gordon D, Ubel FA, Shannon DC, Barger AC, et al. (1981) Power spectrum analysis of heart rate fluctuation: a quantitative probe of beat to beat cardiovascular control. Science 213: 220–222.

57. Appel ML, Berger RD, Saul JP, Smith JM, Cohen RJ (1989) Beat to beat variability in cardiovascular variables: noise or music? J Am Coll Cardiol 14: 1139–1148.

58. Billman GE (2013) The LF/HF ratio does no accurately measure cardiac sympatho-vagal balance. Front Physiol 4: 1–5.

59. Morady F, Kou WH, Nelson SD, de Buitleir M, Schmaltz S, et al. (1988) Accentuated antagonism between beta-adrenergic and vagal effects on ventricular refractoriness in humans. Circulation 77: 289–297.

60. Eckberg DL, Mohanty SK, Raczkowska M (1984) Trigemina-baroreceptor reflex interactions modulate human cardiac vagal efferent activity. J Physiol 347: 75–83.

61. Merri M, Farden DC, Mottley JG, Titlebaum EL (1990) Sampling frequency of the electrocardiogram for spectral analysis of the heart rate variability. IEEE Trans Biomed Eng 37: 99–106.

62. Daskalov I, Christov I (1997) Imprvement of resolution in measurement of electrocardiogram RR intervals by interpolation. Med Eng Phys 19: 375–379.

63. Berntson GG, Bigger Jr JT, Eckberg DL, Grossman P, Kaufmann PG, et al. (1997) Heart rate variability: Origins, methods, and interpretive caveats. Psychophysiology 34: 623–648.

64. Molgaard H, Hermansen K, Bjerregaard P (1994) Spectral components of short-term RR interval variability in healthy subjects and effects of risk factors. Eur Heart J 15: 1174–1183.

65. Bigger JT, Fleiss JL, Rolnitzky LM, Steinman RC (1992) Stability over time of heart period variability in patients with previous myocardial infraction and ventricular arrhythmias. Am J Cardiol 69: 718–723.

66. Stein KM, Borer JS, Hochreiter C, Okin PM, Herrold EM, et al. (1993) Prognostic value and physiological correlates of heart rate variability in chronic severe mitral regurgitation. Circulation 88: 127–135.

67. Welch PD (1967) The use of fast fourier transform for the estimation of power spectra: a method based on time averaging over short, modified periodograms. IEEE Trans on Audio and Electroacoustics AU-15: 70–73.

68. Bolduc C, Daoust A-M, Limoges É, Braun CMJ, Godbout R (2003) Hemispheric lateralization of the EEG during wakefulness and REM sleep in young healthy adults. Brain Cogn 53: 193–196.

69. Robbins TW (1997) Arousal systems and attentional processes. Biol Psychol 45: 57–71.

70. Robbins TW (2005) Chemistry of the mind: neurochemical modulation of prefrontal cortical function. Journal of Computational Neurology 493: 140–146.

71. Hasegawa RP, Blitz AM, Geller NL, Goldberg ME (2000) Neurons in monkey prefrontal cortex that track past or predict future performance. Science 290: 1786–1789.

72. MMVirtual Design L (2004) Imagery testing battery [Computer software]. Newark, New-Jersey.

73. Aftanas LI, Golocheikine SA (2002) Non-linear dynamic complexity of the human EEG during meditation. Neurosci Lett 330: 143–146.

74. Huang HY, Lo PC (2009) EEG dynamics of experienced Zen meditation practitioners probed by complexity index and spectral measure. J Med Eng Technol 33: 314–321.

75. Travis F, Wallace RK (1999) Autonomic and EEG patterns during eyes-closed rest and transcendental meditation (TM) practice: The basis for a neural model of TM practice. Conscious Cogn 8: 302–318.

76. Baijal S, Narayanan S (2010) Theta activity and meditative states: spectral changes during concentrative meditation. Cogn Process 11: 31–38.

77. Klimesch W (1999) EEG alpha and Theta oscillations reflect cognitive and memory performance: a review and analysis. Brain Res Rev 29: 179–195.

78. Strijkstra AM, Beersma DGM, Drayer B, Halbesma N, Daan S (2003) Subjective sleepiness correlates negaively with global alpha (8–12 Hz) and positively with central frontal theta (4–8 Hz) frequencies in the human resting awake electroencephalogram. Neurosci Lett 340: 17–20.

79. Lohman DF, Nochols PD (1990) Training spatial abilities: Effects of practice on rotation and synthesis tasks. Learning and Individual Differences 2: 67–93.

80. Bhasin MK, Dusek JA, Chang B-H, Joseph MG, Denninger JW, et al. (2013) Relaxation response induces temporal transcriptome changes in energy metabolism, insulin secretion and inflammatory pathways. PLoS One 8: 1–13.

81. Kozhevnikov M, Elliott J, Shephard J, Gramann K (2013) Neurocognitive and somatic components of temperature increases during g-Tummo meditation: legend and reality. PLoS One 8: 1–12.

82. Morrison SF, Blessing WW (2011) Central nervous system regulation of body temperature. In: I. J . Llewellyn-Smith and A. J. M . Verberne, editors. Central Regulation of Autonomic Functions. Oxford Scholarship Online. pp. 1–34.

83. Walter C (1932) The wisdom of the body. United States: WW. Norton & Company.

84. Barnett KJ, Cooper NJ (2008) The effects of a poor night sleep on mood, cognitive, autonomic and electrophysiological measures. J Integr Neurosci 7: 405–420.

85. Hall M, Thayer JF, Germain A, Moul D, Vasko R, et al. (2007) Psychological stress is associated with heightened physiologial arousal during NREM sleep in primary insomnia. Behav Sleep Med 5: 178–193.

86. Klaus B, Schafer V, Nissen L, Schenkel M (2013) Heightened Beta EEG activity during nonrapid eye movement sleep in primary insomnia patients with reports of childhood maltreatment. J Clin Neurophysiol 30: 188–198.

87. Silber MH, Ancoli-Israel S, Bonnet MH, Chokroverty S, Grigg-Damberger MM, et al. (2007) The visual scoring of sleep in adults. J Clin Sleep Med 3: 121–131.

88. Engel AK, Fries P (2010) Beta-band oscillations–signalling the status quo? Curr Opin Neurobiol 20: 156–165.

89. Fell J, Axmacher N, Haupt S (2010) From alpha to gamma: electrophysiological corelates of meditation-related states of consciousness. Med Hypotheses 75: 218–224.

90. Yuval-Greenberg S, Tomer O, Keren AS, Nelken I, Deouell LY (2008) Transient induced gamma-band response in EEG as a manifestation of miniature saccades. Neuron 58: 429–441.

91. Gruber T, Muller MM (2005) Oscillatory brain activity dissociates between associative stimulus content in a repetition priming task in the human EEG. Cereb Cortex 15: 109–116.

92. Hassler U, Barreto NT, Gruber T (2011) Induced gamma band responses in human EEG after the control of miniature saccadic artifacts. Neuroimage 57: 1411–1421.

93. Tallon-Baudry C, Bertrand O (1999) Oscillatory gamma activity in humans and its role in object representation. Trends Cogn Sci 3: 151–162.

94. Zion-Golumbic E, Bentin S (2007) Dissociated neural mechanisms for face detection and configural encoding: Evidence from N170 and induced gamma-band oscillation effects. Cereb Cortex 17: 1741–1749.

95. Cantero JL, Atienza M, Salas RM, Gomez CM (1999) Alpha EEG coherence in different brain states: an electrohysiological index of the arousal level in human subjects. Neurosci Lett 271: 167–170.

96. Lipsman N, Kaping D, Westendorff S, Sankar T, Lozano AM, et al. (2013) Beta coherence within human ventromedial prefrontal cortex precedes affective value choices. Neuroimage 85: 769–778.

97. Dalai Lama, Ekman P (2008) Emotional awareness: Overcoming the obstacles to psychological balance and compassion. New York, U.S.A.: Holt Paperbacks. 288 p.

98. Tang YY, Lu Q, Fan M, Yang Y, Posner MI (2012) Mechanisms of white matter changes induced by meditation. Proc Natl Acad Sci U S A 109: 10570–10574.

99. MacLean KA, Ferrer E, Aichele SR, Bridwell DA, Zanesco AP, et al. (2010) Intensive meditation training improves perceptual discrimination and sustained attention. Psychol Sci 21: 829–839.

100. Chiesa A, Seretti A (2009) Mindfulness-based stress reduction for stress management in healthy people: a review and meta-analysis. The Journal of Alternative and Complementary Medicine 15: 593–600.

101. Grossman P, Niemann L, Schmidt S, Walach H (2010) Mindfulness-based stress reduction and health benefits: A meta-analysis. Focus on Alternative and Complementary Therapies 8: 500.

102. Agee JD, Danoff-Burg S, Grant CA (2009) Comparing brief stress management courses in a community sample: Mindfulnes skills and progressive muscle relaxation. Explore (NY) 5: 104–109.

103. Jain S, Shapiro SL, Summer S, Roesch SC, Mills PJ, et al. (2007) A randomized controlled trial of mindfulness meditation versus relaxation training: effects on distress, positive states of mind, rumination, and disraction. Ann Behav Med 33: 11–21.

14

Neural Manifestations of Implicit Self-Esteem: An ERP Study

Lili Wu[1], Huajian Cai[2]*, Ruolei Gu[2], Yu L. L. Luo[2], Jianxin Zhang[1], Jing Yang[2], Yuanyuan Shi[2], Lei Ding[3]

1 Key Laboratory of Mental Health, Institute of Psychology, Chinese Academy of Sciences, Beijing, China, **2** Key Laboratory of Behavioral Science, Institute of Psychology, Chinese Academy of Sciences, Beijing, China, **3** School of Electrical and Computer Engineering, University of Oklahoma, Norman, Oklahoma, United States of America

Abstract

Behavioral research has established that humans implicitly tend to hold a positive view toward themselves. In this study, we employed the event-related potential (ERP) technique to explore neural manifestations of positive implicit self-esteem using the Go/Nogo association task (GNAT). Participants generated a response (Go) or withheld a response (Nogo) to *self* or *others* words and *good* or *bad* attributes. Behavioral data showed that participants responded faster to the *self* paired with *good* than the *self* paired with *bad*, whereas the opposite proved true for *others*, reflecting the positive nature of implicit self-esteem. ERP results showed an augmented N200 over the frontal areas in Nogo responses relative to Go responses. Moreover, the positive implicit self-positivity bias delayed the onset time of the N200 wave difference between Nogo and Go trials, suggesting that positive implicit self-esteem is manifested on neural activity about 270 ms after the presentation of self-relevant stimuli. These findings provide neural evidence for the positivity and automaticity of implicit self-esteem.

Editor: Alexandra Key, Vanderbilt University, United States of America

Funding: This work was supported by the National Natural Science Foundation of China [Grant Nos. 31200789, 31070919], the Scientific Foundation of Institute of Psychology, Chinese Academy of Sciences [Grant No. Y0CX363S01], the Hundred Talents Program [Grant No. Y0C2024002] and the Knowledge Innovation Program of the Chinese Academy of Sciences [Grant No. KSCX2-EW-J-8]. The funders had no role in study design, data collection and analysis, decision to publish, or preparation of the manuscript.

Competing Interests: The authors have declared that no competing interests exist.

* Email: caihj@psych.ac.cn

Introduction

Since Greenwald and Banaji's influential paper [1] was published, implicit social cognition has been extensively studied at the behavioral level. In recent years, burgeoning interest has attracted study of the underlying mechanisms of implicit social cognition through the help of cognitive neuroscience methods [2]. To date, research from a cognitive-neural perspective has addressed racial bias [3–8], prejudice [9,10], political attitudes [11], and many other aspects. Surprisingly, while an important area of implicit social cognition, implicit self-esteem has received little attention among cognitive-neural scientists. In our research, we aimed to study neural manifestations of implicit self-esteem.

Implicit self-esteem reflects a kind of automatic, unconscious, and habitual self-evaluation and is often manifested as positive self-associations [1,12,13]. It is common for people with high implicit self-esteem to automatically associate self or self-associated objects with positive stimuli as a kind of self-positivity bias [1,13]. Based on this understanding, a variety of measures have been employed to measure implicit self-esteem, including the Implicit Association Test (IAT, ref. [14]), semantic or affective priming paradigm [15], and Go/Nogo association task (GNAT, refs [16,17]). Besides disassociation from explicit self-esteem [18], another robust finding about implicit self-esteem so far is its positive nature, that is, people implicitly harbor a positive view about themselves. The positive nature of implicit self-esteem consistently has been demonstrated across different measures [18] and cultures [19], ethnicities [20], and age groups [20], as well as in comparison to different social dynamics (such as others, ingroups, best friends,

etc., refs [19,20]; for a review, see ref. [21]). Given this consistency, interesting questions from the perspective of cognitive neuroscience are how and when this ubiquitous positive implicit self-view manifests on or is reflected in neural activity. We will address this issue using event-related potentials (ERPs) that offer high temporal resolution and enable us to investigate dynamic time courses for neural information processes [22].

Based on our conceptualization of implicit self-esteem, we can see that implicit self-esteem involves processing affective valence or evaluative information of the implicit self. Studies from the cognitive neural perspective about the self are numerous (for reviews, see refs [2,23,24]). Early studies have mainly focused on neural representations of the cognitive self and found that cortical midline structures, such as medial prefrontal and posterior cingulate cortices, are relevant to self-referential processing [25,26]. Recently, research has examined evaluative self-processing [27–29] and implicit self-processing [30,31]. When people explicitly performed self-evaluations, functional magnetic resonance imaging (fMRI) research discovered that the ventral anterior cingulate cortex [28], medial prefrontal cortex, and orbitofrontal cortex were all involved [27]; and ERP research found that the self-positivity bias manifested on the N400 component in the time course measured between 450 ms and 600 ms after stimulus onset [29]. When people processed self-relevant information implicitly, fMRI research found similar regions were involved in processing self-information explicitly, such as the medial prefrontal cortex, posterior cingulate/precuneus, etc. [30]. Similarly, ERP research found that implicit self-processing occurred during a perceptual analysis stage as indicated in P200 [31,32]. In addition, new research showed that self-esteem modulates neural responses when people receive social feedback [33,34] or when people complete special tasks such as self-evaluation [35], implicit self-processing [36], math problems [37], and visual probes [38]. A recent study revealed that multi-modal frontostriatal connectivity underlies individual differences in self-esteem [39]. To date, however, neural studies that examined implicit self-processing rarely have involved affective nature or evaluation of the self [30,31]. Neural studies that involved affective nature and evaluative processes of the self are mostly based on self-report rather than implicit measures [27,28]. Consequently, neural studies that examine implicit self-esteem or self-evaluations tapped by implicit measures are still rare.

Among the various measures for implicit self-esteem, we opted for GNAT in the present study [17]. GNAT is a classical measure of implicit attitude, or the strength of association between a target and *good* vs. *bad* attributes. A self-esteem GNAT involves at least two blocks [16,40]. In one block (*self* + *good* condition), participants respond to *self* and *good* stimuli (Go), but ignore *others* and *bad* stimuli (Nogo) ("Press if a *self* word or *good* word"); in the other block (*self* + *bad* condition), participants respond to *self* and *bad* stimuli (Go), but ignore *others* and *good* stimuli (Nogo) ("Press if a *self* word or *bad* word"). If individuals respond faster and/or make fewer errors in the *self* + *good* condition than in the *self* + *bad* condition, they exhibit implicit self-positivity.

In the area of cognitive neuroscience, the Go/Nogo paradigm has been widely used to study neural mechanisms behind response inhibition, which is typically indicated by the N200 component in ERP [41–45]. As an index of response inhibition, the augmented N200, in particular the fronto-central N200 [46], frequently has been observed in Nogo responses in comparison with Go responses [47,48]. The onset of N200 indicates the time at which the information to determine Go/Nogo decision comes available [48–50]. In an attitude GNAT, both Go and Nogo responses involve congruent or incongruent pairs of stimuli. When a category pair is incongruent (e.g. *self* + *bad*), participants suppress initially activated response tendencies before making a Go/Nogo decision. This inhibition may interfere and set back a Go/Nogo decision, leading to a delayed Nogo N200 component. That is, the attitude would modulate the Nogo N200 negativity [47,48].

A recent electrophysiological study has examined neural activity underlying the attitude GNAT, specifically, a GNAT measuring an implicit attitude toward *fruit* vs. *bugs* [47]. Consistent with previous findings, results revealed an augmented N200 negativity in Nogo responses compared with Go responses. Moreover, the onset latency of this N200 negativity or the N200 difference wave obtained from Nogo minus Go were delayed in an incongruent condition (Press if a "fruit" word or a "bad" word) by a priori *fruit-good* association. Based on the timing of the N200 difference wave, the authors inferred that automatic attitude information (i.e., *fruit-good association*) was available about 250 ms after the onset of the stimuli, which is notably earlier than what was previously derived from behavioral data (i.e., between 600–700 ms). Similarly, in another study, examining the timing of Nogo negativity, van der Lugt et al. [51] found that the implicit attitude toward young vs. old people was activated between 170–230 ms after the onset of the target stimuli. These studies suggested that N200 negativity across Nogo and Go trials is useful in studying the timing of automatic attitude activations.

Based on these studies [47,51], we focused on the N200 in the present study, elicited by *self*-stimulus in a self-esteem GNAT. We aimed to examine how and when the self-positivity association would manifest on the N200 component. We hypothesized that Nogo responses to *self* would elicit a larger (or more negative)

N200 relative to Go responses. Moreover, this self-positivity association would delay the onset of N200 in difference waves obtained from Nogo minus Go in the *self* + *bad* condition compared with the *self* + *good* condition. For purposes of comparison and control, we also used a second GNAT to measure implicit attitude toward *others*. This *others* GNAT used identical stimuli to the self-esteem GNAT, but instead asked participants to "press if an *others* word or a *good* word" in an *others* + *good* condition and "press if an *others* word or a *bad* word" in an *others* + *bad* condition. Previous studies showed that a person's attitude toward *others* is neutral or negative [52,53]. Hence, for the *others* GNAT, the latency changes in the N200 difference wave from Nogo minus Go would be trivial or in the opposite direction across *others* + *good* and *others* + *bad* conditions. As a result, interaction between a target (*self* vs. *others*) and valence (*good* vs. *bad*) would be observed. At a behavioral level, we considered reaction time to *self* and *others* in Go trials and expected a similar interaction between the target (*self* vs. *others*) and valence (*good* vs. *bad*). In particular, we believed participants would respond faster to *self* in the *self* + *good* condition than to *self* in the *self* + *bad* condition. However, the pattern in the *others* GNAT would expect not to hold.

Method

Ethics statement

The Local Ethics Committee at the Institute of Psychology, Chinese Academy of Sciences approved the experimental protocol. All participants gave their informed written consent prior to the experiment.

Participants

Nineteen college students (7 women, mean age 23, all right-handed) participated in this study. Each was paid CNY50 for the compensation of their time. None of them had a demonstrated history of neurological or psychiatric disorders. All possessed normal or corrected-to-normal vision. Data from four participants (three men) were not included in the ERP analysis due to technical problems during EEG data recordings. As a result, the final sample consisted of fifteen participants (6 women; age: Mean = 22.9 years, SD = 2.7 years).

Materials

We selected 170 Chinese words as stimuli: 5 *self* words including self, me, myself, I, and mine; 5 *others* words being he/she, him/her, his/her, other ("他人", meaning other in Chinese) and other ("别人", also meaning other); as well as 80 *good* or *positive* attribute words and 80 *bad* or *negative* attribute words. Most attributes were selected from the Chinese version of the Anderson Word List [54]; the remaining attributes were selected from a Chinese word list developed by a previous study that examined Chinese (implicit and explicit) self-esteem. The visual/perceptual complexity of *self* and *others* words indexed by the number of strokes was comparable, Mean = 10.80, 9.60, SD = 4.38, 3.85, respectively, $t_{(8)} = 0.46$, $p = .66$.

Procedure

Two GNATs included four blocks: *self* + *good*, *self* + *bad*, *others* + *good*, and *others* + *bad*, measuring automatic attitudes toward the self (*self* + *good* and *self* + *bad*) and others (*others* + *good* and *others* + *bad*), respectively. In each block, four identical categories of stimuli were presented, one at a time. Different blocks, however, required participants to respond to different pairs of stimuli (signal) but ignore other stimuli (noise). For example, in the *self* + *good* block, participants were instructed to press the space bar if a stimulus conveyed *self* words or *good* words (e.g., *me* and *delight*), but to do nothing if a stimulus was *other* words or *bad* words (e.g., *he* and *bragging*). The sequence of four blocks was counterbalanced across participants. Before each block, pilot trials were run to enable participants to become familiar with the task.

Each block included 320 trials. For each trial, the stimulus was randomly selected from four categories of stimuli, with equal numbers of stimuli from each category. The target stimuli *self* and *others* were repeatedly used because each of them only comprised five variations. The attribute words, *good* and *bad*, were presented without repetition. The ratio of signal to noise was 1:1 in each block.

Figure 1 shows the sequence of stimuli presentations. At the start of each trial, a fixation cross ('+') was centrally presented with a randomized duration between 500 and 1500 ms. After that, the stimulus was presented in the center of the screen for 1000 ms, and participants were required to press the spacebar if the stimulus belonged to signal categories or otherwise register no response. Next, the second fixation was presented for 500 ms. Finally, another trial started anew with the appearance of another fixation.

EEG data recording and analysis

Continuous electroencephalogram (EEG) was recorded from 64 scalp sites using Ag/AgCl electrodes mounted on an elastic cap (NeuroScan Inc., Herndon, VA, USA) with an online reference to the right mastoid and off-line algebraic re-reference to the average of left and right mastoids. The vertical electrooculogram (VEOG) and horizontal electrooculogram (HEOG) were recorded from two pairs of electrodes, with one placed above and below the left eye and another one 10 mm from the outer canthi of each eye. The impedances of all electrodes were maintained below 5 kΩ. EEG and EOG were filtered using a 0.05–100 Hz bandpass filter and sampled at 500 Hz.

During the offline analysis, EEG data were digitally filtered with a 35 Hz low-pass filter. A regression procedure implemented in the Neuroscan software removed ocular artifacts from filtered EEG data [48]. The onset of stimuli was set as the zero time point, and continuous EEG data were epoched into segments of 1000 ms long, including a 200 ms pre-stimulus baseline. Epochs with artifacts due to eye blinks, amplifier clippings, and bursts of

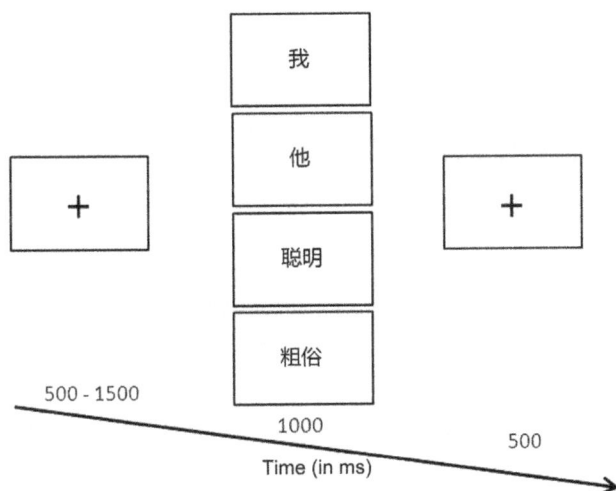

Figure 1. Illustration of the experimental procedure. The stimulus was randomly selected from four categories of stimuli (in this illustration, "我" = *self*, "他" = *others*, "聪明" = *bright*, "粗俗" = *crude*).

electromyographic (EMG) activity exceeding ±100 μV were excluded. ERPs for different word categories and two types of response (*Go* or *Nogo*) were obtained by averaging corresponding epochs from four blocks separately. Data from epochs with incorrect responses and extremely slow responses (i.e., reaction times larger than three standard deviations from mean) were not included during averaging. Finally, eight ERPs for four word categories and two response types were created.

To quantify the Nogo N200 negativity, we measured the mean amplitude of N200 within 250–450 ms at six anterior sites: F3, Fz, F4, FC3, FCz, and FC4, and then conducted a five-way ANOVA with target (*self* vs. *others*), valence (*good* vs. *bad*), response type (*Go* vs. *Nogo*), Anterior-Central (F vs. FC) and Laterality (left vs. midline vs. right) as within-subject variables.

To examine the influence of implicit self-esteem on N200 negativity in the Nogo condition relative to the Go condition, the difference wave from Nogo minus Go was computed first for each participant. Then the onset latencies of N200 negativity or N200 in difference waves were assessed through the jackknife method, which is resistant to individual noise [56,57]. To carry this out, we obtained a new Nogo N200 difference waveform for each participant by averaging the N200 difference waveforms from all other participants in each block. We then measured the total area under the new Nogo N200 difference wave in the time window of 200–500 ms. The onset latency was defined as the time point where a pre-specified fraction (20% in this case) of the total area was reached. Therefore, for each participant, the combination of the jackknife method and fractional area latency measure produced the onset latency of the N200 difference wave. These onset latencies were entered into a 2 (*self* vs. *others*) ×2 (*good* vs. *bad*) ANOVA. The Greenhouse–Geisser correction was used to compensate for sphericity violations. The amended results were then reported in line with previous studies [55,56]. That is, the statistical results (*F*-values and *t*-values) were corrected using the formulas: $F_C = F/(N-1)^2$, and $t_C = t/(N-1)$, where N denotes the number of observations in each condition.

Results

Behavioral Results

To examine whether implicit self-esteem manifested on behavioral data, we performed an ANOVA on reaction time to *self* and *other* words in Go trials with the target (*self* vs. *others*) and valence (*good* vs. *bad*) as two within-subject factors. Participants responded faster to target stimuli paired with *good* words (*Mean* = 502 ms, *SD* = 54 ms) than to those paired with *bad* words (*Mean* = 518 ms, *SD* = 50 ms), $F_{(1, 14)} = 6.51$, $p = .023$. But there was no significant difference in the response speed to *self* (*Mean* = 505 ms, *SD* = 56 ms) and *others* (*Mean* = 514 ms, *SD* = 47 ms), $F_{(1, 14)} = 1.58$, $p = .23$. As expected, the interaction was significant, $F_{(1, 14)} = 31.88$, $p < .001$. Additional simple effect tests showed that participants responded faster to *self* words in the *self* + *good* (*Mean* = 481 ms, *SD* = 53 ms) condition than in the *self* + *bad* condition (*Mean* = 530 ms, *SD* = 50 ms), $t_{(14)} = -5.12$, $p < .001$. In contrast, they responded faster to *other* words in the *others* + *bad* condition (*Mean* = 523 ms, *SD* = 48 ms) than in the *others* + *good* condition (*Mean* = 506 ms, *SD* = 47 ms), $t_{(14)} = 2.39$, $p < .05$. These findings suggest that people implicitly have a positive attitude toward themselves, which is consistent with established implicit self-positivity [21].

ERP Results

Mean amplitude of N200. We first checked if the classical Nogo vs. Go N200 negativity existed. Given individual difference in the appearance of N200, we considered a relatively large time window that was between 250 and 450 ms. The mean N200 amplitudes were measured and submitted to an ANOVA with target (*self* vs. *others*), valence (*good* vs. *bad*), response-type (Go vs. Nogo), Anterior-Central (F vs. FC), and Laterality (left vs. middle vs. right) as the within-subject variables. Consistent with past research [41,47,51], the target, regardless of *self* or *others*, in Nogo trials (*Mean* = 1.87 uV) elicited a larger N200 than in Go trials (*Mean* = 4.11 uV), $F_{(1, 14)} = 34.32$, $p<.001$, suggesting the suppression of motor responses in Nogo trials. No other significant effect was found, all *F*s<4.6 and all *p*s>.05.

Onset latency of Nogo N200. The N200 components elicited by *self* and *other* words with Go responses and Nogo responses as well as their difference waves computed from Nogo minus Go waves are displayed in Figures 2 and 3, respectively. Based on previous suggestions (for a review, see ref [46]), in each of these Figures, we presented the ERP waveforms from only two locations: Fz and FCz. Visual inspection suggests that the Nogo N200 negativity in the *self* + *bad* condition appears later than in the *self* + *good* condition. No visible difference, however, exists between the *others* + *bad* and *others* + *good* conditions. To examine the timing of the Nogo N200 negativity, the onset latencies of the N200 difference waveforms across all four conditions were obtained through the jackknife approach using the 20% criterion and then submitted into a 2 (*self* vs. *others*) ×2 (*good* vs. *bad*) ANOVA.

Results demonstrated that augmented Nogo N200 negativity clocked an earlier onset time (about 275 ms) when targets were paired with *good* attributes than when they were paired with *bad* attributes (about 327 ms), $F_{(1, 14)} = 1572.52$, $F_{C(1, 14)} = 8.02$, $p<.05$. As expected, the interaction was significant, $F_{(1, 14)} = 1291.80$, $F_{C(1, 14)} = 6.59$, $p<.05$. Further simple effect analysis showed that the N200 difference appeared later in the *self* + *bad* condition (347 ms) than in the *self* + *good* condition (271 ms), $t = -46.68$, $t_C = -3.33$, $p<.01$,

whereas no significant difference in Nogo N200 negativity onset latency was recorded between the *others* + *good* (278 ms) and *others* + *bad* (306 ms) conditions, $t = -16.64$, $t_C = -1.19$, $p>.1$. Since the onset time indicated the point in time at which the evaluative information for the attitude target was available, the current findings suggested that after seeing the *self* relevant stimuli, self-evaluative information would be activated and available in less than 271 ms, which is much earlier than behavioral data have been suggested (about 600 ms).

Discussion

Humans implicitly possess a positive view about themselves. We examined how and when this positive implicit self-esteem influences or manifests on brain activity using high temporal resolution ERPs. We measured implicit self-esteem using GNAT and focused on the ERP component of N200 that had been widely studied under the GNAT paradigm. Our behavioral data replicated findings in previous studies [16,40]. Participants responded faster to *self* stimuli paired with *good* words than those paired with *bad* words, whereas they responded slower to *others* stimuli paired with *good* words than those paired with *bad* words, indicating the positive nature of implicit self-esteem. At the neural level, classic Nogo N200 negativity resulted. More important, the *self-positivity* association delayed Nogo N200 negativity in the *self* + *bad* condition as compared with the *self* + *good* condition, suggesting the manifestion of implicit self-esteem on brain activity. Notably, two early ERP components elicited by *self* and *others* words, P100 and N100, were comparable, *F*s<2.87, and *p*s>0.11, suggesting that the influences of the stimuli featured are negligible and that our main findings are not confused by irrelevant factors.

Behavioral evidence for the positivity of implicit self-esteem in humans is sizeable. Greenwald and Banaji [1] have summarized

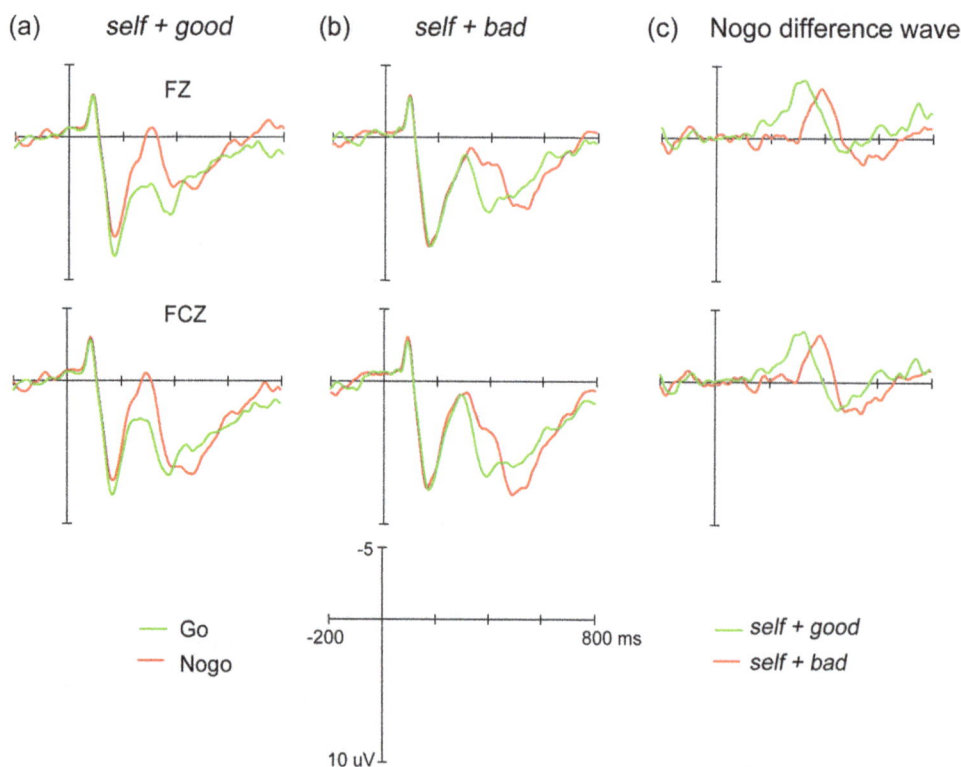

Figure 2. Grand-averaged ERPs for *self* words.

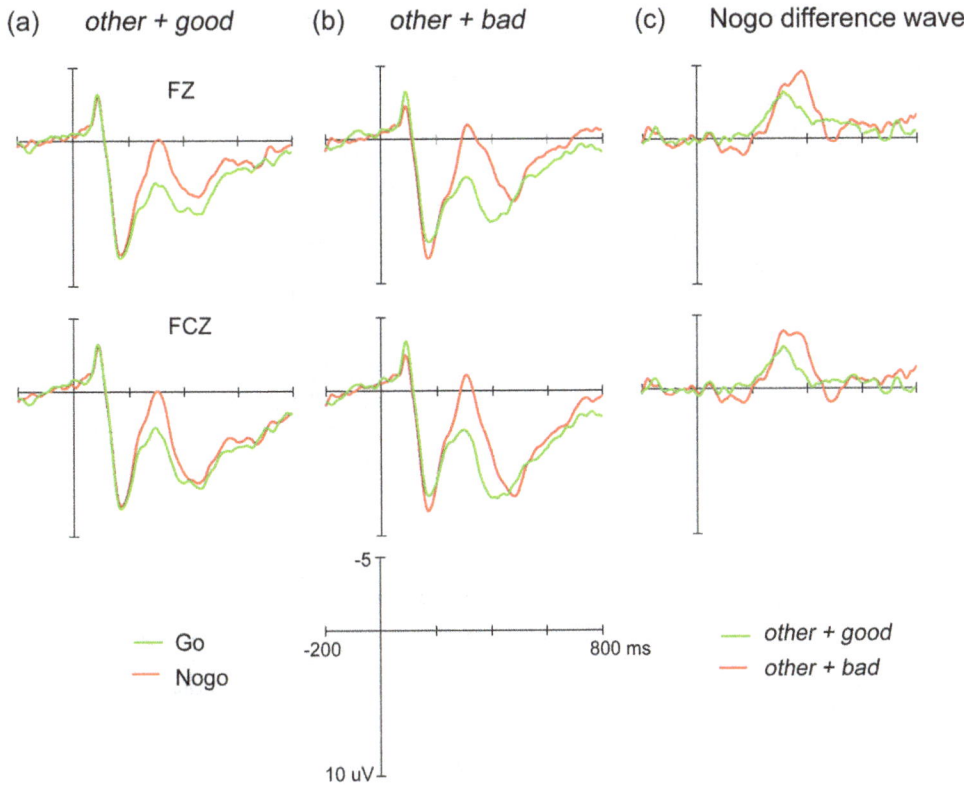

Figure 3. Grand-averaged ERPs for *others* words.

three kinds of evidence: experimental implicit self-esteem (e.g., mere ownership effect); naturally mediated implicit self-esteem (e. g., liking for name-letters); and second-order implicit self-esteem (e. g., self-positivity in judgment). The subsequent large body of research about implicit self-esteem provides further behavioral evidence for the positive nature of implicit self-esteem (for a review, see ref [21]). Our research adds to existing literature by providing novel neural evidence for the positivity of implicit self-esteem. Typical N200 negativity associated with Nogo responses relative to Go responses is delayed in the *self + bad* condition compared with the *self + good* condition, suggesting that activated *self-association* is positive and, moreover, modulates brain activity. This result is consistent with previous findings that show automatic attitudes modulate the onset of N200 [47,51]. People may wonder why humans possess such a positive self-bias. In examining the biological mechanism of another human positive bias, i.e., optimism bias, Sharot and her colleagues suggested that selective registration of more positive than negative self-information is an important cause [58–60]. Similar mechanisms may also explain positive implicit self-esteem because selective updating of self-information may have made self-positive associations more accessible than self-negative associations. These have led to more efficient processing of self-information in *self + good* condition than in *self + bad* condition, which, of course, represents a new direction for future study.

Our study also sheds light on the timing in processing implicit self-associative information. Behavioral responses can only suggest the endpoint of information processing and provide little information about the process of self-associative information. Since the onset of the N200 indicates the time at which attitude information is available [47,51], with the help of the ERP technique, we have identified that implicit self-positivity is

activated and available in less than 270 ms. This time is notably earlier than the time indicated in behavioral response data, i.e., between 600 and 700 ms. Since processing speed is a core indicator of the automaticity of cognitive processes, particularly in the case of implicit social cognition [61], these findings undoubtedly provide convincing evidence about automatic nature of implicit self-esteem. Using a similar methodology, previous studies showed that attitude information about fruit versus bugs and old people versus young people is activated and available in less than 250 ms after the onset of corresponding stimuli [47,51]. This activiation time is somewhat earlier than what we observed for implicit self-esteem, i.e., 270 ms. The difference in activation time might reflect distinct natures of attitude targets (e.g., fruit vs. self) and their representative stimuli in the two studies, or alternatively, might simply suggest random variation. Nevertheless, these findings in toto stand as general evidence for the automaticity of implicit attitude.

In addition, we used the *others* GNAT as a control in this study. Behavioral data replicated past findings [52], whereby humans possess a different implicit attitude toward *others* than toward *selves*. Neural responses in the *others* GNAT, i.e., in *others + good* and *others + bad* blocks, however, exhibit a different pattern. The onset times of Nogo N200 negativity or N200 difference waveform do not differ across conditions. Attitudes toward the *others* factor similarly do not influence neural activity as implicit self-esteem does. These findings provide neural evidence that people's implicit attitudes toward others are distinct from attitudes toward themselves. More importantly, this study also rules out the possibility that the difference between *self + good* and *self + bad* conditions is due to paired attribute valence (*good* vs. *bad*). Thus, utilizing the *others* GNAT as a control, we are more confident that implicit self-esteem (or implicit *self-positivity* bias), rather than the valence of paired categories, modulates the latency of Nogo N200 negativity. People might wonder why an implicit negative bias against *others* manifests in a behavioral index, but not in a neural index. Research has shown that behavioral outcomes of implicit measures, such as GNAT, are the result of cumulative output from many processes, including both automatic and controlled processes [63]. It is possible that some controlled processes have influenced behavioral outputs. Humans have a basic need for a positive self [64,65] and downward social comparison serves as a common way for people to enhance self-positivity [66]. It has also been suggested that automatic social comparison can influence implicit self-evaluation [67]. Therefore, the negative bias manifesting in a behavioral index might be caused by the tendency of enhancing self by looking down on others, which should be further studied in the future.

Recently, implicit self-esteem, particularly as elucidated by the Implicit Assocation Test [14] and Name Letter Preference [12], has been challenged due to its dubious predictive power [21]. In light of this concern, one may question the significance of examining neural substrates of implicit self-esteem. Low predictive capability, however, is not necessarily equated with low validity of a measure or a construct [62], particularly for implicit measures of social cognition [63]. The establishment of predictive validity is usually based on presumed nomological principles in terms of behavioral criteria, which may be misleading due to the limitations of the nomological network as well as the correlational nature of evidence. Hence, the low predictive power of implicit self-esteem may not suggest its low validity and subseqent inefficacy, but rather, highlights the importance of looking into the nature of implicit self-esteem using alternative methodologies. We believe

the cognitive neuroscience approach constitutes a promising new way given its exquisite utility in revealing the cognitive neural basis of a construct or a psychological process. In this sense, our work represents an innovative attempt from the perspective of cognitive neuroscience. We demonstrate that implicit self-esteem is reflected in neural activity by modulating the onset time of the N200 difference wave (Nogo minus Go). We hope that more studies from a cognitive neuroscience perspective will appear in the near future and will help to clarify further the nature of implicit self-esteem.

In conclusion, we demonstrated the electrophysiological signature of implicit self-esteem and revealed relevant timing features for the processing of early self-associative information. These findings provide novel evidence for the positivity and automaticity of implicit self-esteem. Future studies may examine how implicit self-esteem reflects on other neural activities.

Author Contributions

Conceived and designed the experiments: HJC. Performed the experiments: LLW. Analyzed the data: LLW. Wrote the paper: HJC LLW. Helped with the data analysis: LD RLG. Helped with the data collection: JY YYS. Wrote the introduction and discussion sections: HJC. Wrote the method and results sections: LLW. Helped with the revision of the manuscript: YLLL JXZ LD.

References

1. Greenwald AG, Banaji MR (1995) Implicit Social Cognition - Attitudes, Self-Esteem, and Stereotypes. Psychological Review 102: 4–27.
2. Ito TA (2010) Reflections on Social Neuroscience. Social Cognition 28: 686–694.
3. Dickter CL, Bartholow BD (2010) Ingroup categorization and response conflict: Interactive effects of target race, flanker compatibility, and infrequency on N2 amplitude. Psychophysiology 47: 596–601.
4. Ronquillo J, Denson TF, Lickel B, Lu ZL, Nandy A, et al. (2007) The effects of skin tone on race-related amygdala activity: an fMRI investigation. Social Cognitive and Affective Neuroscience 2: 39–44.
5. Ito TA, Urland GR (2003) Race and gender on the brain: electrocortical measures of attention to the race and gender of multiply categorizable individuals. Journal of Personality and Social Psychology 85: 616–626.
6. Lieberman MD, Hariri A, Jarcho JM, Eisenberger NI, Bookheimer SY (2005) An fMRI investigation of race-related amygdala activity in African-American and Caucasian-American individuals. Nature Neuroscience 8: 720–722.
7. McCarthy G, He Y, Johnson MK, Dovidio JF (2009) The relation between race-related implicit associations and scalp-recorded neural activity evoked by faces from different races. Social Neuroscience 4: 426–442.
8. Phelps EA, O'Connor KJ, Cunningham WA, Funayama ES, Gatenby JC, et al. (2000) Performance on indirect measures of race evaluation predicts amygdala activation. Journal of Cognitive Neuroscience 12: 729–738.
9. Gozzi M, Zamboni G, Krueger F, Grafman J (2010) Interest in politics modulates neural activity in the amygdala and ventral striatum. Human Brain Mapping 31: 1763–1771.
10. Wheeler ME, Fiske ST (2005) Controlling racial prejudice: social-cognitive goals affect amygdala and stereotype activation. Psychological Science 16: 56–63.
11. Knutson KM, Wood JN, Spampinato MV, Grafman J (2006) Politics on the brain: an FMRI investigation. Social Neuroscience 1: 25–40.
12. Koole SL, Dijksterhuis A, van Knippenberg A (2001) What's in a name: Implicit self-esteem and the automatic self. Journal of Personality and Social Psychology 80: 669–685.
13. Greenwald AG, Banaji MR, Rudman LA, Farnham SD, Nosek BA, et al. (2002) A unified theory of implicit attitudes, stereotypes, self-esteem, and self-concept. Psychological Review 109: 3–25.
14. Greenwald AG, Farnham SD (2000) Using the implicit association test to measure self-esteem and self-concept. Journal of Personality and Social Psychology 79: 1022–1038.
15. Hetts JJ, Sakuma M, Pelham BW (1999) Two roads to positive regard: Implicit and explicit self-evaluation and culture. Journal of Experimental Social Psychology 35: 512–559.
16. Gregg AP, Sedikides C (2010) Narcissistic Fragility: Rethinking Its Links to Explicit and Implicit Self-esteem. Self Identity 9: 142–161.
17. Nosek BA, Banaji MR (2001) The Go/No-go Association Task. Social Cognition 19: 625–666.
18. Bosson JK, Swann WB, Jr., Pennebaker JW (2000) Stalking the perfect measure of implicit self-esteem: The blind men and the elephant revisited? Journal of Personality and Social Psychology 79: 631–643.
19. Yamaguchi S, Greenwald AG, Banaji MR, Murakami F, Chen D, et al. (2007) Apparent universality of positive implicit self-esteem. Psychological Science 18: 498–500.
20. Baron AS, Banaji MR (2006) The development of implicit attitudes. Evidence of race evaluations from ages 6 and 10 and adulthood. Psychological Science 17: 53–58.
21. Buhrmester MD, Blanton H, Swann WB (2011) Implicit Self-Esteem: Nature, Measurement, and a New Way Forward. Journal of Personality and Social Psychology 100: 365–385.
22. Liotti M, Woldorff MG, Perez R, Mayberg HS (2000) An ERP study of the temporal course of the Stroop color-word interference effect. Neuropsychologia 38: 701–711.
23. Beer JS (2007) The default self: feeling good or being right? Trends in Cognitive Sciences 11: 187–189.
24. Lieberman MD (2007) Social cognitive neuroscience: a review of core processes. Annual Review of Psychology 58: 259–289.
25. Denny BT, Kober H, Wager TD, Ochsner KN (2012) A Meta-analysis of Functional Neuroimaging Studies of Self- and Other Judgments Reveals a Spatial Gradient for Mentalizing in Medial Prefrontal Cortex. Journal of Cognitive Neuroscience 24: 1742–1752.
26. Northoff G, Heinzel A, Greck M, Bennpohl F, Dobrowolny H, et al. (2006) Self-referential processing in our brain - A meta-analysis of imaging studies on the self. Neuroimage 31: 440–457.
27. Beer JS, Lombardo MV, Bhanji JP (2010) Roles of medial prefrontal cortex and orbitofrontal cortex in self-evaluation. Journal of Cognitive Neuroscience 22: 2108–2119.
28. Moran JM, Macrae CN, Heatherton TF, Wyland CL, Kelley WM (2006) Neuroanatomical evidence for distinct cognitive and affective components of self. Journal of Cognitive Neuroscience 18: 1586–1594.
29. Watson LA, Dritschel B, Obonsawin MC, Jentzsch I (2007) Seeing yourself in a positive light: brain correlates of the self-positivity bias. Brain research 1152: 106–110.

30. Moran JM, Heatherton TF, Kelley WM (2009) Modulation of cortical midline structures by implicit and explicit self-relevance evaluation. Social Neuroscience 4: 197–211.

31. Yang J, Guan L, Dedovic K, Qi M, Zhang Q (2012) The neural correlates of implicit self-relevant processing in low self-esteem: An ERP study. Brain research 1471: 75–80.

32. Rameson LT, Satpute AB, Lieberman MD (2009) The neural correlates of implicit and explicit self-relevant processing. Neuroimage 50: 701–708.

33. Eisenberger NI, Inagaki TK, Muscatell KA, Byrne Haltom KE, Leary MR (2011) The Neural Sociometer: Brain Mechanisms Underlying State Self-esteem. Journal of Cognitive Neuroscience 23: 3448–3455.

34. Somerville LH, Kelley WM, Heatherton TF (2010) Self-esteem modulates medial prefrontal cortical responses to evaluative social feedback. Cereb Cortex 20: 3005–3013.

35. Zhang H, Guan LL, Qi MM, Yang J (2013) Self-Esteem Modulates the Time Course of Self-Positivity Bias in Explicit Self-Evaluation. PLoS One 8.

36. Yang J, Qi M, Guan L (2014) Self-esteem modulates the latency of P2 component in implicit self-relevant processing. Biological Psychology 97: 22–26.

37. Yang J, Zhao RF, Zhang QL, Pruessner JC (2013) Effects of self-esteem on electrophysiological correlates of easy and difficult math. Neurocase 19: 470–477.

38. Li HJ, Yang J (2013) Low self-esteem elicits greater mobilization of attentional resources toward emotional stimuli. Neuroscience Letters 548: 286–290.

39. Chavez RS, Heatherton TF (2014) Multi-modal frontostriatal connectivity underlies individual differences in self-esteem. Social Cognitive and Affective Neuroscience doi: 10.1093/scan/nsu063.

40. Boucher HC, Peng KP, Shi JQ, Wang L (2009) Culture and Implicit Self-Esteem Chinese Are "Good" and "Bad" at the Same Time. Journal of Cross-Cultural Psychology 40: 24–45.

41. Falkenstein M, Hoormann J, Hohnsbein J (1999) ERP components in Go Nogo tasks and their relation to inhibition. Acta Psychologica 101: 267–291.

42. Gemba DH, Sasaki K (1989) Potential Related to No-Go Reaction of Go-No-Go Hand Movement Task with Color Discrimination in Human. Neuroscience Letters 101: 263–268.

43. Kok A (1986) Effects of degradation of visual stimulation on components of the event-related potential (ERP) in go/nogo reaction tasks. Biological Psychology 23: 21–38.

44. Nieuwenhuis S, Yeung N, Cohen JD (2004) Stimulus modality, perceptual overlap, and the go/no-go N2. Psychophysiology 41: 157–160.

45. Sasaki K, Gemba H, Nambu A, Matsuzaki R (1993) No-Go Activity in the Frontal Association Cortex of Human-Subjects. Neuroscience Research 18: 249–252.

46. Folstein JR, Van Petten C (2008) Influence of cognitive control and mismatch on the N2 component of the ERP: A review. Psychophysiology 45: 152–170.

47. Banfield JF, van der Lugt AH, Munte TF (2006) Juicy fruit and creepy crawlies: An electrophysiological study of the implicit Go/NoGo association task. Neuroimage 31: 1841–1849.

48. Thorpe S, Fize D, Marlot C (1996) Speed of processing in the human visual system. Nature 381: 520–522.

49. Schiller NO, Schuhmann T, Neyndorff AC, Jansma BM (2006) The influence of semantic category membership on syntactic decisions: a study using event-related brain potentials. Brain Research 1082: 153–164.

50. Schmitt BM, Schiltz K, Zaake W, Kutas M, Munte TF (2001) An electrophysiological analysis of the time course of conceptual and syntactic encoding during tacit picture naming. Journal of Cognitive Neuroscience 13: 510–522.

51. van der Lugt AH, Banfield JF, Osinsky R, Münte TF (2012) Brain potentials show rapid activation of implicit attitudes towards young and old people. Brain Research 1429: 98–105.

52. Karpinski A (2004) Measuring self-esteem using the Implicit Association Test: The role of the other. Personality and Social Psychology Bulletin 30: 22–34.

53. Pinter B, Greenwald AG (2005) Clarifying the role of the "other" category in the self-esteem IAT. Experimental Psychology 52: 74–79.

54. Anderson NH (1968) Likableness ratings of 555 personality-trait words. Journal of Personality and Social Psychology 9: 272–279.

55. Semlitsch HV, Anderer P, Schuster P, Presslich OA (1986) solution for reliable and valid reduction of ocular artifacts, applied to the P300 ERP. Psychophysiology 23: 695–703.

56. Miller J, Patterson T, Ulrich R (1998) Jackknife-based method for measuring LRP onset latency differences. Psychophysiology 35: 99–115.

57. Ulrich R, Miller J (2001) Using the jackknife-based scoring method for measuring LRP onset effects in factorial designs. Psychophysiology 38: 816–827.

58. Sharot T, Shiner T, Brown AC, Fan J, Dolan RJ (2009) Dopamine Enhances Expectation of Pleasure in Humans. Current Biology 19: 2077–2080.

59. Sharot T, Korn CW, Dolan RJ (2011) How unrealistic optimism is maintained in the face of reality. Nature Neuroscience 14: 1475–U1156.

60. Sharot T, Guitart-Masip M, Korn Christoph W, Chowdhury R, Dolan Raymond J (2012) How Dopamine Enhances an Optimism Bias in Humans. Current Biology 22: 1477–1481.

61. De Houwer J, Moors A (2007) How to define and examine the implicitness of implicit measures. In: Wittenbrink B, Schwarz N, editors. Implicit measures of attitudes: Procedures and controversies. New York: Guilford Press. pp. 179–194.

62. Borsboom D, Mellenbergh GJ, van Heerden J (2004) The concept of validity. Psychological Review 111: 1061–1071.

63. De Houwer J, Teige-Mocigemba S, Spruyt A, Moors A (2009) Implicit Measures: A Normative Analysis and Review. Psychological Bulletin 135: 347–368.

64. Cai H, Wu Q, Brown JD (2009) Is self-esteem a universal need? Evidence from The People's Republic of China. Asian Journal of Social Psychology 12: 104–120.

65. Sedikides C, Gaertner L, Toguchi Y (2003) Pancultural self-enhancement. Journal of Personality and Social Psychology 84: 60–79.

66. Wood JV (1989) Theory and research concerning social comparisons of personal attributes. Psychological Bulletin 106: 231–248.

67. Stapel DA, Blanton H (2004) From seeing to being: Subliminal social comparisons affect implicit and explicit self-evaluations. Journal of Personality and Social Psychology 87: 468–481.

15

Conscious Brain-to-Brain Communication in Humans using Non-Invasive Technologies

Carles Grau[1,2], Romuald Ginhoux[3], Alejandro Riera[1,4], Thanh Lam Nguyen[3], Hubert Chauvat[3], Michel Berg[3], Julià L. Amengual[5], Alvaro Pascual-Leone[6], Giulio Ruffini[1,4]*

1 Starlab Barcelona, Barcelona, Spain, 2 Neurodynamics Laboratory, Department of Psychiatry and Clinical Psychobiology, Psychology and Medicine Faculties, University of Barcelona, Barcelona, Spain, 3 Axilum Robotics, Strasbourg, France, 4 Neuroelectrics Barcelona, Barcelona, Spain, 5 Cognition and Brain Plasticity Unit, Department of Basic Psychology, University of Barcelona, Barcelona, Spain, 6 Berenson Allen Center for Noninvasive Brain Stimulation, Beth Israel Deaconess Medical Center, Harvard Medical School, Boston, Massachusetts, United States of America

Abstract

Human sensory and motor systems provide the natural means for the exchange of information between individuals, and, hence, the basis for human civilization. The recent development of brain-computer interfaces (BCI) has provided an important element for the creation of brain-to-brain communication systems, and precise brain stimulation techniques are now available for the realization of non-invasive computer-brain interfaces (CBI). These technologies, BCI and CBI, can be combined to realize the vision of non-invasive, computer-mediated brain-to-brain (B2B) communication between subjects (*hyperinteraction*). Here we demonstrate the conscious transmission of information between human brains through the intact scalp and without intervention of motor or peripheral sensory systems. Pseudo-random binary streams encoding words were transmitted between the minds of emitter and receiver subjects separated by great distances, representing the realization of the first human brain-to-brain interface. In a series of experiments, we established internet-mediated B2B communication by combining a BCI based on voluntary motor imagery-controlled electroencephalographic (EEG) changes with a CBI inducing the conscious perception of phosphenes (light flashes) through neuronavigated, robotized transcranial magnetic stimulation (TMS), with special care taken to block sensory (tactile, visual or auditory) cues. Our results provide a critical proof-of-principle demonstration for the development of conscious B2B communication technologies. More fully developed, related implementations will open new research venues in cognitive, social and clinical neuroscience and the scientific study of consciousness. We envision that hyperinteraction technologies will eventually have a profound impact on the social structure of our civilization and raise important ethical issues.

Editor: Mikhail A. Lebedev, Duke University, United States of America

Funding: This work was partly supported by the EU FP7 FET Open HIVE project (GR, AR, CG, http://hive-eu.org, FET-Open grant 222079, http://cordis.europa.eu/fp7/ict/fetopen/home_en.html), the Starlab Kolmogorov project (GR, CG, SIF-003, http://starlabint.com), the research group 2009SGR00093 from the Generalitat de Catalunya (GR, CG, http://www10.gencat.cat/agaur_web/AppJava/english/a_beca.jsp?categoria = altres&id_beca = 4861), and by the Neurology Department of the Hospital de Bellvitge (JLA). Co-authors CG, AR and GR were employed by Starlab Barcelona during these studies. The funder, Starlab, provided support in the form of salaries for authors CG, AR and GR, but did not have any additional role in the study design, data collection and analysis, decision to publish, or preparation of the manuscript. The specific roles of these authors are articulated in the 'author contributions' section. Co-authors RG, TLN and MB are employed by Axilum Robotics. Co-authors AR and GR are employed by Neuroelectrics Barcelona. Axilum Robotics and Neuroelectrics Barcelona provided support in the form of salaries for authors RG, TLN, MB, AR and GR, but did not have any additional role in the study design, data collection and analysis, decision to publish, or preparation of the manuscript. The specific roles of these authors are articulated in the 'author contributions' section.

Competing Interests: The authors have the following interests: This study was funded in part by Starlab Barcelona. Co-authors Carles Grau, Alejandro Riera and Giulio Ruffini were employed by Starlab Barcelona during these studies. Co-authors Romuald Ginhoux, Thanh Lam Nguyen and Michel Berg are employed by Axilum Robotics. Co-authors Alejandro Riera and Giulio Ruffini are employed by Neuroelectrics Barcelona. Authors affiliated to Starlab or Neuroelectrics have a commercial interest in promoting the EEG/brain-stimulation system described in the paper (Starstim). Authors affiliated to Axilum Robotics have an interest in promoting their robot to automate the positioning of a transcranial magnetic stimulation coil.

* Email: Giulio.Ruffini@Starlab.es

Introduction

The evolution of civilization points to a progressive increase of the interrelations between human minds, where by ''mind'' we mean a set of processes carried out by the brain [1]. Until recently, the exchange of communication between minds or brains of different individuals has been supported and constrained by the sensorial and motor arsenals of our body. However, there is now the possibility of a new era in which brains will dialogue in a more direct way [2]. Previous attempts to realize this vision include demonstrations of bidirectional computer-brain communication [3–5] and cortical-spinal communication [6] in the monkey, and hippocampus-to-hippocampus [7] or social communication [8] in the rat – all of invasive nature. Despite these and other significant advances with human subjects [9–10], invasive methods in humans remain severely limited in their practical usefulness. Pioneering research in the 60's using non-invasive means already demonstrated the voluntary control of alpha rhythm de-synchronization to send messages based on Morse code [11]. Over the last

15 years, technologies for non-invasive transmission of information from brains to computers have developed considerably, and today brain-computer interfaces embody a well-established, innovative field of study with many potential applications [12–16]. Recent work has demonstrated fully non-invasive human to rat B2B communication by combining motor imagery driven EEG in humans on the BCI side with ultrasound brain stimulation on the CBI-rat side [17]. However, the realization of non-invasive CBI in humans remains elusive, and adequate methodologies to provide computer-mediated non-invasive brain conscious interventions are lacking. Here we show how to link two human minds *directly* by integrating two neurotechnologies – BCI and CBI –, fulfilling three important conditions, namely a) being non-invasive, b) cortically based, and c) consciously driven (Fig. 1). In this framework we provide the first demonstration of non-invasive direct communication between human minds.

Materials and Methods

Human Subjects

Four healthy participants (age range 28–50) were recruited, and their informed written consent was obtained. Of the four subjects, one was assigned to the BCI branch (the *emitter* - Subject 1) and the other three to the CBI branch of the experiments (i.e., as *receivers* - Subjects 2, 3 and 4).

Ethics Statement

The Ethics Committee of the University of Barcelona, following the Ethical Principles for Medical Research Involving Human Subjects of the WMA Declaration of Helsinki, approved this study. The TMS part of the experiments was conducted according to TMS safety guidelines [18]. The individuals in this manuscript gave their written informed consent (as outlined in the PLOS consent form) to publish these case details.

Methods Summary

The computer-mediated brain-to-brain transmission from Thiruvananthapuram (Kerala state, India) (BCI side) to Strasbourg, France (CBI) was realized using internet-linked EEG and TMS technologies respectively. On the CBI side, three information *receiver* subjects were stimulated with biphasic TMS pulses at a subject-specific occipital cortex site. The intensity of pulses was adjusted for each subject so that a) one particular orientation of the TMS-induced electric field produced phosphenes [19] (representing the "active direction" and coding the bit value "1"), and b) the orthogonal direction did not produce phosphenes (representing the "silent direction" and coding the bit value "0"). Subjects reported verbally whether or not they perceived phosphenes on stimulation. A fourth subject acted as *emitter* of information using a BCI system based on motor imagery (of moving feet or hands) to select two kinds of states in EEG spectral power in the motor cortex (coding for the bit values of "0" and "1"). We ensured that receiver subjects were not relying on peripheral nervous system (PNS) cues (visual, tactile and auditory sensations produced by the TMS device) to decode the information by blocking sensory cues: we used a force sensor on the coil to maintain a constant contact pressure on the scalp, implemented a coil rotation information encoding strategy (as opposed to one relying on coil location), and had subjects wear eye mask and earplugs. We verified the effectiveness of these means in series of *d-prime* control experiments [20–22] comparing pairs of stimuli delivered either with the same or different orientations of the coil. Finally, as performance measures for the BCI, CBI and B2B system we analyzed error transmission rates and transmission speed (bits per minute).

Brain-Computer Interface

The BCI communication subsystem used in our experiments converted conscious voluntary motor imagery into brain activity changes that could be captured non-invasively as physical signals

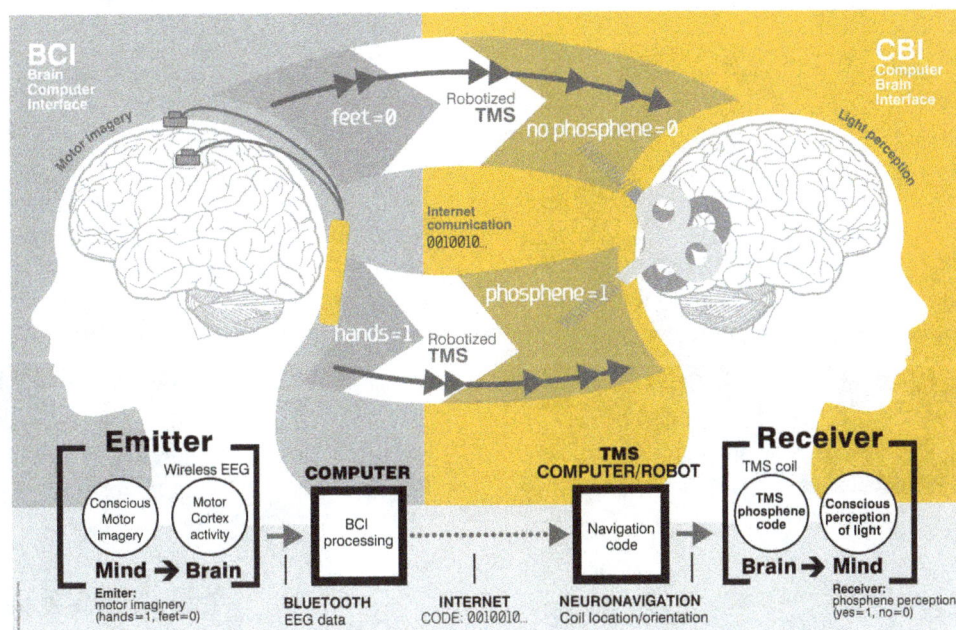

Figure 1. Brain-to-brain (B2B) communication system overview. On the left, the BCI subsystem is shown schematically, including electrodes over the motor cortex and the EEG amplifier/transmitter wireless box in the cap. Motor imagery of the feet codes the bit value 0, of the hands codes bit value 1. On the right, the CBI system is illustrated, highlighting the role of coil orientation for encoding the two bit values. Communication between the BCI and CBI components is mediated by the internet.

conveying information. To monitor EEG activity related with motor imagery tasks we used a wireless (500 S/s, 24 bit) EEG recording system [23] (Starstim tCS/EEG system, by Neuro-electrics, http://www.neuroelectrics.com). Eight Ag/AgCl electrodes were placed at F3, F4, T7, C3, Cz, C4, T8 and Fz scalp sites (10–20 EEG positioning system) and electrically referenced to a clip electrode placed in the right ear lobe. A spatial filter was applied to the electrodes of interest (C3, Cz and C4) by referencing them to the average potential of their neighboring electrodes. To transform EEG signals into binary information we used the BCI-2000 platform [24] implementing the detection of anatomically localized changes in EEG related with voluntary motor imagery. The emitter subject was sequentially shown on the screen a representation of the bits to be transmitted (the message). Each bit was represented either by a target cue in the downright part of the screen (bit value 0) or in the upright part (bit value 1) (Figs. 1 and 2). If the bit to be transmitted was a 1 (0), the emitter was to encode it through motor imagery of the hands (feet). These motor imagery tasks controlled the vertical movement of a ball appearing on the screen from the left with a constant horizontal speed. If the ball hit the displayed target on the right of the screen, the transmitted bit was then correctly encoded. Whatever the outcome the BCI encoded bits were then automatically sent via email to the CBI subsystem. Following a training period, the emitter subject was able to regularly achieve an accuracy of well over 90% in BCI encoding.

Computer-Brain Interface

For the CBI subsystem, we relied on biphasic TMS pulses to encode information. For each receiver subject, we identified first a TMS phosphene-producing hotspot in the right visual occipital cortex (approximately 2 cm anterior and 2 cm right from inion, the precise location depending on the subject), which was used for the *active* condition (to encode the bit value '1'). We achieved the required high precision in relocation and reorientation of the TMS target by using a neuronavigated [25–28], robotized TMS system

(Axilum Robotics TMS-Robot, http://www.axilumrobotics.com, piloted by Localite 2.8 Neuronavigation system using the MagVenture MagPro R30 TMS Stimulator with a "butterfly" coil of type Cool-B65-RO). Subjects went through a familiarization period in which we administered several TMS pulses to the chosen right occipital cortex site using various rotations of the coil, and identified the intensity of TMS pulses (range 57–90% of maximum intensity of the coil) that optimally discriminated *active* (i.e., producing phosphenes) from *silent* (not producing phosphenes) orientations (Fig. 3). Subjects described the sensations of light produced by TMS pulses of the active orientation as having a strong, clear and reliable nature, and located at the bottom of the visual field contralateral to the stimulation site [29]. They were instructed to report verbally the presence of phosphenes immediately after TMS pulse delivery. TMS pulses were administered by the robotized TMS system controlled by a researcher sitting away from the visual field of the subject, or directly programmed into the neuronavigation computer by the BCI message sequence received via email (Fig 2). Sequences of two or three redundant TMS pulses were delivered with an inter-stimulus interval of 2 seconds.

Our first robotized CBI experiments (subject 1) used a position-dependent encoding with the TMS hotspot representing the active condition (bit = 1) and another scalp location (displaced about 2 cm from the first) representing the silent condition (bit = 0). This strategy was used for CBI transmissions of 60 bit messages with a low error rate. An associated first B2B experiment (Barcelona to Strasbourg) – carried out offline (i.e., with the BCI and CBI branches of transmission separated in time by buffering the data after BCI transmission) – resulted in a 15% transmission error rate (5% in the BCI segment and 11% in the CBI one). However, we identified the possibility that the receiver subject at the CBI end was being cued on the (active or silent) stimulation condition by PNS sensory inputs (tactile, auditory or visual) related to the repositioning of the coil at different scalp sites. In order to rule this out, we implemented a series of measures on the next experiments

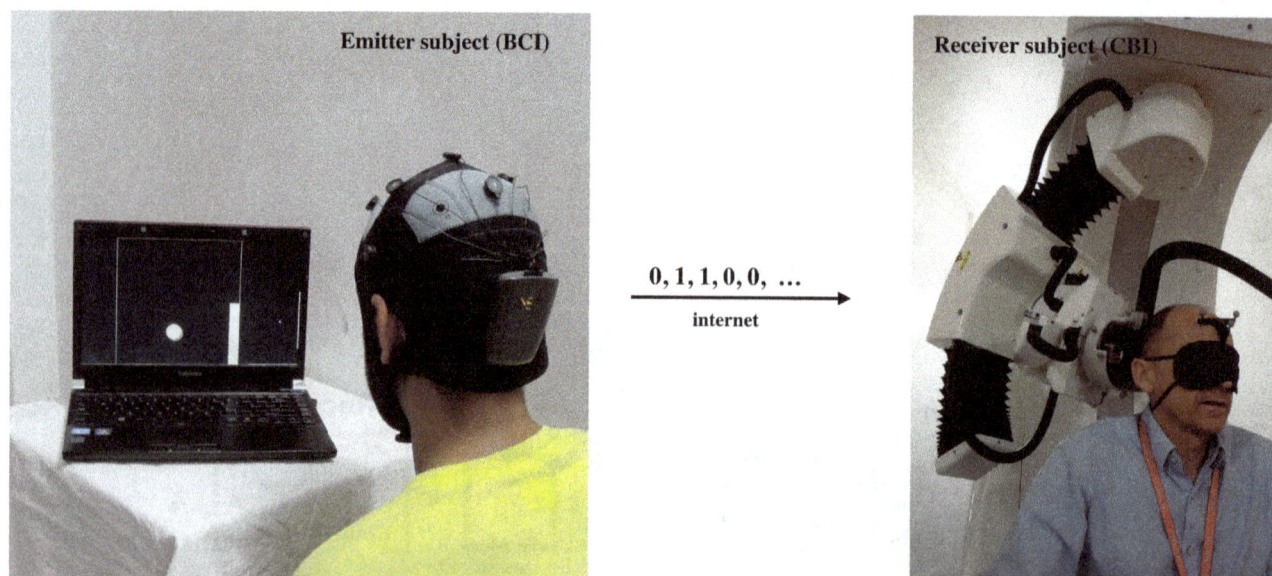

Emitter subject (BCI)

0, 1, 1, 0, 0, ...

internet

Receiver subject (CBI)

Figure 2. View of emitter and receiver subjects with non-invasive devices supporting, respectively, the BCI based on EEG changes driven by motor imagery (left) and the CBI based on the reception of phosphenes elicited by a neuronavigated TMS (right) components of the B2B transmission system. The successfully transmitted code in the particular scenario shown is a '0': the target and ball are at the bottom of the screen (correctly encoding a 0 through motor imagery of the feet) and the TMS coil is in the orientation not producing phosphenes for this particular participant (subject 2, see Figure 3), with the handle pointing upwards.

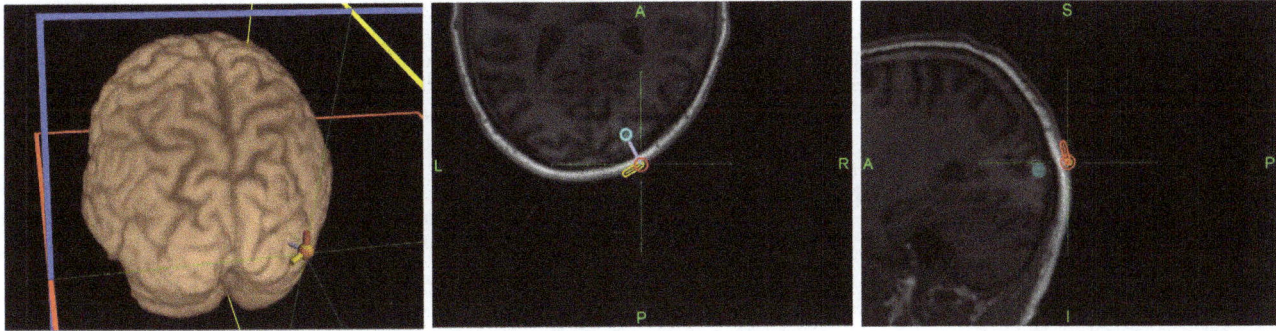

Figure 3. Location and orientation of hot spot for phospene production overlaid on MRI image of the head of subject 2 (see Figure 2). The active direction producing phospenes is highlighted in orange (in red, the orthogonal direction not producing phosphenes).

– including the final B2B transmissions described below. First, to avoid contact related cues and taking advantage of the anisotropic response of the visual cortex to TMS [30], we adopted the strategy of encoding bits through rotation of the TMS coil: the location and "active" orientation of the coil (producing phosphenes in most trials) were chosen with the condition that a 90° rotation of the coil on the same location did not produce phosphenes (Fig. 2). The robot was programmed to move the coil away from the scalp after the delivery of each triad of TMS pulses. A force sensor on the coil surface was used to maintain a constant contact force with the scalp in all conditions. The cable holder on the robot was adjusted to keep the coil's cable at a good distance from the subject's shoulders and back, preventing contact during coil rotation. Second, to avoid identification of coil orientation from auditory information, subjects wore earplugs and the robot moved the coil between each pair or triads of TMS pulses towards a parking site located approximately 1 cm away from the scalp with an intermediate rotation of 45°. This forced the robot to realize a movement of similar duration and with equal noise levels for all bit transmission events, irrespective of coil orientation. Lastly, we blocked visual cues on stimulation configuration by having subjects close their eyes and wear an eye mask.

To assess the effectiveness of these measures, we carried out a series of control studies using the sensitivity index (or *d-prime*) statistic [20–22]. The first control studied TMS noise induced auditory cueing and had subjects (2 and 3) wear an eye mask and earplugs and receive a sequence of 32 balanced pairs of three TMS stimuli randomly interspersed over silent and active conditions. We mimicked the contact of the coil but eliminated the production of phosphenes by interposing, between coil and scalp, a single piece of foam slightly displacing (~1 cm) the center of the coil orthogonally away from the head. After the administration of each pair (of triads) of stimuli, subjects were asked if they were delivered with the equal or different orientations. Then, we performed a second control experiment to evaluate cues from (tactile) skin contact, based on another sequence of 32 balanced pairs, without foam on the coil but setting a null intensity in the magnetic stimulator. Results from these tests indicated with high confidence that, after correct blinding of auditory, visual or tactile cues, the subjects were unable to distinguish coil orientations in the absence of actual phosphene-inducing TMS pulses (Subject 2: $d' = 0.0$ in the auditory task, $d' = -0.1$ in the skin contact task; Subject 3: $d' = 0.6$ in the auditory task, $d' = 0.1$ in the skin task).

Results

The final round of experiments targeted the demonstration of online brain-to-brain transmission of information between remotely located subjects. On March 28th, 2014, 140 bits were encoded by the BCI emitter in Thiruvananthapuram and automatically sent via email to Strasbourg, where the CBI receiver (subject 3) was located. There, a program parsed incoming emails to navigate the robot and deliver TMS pulses precisely over the selected site and with the appropriate coil orientation. A similar transmission with receiver subject 2 took place on April 7th, 2014. In both cases, the transmitted pseudo-random sequences carried encrypted messages encoding a word – "*hola*" ("*hello*" in Catalan or Spanish) in the first transmission, "*ciao*" ("hello" or "goodbye" in Italian) in the second. Words were encoded using a 5-bit Bacon cipher [31] (employing 20 bits) and replicated for redundancy 7 times (for a total of 140 bits). The resulting bit streams were then randomized using random cyphers selected to produce balanced pseudo-random sequences of 0's and 1's (for subject blinding and proper statistical analysis purposes in addition to providing word-coding). On reception, de-cyphering and majority voting from the copies of the word were used to decode the message.

In these experiments, the individual BCI and CBI segments as well as the complete B2B link provided transmission of pseudo-random information with excellent integrity. In the first experiment the transmission error rates were of 6%, 5% and 11% for the BCI, CBI and the combined B2B components respectively, and in the second, error rates were of 2%, 1% and 4% respectively. We note that the probability of transmission of lists of 140 items having occurred with the low observed error rates or less by chance is negligible ($p < 10^{-22}$). For example, the probability of guessing correctly 140 random, balanced bits with an error rate of 20% (28 errors out of 140) or less is extremely low, this being equivalent to obtaining 112 heads or more after 140 tosses of a fair coin ($p < 10^{-13}$).

BCI and CBI transmission rates were of 3 and 2 bits per minute respectively. The overall B2B transmission speed was of 2 bits per minute (limited by the CBI branch). The encoded words were transmitted with full integrity by all links – BCI, CBI and B2B.

Discussion

In these experiments we demonstrated the feasibility of direct brain-to-brain communication in human subjects, with special care taken to ensure the non-participation of sensory or motor systems in the exchange of information (Figure 1). Streams of pseudo-random bits representing the words "*hola*" and "*ciao*" were successfully transmitted mind-to-mind between human subjects separated by a great distance, with a negligible probability of this happening by chance.

We believe these experiments represent an important first step in exploring the feasibility of complementing or bypassing traditional language-based or other motor/PNS mediated means in interpersonal communication. Although certainly limited in nature (e.g., the bit rates achieved in our experiments were modest even by current BCI standards, mostly due to the dynamics of the precise CBI implementation), these initial results suggest new research directions, including the non-invasive direct transmission of emotions and feelings or the possibility of sense synthesis in humans, that is, the direct interface of arbitrary sensors with the human brain using brain stimulation, as previously demonstrated in animals with invasive methods [2].

The main differences of this work relative to previous brain-to-brain research are a) the use of human emitter and receiver subjects, b) the use of fully non-invasive technology and c) the conscious nature of the communicated content. Indeed, we may use the term *mind-to-mind* transmission here as opposed to *brain-to-brain*, because both the origin and the destination of the communication involved the conscious activity of the subjects.

Our findings strengthen the relevance of integrating the CBI branch in human-computer communication using precision technologies for high performance (i.e., a robotized, neuronavigated TMS system). Importantly, we demonstrated the use of rotation-encoding TMS induced phosphenes as a reliable CBI solution, providing methods and controls to exclude PNS involvement.

The proposed technology could be extended to support a bi-directional dialogue between two or more mind/brains (namely, by the integration of EEG and TMS systems in each subject). In addition, we speculate that future research could explore the use of closed mind-loops in which information associated to voluntary activity from a brain area or network is captured and, after adequate external processing, used to control other brain elements in the same subject. This approach could lead to conscious synthetically mediated modulation of phenomena best detected subjectively by the subject, including emotions, pain and psychotic, depressive or obsessive-compulsive thoughts.

Finally, we anticipate that computers in the not-so-distant future will interact directly with the human brain in a fluent manner, supporting both computer- and brain-to-brain communication routinely. The widespread use of human brain-to-brain technologically mediated communication will create novel possibilities for human interrelation with broad social implications that will require new ethical and legislative responses [32].

Acknowledgments

G.R. would like to thank Walter Van de Velde for early initial discussions on the vision of computer mediated mind-to-mind communication, and to Pedro Miranda for technical discussions on the dependence of generated electric field direction on TMS "butterfly" (or "figure of 8") coil orientation. The authors thank Ms. Ana Clapés for illustration graphic design.

Author Contributions

Conceived and designed the experiments: GR CG APL. Performed the experiments: AR RG MB GR CG HC JLA. Analyzed the data: GR RG AR CG HC. Contributed reagents/materials/analysis tools: TLN GR CG AR. Contributed to the writing of the manuscript: GR CG APL RG MB AR.

References

1. Kandel E (2013) The New Science of Mind and the Future of Knowledge. Neuron 80, 546–560.
2. Nicolelis MA (2010) Beyond Boundaries: The New Neuroscience of Connecting Brains with Machines and How It Will Change Our Lives. St. Martin's Griffin. 368 p.
3. Delgado JMR (1969) The physical control of the mind: Toward a Psychocivilized Society. New York: Harper & Row. 288 p.
4. Chapin JK, Moxon KA, Markowitz RS, Nicolelis MA (1999) Real-time control of a robot arm using simultaneously recorded neurons in the motor cortex. Nat Neurosci 2, 664–670.
5. O'Doherty JE, Lebedev M, Ifft PJ, Zhuang KZ, Shokur S, et al. (2011) Active tactile exploration using a brain–machine–brain interface. Nature 479: 228–231.
6. Shanechi MM, Hu RC, Williams ZM (2014) A cortical-spinal prosthesis for targeted limb movement in paralysed primate avatars. Nat Commun 5: 3237.
7. Deadwyler SA, Berger TW, Sweatt AJ, Song D, Chan RH, et al. (2013) Donor/recipient enhancement of memory in rat hippocampus. Front Syst Neurosci 7: 120.
8. Pais-Vieira M, Lebedev M, Kunicki C, Wang J, Nicolelis MAL (2013) Brain-to-Brain Interface for Real-Time Sharing of Sensorimotor Information. Scientific Reports 3, 1319.
9. Hochberg LR, Serruya MD, Friehs GM, Mukand JA, Saleh M, et al. (2006) Neuronal ensemble control of prosthetic devices by a human with tetraplegia. Nature 442: 164–171.
10. Hochberg LR, Bacher D, Jarosiewicz B, Masse NY, Simeral JD, et al. (2012) Reach and grasp by people with tetraplegia using a neurally controlled robotic arm. Nature 485: 372–375.
11. Dewan EM (1967) Occipital alpha rhythm eye position and lens accomodation. Nature 214: 975–977.
12. Birbaumer N (2006) Breaking the silence: Brain–computer interfaces (BCI) for communication and motor control. Psychophysiology 43: 517–532.
13. Wolpaw JR, McFarland DJ (1994) Multichannel EEG-based brain-computer communication. Electroencephalogr Clin Neurophysiol 90, 6: 444–9.
14. Wolpaw JR, Birbaumer N, McFarland DJ, Pfurtscheller G, Vaughan TM (2002) Brain-computer interfaces for communication and control (Review). Clinical Neurophysiology 113, 6: 767–791.
15. Lebedev MA, Nicolelis MAL (2006) Brain machine interfaces: Past, present and future. Trends in Neuroscience 29: 536–46.
16. Allison BZ, Dunne S, Leeb R, Millán JDR, Nijholt A (Eds.) (2013), Towards Practical Brain-Computer Interfaces. Springer-Verlag. 412p.
17. Yoo S-S, Kim H, Filandrianos E, Taghados SJ, Park S (2013) Non-Invasive Brain-to-Brain Interface (BBI): Establishing Functional Links between Two Brains. PLoS ONE 8(4): e60410.
18. Rossi S, Hallett M, Rossini PM, Pascual-Leone A (2009) Safety, ethical considerations, and application guidelines for the use of transcranial magnetic stimulation in clinical practice and research. Clin Neurophysiol 120(12): 2008–39.
19. Taylor PCJ, Walsh V, Eimer M (2010) The Neural Signature of Phosphene Perception, Human Brain Mapping 31, 9: 1408–1417.
20. Green DM, Swets JA (1966) Signal Detection Theory and Psychophysics. New York: Wiley (1966).
21. Wichchukit S, O'Mahony M A (2010) Transfer of Technology from Engineering: Use of ROC Curves from Signal Detection Theory to Investigate Information Processing in the Brain during Sensory Difference Testing. Journal of Food Science, 75 (9): R183–R193.
22. MacMillan N, Creelman C (2005) Detection Theory: A User's Guide. Lawrence Erlbaum Associates. 512 p.
23. Schestatsky P, Morales-Quezada L, Fregni F (2013) Simultaneous EEG Monitoring During Transcranial Direct Current Stimulation. J Vis Exp (76).
24. Schalk G, Mellinger JA (2010) Practical Guide to Brain-Computer Interfacing with BCI2000 (1st ed.). Springer. 264 p.
25. Ginhoux R, Renaud P, Zorn L, Goffin L, Bayle B., et al. (2013) A Custom Robot for Transcranial Magnetic Stimulation: First Assessment on Healthy Subjects. Conf Proc IEEE Eng Med Biol Soc.: 5352–5.

26. Bashir S, Edwards D, Pascual-Leone A (2011) Neuronavigation increases the physiologic and behavioral effects of low-frequency rTMS of primary motor cortex in healthy subjects. Brain Topogr. 24, 1: 54–64.

27. Julkunen P, Säisänen L, Danner N, Niskanen E, Hukkanen T, et al. (2009) Comparison of navigated and non-navigated transcranial magnetic stimulation for motor cortex mapping, motor threshold and motor evoked potentials. NeuroImage 44: 790–795.

28. Ruohonen J, Karhu J (2010) Navigated transcranial magnetic stimulation. Clin Neurophysiol 40: 7–17.

29. Fried PJ, Elkin-Frankston S, Rushmore RJ, Hilgetag CC, Valero-Cabre A (2011) Characterization of Visual Percepts Evoked by Noninvasive Stimulation of the Human Posterior Parietal Cortex. PLoS ONE 6(11): e27204.

30. Kammer T, Vorwerg M, Herrnberger B (2007) Anisotropy in the visual cortex investigated by neuronavigated transcranial magnetic stimulation. Neuroimage 36, 313–321.

31. Fouché Gaines H (1989) Cryptanalysis: a Study of Ciphers and Their Solutions. Dover publications. 256 p.

32. Trimper JB, Wolpe PR, Rommelfanger KS (2014) When "I" becomes "We": ethical implications of emerging brain-to-brain interfacing technologies. Front Neuroeng 7: 4: 1–4.

16

How Listeners Weight Acoustic Cues to Intonational Phrase Boundaries

Xiaohong Yang[1], Xiangrong Shen[1,2], Weijun Li[1]*, Yufang Yang[1]*

1 Key Laboratory of Behavioral Science, Institute of Psychology, Chinese Academy of Sciences, Beijing, China, **2** College of Humanities and Communications, Shanghai Normal University, Shanghai, China

Abstract

The presence of an intonational phrase boundary is often marked by three major acoustic cues: pause, final lengthening, and pitch reset. The present study investigates how these three acoustic cues are weighted in the perception of intonational phrase boundaries in two experiments. Sentences that contained two intonational phrases with a critical boundary between them were used as the experimental stimuli. The roles of the three acoustic cues at the critical boundary were manipulated in five conditions. The first condition featured none of the acoustic cues. The following three conditions featured only one cue each: pause, final lengthening, and pitch reset, respectively. The fifth condition featured both pause duration and pre-final lengthening. A baseline condition was also included in which all three acoustic cues were preserved intact. Listeners were asked to detect the presence of the critical boundaries in Experiment 1 and judge the strength of the critical boundaries in Experiment 2. The results of both experiments showed that listeners used all three acoustic cues in the perception of prosodic boundaries. More importantly, these acoustic cues were weighted differently across the two experiments: Pause was a more powerful perceptual cue than both final lengthening and pitch reset, with the latter two cues perceptually equivalent; the effect of pause and the effects of the other two acoustic cues were not additive. These results suggest that the weighting of acoustic cues contributes significantly to the perceptual differences of intonational phrase boundary.

Editor: Joel Snyder, UNLV, United States of America

Funding: This research was supported by the National Natural Science Foundation of China (31000505). The funders had no role in study design, data collection and analysis, decision to publish, or preparation of the manuscript.

Competing Interests: The authors have declared that no competing interests exist.

* Email: liwj88@gmail.com (WL); yangyf@psych.ac.cn (YY)

Introduction

Spoken language is hierarchically structured into prosodic units divided by prosodic breaks. While researchers disagree on the number and definitions of prosodic units, they generally agree that prosodic units include prosodic words, phonological phrases, and intonational phrases [1–4]. There is a high correspondence of intonational phrase boundaries (IPBs) with major syntactic boundaries such as clause and sentence boundaries, which are central to language comprehension [5,6]. Thus, the phrasing of intonational phrases has been the subject of numerous studies in the areas of speech production and perception [7–10]. In this paper, we will investigate how acoustic correlates are weighted in the perception of IPBs.

Previous studies have established three major acoustic correlates of IPBs: pause, final lengthening, and pitch reset [3,6,8,11–16]. Specifically, pauses are always found to accompany IPBs [17–19]. Furthermore, syllable durations are longer at the end of an intonational phrase than in the middle of it, a phenomenon known as final lengthening or pre-boundary lengthening [3,20–23]. Finally, pitch tends to decline across the course of an utterance and reset to a higher value after an IPB boundary ([24–26]; for a review of the prosodic correlates of IPBs, please see [27]). These prosodic correlates have been found to be helpful for listeners in speech segmentation [5,28,29], and recent studies using Event-Related Potentials (ERPs) have shown that the perception of boundaries accompanied by these prosodic correlates elicited the Closure Positive Shift(CPS), a brain ERP component known to reflect the perception of prosodic boundary [30–32].

Although it is relatively clear that IPBs often coincide with prosodic parameters such as pause, final lengthening, and pitch reset, which help listeners interpret prosodic boundaries, it is still unclear how these three cues are weighted on the perceptual side. Studies on how listeners weight these cues in the perception of IPBs have been scarce, and most findings are based on studies involving only two of the three major acoustic correlates [29,33–35]. Scott [29] tested the effects of pause and phrase-final lengthening by using syntactically ambiguous sentences such as " Kate or Pat and Tony will come." where the position of a phrase boundary after " Kate" represented one meaning, and after "Pat" another meaning. She found that the duration of a pause alone or the combined duration of a pause and final stressed syllable lengthening could provide listeners with a cue to the location of a phrase boundary, even in the absence of a disambiguating pitch contour. Furthermore, the duration of a pause was perceptually equivalent to the same duration of final lengthening and an accompanying pause combined. Similarly, Shen [35] found that in perception, pause seemed to be a more important cue than phrase-final lengthening, since only when the duration of phrase-final syllables was increased to a certain length could it cue syntactic boundaries. Lin and Fon [33] moved one step further by showing that the roles of temporal cues in perception were weighted differently for different purposes: Final lengthening was more important for participants to detect boundaries, while pause duration was more responsible in cuing boundary sizes. These three studies are limited in that only temporal cues are investigated. In Streeter [34], the role of pitch change was compared to other parameters: amplitude and duration pattern. It was found that both pitch contour and duration pattern were reliably used as cues in parsing ambiguous algebraic expressions. Amplitude by comparison appeared to be a less important cue that was only effective in combination with appropriate values of duration.

The studies described above compared either the role of pause or the role of pitch change with that of final lengthening. Thus, there is, as yet, no clear picture of how these three correlates are weighted in the perception of IPBs. This issue has been partially resolved by Zhang [36], who tested the roles of pause, pre-boundary lengthening, and pitch in the perception of prosodic boundaries with expressions such as "turkey salad and coffee" (no-boundary condition) vs. "turkey, salad, and coffee" (boundary condition). She found that for Chinese listeners, pitch reset was weighted more heavily than pause and pre-boundary lengthening. However, it is possible that this finding may have resulted from her experimental design. In the production of her experimental materials, the distinction in pause duration ranged from zero ms in the non-boundary condition to over 300 ms in the boundary condition. However, in the perception task, the maximum pause duration was set at 80 ms in the boundary condition. This manipulation probably reduced the contribution of pause, making pitch reset a much more pronounced acoustic cue for Chinese listeners.

As described above, whereas numerous studies have explored the acoustic correlates of IPBs in production, only a relatively small number have focused on how the acoustic correlates are weighted in the perception of IPBs, and no clear picture of it has emerged yet. In this study, we present two experiments explicitly testing the roles of pause, final lengthening, and pitch reset in Chinese. In line with Lin and Fon [33], we not only tested how these acoustic cues contributed perceptually to the presence of an IPB, but also investigated how they contributed to the perceived boundary strength of an IPB. In Experiment 1, we explored whether listeners' performance in a boundary perception task remained the same or was degraded as a result of the loss of these correlates. In Experiment 2, we examined whether the perceived strength of an IPB was affected by the weighting of the correlates.

Experiment 1

1.1 Materials

Forty-eight sentences that were originally used in Li and Yang [30] were used in this experiment. Each sentence consisted of two intonational phrases with an explicit IPB between them, which was the critical boundary for the present study. We chose these well-formed sentences to allow for a precise acoustic realization of the crucial IPBs. For instance, in example (1a) below, the two intonational phrases were "想保持领先" and "花时间进行练习非常重要." Thus, there was an IPB between the two phrases. The pre-boundary syllable was "先(xian1),"and the post-boundary syllable was "花(hua1)." They were both marked in bold. The presence of the acoustic features of an IPB in these sentences was confirmed by a detailed acoustic analysis carried out in PRAAT. The sentences clearly revealed the three main prosodic boundary cues that were characteristic of IPBs at the crucial boundary position: pause, final lengthening, and pitch reset. Furthermore,

perceptual data from ERPs clearly showed that CPS, a brain component marking speech segmentation, was observed for the crucial IPBs. For details regarding the acoustic parameters and the CPS data, please see Li and Yang [30].

(1a) [想/保持/领**先**/]IPB1 [**花**/时间/进行/练习/非常/重要/]IPB2.

[Xiang3/bao3chi2/ling3**xian1**]IPB1 [**hua1**/shi2jian1/jin4xing2/lian4xi2/feilchang2/bi4yao4]IPB2.
If/you/want to/keep/ahead/, taking/time/to do/exercises/is very/necessary.
'If you want to keep ahead, it is very necessary to take time to do exercises.'

The 48 sentences served as the baseline condition in which no cues were manipulated and all prosodic correlates were preserved intact. Out of these 48 sentences, we created another five conditions. The first condition was a no-cue condition, in which all three acoustic correlates were removed. The following three conditions featured only one cue each: pause, final lengthening, and pitch reset, respectively. For instance, in the second condition, only pause was preserved while the other two acoustic correlates were removed. Likewise, in the third condition, only final lengthening was preserved while the other two acoustic cues were removed. This manipulation allows us to isolate the acoustic correlates and directly examine their relevance to the perception of IPB. The fifth condition featured both pause and final lengthening. We manipulated this condition because some studies have found that the combination of pause and final lengthening was a good indicator of boundary size [22,37]. These five manipulated conditions plus the baseline condition yielded altogether six conditions for the present study.

The crucial procedure for creating the manipulated conditions involved removing one or more of the acoustic features at the critical IPBs. For the removal of pause duration, the silent pauses at the critical boundary position were removed based on visual inspection in PRAAT. The removal of final lengthening and pitch reset was more complicated. Instead of neutralizing the values of final lengthening and pitch reset as has been done in previous studies [12,34], we followed a procedure of exchanging acoustic features to circumvent the problem of determining a priori the neutral value of a specific acoustic feature [36]. Specifically, we exchanged the acoustic features of the words pronounced at the IPBs with the acoustic features of the same words that were not pronounced at a boundary position. This was realized by using another 48 sentences in which the pre- and post-boundary syllables did not span an IPB boundary, but only a syllable boundary (SB).

A SB exists between two syllables that form a word in Chinese. A word in Chinese is usually a bigram (two-syllable word). For instance, the word "鲜花" ('flower') is composed of two syllables: 鲜 and 花. Two syllables that are parts of a word are usually pronounced with a within-word syllable boundary [38]. Syllable boundaries in Mandarin Chinese are pronounced without distinct acoustic correlates and are often used as a no-boundary control condition in the study of prosodic hierarchies [30]. An IPB, however, often exists between two clauses that form a sentence or accompanies the end of a sentence [6]. IPBs are often pronounced with acoustic correlates such as pause, final lengthening, and pitch reset [11–16].

For example, (1a) had the SB counterpart (1b), shown below. In (1b), the pre-boundary syllable "鲜 (xian1)" and the post-boundary syllable "花 (hua1)" had exactly the same pronunciation and location as "先 (xian1)" and "花(hua1)" in the IPB sentences but were pronounced together as a word with only a within-word syllable boundary between them. Of particular importance is that these syllable-boundary sentences were only used for the acoustic-exchanging procedures to create the five manipulated conditions in the present study, but not for the perception experiments as reported below. The syllable-boundary sentences were also materials from Li and Yang [30].

(1b) [商店里的/**鲜花**/散发出/阵阵/浓郁的/芳香]_IPB1.

  [Shang1 dian4 li3 de0/**xian1 hua1**/san4 fa1 chu1/zhen4 zhen4/nong2 yu4 de0/fang1xiang1]_IPB1.
  In the store/the flowers/emit/bouts of/full-bodied/aroma.
  'The flowers in the store emit bouts of full-bodied aroma.'

These SB counterparts were used in the procedures of exchanging acoustic parameters. For the removal of final lengthening at IPBs, the duration patterns of the pre-boundary syllables in the IPB sentences were compressed to conform to the duration patterns of pre-boundary syllables in the SB sentences. For the removal of pitch reset, the fundamental frequency contours for the pre- and post-boundary syllables from the SB sentences were superimposed on the pre- and post-boundary syllables in the IPB sentences. The procedures used to create the experimental conditions are shown in Fig. 1. The three major acoustic features of the critical boundaries in the five manipulated conditions as well as the baseline condition are shown in Table 1.

Through the procedures described above, 48 sentence sets were created out of the original 48 sentences, with each set containing five manipulated sentences and one baseline sentence. Thus, altogether, 288 sentences were used for the perception experiment. The 48 sentence sets were counterbalanced according to a Latin square design and divided into six lists, with each sentence set presented only once within each list. Each list contained eight sentences per condition. To each list, 48 filler sentences with no sentence-internal IPB boundaries were also added. These filler sentences were added to balance the "Yes" and "No" responses of the task.

1.2 Ethics Statement

All participants provided written informed consent in accordance with the Declaration of Helsinki. The ethics committee of the Institute of Psychology, Chinese Academy of Sciences approved this study, including its participant recruitment procedure and methodology.

1.3 Participants

Twenty-four university students (13 women; mean age = 23.0 years; SD = 1.74) participated in the experiment for cash. All were native speakers of Chinese. All of them reported having no hearing problems.

1.4 Procedures and Data Analysis

The participants were tested individually in a sound-attenuating shielded chamber. They were seated in a comfortable chair approximately 60 cm in front of a monitor and were instructed to listen to the sentences attentively to detect speech boundaries. A trial started with a fixation cross, and 1000 ms later, a sentence was presented via headphones. At the end of each sentence, a question appeared on the screen which tested whether the participants had perceived the intended IPBs. For example, the question following sentence (1a) was "Do you perceive a boundary between "xian1" and "hua1"?" The participants were told to

respond to this question by pressing "J" on the keyboard for a "Yes" response and "F" for a "No" response. The next trial began immediately after the participants gave their response. The experiment lasted about 15 minutes.

A repeated-measures analysis of variance (ANOVA) was performed with the factor condition as the independent variable and the mean proportions of boundaries detected by the participants as the dependent variable. Greenhouse-Geisser adjustment was used to correct for violations of sphericity. Post hoc comparisons were adjusted using Bonferroni's correction.

1.5 Results and Discussions

Mean proportions of boundaries detected by the participants are displayed in Fig. 2. A repeated-measures ANOVA showed a main effect of condition, $F(5, 115) = 18.47$, $p < 0.001$, $\eta^2_{partial} = 0.45$. Post hoc comparisons revealed that the proportion of boundaries detected for the no-cue condition was significantly lower than those for all the other five conditions ($ps < 0.05$). The proportion of boundaries detected for the pause condition was significantly higher than those for the final lengthening ($p < 0.05$) and pitch reset condition ($p < 0.05$). Similarly, the proportions of boundaries detected for the pause + final lengthening condition were also significantly higher than those for the final lengthening ($p < 0.01$) and pitch reset condition ($p < 0.01$). This pattern was the same for the baseline condition: A higher proportion was found for the baseline condition than for the final lengthening ($p < 0.05$) and pitch reset condition ($p < 0.05$). There was no significant difference between the pause, pause + final lengthening, and baseline conditions ($ps > 0.05$). The final lengthening and pitch reset conditions did not differ from each other ($p > 0.05$).

The above results showed that participants' responses for boundary detection varied among the experimental conditions. However, note that except for the baseline condition, the five manipulated conditions were not natural speech but synthesized speech created in PRAAT. This could result in different degrees of naturalness, which may confound the effects of the acoustic parameters on the participants' responses for boundary detection. To examine whether the perceived boundary strength was influenced by the degrees of naturalness, we conducted a posttest by asking another 24 participants to rate the naturalness of the sentences on a scale of 1 (very unnatural) to 7 (very natural). The results for the naturalness rating are given in Table 2.

A repeated-measures ANOVA for the rating scores showed a main effect of condition, $F(5, 115) = 25.83$, $p < 0.001$, $\eta^2_{partial} = 0.53$. Post hoc comparisons revealed that the no-cue condition was rated as less natural than all the other five conditions ($ps < 0.05$). Furthermore, the pause condition was rated as more natural than the lengthening condition ($p < 0.01$) and pitch reset condition ($p < 0.05$). The pause + final lengthening condition was also rated as more natural than the lengthening condition ($p < 0.001$) and pitch reset condition ($p < 0.01$). Rating scores were higher for the baseline condition than for the lengthening condition ($p < 0.01$) and pitch reset condition ($p < 0.01$). No other differences were significant ($ps > 0.05$). Thus, it appears that the naturalness of the sentences differed across conditions. To control for the influence of naturalness on the results of boundary detection, we ran a univariate analysis with condition as the independent variable, naturalness rating score as the covariate, and mean proportion of boundaries detected as the dependent variable. The results are shown in Fig. 3.

As shown in Fig. 3, when the influence of naturalness degree was controlled for, the resulting pattern was almost identical to that shown in Fig. 2. This impression was confirmed by statistical analysis. The results of the univariate analysis revealed a main

Features preserved for each condition	Features removed	Procedures to remove the features

Cond. 1: none

Cond.2: pause

Cond.3: final lengthening

Cond.4: pitch reset

Cond.5: pause + Final lengthening

Cond.6: all

Pause

Final lengthening

Pitch reset

Cut the silent pauses at the IPB position

Compress the durations of the pre-boundary words at the IPBs to conform to those at the syllable boundaries.

Replace the pitch contours of the pre- and post-boundary syllables at the IPBs with those at the syllable boundaries.

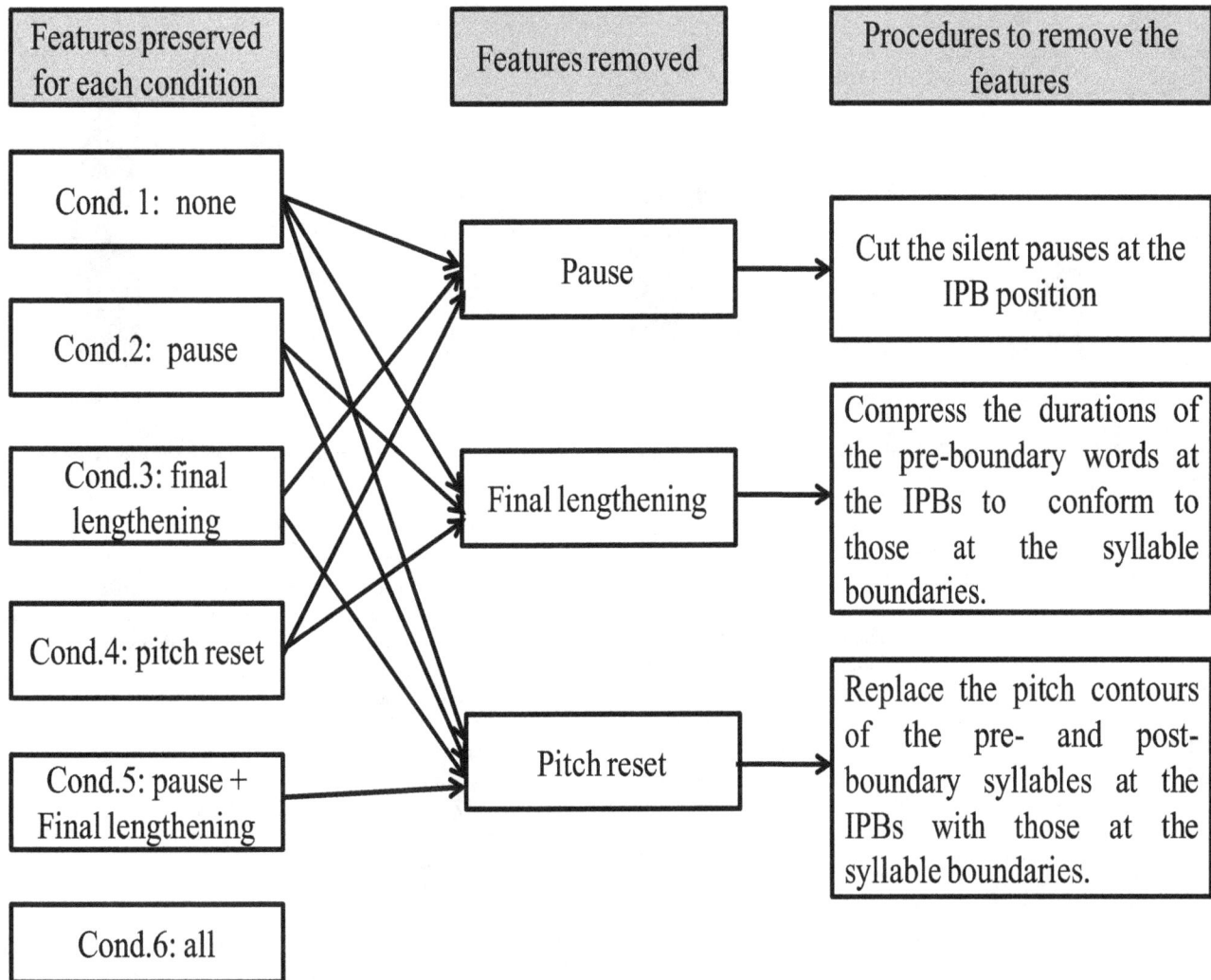

Figure 1. The procedures used to create the experimental conditions.

effect of condition, F $(5, 281) = 16.60$, $p<0.001$, $\eta^2_{partial} = 0.23$. Post hoc comparisons revealed that the proportion of boundaries detected was significantly lower in the no-cue condition than in all the other five conditions ($ps<0.01$). The proportion of boundaries detected for the pause condition was significantly higher than those for the final lengthening condition ($p<0.01$) and pitch reset condition ($p<0.01$). Similarly, the proportion of boundaries detected for the pause + final lengthening condition was significantly higher than those for the final lengthening condition ($p<0.01$) and pitch reset condition ($p<0.01$). Finally, the proportion was also higher for the baseline condition than for the final lengthening condition ($p<0.01$) and pitch reset condition ($p<0.01$).

Table 1. Means of the acoustic parameters for the six conditions (with standard deviations in parentheses).

Conditions	Pause duration(s)	Syllable duration(s)	F0 reset (st)
No-cue	----	0.22 (0.05)	-0.42 (4.82)—
Pause	0.27 (0.11)	0.22 (0.05)	-0.42 (4.82)
Final lengthening	----	0.26 (0.04)	—0.42 (4.82)
Pitch reset	----	0.22 (0.05)	4.55 (4.68)
Pause + final lengthening	0.27 (0.11)	0.26 (0.04)	-0.42 (4.82)
Baseline	0.27 (0.11)	0.26 (0.04)	4.55 (4.68)

Note: Pause duration was measured as the duration of the silent interval at the IPBs. Final lengthening was measured as the duration of the pre-boundary syllable. Pitch reset was measured as the mean f0 differences between the two words before and after the boundaries. Pitch values were transformed into semitones through the following equation: St = 12 $\log_2$ (f0/f0$_{ref}$). F0$_{ref}$ was determined to be 70 Hz since the speaker for the experimental material was male in the present study [39].

Proportions of boundaries detected

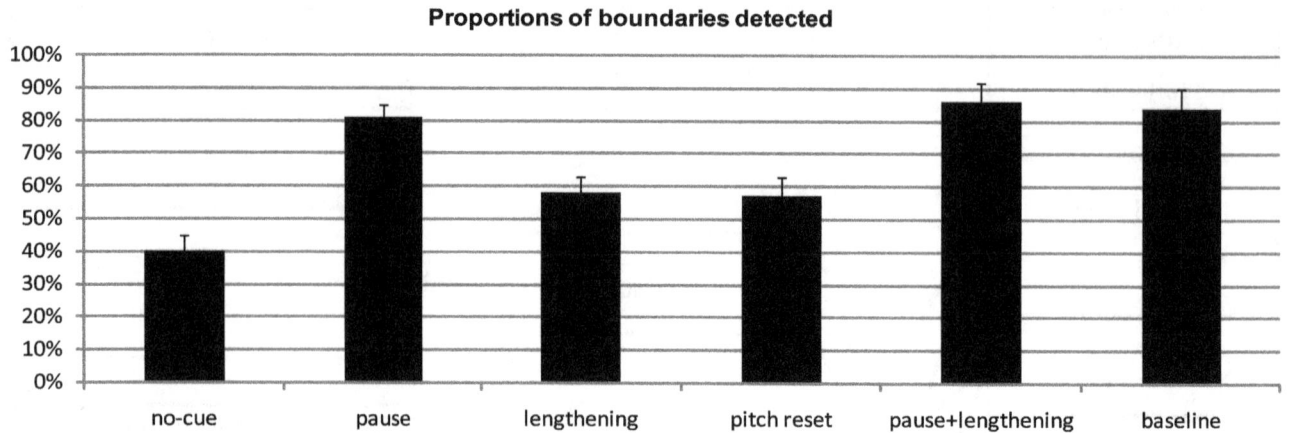

Figure 2. Proportions of the boundaries detected in the six experimental conditions (Error bars represent standard error of the mean).

No significant differences were found between the pause, pause + final lengthening, and baseline conditions ($ps > 0.05$). There was also no significant difference between the final lengthening and pitch reset conditions ($p > 0.05$). These results suggest that naturalness degree was not a confounding factor for the results of boundary detection.

The above results showed that acoustic cues were weighted differently in the detection of IPBs: Pause was the strongest indicator of an IPB; final lengthening was perceptually equivalent to pitch reset; the effect of a pause and the effects of the other two acoustic cues were not additive. However, these results alone cannot provide us with a full picture of how the three acoustic cues are weighted in the perception of IPBs. It has been shown that listeners are sensitive not only to the presence or absence of a boundary, but also to how strong a boundary is [8,33]. We believe that listeners' weighting of acoustic cues is not only displayed in their judgment of boundary presence; instead, perceptual sensitivity to acoustic cues should also be reflected in boundary strength judgments, as has been shown in previous research [33]. Therefore, in Experiment 2, we address the roles of the three acoustic parameters in the perceived strength of an IPB.

Experiment 2

2.1 Materials

The materials of Experiment 1 were used.

2.2 Ethics Statement

All participants provided written informed consent in accordance with the Declaration of Helsinki. The ethics committee of the Institute of Psychology, Chinese Academy of Sciences approved this study, including its participant recruitment procedure and methodology.

2.3 Participants

Twenty-four undergraduate students (12 women; mean age = 22.3 years; SD = 2.61) participated for financial compensation. All were native speakers of Chinese with normal hearing. None of them had participated in Experiment 1.

2.4 Procedures and Data Analysis

The procedures were the same as those of Experiment 1 except that the participants were asked to perform a different task in this experiment. Instead of judging the absence or presence of a boundary, they were asked to indicate how strong a boundary was on a 7-point scale from 1 "no boundary at all" to 7 "a very strong boundary." For example, the question following sentence (1a) was "How strong is the boundary between "xian1" and "hua1?" The participants gave their answers by pressing the appropriate number keys on the keyboard.

A repeated-measures ANOVA was performed with the factor condition as the independent variable and perceived boundary strength as the dependent variable. Greenhouse-Geisser adjustment was used to correct for violations of sphericity. Post hoc comparisons were adjusted using Bonferroni's correction.

Table 2. Naturalness rating scores for the six conditions.

Conditions	Means	Standard deviations
No-cue	3.49	1.23
Pause	5.04	0.77
Final lengthening	4.12	0.97
Pitch reset	4.17	1.03
Pause + final lengthening	5.20	0.63
Baseline	5.45	0.81

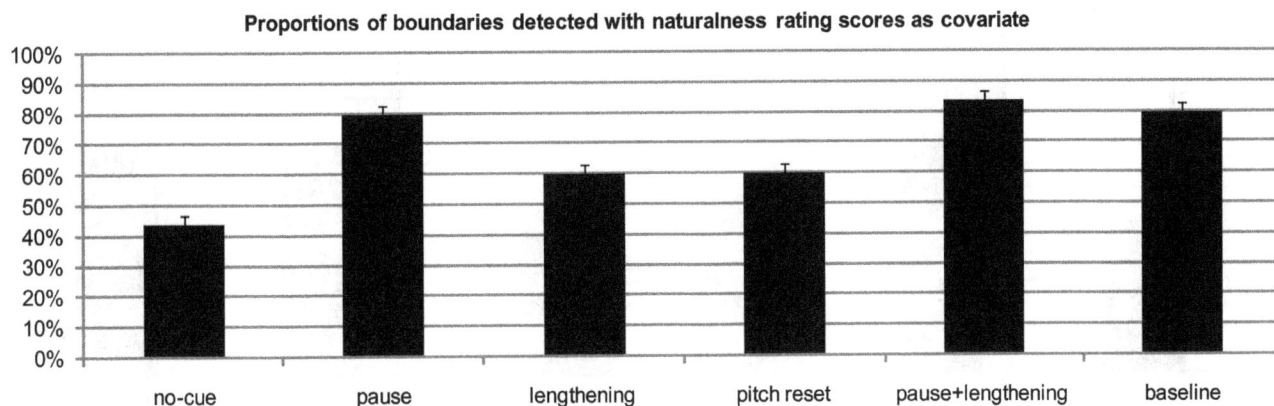

Figure 3. Proportions of the boundaries detected with naturalness rating as covariate.

2.5 Results

As shown in Fig. 4, participants perceived stronger boundaries in the pause, pause + final lengthening, and baseline conditions than in the no-cue, final lengthening, and pitch reset conditions. This indicates that perceived boundary strength was stronger when a pause was present as opposed to absent. This impression was confirmed by statistical analysis. A repeated-measures ANOVA showed a main effect of condition, F (5,115) = 15.39 $p<0.001$, $\eta^2_{partial} = 0.40$. Post hoc comparisons revealed that the perceived strength for the no-cue condition was significantly weaker than for all the other five conditions ($ps<0.05$). Perceived strength for the pause condition was significantly stronger than that for the final lengthening condition ($p<0.05$) and pitch reset condition ($p = 0.05$). Stronger boundary strength was also found for the pause + final lengthening condition than for the final lengthening condition ($p<0.01$) and pitch reset condition ($p<0.05$). Finally, perceived strength was also stronger for the baseline condition than for the final lengthening condition ($p = 0.06$) and pitch reset condition ($p = 0.07$). There was no significant difference between the pause, pause + final lengthening, and baseline conditions ($ps>0.05$). The final lengthening and pitch reset conditions did not differ from each other ($p>0.05$).

These results showed that perceived boundary strength varied among experimental conditions. As with Experiment 1, to test whether the influence of naturalness degree was a confounding factor for the results of perceived boundary strength, we ran a univariate analysis with condition as the independent variable, naturalness rating score as the covariate, and perceived boundary strength as the dependent variable. The results (shown in Fig. 5) again showed a main effect of condition, F (5,281) = 18.97, $p<0.001$, $\eta^2_{partial} = 0.25$. Post hoc comparisons revealed that the no-cue condition was perceived as less strong than all the other five conditions ($ps<0.001$). Perceived strength for the pause condition was significantly stronger than that for the final lengthening condition ($p<0.001$) and pitch reset condition ($p<0.001$). Stronger boundary strength was also found for the pause + final lengthening condition than for the final lengthening condition ($p<0.001$) and pitch reset condition ($p<0.001$). Finally, perceived strength was also stronger for the baseline condition than for the final lengthening condition ($p<0.001$) and pitch reset condition ($p<0.001$). No significant difference was found between the pause, pause + final lengthening, and baseline conditions ($ps>0.05$). There was also no significant difference between the final lengthening and pitch reset conditions ($p>0.05$). These results suggest that naturalness degree was not a confounding factor in

our results. Thus, a strong pattern emerged whereby pause appeared to be a more powerful perceptual cue for the perceived strength of an IPB than final lengthening and pitch reset, with the latter two cues perceptually equivalent.

General Discussion

The aim of the present study was to test listeners' weighting of acoustic cues in their perception of IPB. The roles of three acoustic cues (pause, final lengthening, and pitch reset) were examined in two experiments. In Experiment 1, we examined how listeners weighted these acoustic cues in the detection of prosodic boundaries, while in Experiment 2, we examined how they weighted the same acoustic cues in the perceived strength of prosodic boundaries. The results of the two experiments consistently showed that the three acoustic cues played significant roles in the perception of IPB. More importantly, we found that they were weighted differently: Of the three cues, listeners relied most heavily on pause. Final lengthening and pitch reset were not heavily weighted, and these two cues were perceptually equivalent. Finally, the effect of pause and the effects of the other two acoustic parameters were not additive. These results suggest that acoustic cues are weighted differently not only in the detection of boundary presence, but also in the judgment of boundary strength.

In Experiment 1, we found that the proportions of boundaries detected were significantly lower in conditions where none of the acoustic cues were present than in conditions where one or more of the acoustic cues were present. This suggests an important role of the acoustic cues in speech segmentation. Note that for the no-cue condition, the proportions of prosodic boundaries detected were around 40%. This might be because we used syntactically unambiguous sentences as the experimental material, and the explicit syntactic structure of the sentences probably has a predictive power on where a break is placed, as has been found previously [40]. More importantly, in Experiment 1, we found that the three acoustic cues were weighted differently for the detection of an IPB. Proportions of boundaries detected in conditions where only pause was present (81%) were significantly higher than in conditions where only final lengthening (58%) or pitch reset (57%) was present. This suggests that boundary pause was perceptually more powerful than both final lengthening and pitch reset, while the latter two acoustic cues were perceptually equivalent in terms of the perceptual effects on listeners.

In Experiment 2, we found that the no-cue condition was less natural than all the other five conditions. This suggests that IPBs were perceived as more natural when they were accompanied by

Perceived boundary strength

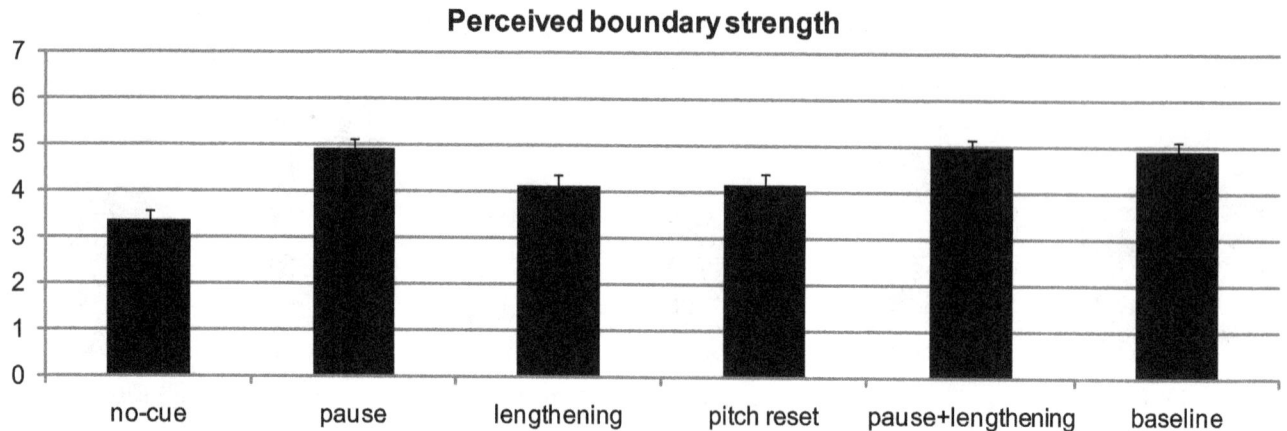

Figure 4. Perceived boundary strength across the six experimental conditions.

acoustic cues. Consistent with Experiment 1, Experiment 2 revealed the same pattern of acoustic weighting in the perceived strength of IPBs: Pause appeared to be a more powerful perceptual cue for the perceived strength of an IPB than final lengthening and pitch reset, with the latter two cues perceptually equivalent. These results suggest that listeners' weighting of acoustic cues is not only displayed in their judgment of boundary presence, but also in their judgment of boundary strength. Previous research has found that pause is more responsible in cueing boundary size than final lengthening [33]. Our results extend this finding by showing that pause is more heavily weighted in cuing boundary size than both final lengthening and pitch reset. The fact that listeners can perceive boundaries of the same prosodic category to be of different strengths has already been noted by prior studies [3,9]. Our results add to the literature by showing that listeners can perceive IPBs to be of different strengths simply based on the acoustic cues presented to them.

The results of both experiments showed that the pause condition was perceptually equivalent to the pause + final lengthening and baseline conditions. This suggests that perception of an IPB is heavily dependent on the presence of pauses, even to the extent that it may overrule the contribution of other parameters such as pre-boundary lengthening and pitch reset. The perceptual equivalence of a grammatical pause and a pause + final lengthening has been noted in Scott [29]. Our results extend this finding by indicating a perceptual equivalence between pause

and pause plus the other two acoustic parameters (final lengthening and pitch reset).

Across both experiments, no significant difference was found between final lengthening and pitch reset in terms of their perceptual effects on the listeners. This implies a discrepancy between production and perception: In the production of an IPB in Chinese, pitch reset was found to be a more reliable cue than final lengthening [41]; however, in perception, we found that pitch reset was only perceptually equivalent to final lengthening. This may have occurred because Chinese is a tonal language, and listeners who speak a tonal language are more sensitive to lexical tones but less sensitive to F0 information at the sentence level [42]. Thus, although in production pitch reset varies more dramatically than final lengthening, for Chinese listeners, these two cues can be perceptually equivalent.

One thing that should be noted is that although we only used IPBs in the present study, it is difficult to know whether an IPB is still perceived as one when cues are removed or manipulated. In studies that have manipulated acoustic cues at IPBs, listeners showed the closure positive shift, a particular ERP component known to reflect the perception of IPBs, independent of the presence of a pause cue, suggesting that the remaining cues in combination were sufficient for successful perception of IPBs [30–32]. In the present study, we found that the presence of a pause was a powerful indicator of an IPB: The proportions of boundaries detected in the pause condition (81%) did not significantly differ

Perceived boundary strength with naturalness rating scores as covariate

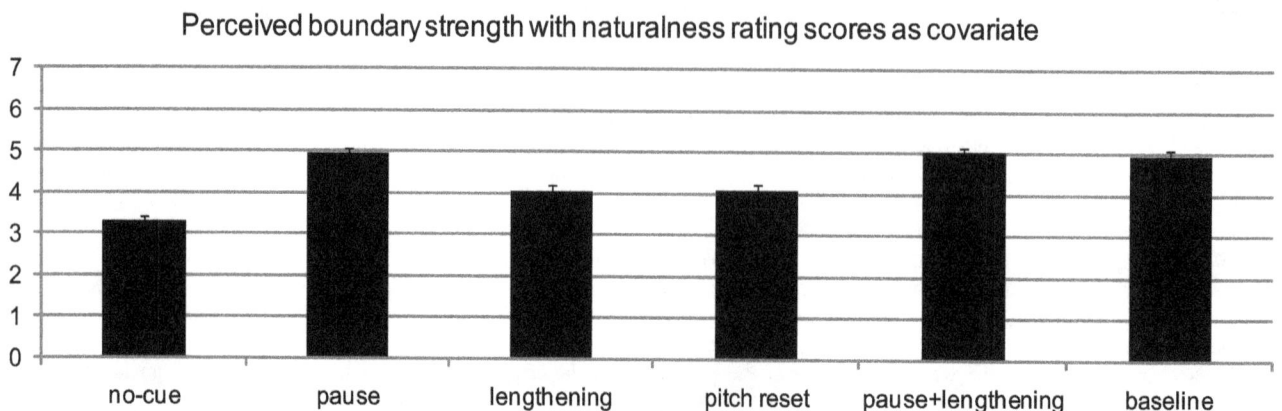

Figure 5. Perceived boundary strength with naturalness rating as covariate.

from those in the baseline condition where all cues were present (84%). This suggests that the removal of final lengthening and pitch reset did not affect the perception of IPBs. However, the presence of a pitch reset or final lengthening was not a strong indicator of an IPB: The proportions of boundaries detected in the pitch reset condition (57%) and in the final lengthening condition (58%) were quite low. This suggests that the removal of pause plus another primary cue (final lengthening or pitch reset) could significantly affect the perception of IPBs. Therefore, it appears that whether an IPB is still perceived as one depends on which cues are present.

It should be noted that one reason listeners might be more affected by the removal of one cue compared to another may have to do with the salience of these variations for listeners. Previous study has suggested that only when the salience of two acoustic cues is comparable can their relative contributions be assessed [43]. In the present study, due to the acoustic-feature exchanging technique that we used to create the experimental materials, we could not equate the salience of the acoustic cues before their contributions were assessed. However, acoustic salience alone could not explain our results. As reflected by our acoustic analysis in Table 1, compared to the values of pitch reset and final lengthening in the no-cue condition, the value of resetting in the pitch reset condition was 4.13 St larger, and the value of lengthening in the final lengthening condition was 40 ms larger. Given that 5St and 100 ms are perceptually comparable [43], it can be argued that the extent of pitch resetting was greater than that of final lengthening in production for our experimental materials. However, across the two experiments, the conditions of final lengthening and pitch reset were perceptually equivalent. Thus, it is unlikely that our results were due to the differences of acoustic salience. Nonetheless, future studies will need to explore

whether changes in acoustic cues modulate phrase perception when the salience of the acoustic cues is experimentally equated, which would require a pre-test to determine how the salience of a change in one cue can be equated with that of other cues.

Conclusions

In summary, the contribution of this research is that it is the first study to systematically manipulate the three acoustic correlates to examine cue weighting in the perception of IPBs. It is clear from the results that acoustic cues were weighted differently for the perception of IPBs: Pause was a more powerful perceptual cue than both final lengthening and pitch reset, with the latter two cues perceptually equivalent. Also, the effect of pause and the effects of the other two acoustic cues were not additive. However, this study is limited in that we only studied acoustic weighting in Chinese. Given that prosodic features vary across languages, which can result in different patterns of cue weighting across languages, future studies are needed to compare the perceptual weighting of the prosodic cues in different languages. Furthermore, note that we chose natural speech with well-formed structures to allow for a more natural acoustic realization of the boundaries. This is important in that it resembles what we encounter in everyday life. However, this could have reduced the effect of acoustic features in cueing boundaries. Thus, future studies are also needed to systematically explore the weighting of the three major acoustic correlates in syntactically ambiguous sentences.

Author Contributions

Conceived and designed the experiments: XY. Performed the experiments: XY XS. Analyzed the data: XY. Contributed reagents/materials/analysis tools: WL. Wrote the paper: XY YY.

References

1. Selkirk E (1984) Phonology and syntax: The relation between sound and structure. MIT Press. Cambridge, MA.
2. Beckman M, Pierrehumbert J (1986) Intonational structure in Japanese and English. Phonology yearbook 3: 5–70.
3. Wightman CW, Shattuck-Hufnagel S, Ostendorf M, Price PJ (1992) Segmental durations in the vicinity of prosodic phrase boundaries. Journal of the Acoustical Society of America 91: 1707–1717.
4. Nesport M, Vogel I (2007) Prosodic phonology: with a new foreword. Walter de Gruyter.
5. Frazier L, Carlson K, Clifton C (2006) Prosodic phrasing is central to language comprehension. Trends in Cognitive Sciences 10: 244–249.
6. Venditti J, Jun S-A, Beckman ME (1996) Prosodic cues to syntactic and other linguistic structures in Japanese, Korean, and English. Signal to syntax: Bootstrapping from speech to grammar in early acquisition: 287–311.
7. Cole J, Mo Y, Baek S (2010) The role of syntactic structure in guiding prosody perception with ordinary listeners and everyday speech. Language and Cognitive Processes 25: 1141–1177.
8. de Pijper JR, Sanderman AA (1994) On the perceptual strength of prosodic boundaries and its relation to suprasegmental cues. The Journal of the Acoustical Society of America 96: 2037–2047.
9. Krivokapić J, Byrd D (2012) Prosodic boundary strength: An articulatory and perceptual study. Journal of phonetics.
10. Vaissière J, Michaud A (2006) Prosodic constituents in French: a data-driven approach. Prosody and syntax: 47–64.
11. Swerts M, Bouwhuis DG, Collier R (1994) Melodic Cues to the Perceived Finality of Utterances. Journal of the Acoustical Society of America 96: 2064–2075.
12. Seidl A (2007) Infants' use and weighting of prosodic cues in clause segmentation. Journal of Memory and Language 57: 24–48.
13. Wellmann C, Holzgrefe J, Truckenbrodt H, Wartenburger I, Höhle B (2012) How each prosodic boundary cue matters: Evidence from German infants. Frontiers in psychology 3: 580.
14. Vaissière J (1983) Language-independent prosodic features. Prosody: Models and measurements: Springer. pp. 53–66.
15. Price PJ, Ostendorf M, Shattuck-Hufnagel S, Fong C (1991) The use of prosody in syntactic disambiguation. The Journal of the Acoustical Society of America 90: 2956.
16. Hirst D, Di Cristo A (1998) A survey of intonation systems. Intonation systems: A survey of twenty languages: 1–44.
17. Smith CL (2004) Topic transitions and durational prosody in reading aloud: production and modeling. Speech Communication 42: 247–270.
18. den Ouden H, Noordman L, Terken J (2009) Prosodic realizations of global and local structure and rhetorical relations in read aloud news reports. Speech Communication 51: 116–129.
19. Krivokapi J (2007) Prosodic planning: Effects of phrasal length and complexity on pause duration. Journal of phonetics 35: 162–179.
20. Berkovits R (1994) Durational effects in final lengthening, gapping, and contrastive stress. Language and Speech 37: 237–250.
21. Byrd D, Krivokapi J, Lee S (2006) How far, how long: On the temporal scope of prosodic boundary effects. The Journal of the Acoustical Society of America 120: 1589–1599.
22. Fon J, Johnson K, Chen S (2011) Durational Patterning at Syntactic and Discourse Boundaries in Mandarin Spontaneous Speech. Language and Speech 54: 5–32.
23. Nakai S, Kunnari S, Turk A, Suomi K, Ylitalo R (2009) Utterance-final lengthening and quantity in Northern Finnish. Journal of phonetics 37: 29–45.
24. Cooper WE, Sorensen JM (1977) Fundamental frequency contours at syntactic boundaries. The Journal of the Acoustical Society of America 62: 683–692.
25. Thorsen NG (1986) Sentence intonation in textual context_Supplementary data. The Journal of the Acoustical Society of America 80: 1041–1047.
26. Sluijter AM, Terken JM (1993) Beyond sentence prosody: paragraph intonation in Dutch. Phonetica. pp. 180–188.
27. Wagner M, Watson DG (2010) Experimental and theoretical advances in prosody: A review. Language and Cognitive Processes 99999: 1–41.
28. Mo Y, Cole J (2010) Perception of prosodic boundaries in spontaneous speech with and without silent pauses. Journal of the Acoustical Society of America 127: 1956–1956.
29. Scott DR (1982) Duration as a cue to the perception of a phrase boundary. The Journal of the Acoustical Society of America 71: 996.
30. Li W, Yang Y (2009) Perception of prosodic hierarchical boundaries in Mandarin Chinese sentences. Neuroscience 158: 1416.
31. Männel C, Friederici AD (2009) Pauses and intonational phrasing: ERP studies in 5-month-old German infants and adults. Journal of Cognitive Neuroscience 21: 1988–2006.
32. Steinhauer K (2003) Electrophysiological correlates of prosody and punctuation. Brain and Language 86: 142–164.
33. Lin H-Y, Fon J. (2009) Perception of temporal cues at discourse boundaries. In INTERSPEECH-2009. pp. 808–811.

34. Streeter LA (1978) Acoustic determinants of phrase boundary perception. The Journal of the Acoustical Society of America 64: 1582–1592.

35. Shen XS (1992) A pilot study on the relation between the temporal and syntactic structures in Mandarin. Journal of the International Phonetic Association 22: 35–43.

36. Zhang X (2012) A comparison of cue-weighting in the perception of prosodic phrase boundaries in English and Chinese. PhD thesis, The University of Michigan.

37. Fon J, Johnson K (2004) Syllable onset intervals as an indicator of discourse and syntactic boundaries in Taiwan Mandarin. Language and Speech 47: 57–82.

38. Chen Y (2006) Durational adjustment under corrective focus in Standard Chinese. Journal of phonetics 34: 176–201.

39. Yang X, Yang Y (2012) Prosodic Realization of Rhetorical Structure in Chinese Discourse. Audio, Speech, and Language Processing, IEEE Transactions on 20: 1196–1206.

40. Carlson R, Hirschberg J, Swerts M (2005) Cues to upcoming Swedish prosodic boundaries: Subjective judgment studies and acoustic correlates. Speech Communication 46: 326–333.

41. Bei W, Shinan L, Yufang Y (2005) The acoustic characteristics of large information units' boundaries in monologue discourse. Acta Acustica 2: 177–183.

42. Liang J, van Heuven VJ (2007) Chinese tone and intonation perceived by L1 and L2 listeners. Tones and tunes 2: 12–12.

43. Ellis RJ, Jones MR (2009) The role of accent salience and joint accent structure in meter perception. Journal of Experimental Psychology: Human Perception and Performance 35: 264–280.

17

The Cerebral Cost of Breathing: An fMRI Case-Study in Congenital Central Hypoventilation Syndrome

Mike Sharman[1,2], Cécile Gallea[3], Katia Lehongre[1,2], Damien Galanaud[3,4,5], Nathalie Nicolas[6], Thomas Similowski[5,7,8,9], Laurent Cohen[1,2,5,10], Christian Straus[5,7,8,9,11,12], Lionel Naccache[1,2,6,10,13]*

1 Institut National de la Santé et de la Recherche Médicale (INSERM), Institut du Cerveau et de la Moelle Épinière (ICM), Unité Mixte de Recherche 1127, PICNIC Lab, Paris, France, **2** Centre National de la Recherche Scientifique (CNRS), Institut du Cerveau et de la Moelle Epinière (ICM), Unité 7225, PICNIC Lab, Paris, France, **3** Institut National de la Santé et de la Recherche Médicale (INSERM), Institut du Cerveau et de la Moelle Epinière (ICM), Unité Mixte de Recherche 1127, (CENIR), Paris, France, **4** Assistance Publique–Hôpitaux de Paris, Groupe hospitalier Pitié- Salpêtrière Charles Foix, Department of Neuroradiology, Paris, France, **5** Université Pierre et Marie Curie-Paris 6, Faculté de Médecine Pitié-Salpêtrière, Paris, France, **6** Assistance Publique–Hôpitaux de Paris, Groupe hospitalier Pitié- Salpêtrière Charles Foix, Centre d'Investigation Clinique 1421, Paris, France, **7** Assistance Publique–Hôpitaux de Paris, Groupe Hospitalier Pitié-Salpêtrière Charles Foix, Service de Pneumologie et Réanimation Médicale (Département "R3S"), Paris, France, **8** Sorbonne Universités, Université Pierre et Marie Curie-Paris 6, Unité Mixte de Recherche 1158 "Neurophysiologie Respiratoire Expérimentale et Clinique", Paris, France, **9** Institut National de la Santé et de la Recherche Médicale (INSERM), Unité Mixte de Recherche 1158 "Neurophysiologie Respiratoire Expérimentale et Clinique", Paris, France, **10** Assistance Publique–Hôpitaux de Paris, Groupe hospitalier Pitié-Salpêtrière Charles Foix, Department of Neurology, Paris, France, **11** Assistance Publique–Hôpitaux de Paris, Groupe Hospitalier Pitié-Salpêtrière Charles Foix, Service des Explorations Fonctionnelles de la Respiration, de l'Exercice et de la Dyspnée (Département "R3S"), Paris, France, **12** Assistance Publique–Hôpitaux de Paris, Groupe Hospitalier Pitié-Salpêtrière Charles Foix, Centre de Référence Maladies Rares "syndrome d'Ondine", Paris, France, **13** Assistance Publique–Hôpitaux de Paris, Groupe hospitalier Pitié-Salpêtrière Charles Foix, Department of Neurophysiology, Paris, France

Abstract

Certain motor activities - like walking or breathing - present the interesting property of proceeding either automatically or under voluntary control. In the case of breathing, brainstem structures located in the medulla are in charge of the automatic mode, whereas cortico-subcortical brain networks - including various frontal lobe areas - subtend the voluntary mode. We speculated that the involvement of cortical activity during voluntary breathing could impact both on the "resting state" pattern of cortical-subcortical connectivity, and on the recruitment of executive functions mediated by the frontal lobe. In order to test this prediction we explored a patient suffering from central congenital hypoventilation syndrome (CCHS), a very rare developmental condition secondary to brainstem dysfunction. Typically, CCHS patients demonstrate efficient cortically-controlled breathing while awake, but require mechanically-assisted ventilation during sleep to overcome the inability of brainstem structures to mediate automatic breathing. We used simultaneous EEG-fMRI recordings to compare patterns of brain activity between these two types of ventilation during wakefulness. As compared with spontaneous breathing (SB), mechanical ventilation (MV) restored the default mode network (DMN) associated with self-consciousness, mind-wandering, creativity and introspection in healthy subjects. SB on the other hand resulted in a specific increase of functional connectivity between brainstem and frontal lobe. Behaviorally, the patient was more efficient in cognitive tasks requiring executive control during MV than during SB, in agreement with her subjective reports in everyday life. Taken together our results provide insight into the cognitive and neural costs of spontaneous breathing in one CCHS patient, and suggest that MV during waking periods may free up frontal lobe resources, and make them available for cognitive recruitment. More generally, this study reveals how the active maintenance of cortical control over a continuous motor activity impacts on brain functioning and cognition.

Editor: Dante R. Chialvo, National Scientific and Technical Research Council (CONICET), Argentina

Funding: This work has been supported by the Fondation pour la Recherche Médicale (FRM) ('Equipe FRM 2010' grant to Lionel Naccache), by the Institut pour le Cerveau et la Moëlle épinière (ICM Institute, Paris, France), by INSERM, by AP-HP, by the program "Investissement d'Avenir ANR-10-AIHU 06 of the French Government", by the IHU-A-ICM ('Investissement d'avenir' program, ANR-10-IAIHU-06), by Assistance Publique - Hôpitaux de Paris (AP-HP) Département de la Recherche Clinique et du Développement (DRCD) ("RESPIRONDINE" project), by Association Française du Syndrome d'Ondine (AFSO). The research leading to these results has received funding from the program "Investissements d'avenir" ANR-10-IAIHU-06. The funders had no role in study design, data collection and analysis, decision to publish, or preparation of the manuscript.

Competing Interests: The authors have declared that no competing interests exist.

* Email: lionel.naccache@gmail.com

Introduction

Breathing belongs to the limited number of behaviors that can operate either under an automatic or a voluntary controlled mode, and the only one in this class of which the interruption poses an immediate vital threat. Schematically, the automatic mode is operated by brainstem respiratory pattern generators involving the Pre-Bötzinger complex and the parafacial/retrotrapezoid nuclei located in the medulla and their associated bulbospinal neurons [1], while the controlled mode depends on the activity of a large cortico-subcortical network including notably the anterior cingulate, supplementary-motor and insular cortices, as well as other regions [2–6].

Although this mapping between brainstem and automatic breathing on the one hand, and cortex and voluntary breathing on the other hand is central to our understanding of breathing, it does not inform us about the neural mechanisms at work, and about how these two modes of breathing interact. This issue, however, conveys major neuro-scientific and medical questions such as: how might the controlled mode network pilots the automatic structures when necessary? Is the controlled mode of breathing a conscious and voluntary reportable activity, or can it proceed unconsciously in conscious subjects, or even in non-conscious patients (e.g.: vegetative state patients)? Can this controlled mode of breathing be automatized? How is it coordinated with other cortically controlled motor processes which impact on breathing, such as speech production (segmentation, prosody) or playing a wind instrument?

This crucial issue is challenging because these two modes of breathing interact permanently in a complex and dynamical way. One way to disentangle them could consist in finding experimental or medical conditions in which awake and conscious subjects can be steadily engaged in each of these modes. To date, several functional neuroimaging and electrophysiological studies conducted in normal controls have used experimentally applied inspiratory constraints, - such as an inspiratory threshold loading -, to elicit a switch from automatic to cortically controlled breathing [7–13]. These works reliably demonstrated that the controlled mode of breathing is associated with cortical activation in many areas including premotor and bilateral insular cortices, and with decreased blood-oxygen-level dependent (BOLD) signal in regions of the DMN [14]. Interestingly, in line with the sustained nature of the respiratory-related cortical activity in response to a breathing difficulty [12], a recent study by Raux and colleagues [13] reported functional magnetic resonance imaging (fMRI) evidence that cortically-mediated breathing could itself be subject to automatization when using a continuous inspiratory load rather than an intermittent inspiratory load. Most of the cortico-subcortical areas associated with voluntary breathing showed a marked decrease of activation during continuous inspiratory loading as compared with intermittent inspiratory loading, in agreement with well-established motor skills automatization [15,16]. A common limitation of the above studies is that experimental constraints used to manipulate breathing mode do not correspond to comfortable, ecological conditions for the subjects involved. Moreover, the impact of controlled and automatic breathing on subjective and objective cognitive measures has never been documented. For these reasons, it is considered extremely valuable to identify a stable, comfortable and regular breathing condition that demonstrates the implementation of the cortico-subcortical network associated with controlled breathing. One such very rare condition is congenital central hypoventilation syndrome (CCHS) in which the automatic control of breathing is irreversibly and massively impaired [17]. CCHS is an extremely rare disease (1/2–300000 births) that is characterized by alveolar hypoventilation and autonomic dysregulation [18]. CCHS patients usually have adequate breathing while awake, but significantly decreased breathing drive during sleep, including monotonous respiratory rates and diminished tidal volumes (shallow breathing). Patients therefore require mechanical ventilatory support (via nasal mask or tracheotomy) during sleep, to avoid life-threatening hypoxia consecutive to hypoventilation. Genetic studies have identified the paired-like homeobox 2B gene (PHOX2B) as the disease-defining gene [19]. Autopsy and structural MRI studies have identified subtle and disseminated white and grey matter impairments, affecting both supra-tentorial an infra-tentorial structures. Of particular interest, - given patients' physiological impairments -, is that several brainstem structures show structural abnormalities, including the locus coeruleus, parabrachial pons, caudal raphe nuclei, and lateral medulla (for a recent review see [20]). Several fMRI studies contributed by the Harper group explored brain responses of controls and of CCHS patients to various experimental conditions such as hypoxia, hyperoxia, cold pressor test, and forced expiratory loading [21–24]. Multiple brain regions responded inappropriately to ventilatory or blood pressure challenges, including forebrain, diencephalic, and brainstem related areas such as cerebellum.

Of importance regarding the issue of "resource competition" between the respiratory-related cortico-subcortical network and other cortical functions, anecdotal reports from parents of CCHS children suggest that mental concentration can deteriorate gas exchange (cyanosis during television watching, video gaming or scholarly exercise). Early publications on CCHS relayed this notion [25–27] that was subsequently challenged [28]. Indeed, Shea et al. showed that mental calculus and videogame playing increased ventilation both in CCHS in normal children. Yet these experiments did not take into account the emotional content of the test situation, and it was subsequently shown that video gaming in a neutral emotional environment induced hypoventilation in normal children [29]. Of note, this issue has not been addressed extensively in adults, although it has been shown that cortically-driven breathing is associated with deteriorated reaction times to an auditory stimulus [30]. Within this frame, adult CCHS patients exhibit a respiratory-related EEG activity during resting breathing [31] that resemble the potentials seen in normal subjects in response to inspiratory loading. It is currently unknown whether or not this respiratory-related cortical activity has an impact on operational and cognitive performances.

In the present study, we explored one patient affected with CCHS using a combination of behavioral and simultaneous electroencephalography (EEG) and fMRI brain-imaging measures both under spontaneous breathing (SB) and mechanical ventilation (MV) during wakefulness. We considered that this very rare medical condition could reveal how the active maintenance of cortical control over a regular motor activity impacts on broader cortical activity and function. More precisely, we designed this study in order to test our main hypothesis that during MV, resources used by the executive brain network would be freed up and hence made available for other cognitive purposes. Interestingly, when explaining the general objective of our experiment to the patient, she spontaneously reported that she had regularly switched to MV during her high-school years when needing to solve difficult problems or attend exams, with the subjective feeling of easier concentration and better cognitive performance as compared with SB. From our main hypothesis, we derived three predictions:

Prediction 1: Executive functions, - including sustained executive attention, working memory, executive control, and the richness of the stream of conscious thoughts-, should be more efficient during MV than during SB.

Prediction 2: Patterns of brain activity recorded during resting state should better match the normal DMN under MV than during SB.

Prediction 3: Patterns of functional brain connectivity should differ notably between SB and MV: a stronger correlation is predicted between the executive network and the brainstem during SB, whereas a stronger correlation within the DMN should be observed during MV than during SB.

This case-report falls within a long tradition of physiological and neuropsychological studies which demonstrate how focus on a single patient, if not necessarily representative of the concerned disease, can be decisive in enriching our understanding of impaired and normal physiology [32–35].

Materials and Methods

Patient

The patient is a 29-year-old woman. She was diagnosed with CCHS at the time of her birth. She carries a 9 alanine expansion mutation of the PHOX 2B gene. The main clinical manifestation of her condition pertains to ventilatory control, without any of the other frequent manifestations of the disease (in particular absence of Hirschprung disease and of cardiac rhythm anomalies). She does not increase ventilation and does not feel dyspnea when exposed to hypercapnia (in contrast to healthy subjects who reflexively hyperventilate and report respiratory discomfort in response to increased carbon dioxide levels), and she depends on mechanical ventilation during sleep. For this reason, she was tracheotomized at birth and until the age of 17, and has been ventilated non-invasively since. However, she does not exhibit hypoventilation during wakefulness, with arterial blood gases in room air within normal limits. Of note, this patient participated in another study that demonstrated that she displayed EEG cortical activity related to spontaneous ventilation [31]. The fMRI study was conducted in the frame of the RESPIRONDINE study (NCT01243697) into which the patient was enrolled. She had given her informed written consent to participate. Assistance Publique – Hôpitaux de Paris sponsored the study that was approved by the appropriate local legal and ethics authority (Comité de Protection des Personnes Ile-de-France 6, Pitié-Salpêtrière, Paris). Psychometric tests were part of the clinical follow up of the patient. Their study was approved by the institutional review board of the French Society for Respiratory Medicine ("Société de Pneumologie de Langue Française" reference number CEPRO2012-012). The patient gave her consent to anonymous use of her data for research purposes.

Behavior

"Stream of consciousness" task. We adapted the task designed by [36]. The patient sat comfortably in a quiet dimly lit room. She was instructed: "During the next minutes, we ask you to keep your eyes closed and to avoid prolonged structured thinking, such as counting or singing. When you hear a beep, please indicate me first the intensity of 'external awareness' ongoing prior to the beep by reporting a number orally from 1 to 4, and then indicate me the intensity of 'internal awareness' ongoing prior to the beep by reporting a number orally from 1 to 4. 'External' is here defined as the perception of environmental sensory stimuli (e.g., auditory, visual, olfactory, or somesthetic). 'Internal' here refers to all environmental stimuli-independent thoughts (e.g., inner speech, autobiographical memories, or wandering thoughts)." This experiment was programmed with E-prime 1.1 software (Psychology Software Tools, Inc. Sharpsburg, PA).

Paced Auditory Serial Addition Test (PASAT). The PASAT was delivered using a 'ABBA' design with four blocks in the following order: SB, MV, MV, SB. The patient used her own home mechanical ventilator and face mask. A pause was offered between blocks, and a longer pause of several minutes was used between the two transitions (SB to MV and MV to SB), so as to ensure that the patient was in a comfortable and steady state of respiration in each of the four blocks. The patient was tested with the 3 seconds version of the PASAT test [37] used to probe working memory and sustained executive attention (for a recent review see [38]). The patient was presented with a series of 60 single digit numbers with a 3 seconds inter-stimulus interval, and she was instructed to continuously sum aloud the last two digits, while the experimenter wrote her answers. In order to enable multiple evaluations, two versions of the task were available (tests A & B). The patient was tested with the following order: SB(A), MV(B), MV(A), SB(B). Each experimental block was preceded by a short training (training A, training B) made of 11 numbers.

EEG recording & processing

Continuous EEG data was recorded at 5 kHz from 63 scalp sites (Easycap electrode cap) using MR-compatible amplifiers (BrainAmp MR and Brain Vision Recorder software; Brain Products). One additional electrode was placed on the collarbone to record the electrocardiogram (ECG). Impedances were kept under 15 kΩ. The EEG signal was corrected for MR related and for pulse artefacts (see SI). Then, for each time sample, we computed the ratio between relative alpha power averaged over occipital electrodes, and theta power averaged over frontal electrodes (see Figure 1A). This alpha/theta EEG power ratio is a common measure of vigilance [39–41].

The data were subsequently downsampled to 250 Hz and re-referenced to a common average reference. Visual inspection of the signal checked for the absence of residual obvious artefacts. Time-frequency (TF) analysis was then computed with a Morlet wavelets approach in Fieldtrip (http://www.ru.nl/fcdonders/fieldtrip). TF was computed for frequency from 0.5 to 15 Hz, with a frequency step of 0.5 Hz, a time step of 0.5 sec, and a wavelet width of 4 cycles. The (posterior alpha)/(theta midfrontal) ratio was computed on the normalized power (normalization across the 0.5–15 Hz frequency range), using the following electrodes (Easycap electrode cap numbers): occipital region of interest (ROI) [9 10 19 20 31 37 38 45 46 64], and mid-frontal ROI [1 2 3 4 17 33 34 39 40 63]. Statistical comparisons across MV and SB were performed using the non-parametric Wilcoxon rank-sum test.

Magnetic resonance (MR) imaging

MR acquisition protocol. The MR protocol was carried out with a 3T whole-body system (Siemens, Erlangen, Germany) at the Center for Magnetic Resonance Research (CENIR), Institute of the Brain and the Spinal Cord (ICM), Paris. The functional images were acquired by T2*-weighted fast echo planar imaging (EPI; flip angle = 90°, echo time = 30 ms, repetition time = 2.26 s) from 36 interleaved axial slices (Field Of View = $100 \times 100 \times 36$, gap = 0.3 mm) with a $2 \times 2 \times 2$ mm3 voxel size for the resting state. The resting-state fMRI experiment consisted of one 10-minute run in which the patient was instructed to relax with her eyes closed, without falling asleep. Each run consisted of 200 EPI volumes. Subsequently, a high-resolution structural volume was acquired using a 3D magnetization prepared rapid gradient echo (MP-RAGE) sequence (144 sagittal images; thickness 1 mm; FOV 256×256 mm2; matrix size 256×256). Immediately before each of the four "resting state" blocks, the patient received the following instructions: "please, keep your eyes closed, stay awake during the entire block, and try to let your mind wander to any particular thought". As for the behavioural tests, we also used an 'ABBA' design with the following order: SB, MV, MV and SB. After each of the 4 scanning blocks a brief interview checked the absence of breathing discomfort, the absence of subjective report of drowsiness, and the effective engagement in the "mind-wandering" state. SpO2 was measured during the fMRI experiment.

(A)

Alpha power (%)

Occipital cluster

Theta power (%)

Frontal cluster

(B)

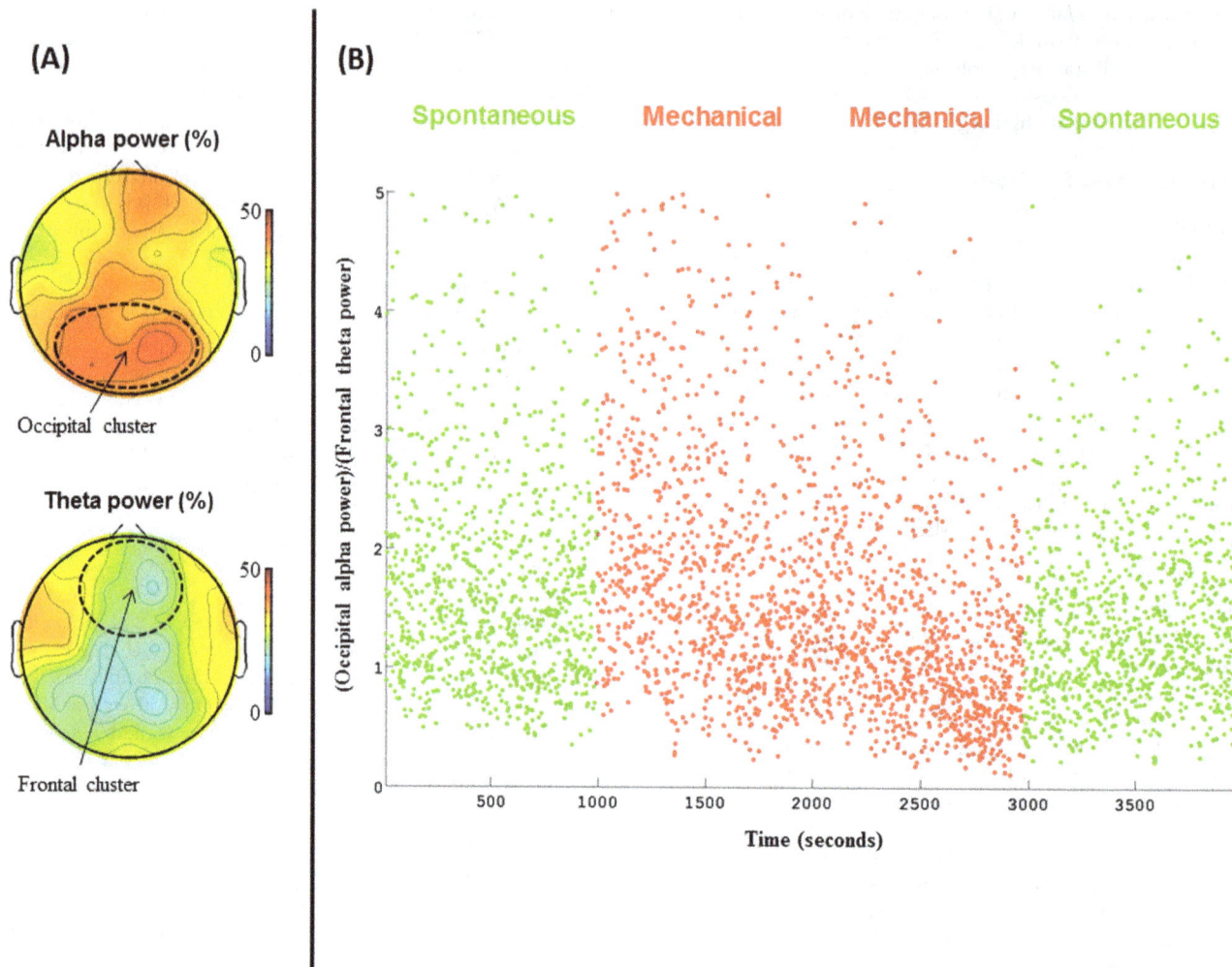

Figure 1. Stability of wakefulness under MV and SB indexed by EEG. (A). Scalp voltage topographies of alpha power (up) and theta (bottom) averaged across the 4 EEG-fMRI sessions reveal a typical pattern of wakefulness characterized by a high posterior alpha power and a low anterior mid-frontal power. (B). Dynamics of the (posterior alpha power)/(mid-frontal theta power) ration is plotted across time for the 4 EEG-fMRI sessions. This index of wakefulness was stable across the 4 sessions, and confirmed a stable level of wakefulness all along the fMRI experiments, with no difference between SB and MV.

fMRI data processing & analysis. A correction was applied to reduce physiological noise (see SI) using a retrospective estimation and correction of respiration and heart beat [42].

General linear model. A general linear model was created, which included the 4 sessions, each modeled by the canonical hemodynamic response function and its first-order time derivative, and 6 individual motion parameters to capture remaining signal variations due to head movements. T-test based contrasts of interests were then defined in SPM8. We reported significant results at the cluster-level (all SPM results are reported with the following significance threshold: p FWE-correction ≤0.05). For significant clusters we also report the peak-level T value as well as the cluster volume (number of voxels).

Functional connectivity assessed with an fMRI or EEG ROI based analysis. Three ROIs were selected: (1) the precuneus which is major hub of normal DMN, (2) the brainstem which is in charge of automatic control of breathing, and (3) auditory cortex as a control region not primarily implicated in the control of breathing. The precuneus ROI (seed region 1) was defined using A canonical template (automatic anatomical labeling

from WFU PickAtlas toolbox of SPM, http://fmri.wfubmc.edu/software/PickAtlas), from which the time course was extracted. We looked at the brain areas that showed a stronger correlation of their time course with the seed region during MV than during SB. We then used a brainstem ROI (seed region 2) manually defined as corresponding to the medulla oblongata: it was delineated from the pons by a horizontal boundary, and occupying a region extending distance ventrally to the estimated boundary with the spinal cord. The third control ROI (seed region 3) was defined using the Automated Anatomical Labelling atlas in regions of the left and right hemisphere considered to closely represent the auditory cortex, namely Herschl's gyrus [43]. The same approach was used to compute correlation of BOLD signal with the posterior EEG alpha-power time series.

Functional connectivity assessed with a spatial ICA based analysis. We used a spatial independent component analysis (ICA) approach to extract group representative functional large-scale networks across the whole brain (see Materials & Methods S1 and [44] for details).

Results

Behavior

The patient was tested in three tasks exploring various aspects of executive functions as well as the reportability of conscious contents.

"Stream of consciousness" test. This task aimed at comparing both the type and the subjective intensity of current conscious contents during the two modes of breathing. As previously showed by [36] internally and externally oriented contents were anti-correlated (correlation coefficient = −0.21; p-value = 0.1). The small number of trials (N = 34) probably explains the weak significance of this anti-correlation. During MV we observed higher values of both internal and external awareness contents as compared with SB (both p values = 0.02 in Wald-Wolfowitz runs tests). This pattern, affecting both external and internal reportable contents, is compatible with our prediction that MV would act by "releasing" attentional and executive resources available for other cognitive activities and contents.

Paced Auditory Serial Addition Test (PASAT). The patient was engaged in this classical test probing both working memory and sustained executive attention. Error rate remained constant across the four experimental blocks (43/60 & 43/60 for the two SB sessions, and 45/60 & 43/60 for the two MV sessions; Chi 2 value = 0.8; p = 0.8). However, a post-hoc analysis revealed that when analyzing the length of chunks of consecutive correct answers, we observed a clear advantage for the MV condition: sequences ranged from 1 to 6 under SB (mean = 3.3), and from 1 to 16 under MV (mean = 4.4). In particular a non-parametric ranking test showed that sequences superior to 5 consecutive correct trials were longer in the MV condition than in the SB condition (p = 0.02 in Mann-Whitney U test).

Taken together, these results support our initial prediction by showing an impact of cortically-controlled breathing on several facets of executive functions. As compared with performances obtained during SB, the patient showed an improvement of sustained attention during MV, and her conscious reports revealed more intense contents during MV than during SB.

EEG-fMRI sessions

After each of the four scanning blocks patient debriefings did not reveal any breathing discomfort, or any subjective report of drowsiness. She confirmed having been engaged in the "mind-wandering" state in each of the 4 blocks. Pulse oximetry saturation (SpO2) ranged from 93% to 100%, with no significant difference across blocks.

EEG

Recording EEG during fMRI acquisition was motivated by the need for an objective physiological marker of vigilance during the resting state sessions, in particular to ensure the absence of drowsiness under mechanical breathing. Even if the patient did not report any drowsiness during the four blocks, subtle variations in vigilance may contribute to differences in fMRI patterns. An EEG index of vigilance (ratio of occipital alpha/frontal theta; see M&M and Figure 1A) did not reveal any difference between the four blocks (see Figure 1B; Wilcoxon rank sum test rank p value = 0.33). In order to better assess the validity of our single subject EEG-fMRI measures, we also analyzed which brain areas (fMRI signal) were correlated with the alpha-power averaged across posterior electrodes (EEG signal). While no positive correlation was observed, this analysis revealed a large fronto-parietal network negatively correlated with alpha-power (see Figure S1 and Table S1), as previously reported by [45] and

many other teams during wakefulness (see [46] for a review). The results hence confirmed that levels of vigilance were consistent across the four blocks tested.

fMRI

Brain areas more activated during MV than during SB corresponded to the typical DMN including parietal-occipital mesial areas (precuneus and posterior cingulate cortices) and anterior mesial-frontal areas (see Figure 2A and Table 1). Interestingly, no brain area showed any increase of activation in the reverse contrast (SB>MV).

In order to better understand the mechanisms at work during the two breathing conditions, we performed complementary analyses exploring patterns of functional connectivity. We defined a ROI in the precuneus (seed region 1) and looked for brain areas showing a stronger correlation of their time course with the seed region during MV than during SB. Only the posterior mesial structures, belonging to the normal DMN showed such a profile (see Figure 3B), whereas a set of subcortical and frontal structures showed a reverse profile (SB>MV). These last structures included superior frontal gyrus and inferior orbito-frontal cortex, as well as thalami and caudate nuclei, cerebellum and brainstem regions (see Table 1). This ROI analysis confirms that a major hub of normal DMN, - the precuneus -, varies its functional connectivity in relation with the respiratory condition. Whereas precuneus was connected with other postero-mesial normal DMN structures under MV, it showed an unusual connectivity during SB with an anterior network suggestive of a frontal-subcortical control of brainstem breathing structures.

We then used a brainstem ROI (seed region 2), which showed a stronger functional connectivity with a cortico-subcortical anterior network during SB than during MV (see Figure 2C). This network included several frontal lobe and anterior cingulate areas, as well as insular regions and the caudate nuclei, which have been previously implicated in effortful breathing [7–9,13]. A control ROI (seed region 3) defined in the primary auditory cortex did not show any modulation of functional connectivity when comparing SB and MV blocks.

Finally, we used a non-arbitrary method based on spatial independent component analysis to quantify functional connectivity within brain-scale networks. Hierarchical integration was significantly larger within the DMN during MV than during SB (p = 0.997 considered as significant using Bayesian statistics with p>0.909 as the threshold of significance; see methods and Figure 3A & 3B). A non-significant trend in the opposite comparison (SB>MV) was observed within the SMN (p = 0.818, see Figure 3C & 3D).

Discussion

The goal of this study was to take advantage of a very rare syndrome, - characterized by a massive impairment of the automatic control of breathing-, to explore how the active maintenance of cortical control over an enduring motor activity impacts on cortical activity and function. In a CCHS patient, we tested the general hypothesis that the executive brain network, whose intervention is required for controlling breathing during SB, should be released and made more available for other cognitive purposes during MV. We will now discuss these results by addressing each of our three empirical predictions.

Prediction 1: Better executive functioning during MV than during SB

We tested the patient in two behavioral experiments. First, the PASAT revealed a significant increase in the length of sequences

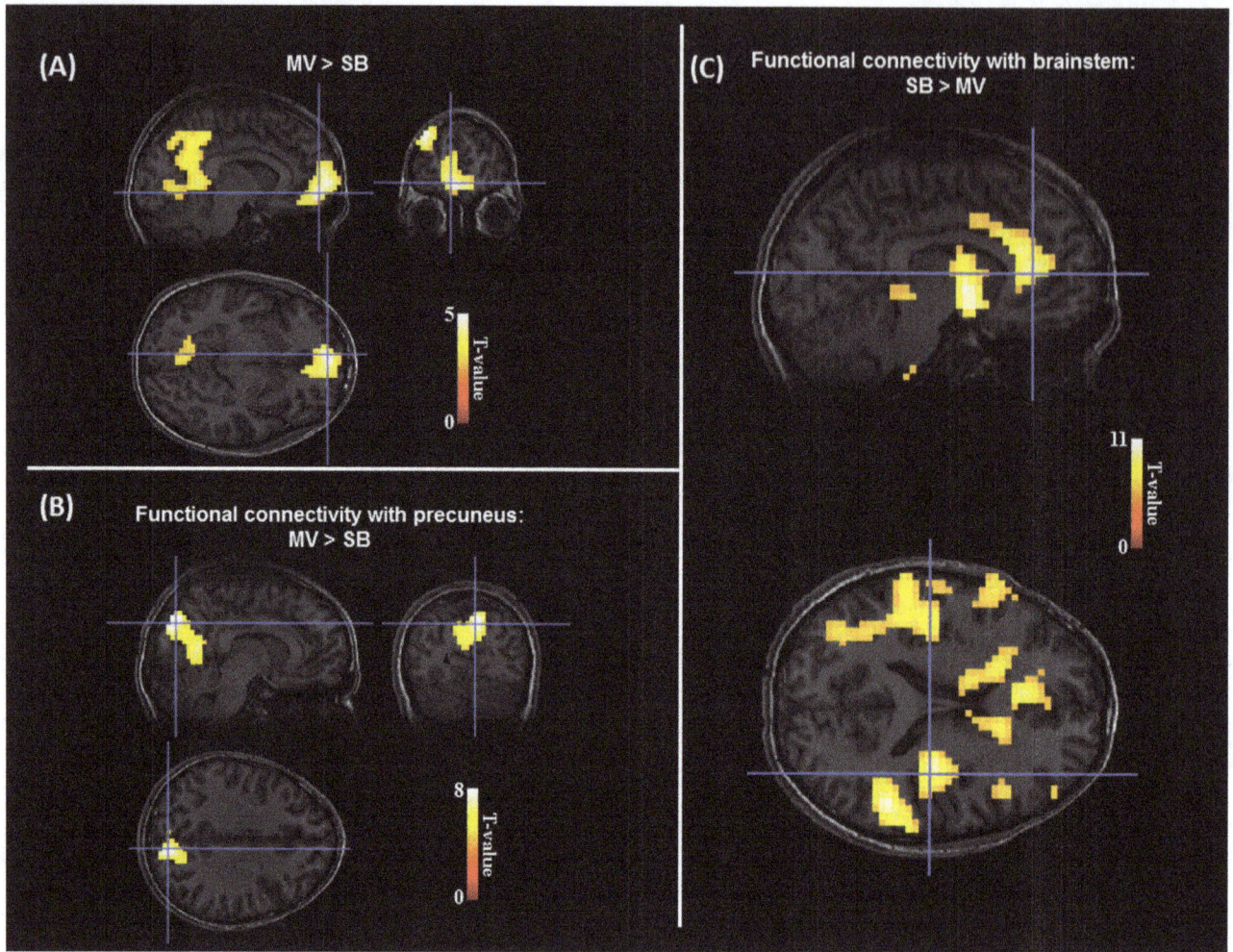

Figure 2. Restoration of DMN under mechanical ventilation. (A). Comparison of BOLD signal between MV and SB revealed a specific increase of activation in the default-mode network associated in awake controls in introspection and self-consciousness. No significant result was observed in the opposite contrast. See Table 1 for detailed fMRI results. (B&C). Functional connectivity assessed with a hypothesis-driven approach revealed a larger correlation with precuneus activity in posterior mesial areas during MV than during SB (B), and a larger correlation between brainstem activity and a large anterior cortico-subcortical network during SB than during MV (C). This large network resembles the executive attention network.

of correct responses during MV as compared to SB. The 'ABBA' design prevented a systematic confound of breathing condition with time, and this result therefore confirms the prediction that working memory and sustained executive attention were improved during MV. We also observed a general increase in the subjective intensity of spontaneous conscious contents under MV, as compared to SB, during a resting state experiment. We regret the absence of 'ABBA' design for this last experiment, but this was due to a schedule constraint of the patient. One may have expected internally-related thoughts to be more frequent than externally-related ones during MV by releasing executive resources from breathing control. The fact that we did not observe such a trend may call for more subtle probing of conscious thoughts, to check specifically if breathing related thoughts decreased during MV. Note also that even if we had tried to clearly categorize sensory-motor and somesthesic thoughts as being related to the external world, breathing may have a special status, intermediate between our external and internal categories. A complementary way to test this possibility would consist in replicating this experiment during an fMRI scan, and to check the respective correlates of internal and external thoughts under SB

and MV. Taken together, both objective (PASAT) and subjective behavioral measures tended to confirm our prediction that the engagement of executive functions in various cognitive tasks increased under MV in comparison with SB. In addition to our main goal, this result may prove relevant to explain the mild cognitive disabilities presented by most CCHS patients [47,48]. If this result was confirmed on a larger cohort of patients and in a larger set of tasks, one may consider prescribing MV in these patients for cognitive purposes such as in academic study, in addition to preventing sleep hypoventilation.

Prediction 2: Restoration of DMN networks during MV as compared to SB

The most impressive result of this study is the specific increase of DMN activity during MV as compared to SB. We checked the absence of several potential confounds and caveats. First, the 'ABBA' design we used discarded a possible confound with time, which may be interpreted in terms of habituation. Second, we ensured the absence of a confound with drowsiness under MV during which the patient may have relaxed and decreased her level

Table 1. Synthesis of fMRI results.

Anatomical localization of cluster	Coordinates [x,y,z]			T score	Number of voxels
Activation: MV>SB					
Medial orbito-frontal cortex (BA11)	−7	59	−9	4,43	380
Middle frontal gyrus (BA8)	−51	19	43	4,35	292
Calcarine sulcus	−11	−51	4	4,19	473
Precuneus, posterior cingulate cortex	−8	−55	15	3,75	473
Connectivity Precuneus: MV>SB					
Cuneus (BA19)	11	−82	35	7,95	426
Lingual gyrus (BA19)	11	−54	−3	6,63	426
Calcarine sulcus	−15	−60	6	6,39	426
Middle frontal gyrus (BA6)	50	−3	52	5,65	42
Connectivity Precuneus: SB>MV					
Thalamus, tectum	−7	−29	4	7,33	319
Caudate tail	−17	−15	22	6,1	
Cerebellum (Crus 1)	35	−53	−32	6,07	39
Brainstem	8	−39	−3552	5,94	22
Cerebellum (lobule 7b)	24	−78	−49	5,82	54
Superior frontal gyrus	24	25	62	5,7	33
Inferior orbito-frontal cortex (BA11)	−31	36	−12	5,36	36
Connectivity Brainstem: SB>MV					
Pallidum	−9	1	−6	10,69	1347
Anterior cingulate cortex (BA32)	−6	42	7	9,41	1347
Posterior insula	−39	−22	14	9,36	1347
Posterior insula	36	−17	14	10,51	99
Anterior insula	38	0	5	9,44	343
Brainstem	−3	−31	−50	8,08	13
Tectum	−5	−31	−7	6,89	29
Precentral gyrus, inferior frontal gyrus	61	8	20	6,36	10
Pars triagularis frontalis	−49	41	7	6,12	17
Anterior insula	−30	27	−3	6,03	11
Connectivity Brainstem: SB>MV					
Cerebellum (lobule 9)	−14	−43	−51	7,72	32

of vigilance. Verifying the level of vigilance was particularly important to check because CCHS patients often associate MV with a secure feeling of riskless sleep. For this purpose, the combination of clear instructions, of post-block subjective debriefing and most importantly of continuous EEG recording during fMRI acquisition permitted us to discard any difference in level of wakefulness between MV and SB. Third, we checked that raw parameters of breathing (blood oxygenation, respiratory rate and subjective breathing comfort) were comparable in both conditions. All these controls suggest that a correct interpretation of this fMRI result fits with our prediction: under MV the anterior executive network activity is released from breathing, and is then available to contribute to the normal neuronal signature of awake resting state. This observation is reminiscent of the decrease in DMN activity that occurs shortly after the application of an inspiratory load in normal controls [13]. It would be very valuable to verify whether this result could apply on a larger group of CCHS patients, and to combine it with subjective measures of conscious content in order to more precisely describe the nature of cognitive processes at work in these patients during MV. The raw debriefing we used

only confirmed that the patient really engaged in mind-wandering in both breathing conditions, but more precise measures would certainly be valuable. Finally, the absence of a significant result in the reverse contrast (SB>MV) suggests that frontal areas presumably implicated in the control of breathing during SB were engaged in other tasks during MV with a globally similar level of neural activity. Actually, when we decreased the statistical thresholds (p<0.1, 30 voxels), activated regions began to include frontal areas including dorsolateral prefrontal and anterior cingulate cortices, striatum, as well as a right parietal region. This last finding further strengthens the utility of functional connectivity measures.

Prediction 3: Functional connectivity patterns of brain activity differ during SB and MV

In order to better explore the previous prediction, we used two complementary approaches to evaluate how the breathing modality affected brain-scale functional connectivity in this patient. Using a hypothesis-driven seed approach, we first showed

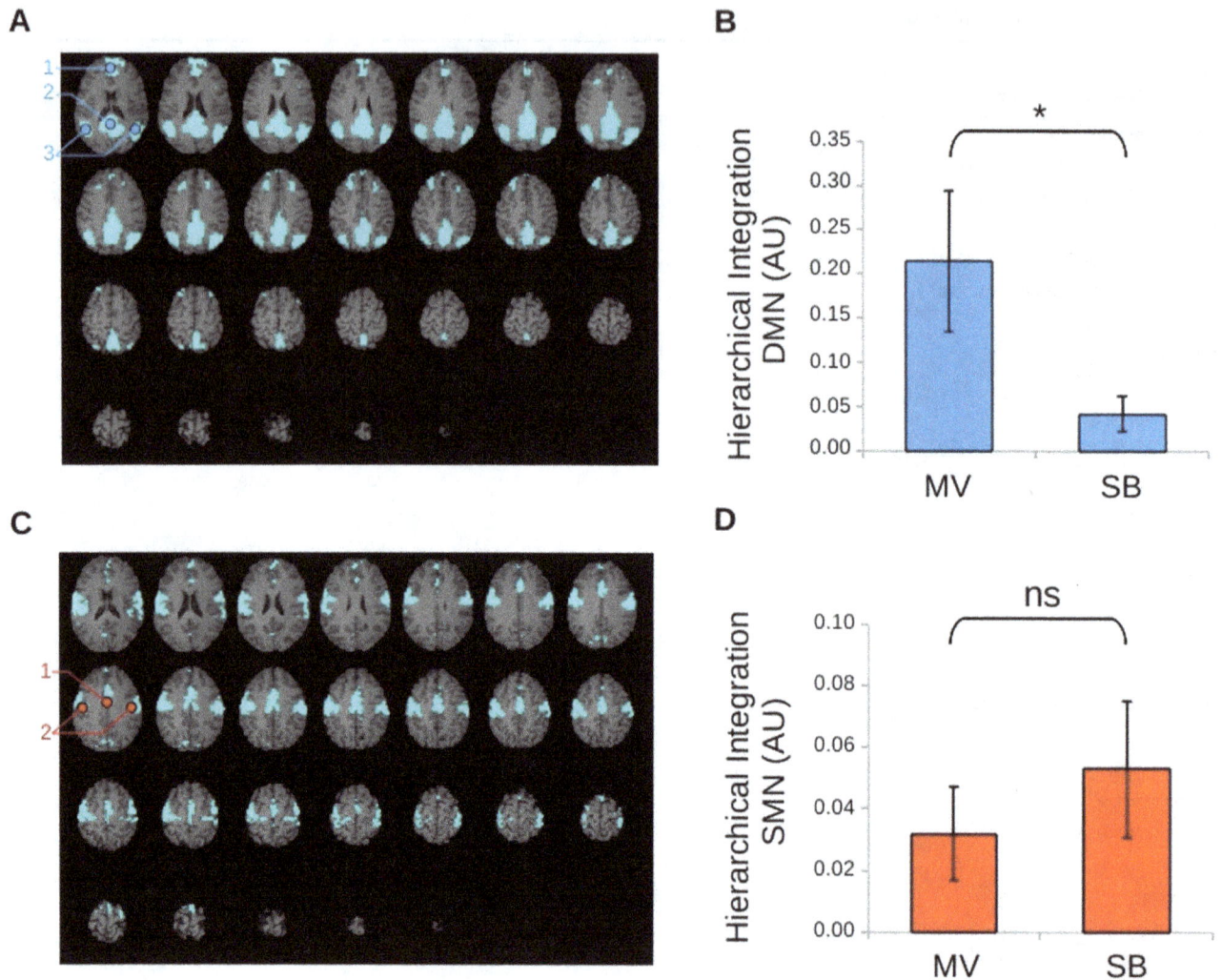

Figure 3. Functional MR connectivity assessed with an ICA method. (A).Default mode network (DMN): bilateral medial prefrontal and anterior cingulate cortices (1), bilateral precuneus (2), bilateral superior parietal cortices (3). (B).Mean values ± standard deviation of DMN integrations for the mechanical (MV) and the spontaneous (SB) breathing blocks of resting state. The asterisk indicates a significant difference between conditions. (C). Sensorimotor network (SMN): bilateral supplementary motor area (1) and bilateral sensorimotor cortices (2). (D).Mean values ± standard deviation of SMN integrations for the mechanical (MV) and the spontaneous (SB) breathing blocks of resting state. NS = non-significant difference between conditions; AU = arbitrary unit.

that one hub of the DMN, - namely the precuneus region -, did increase its functional connectivity with other posterior mesial areas under MV as compared with SB. One may have expected an increase of functional connectivity with anterior regions of the DMN. Actually, when statistical thresholds were decreased (p< 0.1; 30 voxels), we were able to identify such frontal areas. Interestingly, the reverse contrast (SB>MV) revealed an increased functional connectivity of precuneus with frontal and subcortical regions suggestive of a motor control network. Using a data-driven approach we showed that the DMN network was more strongly integrated (as measured by the hierarchical integration index) under MV than under SB. These two functional connectivity results added coherence to the larger BOLD activation we observed in DMN hubs during MV than during SB (see Prediction 2). The last result we obtained confirmed the existence of a stronger correlation between the executive network and the brainstem during SB in comparison with MV. It supports previous reports of co-activation of cortical and brainstem areas in response

to breathing loads in normal subjects [7,8,13,49], and of a recent transcranial magnetic stimulation (TMS) study showing that SMA modulates the cortico-spinal pathway piloting brainstem structures [50].

Overall, this study revealed some important cues related both to the neural mechanism subtending cortical control of brainstem activity during breathing, and to the consequences of such control in terms of functional connectivity and of cognitive processing. These results strengthen the plausibility of our general hypothesis according to which MV would act as freeing up executive resources available for other cognitive purposes (e.g.: introspection during resting state; executive control during the PASAT). A full demonstration of this hypothesis would require additional works including: a replication of these results in a larger population of CCHS patients taking into account the various possible genotypes (e.g.: alanine expansion lengths, various PHOX2B gene mutations), as well as more causal evidence such as for instance the perturbation of SB in CCHS patients in response to TMS inhibition of executive control network. Among the many issues that remain to be addressed, two are considered to be of particular importance: consciousness of cortically-driven breathing, and the value of our findings to the management of CCHS.

The brainstem-driven versus cortex-driven dichotomy of breathing modes is frequently associated with another dichotomy originating from the field of cognitive psychology and information processing: unconscious automatic versus conscious voluntary types of neural processing. However, if many arguments support the unconscious nature of brainstem reflexive breathing, the conscious and voluntary nature of cortex-driven controlled mode of breathing is less evident. In our study, the patient did not report any feeling of voluntary control of breathing (agentivity) during SB. However, we did show that SB was associated with a controlled mode of breathing correlated with the activity of an extended anterior cortical network in this patient. This is coherent with previous observations in the same patient having evidenced the presence of pre-inspiratory potentials during SB, a phenomenon normally absent in healthy subjects [31]. Therefore the contribution of an extended cortical network to breathing control does not guarantee that this form of control is a consciously reportable process. This intriguing possibility of a non-conscious form of cortical control of breathing is even more compelling given that it seems to require cognitive resources typically associated with consciousness such as working memory and dynamic executive control [51]. Interestingly, current cognitive neuroscience studies suggest that some complex cognitive processes of external stimuli (e.g.: dynamic regulation of control; metacognitive effects) may operate unconsciously but still require conscious processing of the stimuli to occur. For instance, in the field of visual perception many studies reported that only consciously visible stimuli can elicit sustained strategical changes [52,53], or dynamic regulation of executive control such as the Gratton effect ([54,55], but see [56]). In sharp contrast, when the very same stimuli are presented under conditions of invisibility (e.g.: subliminal stimuli using visual masking), they are still processed unconsciously but without eliciting such complex effects [51]. However, in these studies most subjects don't have any introspection or conscious agentivity of these strategical changes that were present only when they were conscious of the stimuli [57,58]. This set of findings may be relevant for the case of breathing: it is possible that the cortically-controlled breathing (or, more generally, a cortical contribution to the overall drive to breathe) would require the subject to be awake and conscious, even if the subject was not necessarily conscious of breathing itself. One consequence of this hypothesis would be that no cortical control of breathing should be observed in awake but non conscious patients such as vegetative state patients. Interestingly, the recent fMRI study by Raux et al. [13] suggests that cortically-controlled breathing may itself be automatized. Future studies should combine functional neuroimaging measures with fine subjective reports under various breathing conditions in order to better explore this complex issue.

We will conclude by briefly discussing the value of our finding in regard to the pathophysiology of CCHS. Obviously, a single-patient report can only contribute at opening new research perspectives. Still, if our findings were to be replicated on additional CCHS patients they may suggest that MV could be useful for enhancing cognition during wakefulness, in addition to its current use to prevent hypoxia and death during sleep. Indeed, both spontaneous subjective reports of this patient, as well as our fMRI and behavioral results suggest that MV improves executive function. Given the frequent mild cognitive disabilities of CCHS patients from early childhood, prescription of MV during school time or similar cognitively oriented activities may be particularly relevant to optimize their learning processes, and to improve durably their intellectual abilities.

Acknowledgments

We thank the patient for her active collaboration to this research. This work has been supported by the Fondation pour la Recherche Médicale (FRM) ('Equipe FRM 2010' grant to Lionel Naccache), by the Institut pour le Cerveau et la Moëlle épinière (ICM Institute, Paris, France), by INSERM, by AP-HP, by the program "Investissement d'Avenir ANR-10-AIHU 06 of the French Government", by the IHU-A-ICM ('Investissement d'avenir' program, ANR-10-IAIHU-06), by Assistance Publique - Hôpitaux de Paris (AP-HP) Département de la Recherche Clinique et du Développement (DRCD) ("RESPIRONDINE" project), by Association Française du Syndrome d'Ondine (AFSO). We thank Dr. Marjolaine Georges, Dr. Jésus Gonzales-Bermejo, and Dr. Elise Morawiec for managing mechanical ventilation during MRI. The research leading to these results has received funding from the program "Investissements d'avenir" ANR-10-IAIHU-06. This study is dedicated to CCHS patients. In memoriam of our colleague Dr. Nathalie Nicolas.

Author Contributions

Conceived and designed the experiments: MS TS CS LN. Performed the experiments: MS KL DG NN CS LN. Analyzed the data: MS CG KL LN. Contributed reagents/materials/analysis tools: MS KL DG LN. Wrote the paper: MS CG KL TS LC CS LN.

References

1. Smith JC, Abdala AP, Borgmann A, Rybak IA, Paton JF (2013) *Brainstem respiratory networks: building blocks and microcircuits.* Trends Neurosci. 36(3): p. 152–62.

2. Colebatch JG, Adams L, Murphy K, Martin AJ, Lammertsma AA, et al. (1991) *Regional cerebral blood flow during volitional breathing in man.* J Physiol. 443: p. 91–103.

3. Ramsay SC, Adams L, Murphy K, Corfield DR, Grootoonk S, et al. (1993) *Regional cerebral blood flow during volitional expiration in man: a comparison with volitional inspiration.* J Physiol. 461: p. 85–101.

4. Evans KC, Shea SA, Saykin AJ (1999) *Functional MRI localisation of central nervous system regions associated with volitional inspiration in humans,* in *J Physiol.* England. p. 383–92.

5. Smejkal V, Druga R, Tintera J (2000) *Brain activation during volitional control of breathing.* Physiol Res. 49(6): p. 659–63.

6. McKay LC, Adams L, Frackowiak RS, Corfield DR (2008) *A bilateral cortico-bulbar network associated with breath holding in humans, determined by functional magnetic resonance imaging,* in *Neuroimage:* United States. p. 1824–32.

7. Gozal D, Omidvar O, Kirlew KA, Hathout GM, Hamilton R, et al. (1995) *Identification of human brain regions underlying responses to resistive inspiratory loading with functional magnetic resonance imaging.* Proc Natl Acad Sci U S A. 92(14): p. 6607–11.

8. Gozal D, Omidvar O, Kirlew KA, Hathout GM, Lufkin RB, et al. (1996) *Functional magnetic resonance imaging reveals brain regions mediating the response to resistive expiratory loads in humans.* J Clin Invest. 97(1): p. 47–53.

9. Isaev G, Murphy K, Guz A, Adams L (2002) *Areas of the brain concerned with ventilatory load compensation in awake man,* in *J Physiol:* England. p. 935–45.

10. Raux M, Ray P, Prella M, Duguet A, Demoule A, et al. (2007) *Cerebral cortex activation during experimentally induced ventilator fighting in normal humans receiving noninvasive mechanical ventilation*, in *Anesthesiology*: United States. p. 746–55.

11. Raux M, Straus C, Redolfi S, Morelot-Panzini C, Couturier A, et al. (2007) *Electroencephalographic evidence for pre-motor cortex activation during inspiratory loading in humans*, in *J Physiol*: England. p. 569–78.

12. Tremoureux L, Raux M, Jutand L, Similowski T, (2010) *Sustained preinspiratory cortical potentials during prolonged inspiratory threshold loading in humans*, in *J Appl Physiol (1985)*: United States. p. 1127–33.

13. Raux M, Tyvaert L, Ferreira M, Kindler F, Bardinet E, et al. (2013) *Functional magnetic resonance imaging suggests automatization of the cortical response to inspiratory threshold loading in humans*. Respir Physiol Neurobiol. 189(3): p. 571–80.

14. Raichle ME, MacLeod AM, Snyder AZ, Powers WJ, Gusnard DA, et al. (2001) *A default mode of brain function*. Proc Natl Acad Sci U S A. 98: p. 676–682.

15. Lehericy S, Benali H, Van de Moortele PF, Pelegrini-Issac M, Waechter T, et al. (2005) *Distinct basal ganglia territories are engaged in early and advanced motor sequence learning*, in *Proc Natl Acad Sci U S A*: United States. p. 12566–71.

16. Poldrack RA, Sabb FW, Foerde K, Tom SM, Asarnow RF, et al. (2005) *The neural correlates of motor skill automaticity*, in *J Neurosci*: United States. p. 5356–64.

17. Mellins RB, Balfour HH Jr, Turino GM, Winters RW (1970) *Failure of automatic control of ventilation (Ondine's curse). Report of an infant born with this syndrome and review of the literature*. Medicine (Baltimore). 49(6): p. 487–504.

18. Weese-Mayer DE, Berry-Kravis EM, Ceccherini I, Keens TG, Loghmanee DA, et al. (2010) *An official ATS clinical policy statement: Congenital central hypoventilation syndrome: genetic basis, diagnosis, and management*, in *Am J Respir Crit Care Med*: United States. p. 626–44.

19. Amiel J, Laudier B, Attie-Bitach T, Trang H, de Pontual L, et al. (2003) *Polyalanine expansion and frameshift mutations of the paired-like homeobox gene PHOX2B in congenital central hypoventilation syndrome*, in *Nat Genet*: United States. p. 459–61.

20. Patwari PP, Carroll MS, Rand CM, Kumar R, Harper R, et al. (2010) *Congenital central hypoventilation syndrome and the PHOX2B gene: a model of respiratory and autonomic dysregulation*, in *Respir Physiol Neurobiol*: Netherlands. p. 322–35.

21. Macey KE, Macey PM, Woo MA, Harper RK, Alger JR, et al. (2004) *fMRI signal changes in response to forced expiratory loading in congenital central hypoventilation syndrome*, in *J Appl Physiol (1985)*: United States. p. 1897–907.

22. Macey PM, Macey KE, Woo MA, Keens TG, Harper RM (2005) *Aberrant neural responses to cold pressor challenges in congenital central hypoventilation syndrome*, in *Pediatr Res*: United States. p. 500–9.

23. Macey PM, Woo MA, Macey KE, Keens TG, Saeed MM, et al. (2005) *Hypoxia reveals posterior thalamic, cerebellar, midbrain, and limbic deficits in congenital central hypoventilation syndrome*, in *J Appl Physiol (1985)*: United States. p. 958–69.

24. Woo MA, Macey PM, Macey KE, Keens TG, Woo MS, et al. (2005) *FMRI responses to hyperoxia in congenital central hypoventilation syndrome*, in *Pediatr Res*: United States. p. 510–8.

25. Guilleminault C, McQuitty J, Ariagno RL, Challamel MJ, Korobkin R, et al. (1982) *Congenital central alveolar hypoventilation syndrome in six infants*. Pediatrics. 70(5): p. 684–94.

26. Paton JY, Swaminathan S, Sargent CW, Keens TG (1989) *Hypoxic and hypercapnic ventilatory responses in awake children with congenital central hypoventilation syndrome*. Am Rev Respir Dis. 140(2): p. 368–72.

27. Paton JY, Swaminathan S, Sargent CW, Hawksworth A, Keens TG (1993) *Ventilatory response to exercise in children with congenital central hypoventilation syndrome*. Am Rev Respir Dis. 147(5): p. 1185–91.

28. Shea SA, Andres LP, Paydarfar D, Banzett RB, Shannon DC (1993) *Effect of mental activity on breathing in congenital central hypoventilation syndrome*. Respir Physiol. 94(3): p. 251–63.

29. Denot-Ledunois S, Vardon G, Perruchet P, Gallego J (1998) *The effect of attentional load on the breathing pattern in children*, in *Int J Psychophysiol*: Netherlands. p. 13–21.

30. Gallego J, Perruchet P, Camus JF (1991) *Assessing attentional control of breathing by reaction time*. Psychophysiology. 28(2): p. 217–24.

31. Tremoureux L, Raux M, Hudson AL, Ranohavimparany A, Straus C, et al. (2014) *Does the Supplementary Motor Area Keep Patients with Ondine's Curse Syndrome Breathing While Awake?* PLoS One. 9: p. e84534.

32. Shallice T (1988) *From neuropsychology to mental structure*.

33. McCarthy RA, Warrington EK (1990) *Cognitive neuropsychology: a clinical introduction*.

34. Weiskrantz L (1997) *Consciousness lost and found: A neuropsychological exploration*.

35. Pizoli CE, Shah MN, Snyder AZ, Shimony JS, Limbrick DD, et al. (2011) *Resting-state activity in development and maintenance of normal brain function*, in *Proc Natl Acad Sci U S A*: United States. p. 11638–43.

36. Vanhaudenhuyse A, Demertzi A, Schabus M, Noirhomme Q, Bredart S, et al. (2011) *Two distinct neuronal networks mediate the awareness of environment and of self*. J Cogn Neurosci. 23(3): p. 570–8.

37. Gronwall DM (1977) *Paced auditory serial-addition task: a measure of recovery from concussion*. Percept Mot Skills. 44(2): p. 367–73.

38. Tombaugh TN (2006) *A comprehensive review of the Paced Auditory Serial Addition Test (PASAT)*, in *Arch Clin Neuropsychol*: United States. p. 53–76.

39. Goldenberg F (1986) *[Refinement of an EEG diurnal vigilance index. Application to drug trials]*. Rev Electroencephalogr Neurophysiol Clin. 16(1): p. 39–48.

40. Goldenberg F, Weil JS, Von Frenckell R (1988) *[Utilization of theta/alpha spectral range as an indicator of vigilance: pharmacological applications during repeated sleep latency tests]*. Neurophysiol Clin. 18(5): p. 433–45.

41. Cajochen C, Brunner DP, Krauchi K, Graw P, Wirz-Justice A (1995) *Power density in theta/alpha frequencies of the waking EEG progressively increases during sustained wakefulness*. Sleep. 18(10): p. 890–4.

42. Hu X, Le TH, Parrish T, Erhard P, (1995) *Retrospective estimation and correction of physiological fluctuation in functional MRI*. Magn Reson Med. 34(2): p. 201–12.

43. Tzourio-Mazoyer N, Landeau B, Papathanassiou D, Crivello F, Etard O, et al. (2002) *Automated anatomical labeling of activations in SPM using a macroscopic anatomical parcellation of the MNI MRI single-subject brain*, in *Neuroimage*: United States. p. 273–89.

44. Perlbarg V, Marrelec G (2008) *Contribution of exploratory methods to the investigation of extended large-scale brain networks in functional MRI: methodologies, results, and challenges*. Int J Biomed Imaging. 2008: p. 218519.

45. Laufs H, Krakow K, Sterzer P, Eger E, Beyerle A, et al. (2003) *Electroencephalographic signatures of attentional and cognitive default modes in spontaneous brain activity fluctuations at rest*, in *Proc Natl Acad Sci U S A*: United States. p. 11053–8.

46. Laufs H, Daunizeau J, Carmichael DW, Kleinschmidt A (2008) *Recent advances in recording electrophysiological data simultaneously with magnetic resonance imaging*, in *Neuroimage*: United States. p. 515–28.

47. Oren J, Kelly DH, Shannon DC (1987) *Long-term follow-up of children with congenital central hypoventilation syndrome*. Pediatrics. 80(3): p. 375–80.

48. Zelko FA, Nelson MN, Leurgans SE, Berry-Kravis EM, Weese-Mayer DE (2010) *Congenital central hypoventilation syndrome: neurocognitive functioning in school age children*. Pediatr Pulmonol. 45(1): p. 92–8.

49. Pattinson KT, Mitsis GD, Harvey AK, Jbabdi S, Dirckx S, et al. (2009) *Determination of the human brainstem respiratory control network and its cortical connections in vivo using functional and structural imaging*, in *Neuroimage*: United States. p. 295–305.

50. Laviolette L, Nierat MC, Hudson AL, Raux M, Allard E, et al. (2013) *The supplementary motor area exerts a tonic excitatory influence on corticospinal projections to phrenic motoneurons in awake humans*, in *PLoS One*: United States. p. e62258.

51. Dehaene S, Naccache L (2001) *Towards a cognitive neuroscience of consciousness: Basic evidence and a workspace framework*. Cognition. 79: p. 1–37.

52. Merikle PM, Joordens S, Stolz JA (1995) *Measuring the relative magnitude of unconscious influences*. Consciousness and Cognition. 4: p. 422–439.

53. El Karoui I, Christoforidis K, Naccache L (2013) *Do acquisition and transfer of a new strategy require conscious perception?* in *CNS Annual meeting*. San Francisco.

54. Kunde W (2003) *Sequential modulations of stimulus-response correspondence effects depend on awareness of response conflict*. Psychon Bull Rev. 10: p. 198–205.

55. van Gaal S, de Lange FP, Cohen MX (2012) *The role of consciousness in cognitive control and decision making*. Front Hum Neurosci. 6: p. 121.

56. Van Gaal S, Lamme VA, Ridderinkhof KR (2010) *Unconsciously triggered conflict adaptation*. PLoS One. 5(7): p. e11508.

57. Naccache L (2008) *Conscious influences on subliminal cognition exist and are asymmetrical: Validation of a double prediction*. Conscious Cogn. 17: p. 1359–1360.

58. Naccache L (2009) *Contrôle exécutif et processus inconscients: une relation subtile*. Revue de Neuropsychologie. 1: p. 42–50.

18

Attentional Demands Influence Vocal Compensations to Pitch Errors Heard in Auditory Feedback

Anupreet K. Tumber, Nichole E. Scheerer, Jeffery A. Jones*

Psychology Department and Laurier Centre for Cognitive Neuroscience, Wilfrid Laurier University, Waterloo, Ontario, Canada

Abstract

Auditory feedback is required to maintain fluent speech. At present, it is unclear how attention modulates auditory feedback processing during ongoing speech. In this event-related potential (ERP) study, participants vocalized/a/, while they heard their vocal pitch suddenly shifted downward a ½ semitone in both single and dual-task conditions. During the single-task condition participants passively viewed a visual stream for cues to start and stop vocalizing. In the dual-task condition, participants vocalized while they identified target stimuli in a visual stream of letters. The presentation rate of the visual stimuli was manipulated in the dual-task condition in order to produce a low, intermediate, and high attentional load. Visual target identification accuracy was lowest in the high attentional load condition, indicating that attentional load was successfully manipulated. Results further showed that participants who were exposed to the single-task condition, prior to the dual-task condition, produced larger vocal compensations during the single-task condition. Thus, when participants' attention was divided, less attention was available for the monitoring of their auditory feedback, resulting in smaller compensatory vocal responses. However, P1-N1-P2 ERP responses were not affected by divided attention, suggesting that the effect of attentional load was not on the auditory processing of pitch altered feedback, but instead it interfered with the integration of auditory and motor information, or motor control itself.

Editor: Donald A. Robin, University of Texas Health Science Center at San Antonio, Research Imaging Institute, United States of America

Funding: This research was funded by a Natural Sciences and Engineering Research Council of Canada (http://www.nserc-crsng.gc.ca/index_eng.asp) Discovery Grant awarded to JAJ. The funders had no role in study design, data collection and analysis, decision to publish, or preparation of the manuscript.

Competing Interests: The authors have declared that no competing interests exist.

* Email: jjones@wlu.ca

Introduction

Proficient motor control is achieved by using sensory feedback to plan, execute, and regulate motor movements [1]. This is particularly true for speech motor control, which relies on auditory feedback for the regulation of ongoing and future speech motor commands [2,3]. In everyday life, speakers receive auditory feedback while simultaneously processing information from other modalities. Since attention is a limited resource, it must be divided amongst the input from different sensory modalities based on the processing demands and encoding requirements imposed by these sensory modalities [4]. In order to understand how auditory feedback facilitates fluent speech motor control, particularly when speech errors are encountered, it is important to understand how attention modulates the processing of auditory feedback during ongoing speech.

The multiple resource theory of divided attention states that when performing two tasks simultaneously, the degree to which performance will decline on each task, compared to when each task is completed in isolation depends on: the resource demands of each of the two tasks, the similarity between the two tasks, and the allocation of resources between the two tasks [5]. Studies examining cross-modal (e.g., visual and auditory) attention have argued for separate, but linked attentional systems [6,7]. When simple stimuli are being processed, separate attentional resources are utilized by each modality, eliminating any interference that

may occur as a result of simultaneously processing stimuli in different modalities [8,9,10]. However, when cross-modal stimuli are complex, and the attentional load is increased, attending to one stimulus modality may interfere with the processing of a second stimulus in a different modality. For example, when participants performed a visual discrimination task where they were required to adjust the length of the arms of a cross-shape, they were less likely to notice a binaurally presented tone [11]. Together, these theories suggest that increasing one's attentional load during ongoing speech, by introducing a secondary task, may interfere with the processing of auditory feedback.

The importance of auditory feedback for maintaining fluent speech has been demonstrated by individuals who have been deafened post-lingually, and experienced a gradual deterioration in the quality of their speech [12]. However, since there are inherent delays involved in processing auditory feedback, a feedforward system driven by internal models must also play a role in fluent speech production, as strict reliance on auditory feedback would result in delayed and inarticulate speech [2,3]. That being said, in order to ascertain the role of auditory feedback during ongoing speech, the frequency-altered feedback (FAF) paradigm is often utilized [13,14,15]. As part of this paradigm, participants produce vocalizations while their fundamental frequency (F0), or vocal pitch, is shifted upwards or downwards and instantaneously presented back to them through headphones.

When the F0 of an individual's auditory feedback is altered, they tend to compensate, or shift their voice in the opposite direction of the manipulation. Since the compensatory response is often only a fraction of the size of the manipulation [13,14,16,17,18,19], it has been suggested that it is an automatic response intended to correct for small production errors [20,21]. However, it is currently unclear whether attention load modulates this reflexive-like response.

In addition to investigating vocal responses, auditory cortical responses to FAF recorded using electroencephalography (EEG) can provide information regarding the underlying neural mechanisms of speech motor control. The P1, N1, and P2 event-related potentials (ERPs) are reliably elicited by FAF [18,19,22]. The P1 is proposed to reflect the early detection of changes in auditory feedback, as previous research has demonstrated that it is elicited in an all-or-nothing manner when FAF perturbations are under 400 cents (100 cents is equivalent to a semitone) [18,22]. On the other hand, the N1 is thought to reflect pre-attentive error-detection, where auditory feedback is compared to a sensory prediction produced by the motor system during the execution of speech motor commands [23]. In line with this notion, Scheerer et al. [18] found that smaller feedback perturbations (less than 250 cents) evoked similarly sized N1 responses, while larger (400 cent) perturbations resulted in significantly larger N1 responses. Based on these findings, it was suggested that the N1 ERP component specifically reflects whether a feedback error is physiologically feasible, and thus likely to be internally generated, or excessively deviant, and thus likely to be externally generated. All feedback alterations perceived as physiologically feasible, elicit small N1 responses, compared to feedback alterations perceived as physiologically implausible, which generate larger N1 responses [18]. The third ERP component commonly elicited by FAF, the P2, has been shown to increase linearly as the size of the feedback perturbations increases [18], leading to the suggestion that the amplitude of the P2 component reflects the size of the speech production error [22,24]. Although researchers are just beginning to understand how FAF modulates the P1, N1, and P2 ERP components, their sensitivity to FAF makes them ideal for assessing the influence of attention on the processing of auditory feedback during ongoing speech.

Although it is unclear how FAF modulates these ERPs under divided attention, when elicited by other forms of auditory stimuli, auditory ERPs have shown sensitivity to divided attention. In particular, the N1 component is often enhanced when participants attend to an auditory stimulus, relative to passive listening of the same stimulus [25,26,27,28,29]. Specifically, Choi and colleagues [25] found that when comparing attended and unattended auditory streams, attentional gains to attended auditory stimuli were associated with an approximate 10 dB increase in loudness, compared to auditory stimuli in the unattended auditory stream. These findings suggest that focused auditory attention results in larger N1 responses to auditory stimuli, and increases the perceived loudness of auditory stimuli. On the other hand, P1 and P2 amplitudes are rarely modulated by selective attention toward an auditory channel (e.g., Choi et al., [24], Coch et al., [26]). Increases in the latency of slow negative ERPs related to the N1 have also been found when attention is divided between two auditory channels, compared to when attention is oriented to a specific channel, which has been attributed to increased processing demands under divided attention [30]. Together these results suggest that the P1-N1-P2 ERP responses may be modulated by divided attention.

For the current experiment, we used a dual-task paradigm to investigate whether divided attention impacts the compensatory vocal responses and ERPs elicited by FAF. In order to reduce the allocation of attentional resources to auditory feedback during the FAF task, participants simultaneously monitored a rapid serial visual presentation (RSVP) of letters. The RSVP contained target letters, which participants identified and later reported. Attentional load was manipulated by varying the rate of the RSVP. Increasing the rate of the RSVP decreased the inter-stimulus interval (ISI) between letters, which modulated the perceptual load by increasing the number of stimuli. As a result of the increased number of stimuli, participants had to process more irrelevant information, which directly impacted the perceptual selection of relevant information, and thus increased the overall attentional demand of the task (see Chun & Wolfe, [31] and Lavie, Hirst, de Fockert, & Viding, [32], for a review).

Since decreasing the ISI of a RSVP of letters has been shown to increase attentional load, we expected that increasing the rate of the RSVP, would reduce participants' abilities to identify the target letters. Furthermore, we expected that as the rate of the RSVP increased, more attention would be allocated to the visual task, which would reduce the saliency of the FAF, and result in smaller and slower compensatory responses. With regard to the ERP responses, since the P1 is thought to reflect the basic detection of FAF [18], we expected that as attentional load increased, and the FAF became less salient, P1 amplitudes would decrease. Similarly, since previous research has shown that attending to an auditory stimulus results in larger N1s, we expected that N1s would be larger in the single-task condition as more attention would be allocated to the processing of auditory feedback, relative to the dual-task, where attention would be divided between the auditory feedback and the visual stream. On the other hand, since the size of the FAF perturbations were not manipulated in this experiment, and the P2 component is thought to play a role in assessing the size of FAF perturbations, we did not predict changes in P2 amplitudes as a function of attention load. However, we did predict that P1-N1-P2 latencies would be later under divided attention, reflecting slower processing under increased attentional load.

Methods

Participants

Sixty-five participants between the ages of 16 and 38 years ($M = 21.51$ years, $SD = 4.81$; 42 females and 23 males) participated. Vocal and behavioural responses were recorded from all 65 participants, while ERP responses were also recorded from a subset of 33 right-handed participants ($M = 19$ years, $SD = 1.37$; 21 females and 12 males). All participants were Canadian-English speakers who did not speak a tonal language, with the exception of one participant who spoke a tonal language, but identified English as their primary language. This tonal language speaker did not show any differences in vocal compensations nor ERP responses to the FAF perturbations compared to the other non-tonal language-speaking participants. All participants also had normal or corrected to normal vision, had not been diagnosed with attention deficit (hyperactivity) disorder (ADD, ADHD), epilepsy (or had a family history of seizures), visual deficits that could not be amended by corrective lenses, and did not have a speech or language disorder.

Ethics Statement

All participants provided written informed consent and received financial compensation or course credit for their participation in this study. All procedures were approved by the Wilfrid Laurier

University Research Ethics Board and were in accordance with the World Medical Association 2013 Declaration of Helsinki.

Procedure

Participants produced 198 vocalizations of the vowel sound/a/, across two conditions, while exposed to a RSVP. Each vocalization was randomly perturbed downward 50 cents for 200 ms. During the single-task condition, participants produced nine practice vocalizations, followed by a block of 45 vocalizations where the participants' only goal was to produce a steady/a/ sound. During the dual-task condition, participants produced nine practice vocalizations, followed by 3 blocks of 45 vocalizations, where participants were also required to attend to a RSVP and answer questions about the visual stream.

For both experimental conditions, each visual stream had two targets: 1. a randomly selected white letter from the alphabet (excluding letter "X"); and 2. an "X," that occurred pseudor-andomly before or after the white letter. All letters in the stream were capitalized and in black font with the exception of the white target letter. Each letter was displayed at the same location in the center of a grey field, where the varied ISI was seen as a uniform grey field. For the single-task trials, each letter stream ended with a blank grey field.

The presentation rate of the RSVP was manipulated to impose a high, intermediate, and low attentional load. The RSVP started with a green fixation cross that lasted for 750 ms, followed by a stream of successively presented letters. Each trial was approximately 5.5 s in duration. Each letter appeared for 50 ms, and each trial occurred with an ISI of either 100, 300, or 500 ms (high, intermediate, or low attentional load, respectively). High attentional load trials were 5.4 s in duration and consisted of 37 letters, with an ISI of 100 ms. The white letter appeared at random between the 4th and the 37th letter, and the "X" randomly occurred between the 1st and 15th letter before or after the white letter (minimum 2nd place, maximum 36th place in the visual stream). Intermediate attentional load trials were 5.4 s in duration and consisted of 16 letters in the visual stream, with an ISI of 300 ms. The white letter appeared at random between the 4th and 16th place in the letter stream, while the "X" occurred at random between the 1st and 12th letter before or after the white letter (minimum 2nd letter and maximum 16th letter). Low attentional load trials were 5.5 s in duration, with 11 letters in the stream and an ISI of 500 ms. The white letter occurred randomly between the 4th and 11th place in the visual stream, and the "X" occurred at random between the 1st and 15th letters from the white letter (minimum 2nd letter in the stream, maximum 11th). Figure 1 depicts the paradigm. Each presentation rate occurred an equal number of times in both the single- and dual-task trials, but was pseudo-randomly presented throughout the experiment. The arrangement of the dual-task condition and the single-task condition was counterbalanced across participants.

During the single-task condition, participants were instructed to attend to the RSVP, as the start of the RSVP was their cue to start vocalizing, and the termination of the RSVP was their cue to stop vocalizing. During the dual-task condition, participants were instructed to attend to the RSVP and monitor the letter stream for their cue to start and stop vocalizing, but also so they could identify two targets: a white letter, and an "X." At the end of the letter stream, participants were required to answer two questions about the target letters. The first question appeared on the screen at the end of the trial and stated, "Identify the WHITE letter. If you are unsure, please guess." The second question, which appeared immediately after the participant's response to the first question stated, "indicate when the "X" appeared with reference

to the white letter." The participant was required to press a key labelled "YES" if they believed that the "X" appeared before the white letter, and a key labelled "NO" if the believed that the "X" appeared after the white letter. During each vocalization, the FAF perturbation occurred either 250–1000 ms before the "X," or 100–1000 ms after the "X." Emphasis was placed on both maintaining a steady vocalization and on responding accurately to the two questions at the end of the trial. Since participants could take as much time as they needed to respond to the two questions, participants moved on to subsequent trials at their own pace during the dual-task trials, whereas single-task trials occurred with an inter-trial interval of 3000 ms. The total duration of the experiment ranged from 40 to 60 minutes, and depended on the participant's reaction time to the questions during the dual-task blocks, and the duration of breaks between blocks.

Apparatus

Participants were seated 76 cm from a 15-inch LCD monitor in an electrically shielded booth (Raymond EMC, Ottawa, ON, Canada) and were fitted with a HydroCel GSN 64 1.0 Cap (Electrical Geodesics Inc., Eugene, OR, USA), Etymotic ER-3 insert earphones (Etymotic Research, Elk Grove Village, IL, USA), and an earset microphone (Countryman Isomax, IL, USA). The presentation of visual stimuli and shift onsets and offsets were controlled by Max/MSP 6 (Cycling' 74, San Francisco, CA). Keyed behavioral responses to questions were also recorded using Max/MSP 6, using a standard keyboard with labeled keys. During the experiment, voice signals were sent to a mixer (Mackie Onyx 1200, Loud Technologies, Woodinville, WA, USA), then to a digital signal processor (DSP; VoiceOne, T.C. Helicon, Victoria, BC, Canada), which altered the F0 of the voice signal. This process introduced a ∼10 ms delay in the feedback signal, that was then presented back to the participant through headphones as auditory feedback. The unaltered voice signal was digitally recorded (TASCAM HD-P2, Montebello, CA, USA) at a sampling rate of 44.1 kHz for later analysis.

Analysis

Behavioural Analysis. For each trial, records were kept of the trial's attentional load condition, the white letter in the stream, whether the "X" appeared before or after the white letter, the participants' keyed responses and reaction time to question one, as well as the participants' keyed responses and reaction time to question two. Participants who did not answer either of the questions according to the instructions were excluded from the analysis. One participant's answers were excluded from the white letter identification analyses for this reason. Accuracy and reaction time for questions one and two were averaged for each of the three categories of attentional load in the dual-task condition (i.e., low, intermediate, and high attentional load trials). Accuracy for high, intermediate, and low attentional load trials were then averaged across all participants for each question. Only accuracy data were examined since response accuracy was emphasized during the participant instructions.

Vocal Analysis. Each participant's unaltered voice recording was segmented into separate vocalizations. The swipe algorithm [33] was used to determine F0 values for each vocalization. The vocalizations were then segmented based on the onset of the perturbation, where F0 values were normalized to a baseline period 200 ms prior to the onset of the perturbation. This normalization was achieved by converting Hertz values to cents using the formula: cents $= 1200$ (LOG2(F/B)), where F is the F0 value in Hertz, and B is the mean frequency of the baseline period. Cents values were calculated for the baseline period (200 ms prior

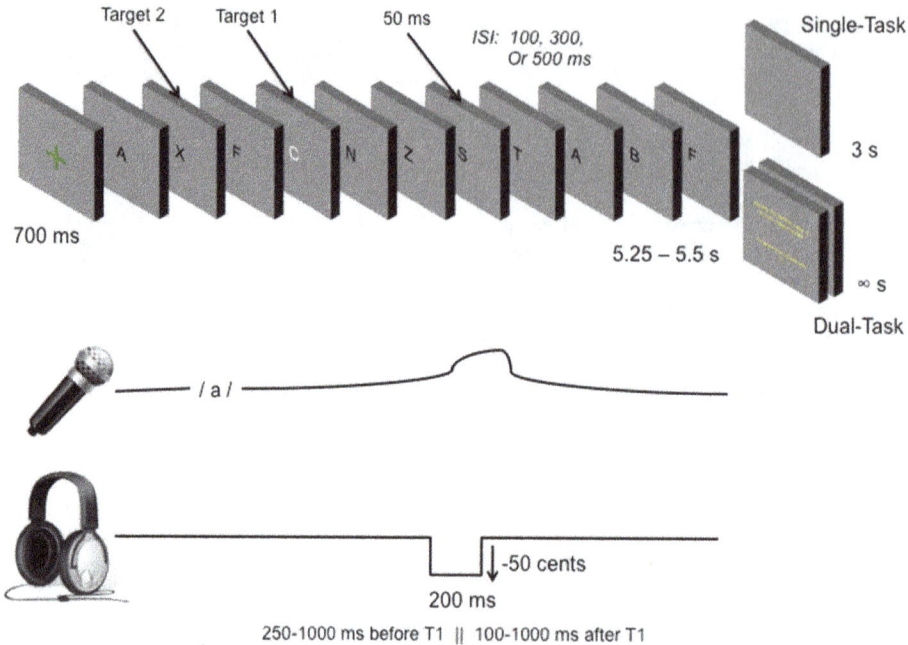

Figure 1. Experimental paradigm. Participants observed a rapid serial visual presentation (RSVP) of letters with two targets (a white letter, and an "X"). In the single-task condition, participants observed a blank screen for 3 s before the next trial. For the dual task condition, participants answered two questions at the end of each trial; they were asked to identify the white letter and whether the "X" appeared before or after the white letter. Attentional load was manipulated by varying the inter-stimulus-interval across trials: 500 ms for the low attentional load, 300 ms for the intermediate attentional load, and 100 ms for the high attentional load. All trials were approximately 5.5 s long. Participants vocalized the/a/sound during the letter stream in both conditions, while listening to their auditory feedback, which was perturbed downward 50 cents for 200 ms either 250–1000 ms before target 1, or 100–1000 ms after target 1.

to the start of the perturbation), and 1000 ms after the perturbation.

Missing and incomplete vocalizations were excluded from the statistical analysis. Participants with more than 67% (i.e., 30 out of 45) rejected trials for any of the four attentional load conditions (i.e., dual task-high, dual task-intermediate, dual task-low, and single task attentional load trials) were removed from further analysis. A total of 11 participants were excluded from the experiment due to F0 tracking issues. For the 54 remaining participants, an averaged F0 trace for retained trials was constructed for each of the four attentional load conditions. The average number of trials in each condition was 42 for the dual task-high, 40 for the dual task-intermediate, 41 for the dual task-low, and 39 for the single task attentional load trials. Traces were averaged across all participants, for each condition. For each participant, the magnitude of the compensatory response and the latency of the response were assessed. The amplitude of the compensatory response was determined by finding the maximum point at which the participants' average F0 trace deviated from the baseline mean. Latency was determined as the time at which the maximum peak in the compensatory response occurred.

EEG Analysis. EEG signals were recorded from 64-electrodes on the scalp, and referenced online to the vertex (Cz). Signals were bandpass filtered (1–30 Hz) and digitized (12-bit precision) at 1000 samples per second. Impedances were maintained below 50 kΩ for the experiment [34]. EEG-voltage values were re-referenced to the average voltage across all electrodes and then epoched into segments from 100 ms before to 500 ms after the onset of the auditory feedback perturbation. Segments were then analyzed for artifacts and rejected if changes in voltage values exceeded 55 uV over a moving average of 80 ms. A visual inspection of the data was also completed to ensure that

segments containing artifacts were excluded from further analysis. Participants with more than 67% (i.e., 30 out of 45) of their trials rejected for any of the four conditions were removed from further analysis. For this reason, three participants were excluded from further analyses, leaving 30 participants for the EEG analysis. For the remaining participants, the average number of trials in each condition was 42 for the dual task-high, 42 for the dual task-intermediate, 41 for the dual task-low, and 41 for the single task attentional load trials. Averaged waveforms were created for each of the four conditions for these participants. All participants' epochs were then grand-averaged for each condition and baseline corrected.

Six electrodes were included in the analysis: Fz, Cz, F3, C3, C4, and F4. These six electrodes were selected for analysis through visual inspection, having demonstrated the most robust P1-N1-P2 components, and based on previous research, which suggests that front-medial and centro-frontal regions display the most robust responses to pitch shifts [16,18,22,35]. These electrodes were grouped into left (average of F3 and C3), medial (average of Fz and Cz), and right (average of F4 and C4) regions for further analysis. The peak amplitude of the P1 component was extracted from a window between 50 and 100 ms, while the peak amplitude of the N1 component was extracted from a window between 100 and 200 ms, and the peak amplitude of the P2 component was extracted from a time window between 200 and 300 ms. These time windows were determined by visual inspection, based on the latency of the most prominent ERP peaks.

Statistical Analysis

Statistical Analysis of the Behavioural Data. Two separate repeated-measures analysis of variances (RM-ANOVAs) were conducted to look at the influence of attentional load (dual-task high, dual-task intermediate, dual-task low) with block-order (single-task first, dual-task first) as a between-subjects factor, on response accuracy for the identification of the white letter and the placement of the "X". The Greenhouse-Geisser [36] correction was used in cases where violations of Mauchley's Assumptions of Sphericity were present. In these cases, the original degrees of freedom were reported for ease of interpretation. Separate Pearson product moment correlations were also conducted for dual-task high, dual-task intermediate, and dual-task low attentional load conditions at an alpha of 0.05 (two-tailed). For each attentional load condition, vocal response magnitude and latency were each correlated with the average accuracy for white letter identification and the average accuracy for "X"-placement.

Statistical Analysis of the Vocal Data. Two separate RM-ANOVAs were conducted to assess the influence of attentional load (dual–task high, dual-task intermediate, dual-task low, and single-task) and block-order (single-task first, dual-task first) on vocal response magnitudes and response latencies. Follow-up RM-ANOVAs were run to investigate significant interactions. The Greenhouse-Geisser [36] correction was used in cases where violations of Mauchley's Assumption of Sphericity were present. In these cases, the original degrees of freedom were reported for the ease of interpretation.

Statistical Analysis of EEG Data. Separate two-way RM-ANOVAs were conducted to look at the impact of attentional load (dual-task high, dual-task intermediate, dual-task low, and single-task) and electrode site (left, medial, and right) with the between subject factor of block-order (single-first, dual-first) on P1-, N1-, and P2- amplitudes, and P1-, N1-, P2- latencies. The Greenhouse-Geisser [36] correction was used in cases where violations of Mauchley's Assumption of Sphericity were identified. In these cases, the original degrees of freedom were reported for ease of interpretation.

Results

Behavioural Results

A RM-ANOVA was conducted to look at the effect of attentional load on white-letter identification accuracy with block-order as a between subjects factor. There was a main effect of attentional load, $F(2,102) = 78.662$, $p<0.001$, $\eta^2 = 0.607$, where white-letter identification was significantly more accurate for the dual-task low attentional load condition, relative to the dual-task high attentional load condition, $p<0.001$. While the dual-task intermediate attentional load condition also elicited higher response accuracy for the white-letter identification, relative to the dual-task high attentional load condition, $p<0.001$ (see Figure 2). The main effect of block-order, $F(1,51) = 0.686$, $p = 0.411$, $\eta^2 = 0.013$, and the interaction between attentional load and block-order were not significant, $F(2,102) = 0.107$, $p = 0.819$, $\eta^2 = 0.002$.

A RM-ANOVA was conducted to look at the effect of attentional load on "X"-placement accuracy, with block-order as a between subjects factor. There was a main effect of attentional load, $F(2,104) = 106.443$, $p<0.001$, $\eta^2 = 0.672$, where accuracy was much higher for the dual-task low attentional load condition, compared to the dual-task intermediate, and dual-task high attentional load conditions, $p<0.01$. In addition, "X"-placement accuracy was also greater for the dual-task intermediate attentional load condition, compared to the dual-task high attentional load condition, $p<0.001$ (see Figure 3). The main effect of block-order, $F(1,52) = 0.159$, $p = 0.691$, $\eta^2 = 0.003$, and the interaction between attentional load and block-order were not significant, $F(2,104) = 2.454$, $p = 0.107$, $\eta^2 = 0.045$.

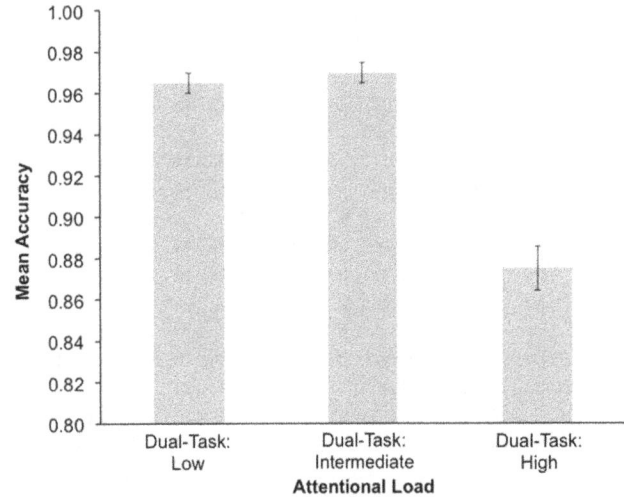

Figure 2. Mean response accuracy for white letter identification during low, intermediate, and high attentional load. Error bars represent standard error.

Pearson-product moment correlations were conducted to look for potential relationships between the magnitude and latency of vocal responses, and the accuracy with which the white-letter and "X"-placement were identified, for the dual-task high, dual-task intermediate, dual-task low attentional load conditions. The correlations between white letter identification accuracy and vocal response magnitude, and white letter identification accuracy and vocal response latency, were not significant, both p>.05. Similarly, the correlations between accuracy for "X"-placement and vocal response magnitude, and accuracy for "X"-placement and vocal response latency, were also not significant, both p>.05.

Vocal Results

A RM-ANOVA was conducted looking at the effect of attentional load on vocal response magnitudes, with block-order as a between subjects factor. The main effect of attentional load on

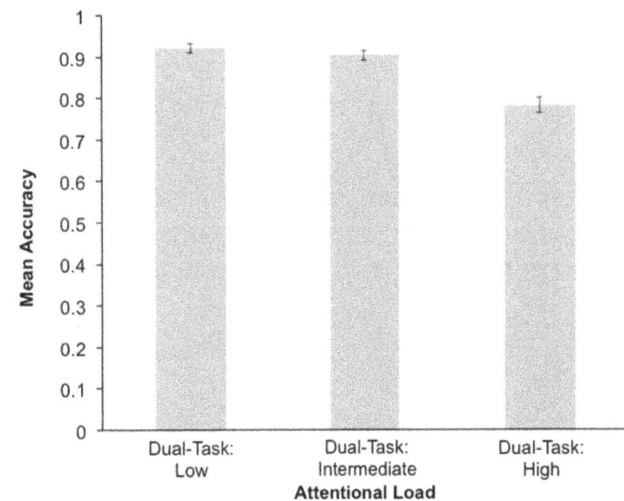

Figure 3. Mean "X"-placement accuracy during low, intermediate, and high attentional load. "X"-placement refers to whether the second target ("X") in the RSVP was presented before or after the white letter. Error bars represent standard error.

vocal response magnitudes was not significant, $F(3,156) = 1.175$, $p = 0.321$, $\eta^2 = 0.022$ (see Figure 4), nor was the main effect of block-order, $F(1,52) = 0.573$, $p = 0.453$, $\eta^2 = 0.011$. However, a significant interaction was found between attentional load and block-order, $F(3,156) = 5.782$, $p = 0.003$, $\eta^2 = 0.1$ (see Figure 5). Follow-up RM-ANOVAs were conducted to investigate the effect of attentional load on vocal response magnitudes for each block order. A significant main effect of attentional load was found for the single-task first block order, $F(3,84) = 7.303$, $p = 0.001$, $\eta^2 = 0.207$, where the vocal response magnitudes were significantly larger in the single-task condition, compared to all attentional load conditions, $p < 0.02$. However, the effect of attentional load on vocal response magnitudes in the dual-task first condition was not significant, $F(3,72) = 1.083$, $p = 0.362$, $\eta^2 = 0.043$.

A RM-ANOVA was conducted to look at the effect of attentional load on vocal response latencies, with block-order as a between subjects factor. The main effect of attentional load was not significant, $F(3,156) = 1.684$, $p = 0.173$, $\eta^2 = 0.031$, nor was the main effect of block-order, $F(1,52) = 0.542$, $p = 0.465$, $\eta^2 = 0.01$, or the attentional load by block-order interaction $F(3,156) = 0.739$, $p = 0.53$, $\eta^2 = 0.014$.

EEG Results

See Figure 6 for the averaged ERP waveforms across all electrode sites, at dual-task high, dual-task intermediate, dual-task low, and single-task attentional load conditions.

P100. A RM-ANOVA was conducted to look at the effect of attentional load, electrode site, and block-order on P100 amplitudes. There was no main effect of attentional load, $F(3,75) = 1.438$, $p = 0.238$, $\eta^2 = 0.054$, no main effect of electrode site, $F(2,50) = 1.375$, $p = 0.261$, $\eta^2 = 0.052$, and no main effect of block-order, $F(1,25) = 0.009$, $p = 0.926$, $\eta^2 < 0.001$. The attentional load by block-order interaction was also not significant, $F(3,75) = 0.979$, $p = 0.407$, $\eta^2 = 0.038$, as was the electrode site by block-order interaction, $F(2,50) = 2.067$, $p = 0.15$, $\eta^2 = 0.076$, the attentional load by electrode site interaction, $F(6,150) = 0.281$, $p = 0.945$, $\eta^2 = 0.011$, and the three-way interaction between attentional load, electrode site, and block-order, $F(6,150) = 0.853$, $p = 0.531$, $\eta^2 = 0.033$.

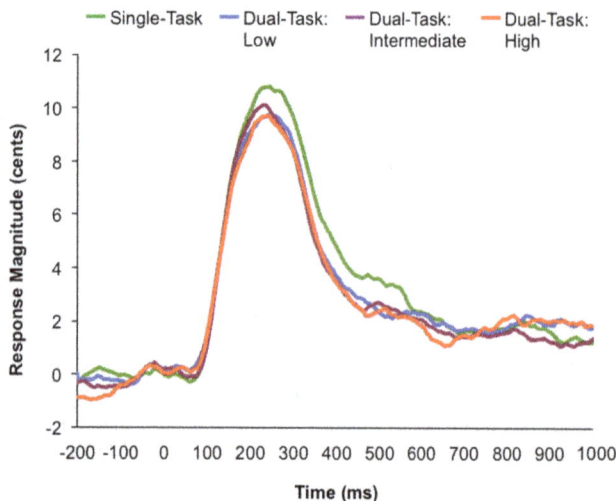

Figure 4. Averaged F_0 traces for each attentional load condition. Time zero represents the onset of the feedback perturbation.

A RM-ANOVA was conducted to look at the effect of attentional load, electrode site, and block-order on P100 latencies. There was no main effect of attentional load, $F(3,75) = 1.349$, $p = 0.265$, $\eta^2 = 0.051$, no main effect of electrode site, $F(2,50) = 0.299$, $p = 0.695$, $\eta^2 = 0.012$, and no main effect of block-order, $F(1,25) = 0.885$, $p = 0.356$, $\eta^2 = 0.034$. The attentional load by block-order interaction was not significant, $F(3,75) = 0.034$, $p = 0.992$, $\eta^2 = 0.001$, as was the electrode site by block-order interaction, $F(2,50) = 0.753$, $p = 0.45$, $\eta^2 = 0.029$, the attentional load by electrode site interaction, $F(6,150) = 0.338$, $p = 0.916$, $\eta^2 = 0.013$, and the three-way interaction between attentional load, electrode site, and block-order, $F(6,150) = 1.246$, $p = 0.286$, $\eta^2 = 0.047$.

N100. A RM-ANOVA was performed to look at the effect of attentional load, electrode site, and block-order on N100 amplitudes. There was no significant main effect of attentional load, $F(3,75) = 2.05$, $p = 0.114$, $\eta^2 = 0.076$, nor a significant main effect of block-order, $F(1,25) = 1.065$, $p = 0.312$, $\eta^2 = 0.041$. However, the main effect of electrode site was significant, $F(2,50) = 4.057$, $p = 0.023$, $\eta^2 = 0.14$, such that the right electrode site recorded smaller N1 amplitudes (absolute value) than the medial electrode site, $p < 0.01$ (see Figure 7). Furthermore, the attentional load by block-order interaction was not significant, $F(3,75) = 1.22$, $p = 0.308$, $\eta^2 = 0.047$, as was the electrode site by block-order interaction, $F(2,50) = 0.747$, $p = 0.479$, $\eta^2 = 0.029$, the attentional load by electrode site interaction, $F(6,150) = 0.795$, $p = 0.523$, $\eta^2 = 0.031$, and the interaction between attentional load, electrode site, and block-order, $F(6,150) = 0.989$, $p = 0.413$, $\eta^2 = 0.038$.

A RM-ANOVA was performed to look at the effect of attentional load, electrode site, and block-order on N100 latencies. There was no main effect of attentional load, $F(3,75) = 0.588$, $p = 0.625$, $\eta^2 = 0.023$, no main effect of electrode site, $F(2,50) = 1.367$, $p = 0.265$, $\eta^2 = 0.052$, and no main effect of block-order, $F(1,25) = 2.225$, $p = 0.148$, $\eta^2 = 0.082$. Furthermore, the attentional load by block-order interaction was not significant, $F(3,75) = 1.061$, $p = 0.371$, $\eta^2 = 0.41$, nor was the electrode site by block-order interaction, $F(2,50) = 2.644$, $p = 0.081$, $\eta^2 = 0.096$, the attentional load by electrode site interaction, $F(6,150) = 1.534$, $p = 0.195$, $\eta^2 = 0.058$, and the interaction between attentional load, electrode site, and block-order, $F(6,150) = 1.649$, $p = 0.164$, $\eta^2 = 0.062$.

P200. A RM-ANOVA was conducted to look at the effect of attentional load, electrode site, and block-order on P200 amplitudes. There was no main effect of attentional load, $F(3,75) = 0.603$, $p = 0.615$, $\eta^2 = 0.024$, no main effect of electrode site, $F(2,50) = 2.013$, $p = 0.144$, $\eta^2 = 0.075$, and no main effect of block-order, $F(1,25) = 0.016$, $p = 0.9$, $\eta^2 = 0.001$. The attentional load by block-order interaction was nonsignificant, $F(3,75) = 0.055$, $p = 0.983$, $\eta^2 = 0.002$, as was the electrode site by block-order interaction, $F(2,50) = 2.259$, $p = 0.115$, $\eta^2 = 0.083$, the attentional load by electrode site interaction, $F(6,150) = 0.311$, $p = 0.93$, $\eta^2 = 0.012$, and the three-way interaction between attentional load, electrode site, and block-order, $F(6,150) = 1.354$, $p = 0.237$, $\eta^2 = 0.051$.

Similar results were obtained from the RM-ANOVA performed to determine whether an effect of attentional load and electrode-site, with block-order as a between-subjects factor, existed for the latency of the P200. There was no main effect of attentional load, $F(3,75) = 2.066$, $p = 0.112$, $\eta^2 = 0.076$, no main effect of electrode site, $F(2,50) = 0.991$, $p = 0.378$, $\eta^2 = 0.038$, and no main effect of block-order $F(1,25) = 1.181$, $p = 0.288$, $\eta^2 = 0.045$. Furthermore, the attentional load by block-order interaction was not significant, $F(3,75) = 1.294$, $p = 0.283$, $\eta^2 = 0.049$, as was the electrode site by

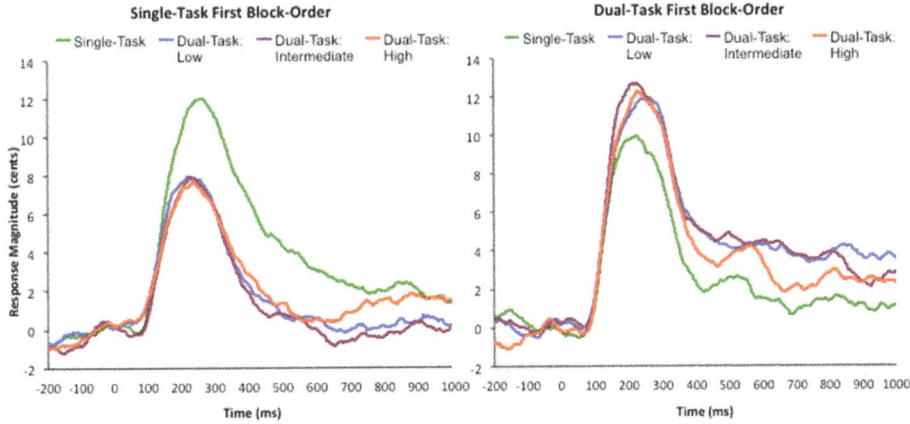

Figure 5. Block-order specific F_0 traces for each attentional load condition. Left: single-task first block-order; averaged F_0 traces for the single-task, and dual-task low, intermediate, and high attentional load conditions. Right: dual-task first block-order; averaged F_0 traces for the single-task, and dual-task low, intermediate, and high attentional load conditions. Time zero on both graphs represents the onset of the feedback perturbation.

block-order interaction, $F(2,50) = 0.204$, $p = 0.816$, $\eta^2 = 0.008$, the attentional load by electrode site interaction, $F(6,150) = 0.369$, $p = 0.898$, $\eta^2 = 0.015$, and the interaction between attentional load, electrode site, and block-order, $F(6,150) = 0.802$, $p = 0.57$, $\eta^2 = 0.031$.

Discussion

The aim of this study was to investigate whether increases in attentional load modulate vocal and neural responses to FAF perturbations. Participants produced vocalizations while exposed to FAF in both single and dual-task conditions. To manipulate participants' attentional load, participants produced vocalizations while they either passively viewed a RSVP of letters, or while they attended to a RSVP of letters that was either presented at a low, intermediate, or high rate, in order to later identify target stimuli. A main effect of attentional load on both white letter identification accuracy, and "X"-placement accuracy was found, as target

identification was better following the dual-task low and dual-task intermediate attentional load trials, relative to the dual-task high attentional load trials. These results suggest that the participants' attentional load was successfully manipulated by increasing the stimulus presentation rate. Despite the differences in accuracy found across the different presentation rates, even in the highest attentional load condition participants accurately identified the white letter 87.5% of the time, while the "X"-placement was correctly identified 78.2% of the time. The high level of accuracy found even in the most attentionally demanding condition, suggests that while the attentional load manipulation was successful, participants were still able to maintain a high level of performance.

Examination of speakers' compensatory responses to the brief FAF perturbations revealed that vocal response magnitudes were modulated by an attentional load by block order interaction. Participants who were exposed to the single-task condition, prior

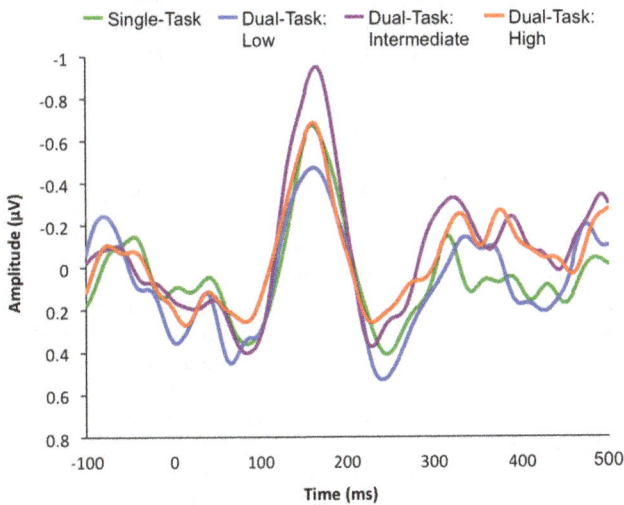

Figure 6. ERP waveforms averaged across all electrode sites for each attentional load condition. The six averaged electrode sites are: F3, C3, Fz, Cz, F4 and C4. Time zero represents the onset of the feedback perturbation.

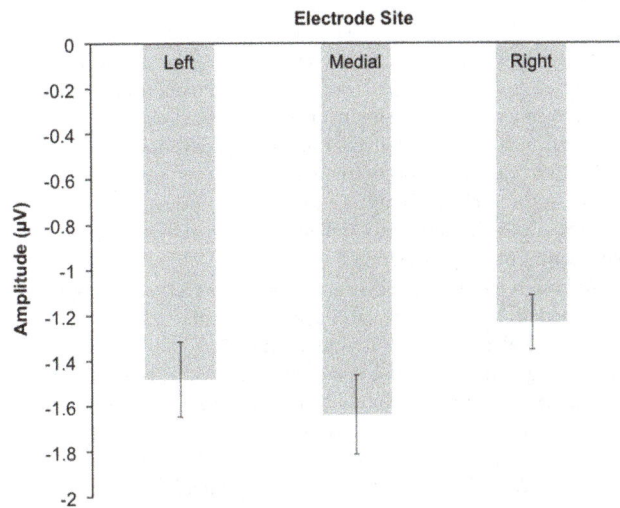

Figure 7. Mean N1 amplitudes for the each electrode site. The left electrode site is the average of the F3 and C3 electrodes; the medial electrode site is the average of the Fz and Cz electrodes; and right electrode site is the average of the F4 and C4 electrodes. Error bars represent standard error.

to the dual-task condition, produced larger vocal responses in the single-task condition, relative to the dual-task condition. However, participants who were exposed to the dual-task condition, prior to the single-task condition, produced similar vocal responses in both conditions. This interaction suggests that when participants completed the single-task prior to the dual-task, they were able to passively view the visual stream during the single-task, with sufficient attentional resources remaining to monitor their auditory feedback and correct for production errors. In contrast, when attentional resources were then split between the vocalization task and the target identification task, fewer attentional resources were available for participants to monitor their auditory feedback, resulting in smaller vocal responses. Although divided attention modulated responses to FAF when the single-task condition occurred prior to the dual-task condition, this was not the case when the dual-task condition occurred prior to the single-task condition. When the dual-task condition was completed prior to the single-task condition, vocal responses in the single-task condition were no different than those in the dual-task condition. We suggest that when participants were exposed to the dual-task, prior to the single-task, the single-task demanded more attentional resources as participants were unable to passively view the visual stream. Previous research has shown that extensive and consistent training on a task can lead to automatic processing of stimuli [37]. We suggest that after exposure to the dual-task, despite no longer being required to identify the target stimuli, participants continued to actively monitor the visual stream for targets, which resulted in fewer attentional resources for monitoring their auditory feedback. As a result, both the single-task and the dual-task resulted in divided attention, making vocal responses across these conditions indistinguishable. Although there was no effect of divided attention when the dual-task occurred first, the fact that vocal responses were larger in the single-task condition, when the single-task occurred first, suggests that divided attention modulates vocal responses to FAF.

The results of this study suggest that when attention is divided, smaller vocal responses to FAF are produced. One possible explanation for these smaller responses is that under divided attention auditory feedback is less salient. Previous research has shown that under visual attentional load, the loudness of tones is attenuated by 7 dB [38], which may be a consequence of reduced cochlear sensitivity [39], or decreased activation of the auditory cortex (e.g., Johnson & Zatorre, [40]). Furthermore, focused attention to an auditory channel has been associated with a 10 dB increase in loudness relative to an unattended auditory channel [25]. If divided attention decreased participants' perception of the loudness of their auditory feedback, it is likely that the FAF perturbations became less salient, which resulted in smaller compensatory responses.

Although the size of the vocal responses to FAF were modulated by divided attention, vocal response latencies were not. We hypothesized that increasing attentional load would increase the processing demands of the visual task, and reduce the amount of attentional resources allocated to the processing of auditory feedback, resulting in later vocal responses. Although it is possible that vocal response latency is not affected by divided attention, it is also possible that the attentional load manipulation was not strong enough to affect the vocal response latencies recorded in this study. As previously mentioned, response accuracy was quite high, even for the highest level of attention load. This being said, while it appears as though attention can be divided without influencing the timing of vocal responses, this may not be the case in situations where attentional resources are more heavily taxed.

Divided attention resulted in the modulation of compensatory vocal responses to FAF; however, divided attention did not modulate the amplitude or latency of the P1-N1-P2 ERP components elicited by the FAF in this study. Although vocal responses were smaller under divided attention, they were still produced. This suggests that the FAF perturbations were detected by the auditory system in both the single- and dual-task conditions. Based on these results, we suggest that the effect of attentional load was not on the auditory processing of FAF, but instead it interfered with the integration of auditory and motor information, or motor control itself. It has previously been suggested that speech motor control may be disrupted under divided attention. For example, when participants were required to read sentences while also completing a secondary motor task, divided attention resulted in decreased displacement and velocity of labial movements [41], as well as increased sound pressure level [42]. Together with the results of this study, these findings suggest that speech motor control is susceptible to divided attention.

Even though divided attention was not found to modulate ERP responses to FAF, the amplitude of the N1 component was found to vary as a function of electrode site. N1 amplitudes were smaller (absolute value) at the right electrodes sites, relative to medial electrode sites. This result is unsurprising, as N1 responses elicited by FAF are generally largest at medial sites [18,22].

Much like the size of the ERPs elicited by the FAF perturbations, and the vocal response latencies, the latencies of the ERP components were not found to differ when attention was divided. We hypothesized that divided attention may result in later ERP latencies as a result of increased processing demands. Although this hypothesis was not confirmed, it is possible that the dual-task condition was not demanding enough to increase processing demands to the extent that ERP latencies were affected. As mentioned previously, even during the most demanding attentional load condition, accuracy was still quite high, thus a more demanding task may be required to produce changes in ERP latencies as a function of attentional load.

Fluent speech production relies on auditory feedback for the regulation of ongoing and future speech motor commands. The aim of the current study was to investigate how attention modulates the processing of auditory feedback during ongoing speech. The results of this study suggest that divided attention can reduce the size of compensatory motor responses to FAF. However, the results of this study also suggest that the P1-N1-P2 ERP components elicited by FAF are less sensitive to divided attention. While the attentional load manipulation utilized in this study was successful at reducing target identification accuracy as the attentional load increased, accuracy was still quite high, even at the highest level of attentional load. With this being said, it is possible that auditory-cortical responses are less sensitive to increases in attention load, but may show attentional modulation if a secondary task is utilized that imposes a higher attentional load. Alternatively, sensorimotor integration, or motor control itself, may be more susceptible to increases in attentional load.

Throughout a typical day, we often encounter situations where we must speak while also performing other tasks. Recently, there has been a focus on assessing the impact of conversation on the performance of secondary tasks such as driving. We instead assessed the impact of divided attention on low level control of speech and found that our ability to use auditory feedback to monitor and regulate our speech may be compromised during many of our daily encounters. While typically developed adults have internal models that can execute fluent speech in a feedforward manner, previous research has suggested that children rely more on auditory feedback [19]. Future research should address how increases in attentional load may modulate sensory-motor integration, and speech motor control in this population, particularly in young children where auditory feedback may be particularly important for acquiring speech [2]. Furthermore, previous research has suggested that individuals who stutter may have an overreliance on auditory feedback [2]. Future research should assess stuttering severity under conditions of divided attention in these individuals, as divided attention may reduce

their reliance on auditory feedback, and help to promote fluent speech.

Author Contributions

Conceived and designed the experiments: JAJ AKT NES. Performed the experiments: AKT NES. Analyzed the data: AKT NES JAJ. Contributed to the writing of the manuscript: AKT NES JAJ.

References

1. Bays PM, Wolpert DM (2006) Computational principles of sensorimotor control that minimize uncertainty and variability. J Physiol 578: 387–396. doi:10.1113/jphysiol.2006.120121.
2. Civier O, Tasko SM, Guenther FH (2010) Overreliance on auditory feedback may lead to sound/syllable repetitions: simulations of stuttering and fluency-inducing conditions with a neural model of speech production. J Fluency Disord 35: 246–279. doi:10.1016/j.jfludis.2010.05.002.
3. Guenther FH (2006) Cortical interactions underlying the production of speech sounds. J Commun Disord 39: 350–365. doi:10.1016/j.jcomdis.2006.06.013.
4. Wickens CD (2002) Multiple resources and performance prediction. Theor. Issues Ergonomics Sci 3: 159–177. doi:10.1080/14639220210123806.
5. Wickens CD (2007) Attention to the second language. IRAL 45. doi:10.1515/iral.2007.008.
6. Ferlazzo F, Couyoumdjian A, Padovani T, Belardinelli MO (2002) Head-centred meridian effect on auditory spatial attention orienting. Q J Exp Psychol-A 55: 937–963. doi:10.1080/02724980143000569.
7. Spence C, Driver J (1996) Audiovisual links in endogenous covert spatial attention. J Exp Psychol Human 22: 1005–1030. doi:10.1037/0096-1523.22.4.1005.
8. Alais D, Morrone C, Burr D (2006) Separate Attentional Resources for Vision and Audition. P Roy Soc B-Biol Sci 273: 1339–1345.
9. Recanzone GH, Schreiner CE, Merzenich MM (1993) Plasticity in the frequency representation of primary auditory cortex following discrimination training in adult owl monkeys. J Neurosci 13: 87–103.
10. Zenger-Landolt B, Heeger DJ (2003) Response Suppression in V1 Agrees with Psychophysics of Surround Masking. J Neurosci 23: 6884–6893.
11. Macdonald JSP, Lavie N (2011) Visual perceptual load induces inattentional deafness. Atten Percept Psychophys 73: 1780–1789. doi:10.3758/s13414-011-0144-4.
12. Waldstein RS (1990) Effects of postlingual deafness on speech production: Implications for the role of auditory feedback. J Acoust Soc Am 88: 2099–2114. doi:10.1121/1.400107.
13. Burnett TA, Senner JE, Larson CR (1997) Voice Fo Responses to Pitch-Shifted Auditory Feedback: A Preliminary Study. J Voice 11: 202–211. doi:10.1016/S0892-1997(97)80079-3.
14. Burnett TA, Freeland MB, Larson CR, Hain TC (1998) Voice F0 responses to manipulations in pitch feedback. J Acoust Soc Am 103: 3153–3161. doi:10.1121/1.423073.
15. Elman JL (1981) Effects of frequency-shifted feedback on the pitch of vocal productions. J Acoust Soc Am 70: 45. doi:10.1121/1.386580.
16. Korzyukov O, Sattler L, Behroozmand R, Larson CR (2012) Neuronal Mechanisms of Voice Control Are Affected by Implicit Expectancy of Externally Triggered Perturbations in Auditory Feedback. PLoS ONE 7: e41216. doi:10.1371/journal.pone.0041216.
17. Liu H, Meshman M, Behroozmand R, Larson CR (2011) Differential effects of perturbation direction and magnitude on the neural processing of voice pitch feedback. Clin Neurophysiol 122: 951–957. doi:10.1016/j.clinph.2010.08.010.
18. Scheerer NE, Behich J, Liu H, Jones JA (2013) ERP correlates of the magnitude of pitch errors detected in the human voice. Neurosci 240: 176–185. doi:10.1016/j.neuroscience.2013.02.054.
19. Scheerer NE, Liu H, Jones JA (2013) The developmental trajectory of vocal and event-related potential responses to frequency-altered auditory feedback. Eur J Neurosci 38: 3189–3200. doi:10.1111/ejn.12301.
20. Hain TC, Burnett TA, Kiran S, Larson CR, Singh S, et al. (2000) Instructing subjects to make a voluntary response reveals the presence of two components to the audio-vocal reflex. Exp Brain Res 130: 133–141. doi:10.1007/s002219900237.
21. Hawco CS, Jones JA (2009) Control of vocalization at utterance onset and mid-utterance: Different mechanisms for different goals. Brain Res 1276: 131–139. doi:10.1016/j.brainres.2009.04.033.
22. Behroozmand R, Karvelis L, Liu H, Larson CR (2009) Vocalization-induced enhancement of the auditory cortex responsiveness during voice F0 feedback perturbation. Clin Neurophysiol 120: 1303–1312. doi:10.1016/j.clinph.2009.04.022.
23. Näätänen R (1991) The role of attention in auditory information-processing as revealed by event-related potentials and other brain measures of cognitive function. Behav Brain Sci 14: 761–761.
24. Behroozmand R, Liu H, Larson CR (2011) Time-dependent Neural Processing of Auditory Feedback during Voice Pitch Error Detection. J Cogn Neurosci 23: 1205–1217. doi:10.1162/jocn.2010.21447.
25. Choi I, Rajaram S, Varghese LA, Shinn-Cunningham BG (2013) Quantifying attentional modulation of auditory-evoked cortical responses from single-trial electroencephalography. Front Hum Neurosci 7. doi:10.3389/fnhum.2013.00115.
26. Coch D, Skendzel W, Neville HJ (2005) Auditory and visual refractory period effects in children and adults: An ERP study. Clin Neurophysiol 116: 2184–2203. doi:10.1016/j.clinph.2005.06.005.
27. Hillyard SA, Hink RF, Schwent VL, Picton TW (1973) Electrical Signs of Selective Attention in the Human Brain. Science 182: 177–180.
28. Hink RF, Hillyard SA, Benson PJ (1978) Event-related brain potentials and selective attention to acoustic and phonetic cues. Biol Psychol 6: 1–16. doi:10.1016/0301-0511(78)90002-9.
29. Hink RF, Van Voorhis ST, Hillyard SA, Smith TS (1977) The division of attention and the human auditory evoked potential. Neuropsychologia 15: 597–605. doi:10.1016/0028-3932(77)90065-3.
30. Parasuraman R (1980) Effects of information processing demands on slow negative shift latencies and N100 amplitude in selective and divided attention. Biol Psychol 11: 217–233. doi:10.1016/0301-0511(80)90057-5.
31. Chun MM, Wolfe JM (2008) Visual Attention. In B. Goldstein (Ed.), Blackwell Handbook of Perception. Oxford, UK: Blackwell Publishers Ltd. 272–310.
32. Lavie N, Hirst A, De Fockert JW (2004) Load theory of selective attention and cognitive control. J Exp Psychol 133: 339–354.
33. Camacho A, Harris JG (2007) Computing pitch of speech and music using a sawtooth waveform inspired pitch estimator. J Acoust Soc Am 122: 2960–2961. doi:10.1121/1.2942550.
34. Ferree TC, Luu P, Russell GS, Tucker DM (2001) Scalp electrode impedance, infection risk, and EEG data quality. Clin Neurophysiol 112: 536–544. doi:10.1016/S1388-2457(00)00533-2.
35. Chen Z, Chen X, Liu P, Huang D, Liu H (2012) Effect of temporal predictability on the neural processing of self-triggered auditory stimulation during vocalization. BMC Neurosci 13: 1–10. doi:10.1186/1471-2202-13-55.
36. Greenhouse SW, Geisser S (1959) On methods in the analysis of profile data. Psychometrika 24: 95–112. doi:10.1007/BF02289823.
37. Schneider W (2003) Controlled & automatic processing: behavior, theory, and biological mechanisms. Cognitive Sci 27: 525–559. doi:10.1016/S0364-0213(03)00011-9.
38. Dai H (1991) Effective attenuation of signals in noise under focused attention. J Acoust Soc Am 89: 2893. doi:10.1121/1.400721.
39. Delano PH, Elgueda D, Hamame CM, Robles L (2007) Selective Attention to Visual Stimuli Reduces Cochlear Sensitivity in Chinchillas. J Neurosci 27: 4146–4153. doi:10.1523/JNEUROSCI.3702-06.2007.
40. Johnson JA, Zatorre RJ (2005) Attention to Simultaneous Unrelated Auditory and Visual Events: Behavioral and Neural Correlates. Cereb Cortex 15: 1609–1620. doi:10.1093/cercor/bhi039.
41. Dromey C, Benson A (2003) Effects of Concurrent Motor, Linguistic, or Cognitive Tasks on Speech Motor Performance. J Speech Lang Hear Res 46: 1234–1246. doi:10.1044/1092-4388(2003/096).
42. Dromey C, Shim E (2008) The Effects of Divided Attention on Speech Motor, Verbal Fluency, and Manual Task Performance. J Speech Lang Hear Res 51: 1171–1182. doi:10.1044/1092-4388(2008/06-0221).

19

Reproducibility of Functional Connectivity and Graph Measures based on the Phase Lag Index (PLI) and Weighted Phase Lag Index (wPLI) Derived from High Resolution EEG

Martin Hardmeier[1], Florian Hatz[1], Habib Bousleiman[1,2], Christian Schindler[2], Cornelis Jan Stam[3], Peter Fuhr[1]*

1 Department of Neurology, Hospital of the University of Basel, Basel, Switzerland, 2 Swiss Tropical and Public Health Institute, University of Basel, Basel, Switzerland, 3 Department of Clinical Neurophysiology and Magnetoencephalography, VU University Medical Center, Amsterdam, The Netherlands

Abstract

Functional connectivity (FC) and graph measures provide powerful means to analyze complex networks. The current study determines the inter-subject-variability using the coefficient of variation (CoV) and long-term test-retest-reliability (TRT) using the intra-class correlation coefficient (ICC) in 44 healthy subjects with 35 having a follow-up at years 1 and 2. FC was estimated from 256-channel-EEG by the phase-lag-index (PLI) and weighted PLI (wPLI) during an eyes-closed resting state condition. PLI quantifies the asymmetry of the distribution of instantaneous phase differences of two time-series and signifies, whether a consistent non-zero phase lag exists. WPLI extends the PLI by additionally accounting for the magnitude of the phase difference. Signal-space global and regional PLI/wPLI and weighted first-order graph measures, i.e. normalized clustering coefficient (gamma), normalized average path length (lambda), and the small-world-index (SWI) were calculated for theta-, alpha1-, alpha2- and beta-frequency bands. Inter-subject variability of global PLI was low to moderate over frequency bands ($0.12<CoV<0.28$), higher for wPLI ($0.25<CoV<0.55$) and very low for gamma, lambda and SWI ($CoV<0.048$). TRT was good to excellent for global PLI/wPLI ($0.68<ICC<0.80$), regional PLI/wPLI ($0.58<ICC<0.77$), and fair to good for graph measures ($0.32<ICC<0.73$) except wPLI-based lambda in alpha1 ($ICC=0.12$). Inter-electrode distance correlated very weakly with inter-electrode PLI ($-0.06<rho<0$) and weakly with inter-electrode wPLI ($-0.22<rho<-0.18$). Global PLI/wPLI and topographic connectivity patterns differed between frequency bands, and all individual networks showed a small-world-configuration. PLI/wPLI based network characterization derived from high-resolution EEG has apparently good reliability, which is one important requirement for longitudinal studies exploring the effects of chronic brain diseases over several years.

Editor: Lawrence M. Ward, University of British Columbia, Canada

Funding: The study has been supported by the Swiss National Science Foundation (grants 33CM30_124115, 326030_128775 and 33CM30_140338), Novartis Research Foundation (grant 09B35), and the Swiss Multiple Sclerosis Society. The funders had no role in study design, data collection and analysis, decision to publish, or preparation of the manuscript.

* Email: peter.fuhr@usb.ch

Introduction

Functional connectivity (FC), graph and nodal network measures are powerful tools to characterize brain function in healthy subjects as well as in neurological and psychiatric diseases [1,2,3]. Based on the concept of the brain as a large complex network of interconnected elements [4], different brain regions interact in the resting state as well as in response to a stimulus or task by synchronization of oscillatory activity [5,6]. Besides structural and functional MRI, magneto- and electro-encephalography (MEG/EEG) have been used to determine FC [7,8].

Scalp signals of EEG are an admix of source activity, volume conduction, i.e. the spatial spread of the electric field during its way from its source through the cerebro-spinal fluid and skull [9], and the influence of the reference electrode [10]. These latter two properties may artificially induce FC as the same signal is measured at different electrodes [11]. In order to circumvent these problems, measures as the imaginary coherence [11] and the phase-lag-index (PLI) [8] have been proposed. The FC estimation by the PLI is based on a consistent lag between the instantaneous phases of two electrodes and is less sensitive to zero-lag phase-relations typical for common sources. The weighted PLI (wPLI) is an extension to the PLI and is reported to be less sensitive to noise [12].

Graph theory provides metrics to characterize complex networks [2,13]. Based on the functional connectivity matrix, indices of functional segregation and integration have been established [14]. Two basic measures are the clustering coefficient describing the connectedness of direct neighbors of a node and the minimum path length describing the average minimal distance of a node to all other nodes in the network. The ratio between the mean normalized clustering coefficient and mean normalized path length indicates whether a network displays an efficient small-world-configuration; i.e. a combination of high local connectedness and short paths to all other nodes in the network minimizing costs for information processing [15].

In order to be useful for characterizing disease states and for capturing disease progression, FC estimates and graph measures should have low inter-subject variability and high test-retest-reliability (TRT) in healthy controls. Only few studies reported on these properties so far, mainly at short-term retest intervals of several weeks. Using MEG and mutual information (MI) as the measure of FC, Deuker et al. [16] reported good TRT for FC and moderate to good TRT for graph measures in the delta to beta-band during an n-back task and considerably lower TRT during an eyes-open resting state condition. Also using MEG and MI, Jin et al. [17] found moderate to good TRT for nodal network measures in eyes-open and eyes-closed resting state, respectively.

The current study reports on the inter-subject variability and long-term test-retest-reliability of the PLI and the wPLI (PLI/wPLI) derived from high-resolution eyes-closed resting state EEG and of first-order graph measures in the signal-space. Additionally, the relation between inter-electrode distance and PLI/wPLI is explored to empirically probe susceptibility to volume conduction; furthermore, the PLI/wPLI connectomes are displayed.

Material and Methods

Subjects

The study was approved by the local ethics committee (Ethikkommission beider Basel, Basel; Switzerland; EK 74/09), and all participants gave written informed consent before study inclusion. At baseline, 48 healthy subjects (median age: 36.0 years, range: 20.0–49.5; female: 73%) were examined. Inclusion criteria comprised unremarkable personal history, normal neurological exam and an EEG-recording without pathological alterations as judged from clinical EEG reading; no concurrent medical treatment was allowed. Four subjects had to be excluded from analysis due to artifactual or low-voltage EEG signal. Thirty-five subjects had a follow-up after one and two years with technically satisfying EEGs.

EEG recording

Subjects were seated comfortably in a reclining chair in a dimly lit, sound attenuated and electromagnetically shielded room. They were instructed to relax, but to stay awake and to minimize eye and body movements. A continuous EEG during an eyes-closed resting state condition was recorded for 12 min with a 256-channel EEG system (Netstation 200 with HydroCel Geodesic Sensor Net, Electrical Geodesics, Inc., Oregon, USA). The electrode net was placed with Fz, Cz, Oz, and the preauricular points as landmarks. Electrode impedances were kept below 40 kOhm. Recording band-pass was 0.1–100 Hz, sampling frequency 1 kHz, and the vertex was used as the recording reference. During data acquisition, a subset of electrodes was monitored online to check for vigilance and artifacts by a technician. Inter-electrode distances were calculated based on a template electrodes cap with dimensions 15.3×19.5×19.3 cm.

EEG processing

Several semi-automated, visually controlled pre-processing steps were employed using customized MATLAB code optimized for

epoch selection in resting-state EEG (TAPEEG, https://sites.google.com/site/tapeeg/[18]). In brief, all EEG were first visually inspected by an experienced neurophysiologist (MH) and segments of 25 to 200 sec containing the least amount of artifacts and sleepiness were selected. Data of 214 electrodes (excluding cheek and neck electrodes) were filtered (0.5–70 Hz; high order least-squares filter) and automatic detection of bad channels using Faster- and Fieldtrip-algorithms [19,20] was applied (median number of interpolated channels per subject: 1, range: 0–3). Thereafter, the EEG was decomposed by independent component analysis (EEGLAB; [21]) and reconstructed after excluding components loading on the electro-cardiogramm, line noise in single electrodes or single gross artifacts; at maximum 5% of components were excluded. For epoch selection, the EEG was re-referenced to average reference, bad channels were interpolated using spherical splines [22] and a combined segment of at least 120 sec length was created; at intersections an inverse hanning window was applied. By a second visual inspection, remaining periods of drowsiness and artifacts as well as intersections were labeled as "bad". Finally, an automatic epoch selection was performed in which one second periods labeled as "bad" (manually or by algorithm) had a very low probability to be included into a final epoch. Based on previous results, twelve 4-sec-epochs were used for further analysis, as they have been shown to be more reliable than four 12-second-epochs of identical total length in the same dataset [23].

Measures of functional connectivity

The phase-lag-index (PLI; [8]) and the weighted PLI (wPLI; [12]) were used as measures of functional connectivity and were calculated using TAPEEG [18]. Shortly, the PLI is an index of the asymmetry in the distribution of phase differences calculated from the instantaneous phases of two time-series, here the signal of a pair of electrodes:

$$PLI = |\langle sign[\sin(\Delta\varphi(tk))]\rangle| \qquad (1)$$

$\Delta\Phi$ is the phase difference at time-point k between two time series and is determined for all time-points (k = 1 ... N) per epoch (N = 4096), sign stands for signum function, <> denotes the mean value and || indicates the absolute value. Instantaneous phases were determined by the Hilbert transformation, applying a Hanning window on the concurrent fast Fourier transform. PLI ranges between 0 and 1. Common sources as volume conduction and the reference electrode do not generate a phase-lag between the time-series of two electrodes, thus phase differences center around 0 or +/− π, resulting in a PLI near or equaling 0; time-series without coupling ("noise") generate a symmetric uniform phase distribution also resulting in a PLI near or equaling 0. In contrast, a consistent phase-lag between two time-series generates an asymmetric distribution of phase differences reflecting true interactions, and a completely asymmetric distribution results in a PLI of 1.

The wPLI is an extension of the PLI [12]. By weighing each phase difference according to the magnitude of the lag, phase differences around zero only marginally contribute to the calculation of the wPLI. This procedure reduces the probability of detecting "false positive" connectivity in the case of volume conducted noise sources with near zero phase lag and increases the sensitivity in detecting phase synchronization [12].Weighing is achieved by using the imaginary component of the cross-spectra as a factor. We employ here the debiased wPLI estimator according to formulas 26 and 32 in Vinck et al. [12].

For further analysis, PLI/wPLI was first calculated for each pair of electrodes per epoch based on N = 4096 phase difference vectors, thereafter twelve replicates were averaged to generate the average PLI/wPLI weight matrix per subject.

Analysis was done on a global and on a regional level of spatial resolution. Global PLI/wPLI equals the average of all PLI/wPLI values of the average weight matrix per subject. Regional PLI/wPLI is based on 22 anatomically defined regions comprising 7 or 8 electrodes (n = 170, excluding electrodes in the midline and at the outer border, see Figure S1). For each region, the average connectivity of all its electrodes to all other regional groups of electrodes was determined, i.e. the regional degree (row average of respective electrodes of the weight matrix). In addition, the connectivity between each two regions was calculated (average over cells of the weight matrix belonging to respective electrodes of two regions) resulting in n = 231 links. For correlation to distance, PLI/wPLI values of pairs of electrodes and their respective inter-electrode distances were used. To display the connectomes, the grand means over all average PLI/wPLI weight matrices at baseline were plotted. PLI/wPLI was calculated for the theta-(4–8 Hz), alpha1-(8–10 Hz), alpha2-(10–13 Hz) and beta-(13–30 Hz) band using a butterworth bandpass-filter.

Graph measures

Graph measures were calculated based on the average PLI/wPLI weight matrix of the twelve epochs per subject in each frequency band (n = 214 nodes). Regional weight matrices (n = 22 nodes) were not used, as it is disputable whether graph measures in small networks are meaningful [24]. Calculation of graph measures on each single epoch weight matrix and subsequent averaging had resulted in lower test-retest reliability (see Table S1). This is probably due to the fact that averaging the single epoch weight matrices diminishes momentary connectivity patterns and spurious connectivity due to noise resulting in the individual "core" connectivity. However, momentary connectivity patterns and subsequent network characterization by graph measures may show different aspects than the network characterization based on the average connectivity matrix. In order to avoid arbitrary thresholds and unconnected nodes, weighted network analysis was employed in which each edge is equivalent to the measured PLI/wPLI of two interconnected nodes. Undirected measures of functional segregation and integration were calculated according to the definitions given in Stam et al. [25]; respective formulas were implemented in TAPEEG [18].

The weighted clustering coefficient C quantifies the intensities of the subgraphs of a node and is equivalent to the unweighted clustering coefficient normalized by the average intensities of triangles at the node, if the weight matrix is symmetric and weights ranging between 0 and 1 [25,26]. The weighted clustering coefficient at node i is defined as:

$$C_i = \frac{\sum_{k \neq i} \sum_{\substack{l \neq i \\ l \neq k}} W_{ik} W_{il} W_{kl}}{\sum_{k \neq i} \sum_{\substack{l \neq i \\ l \neq k}} W_{ik} W_{il}} \quad (2)$$

in which w is defined as the weight between two nodes. The average over all C_i is the mean clustering coefficient (Cw), a global measure of functional segregation of the network [14,27].

The weighted shortest path length L_{ij} gives the average of the shortest distances of one node to each other node in the network, where shortest distance in the weighted case is defined as the smallest inverse of the sum of PLI values of connecting edges between i and j if w_{ij} unequals zero, and L_{ij} is infinity if w_{ij} equals

zero. The average over all L_{ij} is the weighted average path length (Lw), a global measure of functional integration of the network [14,28] and is defined as:

$$Lw = \frac{1}{\frac{1}{N(N-1)} * \sum_{i=1}^{N} \sum_{j \neq i}^{N} (1/L_{ij})} \quad (3)$$

in which N is defined as the number of nodes in the network. Using the harmonic mean instead of the arithmetic mean handles infinitive path lengths from unconnected nodes [25].

In order to make graph measures independent of network size and better comparable between subjects, they were normalized [25]. Edge weights of an original network were randomly reshuffled preserving network size but destroying network structure, and Cw and Lw were calculated for this random network. Using the average Cw and Lw of 50 surrogate random networks iterated five times in the denominator and Cw and Lw in the nominator, the normalized Cw or *gamma* and the normalized Lw or *lambda* were calculated.

To determine whether networks show a small-world-configuration, the small-world-index (SWI; [29]) was calculated as the ratio between gamma and lambda for each subject. An index >1 signifies efficient small-world topology, i.e. the combination of high local clustering, as typical for regular networks and short path length, as typical for random networks; small-world topology has been shown to be a salient feature of many real-world networks [15] including the human brain [30].

Statistical analysis

Cross-sectional inter-subject variability was expressed as the coefficient of variation (CoV) calculated as the ratio between the standard deviation and the mean of global PLI/wPLI, gamma, lambda and SWI at baseline. TRT over three time points was estimated for the same measures as well as for regional degree and regional links using the intra-class-correlation coefficient (ICC [3,1]; [31]). A bootstrapping procedure with replacements and 10000 permutations was performed to estimate the 95% confidence interval (95% CI) for both indices. In accordance with previous studies, TRT was categorized as "excellent" if ICC> 0.75, as "good" if ICC: 0.60–0.75, as "fair" if ICC: 0.40–0.60 and as "poor" if ICC<0.40 [16,17,32].

Spearman's rank correlation coefficient was used to measure associations between inter-electrode distance and PLI/wPLI within subjects. ANOVAs were used to compare global PLI/wPLI values between frequency bands at baseline and within frequency bands between time points. The topographies of the mean connectivity distribution (connectome) were compared between frequency bands by using the average nodal degree over all subjects at baseline in permutation tests on ANOVA with frequency band as factor. Permutation statistics were used to control for multiple comparisons and non-Gaussian distributions [33].

Results

Inter-subject variability of global PLI was low to moderate over frequency bands (0.12<CoV<0.28; Table 1) and very low for PLI based gamma, lambda and SWI (CoV<0.022, CI 95%: 0.01–0.027). Global wPLI showed higher inter-subject variability (0.25<CoV<0.55, Table 1) but comparable values for wPLI based graph measures (CoV<0.048, CI 95%: 0.012–0.059).

TRT was good to excellent for global PLI over frequency bands (0.68<ICC<0.79), and moderate to good for PLI-based graph

Table 1. Inter-subject variability of global PLI and wPLI at baseline by frequency band expressed by the coefficient of variation (CoV; CI: confidence interval estimated from bootstrapping).

		theta	alpha1	alpha2	beta
PLI		**0.12**	**0.23**	**0.28**	**0.15**
	95% CI	0.08–0.20	0.17–0.31	0.21–0.38	0.12–0.17
wPLI		**0.25**	**0.44**	**0.55**	**0.29**
	95% CI	0.14–0.41	0.33–0.56	0.39–0.76	0.25–0.33

measures (gamma: $0.48 < ICC < 0.65$; lambda: $0.51 < ICC < 0.73$; SWI: $0.33 < ICC < 0.63$; see Table 2). Global wPLI had comparable TRT ($0.70 < ICC < 0.80$) but lower values for wPLI-based graph measures (gamma: $0.43 < ICC < 0.57$; lambda: $0.12 < ICC < 0.47$; SWI: $0.32 < ICC < 0.51$; Table 3).

On the regional level, ICC values are given as medians of the 22 ICC values per regional degrees and 231 ICC-values per interregional links over frequency bands. PLI had good TRT for regional degree ($0.58 < ICC < 0.75$) and fair to good TRT for interregional links ($0.42 < ICC < 0.61$; Table 4). TRT of wPLI were comparable for regional degree ($0.59 < ICC\ 0.77$) and interregional links ($0.41 < ICC < 0.64$; Table 5). Figure S2 and Figure S3 show the topographic distribution of ICC values per frequency band and electrode for PLI/wPLI, respectively.

The correlation of inter-electrode distance with inter-electrode PLI was very weak in all subjects at all frequency bands (median rho over frequency bands: $-0.06 < rho < 0$) with no clear direction, albeit highly significant in single subjects (maximal positive correlation: rho $= 0.15$, maximal negative correlation: rho $= -0.19$; $p < 0.0001$) due to the high number of values (214*213/2 data points per subject). For inter-electrode wPLI, a weak negative correlation to inter-electrode distance was found (median rho over frequency bands: $-0.22 < rho < -0.18$) and in single subjects maximal negative correlation was rho $= -0.4$, maximal positive correlation was rho $= 0.03$, $p < 0.0001$).

Global PLI and wPLI were significantly different between frequency bands at baseline (PLI: $F = 127$, $p < 0.0001$; wPLI: $F = 75$, $p < 0.0001$; Figure 1a and 1b); in post-hoc t-tests, all bands were significantly different to each other ($p < 0.05$ for alpha1 vs. alpha2, $p < 0.0001$ for all other comparisons). Within frequency bands global PLI/wPLI showed no significant differences over time (PLI: $F < 0.45$, $p > 0.5$; wPLI: $F < 0.33$, $p > 0.5$). Topographic connectivity patterns differed significantly between frequency

bands at the single electrode level, i.e. in nodal degree (PLI: $F > 73$, $p_{corrected} < 0.001$; wPLI: $F > 45$, $p_{corrected} < 0.001$; respective connectomes are displayed in Figure 2 and Figure 3 and in Figure S4 and Figure S5 for regional connectomes).

All individual networks showed a small-world-configuration (medians over frequency bands; PLI-based SWI: $1.024 < SWI < 1.029$, range: $1.016 – 1.078$; wPLI-based SWI: $1.053 < rho < 1.069$, range: $1.017 – 1.200$).

Discussion

Characterization of functional connectivity by PLI shows good to excellent long-term test-retest-reliability over two years, and mainly good long-term test-retest-reliability of PLI-based graph measures; inter-subject variability is acceptably low. Functional connectivity determined by the wPLI shows comparable TRT as the PLI, wPLI-based graph measures are slightly less reliable and inter-subject variability is higher. High-resolution EEG is a suitable recording modality when care is taken that the measure of functional connectivity is not relevantly influenced by common sources as volume conduction and the reference electrode. The weak negative correlation between inter-electrode distance and inter-electrode wPLI is presumably due to the weighing factor, as short range connections are more likely to have large consistent phase difference than long range connections; volume conduction defined as zero-lag phase difference is neither detected by PLI nor by wPLI.

Only a few studies report so far on test-retest-reliability of functional connectivity and network measures, mainly at short-term test-retest intervals of several weeks. In fMRI-studies using correlations between BOLD-signal time series to estimate functional connectivity, test-retest-reliability was only moderate in one study [34], and even low to poor in another [32]. Using MEG and

Table 2. Test-retest-reliability of global PLI and PLI-based graph measures over time by frequency band expressed by the intraclass-correlation coefficient (ICC; CI: confidence interval estimated from bootstrapping; SWI: small-world-index).

		theta	alpha1	alpha2	beta
PLI		**0.72**	**0.79**	**0.74**	**0.68**
	95% CI	0.49–0.92	0.69–0.90	0.63–0.87	0.46–0.81
gamma		**0.65**	**0.64**	**0.48**	**0.58**
	95% CI	0.43–0.85	0.39–0.88	0.24–0.67	0.36–0.76
lambda		**0.73**	**0.57**	**0.56**	**0.51**
	95% CI	0.52–0.90	0.23–0.87	0.32–0.73	0.18–0.80
SWI		**0.56**	**0.63**	**0.33**	**0.56**
	95% CI	0.34–0.79	0.40–0.86	0.16–0.60	0.40–0.69

Table 3. Test-retest-reliability of global wPLI and wPLI-based graph measures over time by frequency band expressed by the intraclass-correlation coefficient (ICC; CI: confidence interval estimated from bootstrapping; SWI: small-world-index).

		theta	alpha1	alpha2	beta
wPLI		**0.78**	**0.80**	**0.74**	**0.70**
	95% CI	0.56–0.94	0.69–0.90	0.63–0.88	0.50–0.83
gamma		**0.57**	**0.43**	**0.49**	**0.53**
	95% CI	0.33–0.81	0.14–0.78	0.21–0.70	0.28–0.75
lambda		**0.47**	**0.12**	**0.41**	**0.38**
	95% CI	0.27–0.66	−0.02–0.30	0.14–0.62	0.11–0.64
SWI		**0.49**	**0.50**	**0.32**	**0.51**
	95% CI	0.21–0.75	0.24–0.81	0.11–0.55	0.38–0.65

mutual information as the measure of functional connectivity, Deuker et al. [16] found good test-retest-reliability for FC as well as several global graph measures during an eyes-open n-back task at a test-retest interval of 6–8 weeks. In higher frequency bands (beta- and gamma-band), during eyes-open resting state and in second-order graph measures as for example the small-world-index, the TRT was comparably lower. Using as well MEG and mutual information, Jin et al. [17] reported fair to moderate TRT for different nodal centrality measures at a test-retest-interval of two weeks, which was partly higher in the eyes-open as compared to the eyes-closed resting state, and much lower in the gamma-band.

In the current study, beta-band TRT as well as small-world-index TRT also tends to be lower compared to lower frequency bands and first-order graph-measures, respectively. As pointed out previously this is probably due to the different physiological function as higher frequencies may serve to establish cognitive representation, whereas lower frequency bands are more anatomically constrained [35,36]. The gamma-band has not been studied here due to its sensitivity to muscle artifacts, which partly also applies for the beta-band [37]. The level of spatial resolution on which connectivity is determined influences the TRT with highest TRT on the global level and slightly lower TRT for regional degree. On the level of inter-regional links TRT is highly variable ranging from poor for some links to good and excellent in others. Regional connectivity analysis may, on the one hand, better catch more localized group differences in for example parietal hub regions than global measures, and, on the other hand, is more robust to slight variations of local maxima and outliers in connectivity compared to analyses on the single electrode level.

Several methodological differences may explain the higher TRT of eyes-closed resting state reported in the current study as compared to previous studies. First, MEG mainly picks up signals

from sources within sulci, whereas the EEG-signal is mostly driven by sources on the gyri [38,39]; second, mutual information depicts a different aspect of connectivity than measures based on phase synchronization as the PLI and wPLI [7], and third, the way of band-pass-filtering, bandwidth and the choice of unweighted [16] or weighted networks ([17], current study) may play a critical role.

For chronic brain diseases evolving over years, long-term TRT as shown in the current study for the PLI/wPLI is paramount since ageing may influence networks as well [40,41]. Whether networks constitute a stable trait over many years up to a certain age in analogy to the spectral "fingerprint" of the EEG [42,43] and as suggested by a stable association of genetic features and functional connectivity [44,45] remains to be elucidated. However, in a small group of elderly healthy controls around 60 years, the PLI-based normalized clustering coefficient decreased in the alpha-bands over a four year period, whereas path length and other frequency bands did not change significantly [46].

The current study does not allow conclusions on the validity of the PLI/wPLI and PLI/wPLI-based graph measures derived from EEG with respect to characterization and monitoring of diseases of the central nervous system. Currently it is far from clear how tight measures of functional connectivity, which express a mere statistical interdependency [47], are associated with the known thalamo-cortical and other networks involved in the generation of oscillatory brain activity [36]. In particular the resting state scalp signal is difficult to interpret, albeit several studies have shown a complex relationship between resting state brain oscillations and resting state networks derived from functional MRI [48,49]. However, PLI/wPLI networks show a clear dominance in connectivity in parieto-occipital regions, corresponding to the topography of structural and functional connectomes derived from MRI studies [30,50]. Additionally, they show clear differences between frequency bands as would be expected by the known

Table 4. Test-retest-reliability of regional PLI over time by frequency band.

		theta	alpha1	alpha2	beta
regional degree	median	**0.66**	**0.75**	**0.71**	**0.58**
	range	0.51–0.78	0.57–0.83	0.63–0.76	0.42–0.64
inter-regional links	median	**0.47**	**0.61**	**0.60**	**0.42**
	range	0.08–0.83	0.24–0.85	0.41–0.79	0.01–0.82

The median (range) intraclass-correlation coefficients over 22 regional degrees and 231 inter-regional links are given.

Table 5. Test-retest-reliability of regional wPLI over time by frequency band.

		theta	alpha1	alpha2	beta
regional degree	median	0.71	0.77	0.72	0.59
	range	0.57–0.84	0.60–0.85	0.62–0.78	0.49–0.67
inter-regional links	median	0.53	0.64	0.61	0.41
	range	0.14–0.84	0.23–0.87	0.34–82	0.05–0.79

The median (range) intraclass-correlation coefficients over 22 regional degrees and 231 inter-regional links are given.

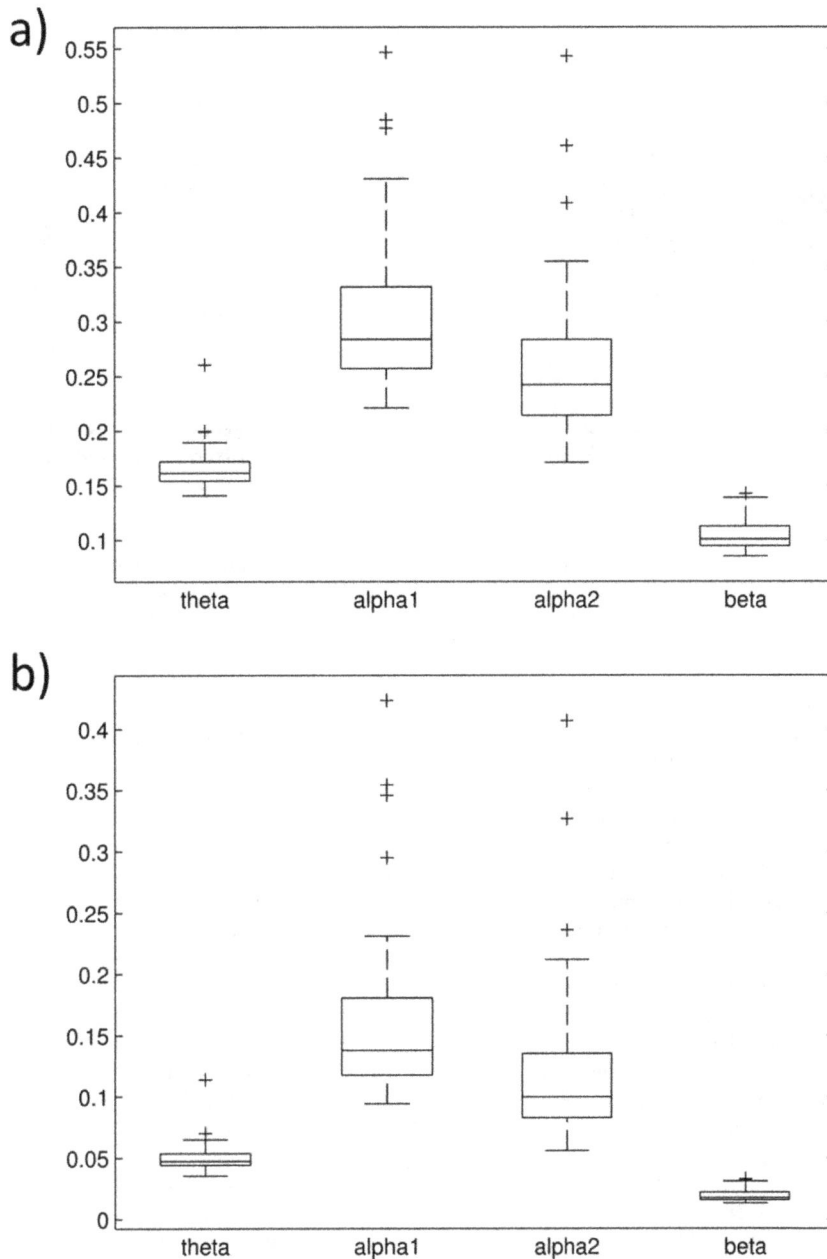

Figure 1. Distribution of a) global PLI values and b) global wPLI values between subjects at baseline in different frequency bands; all bands are significantly different (see text).

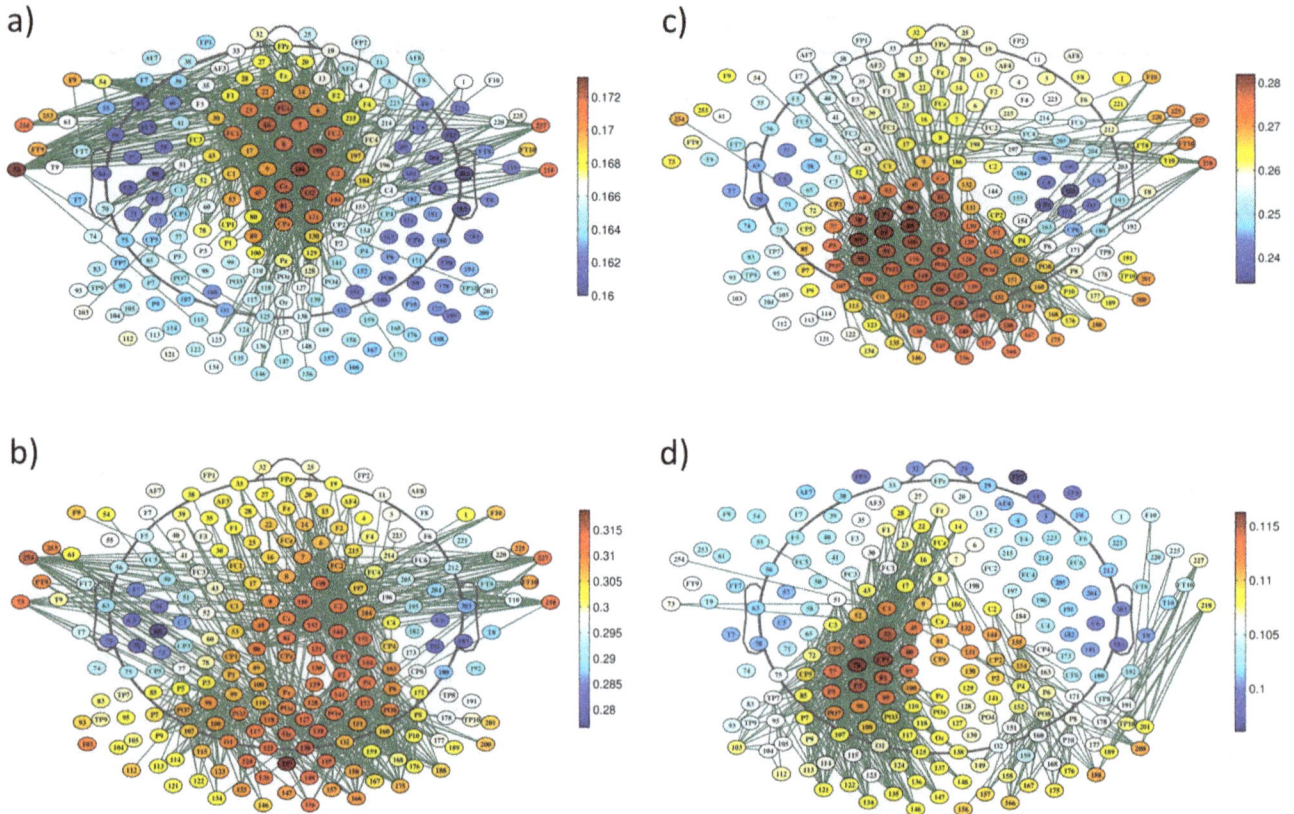

Figure 2. Topographic plots of the grand mean PLI connectomes (green: 3% strongest links are plotted) and grand mean PLI value per electrode (nodal degree, values are color-coded) over all subjects at baseline by frequency band: a) theta, b) alpha1, c) alpha2, d) beta.

physiological differences between frequency bands in spectral analysis [51,52,53,54,55] and as noted in previous MEG studies [17,56]. Smallworldness, a feature apparent in PLI/wPLI-based networks in the current study is more difficult to interpret; in particular as weighted network analysis was used [24]. Furthermore, the concept of smallworldness is challenged by a recent anatomical study [57] and has even been reported to be artificially induced in EEG-model data [58] (see below). However, PLI and PLI-based graph measures have been shown to differentiate between healthy controls and patients with Alzheimer's diseases (AD) [25], Parkinson's disease [46], Multiple Sclerosis [59], and even demonstrated group differences in a clinical trial on a medical food in AD [60]. The wPLI has only been applied in rodent local field potentials showing clear differences in a task related paradigm [12].

Volume conduction is one of the main methodological problems in functional connectivity studies using EEG or MEG [9,11]. The PLI has explicitly been developed to be insensitive to zero-lag phase differences [8], which are a hallmark of volume conduction. In the current study, there was no consistent relation between PLI and inter-electrode distance, confirming robustness against volume conduction. However, using signal modeling Peraza et al. [58] report that volume conduction may influence the PLI when multiple independent sources are present and in turn biases graph measures. The study compared unweighted networks based on 64 uncorrelated sources to networks based on the same sources multiplied by a forward solution to simulate volume conducted scalp signal. Both models were expected to generate random networks but this was not true for the simulated scalp signal and

even small-worldness was found [58]. To reduce such spurious connectivity due to uncorrelated noise, Vinck et al [12] proposed the wPLI. Still, in real data, PLI/wPLI may detect both, physiological and spurious connectivity, in particular on the single subject level. Averaging over epochs reduces noise but is constrained by the availability of a sufficient number of good quality epochs. Applying rigorous ICA filtering by selecting only components of interest harbours the risk to exclude important information systematically. However, given all these caveats, several studies have shown that resting state connectivity and graph measures differ between healthy controls and patients with brain disease [25,46,59,60]. Another relevant limitation of the PLI/wPLI is the downside of its insensitivity to volume conduction: physiological connectivity with zero phase-lag may remain undetected, and thus, PLI/wPLI may underestimate short-range connections and, in terms of networks, local segregation or clustering [56].

The influence of the recording electrode can be greatly diminished by re-referencing to the average of all electrodes when using high-resolution EEG with 128 or more electrodes, as in a closed system the average signal sums up to zero [9]. Another way to deal with common sources would be the reconstruction of the signal in the source space; however, the translation matrix may itself induce artificial functional connectivity [61] and methodology is only going to be developed [56].

Regarding quantification of TRT, the intra-class correlation coefficient is widely used but has been criticized as being susceptible to bias [62,63], as it is only a relative index of reliability and can be inflated by few subjects with high within-

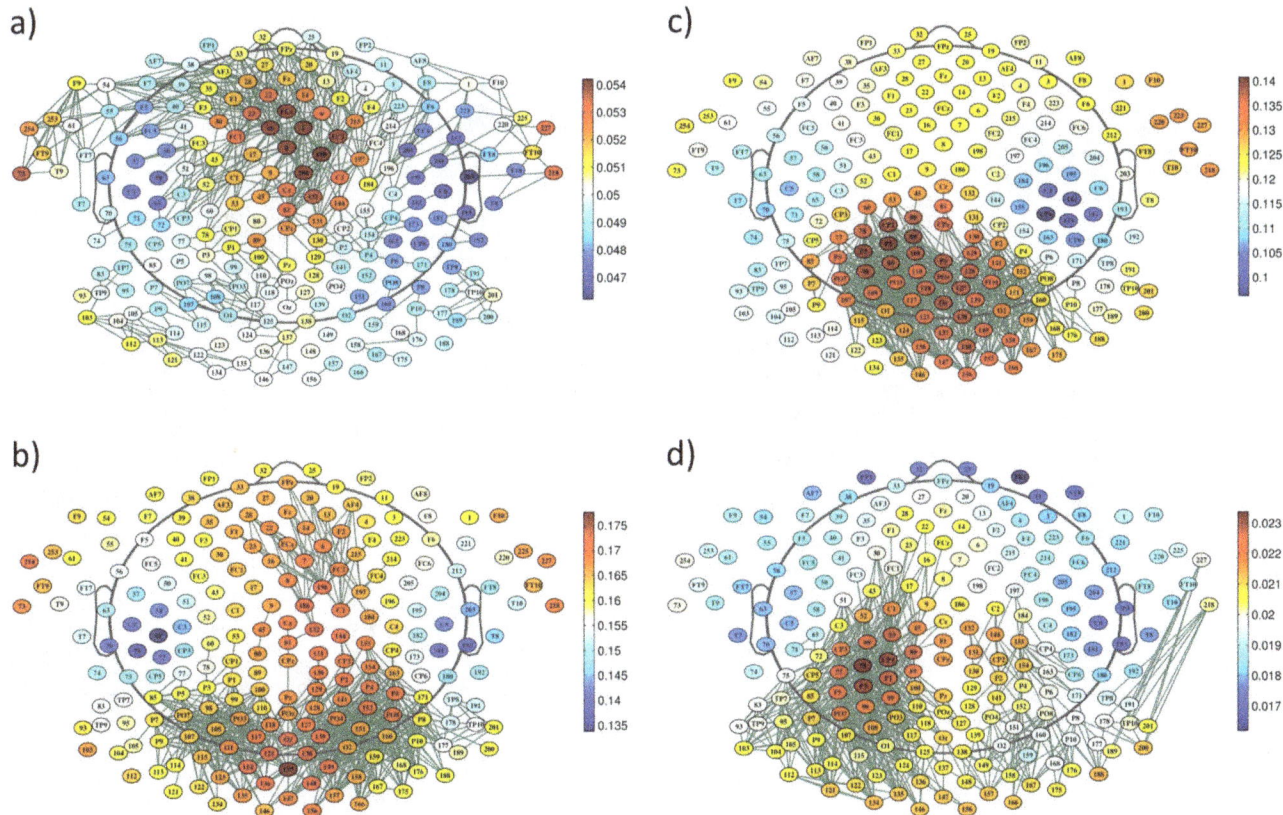

Figure 3. Topographic plots of the grand mean wPLI connectomes (green: as in Figure 2) and grand mean wPLI value per electrode (color-codes as in Figure 2): a) theta, b) alpha1, c) alpha2, d) beta.

subjects variability. Using the bootstrapping technique to estimate 95% confidence intervals, we partly diminished this bias. Still, comparisons to studies not indicating confidence intervals remain difficult, as the ICC-value alone may only be a rough estimate of TRT.

Conclusions

PLI/wPLI based network characterization derived from high-resolution EEG-recordings is apparently reliable over two years on a global and regional level of spatial resolution. Which physiological mechanisms are exactly reflected by these measures in the resting state is currently far from clear, but beyond the scope of the current study. However, good long-term test-retest-reliability is one important requirement for a biomarker. Network characterization may help to explore the effects of chronic disorders on the functional organization of the brain. Long-term TRT in older subjects in whom effects of ageing may have more impact remains to be studied. As high-resolution EEG is widely available and easy to administer data may even be gathered in a multicenter setting, allowing to reach appropriate sample sizes for testing hypotheses on functional reorganization in brain diseases in due time.

Supporting Information

Figure S1   Topography of groups of electrodes used for regional analysis.

Figure S2   Topography of test-retest-reliability (ICC) of mean PLI per electrode (nodal degree).

Figure S3   Topography of test-retest-reliability (ICC) of mean wPLI per electrode (nodal degree).

Figure S4   Connectomes of regional PLI.

Figure S5   Connectomes of regional wPLI.

Table S1   Test-retest-reliability of graph measures calculated in single weight matrices.

Acknowledgments

The authors thank Claudia Baumann, Beatrice Wessner, Darren Hight, Boris Sperisen and the EEG team for technical assistance, and Silke Purschke (Clinical Trial Unit, University Hospital Basel) for assistance in onsite management.

Author Contributions

Conceived and designed the experiments: MH FH CS PF. Performed the experiments: MH FH. Analyzed the data: MH FH HB CS PF. Contributed reagents/materials/analysis tools: CJS FH. Wrote the paper: MH FH HB CS CJS PF.

References

1. Bassett DS, Bullmore ET (2009) Human brain networks in health and disease. Curr Opin Neurol 22: 340–347.

2. Bullmore E, Sporns O (2012) The economy of brain network organization. Nat Rev Neurosci 13: 336–49.

3. Stam CJ, van Straaten EC (2012) The organization of physiological brain networks. Clin Neurophysiol 123: 1067–87.

4. Nunez PL (2010) Brain, mind, and the structure of reality. New York Oxford: Oxford University Press

5. Varela F, Lachaux JP, Rodriguez E, Martinerie J (2001) The brainweb: phase synchronization and large-scale integration. Nat Rev Neurosci 2: 229–39.

6. Fell J, Axmacher N (2011) The role of phase synchronization in memory processes. Nat Rev Neurosci 12: 105–18.

7. David O, Cosmelli D, Friston KJ (2004) Evaluation of different measures of functional connectivity using a neural mass model. Neuroimage 21: 659–73.

8. Stam CJ, Nolte G, Daffertshofer A (2007) Phase lag index: assessment of functional connectivity from multichannel EEG and MEG with diminished bias from common sources. Hum Brain Mapp 28: 1178–93.

9. Nunez PL, Srinivasan R, Westdorp AF, Wijesinghe RS, Tucker DM, et al. (1997) EEG coherency I: statistics, reference electrode, volume conduction, Laplacians, cortical imaging, and interpretation at multiple scales. Electroenceph Clin Neurophysiol 103: 499–515.

10. Guevara R, Velazquez JL, Nenadovic V, Wennberg R, Senjanovic G, et al. (2005) Phase synchronization measurements using electroencephalographic recordings: what can we really say about neuronal synchrony? Neuroinformatics 3: 301–14.

11. Nolte G, Bai O, Wheaton L, Mari Z, Vorbach S, et al. (2004) Identifying true brain interaction from EEG data using the imaginary part of coherency. Clin Neurophysiol 115: 2292–307.

12. Vinck M, Oostenveld R, van Wingerden M, Battaglia F, Pennartz CM (2011) An improved index of phase-synchronization for electrophysiological data in the presence of volume-conduction, noise and sample-size bias. Neuroimage 55: 1548–65.

13. Bullmore E, Sporns O (2009) Complex brain networks: graph theoretical analysis of structural and functional systems. Nat Rev Neurosci 10: 186–198.

14. Rubinov M, Sporns O (2010) Complex network measures of brain connectivity: uses and interpretations. Neuroimage 52: 1059–69.

15. Watts DJ, Strogatz SH (1998) Collective dynamics of 'small-world' networks. Nature 393: 440–442.

16. Deuker L, Bullmore ET, Smith M, Christensen S, Nathan PJ, et al. (2009) Reproducibility of graph metrics of human brain functional networks. Neuroimage 47: 1460–8.

17. Jin SH, Seol J, Kim JS, Chung CK (2011) How reliable are the functional connectivity networks of MEG in resting states? J Neurophysiol 106: 2888–95.

18. Hatz F, Hardmeier M, Bousleiman H, Rueegg S, Schindler C, et al. (2014) Reliability of fully automated versus visually controlled pre- and post-processing of resting-state EEG. Clin Neurophysiol Epub ahead of print.

19. Nolan H, Whelan R, Reilly RB (2010) FASTER: Fully Automated Statistical Thresholding for EEG artifact Rejection. J Neurosci Methods 192: 152–62.

20. Oostenveld R, Fries P, Maris E, Schoffelen JM (2011) FieldTrip: Open source software for advanced analysis of MEG, EEG, and invasive electrophysiological data. Comput Intell Neurosci 2011: 156869.

21. Delorme A, Makeig S (2004) EEGLAB: an open source toolbox for analysis of single-trial EEG dynamics including independent component analysis. J Neurosci Methods 134: 9–21.

22. Perrin F, Pernier J, Bertrand O, Echallier JF (1989) Spherical splines for scalp potential and current density mapping. Electroencephalogr Clin Neurophysiol 72: 184–189.

23. Hardmeier M, Hatz F, Bousleiman H, Schindler C, Stam CJ, et al. (2014) Test-retest reliability and inter-subject variability of the Phase Lag Index (PLI), a measure of functional connectivity in EEG analysis. Poster ICCN, Berlin 2014; Clin Neurophysiol 125:S56–S57.

24. van Wijk BC, Stam CJ, Daffertshofer A (2010) Comparing brain networks of different size and connectivity density using graph theory. PLoS One 5:e13701.

25. Stam CJ, de Haan W, Daffertshofer A, Jones BF, Manshanden I, et al. (2009) Graph theoretical analysis of magnetoencephalographic functional connectivity in Alzheimer's disease. Brain 132: 213–24.

26. Onnela JP, Saramaki J, Kertesz J, Kaski K (2005) Intensity and coherence of motifs in weighted complex networks. Phys Rev E Stat Nonlinear Soft Matter Phys 71: 065103

27. Newman ME (2003) Properties of highly clustered networks. Phys Rev E Stat Nonlin Soft Matter Phys 68: 026121.

28. Latora V, Marchiori M (2001) Efficient behavior of small-world networks. Phys Rev Lett 87: 198701.

29. Humphries MD, Gurney K (2008) Network 'small-world-ness': a quantitative method for determining canonical network equivalence. PLoS One 3: e0002051.

30. Hagmann P, Cammoun L, Gigandet X, Meuli R, Honey CJ, et al. (2008) Mapping the structural core of human cerebral cortex. PLoS Biol 6: e159.

31. Shrout PE, Fleiss JL (1979) Intraclass correlations: uses in assessing rater reliability. Psychol Bull 86: 420–428.

32. Wang JH, Zuo XN, Gohel S, Milham MP, Biswal BB, et al. (2011) Graph theoretical analysis of functional brain networks: test-retest evaluation on short- and long-term resting-state functional MRI data. PLoS One 6: e21976.

33. Nichols TE, Holmes AP (2001) Nonparametric Permutation Tests For Functional Neuroimaging: A Primer with Examples. Hum Brain Mapp 15: 1–25.

34. Braun U, Plichta MM, Esslinger C, Sauer C, Haddad L, et al. (2012) Test-retest reliability of resting-state connectivity network characteristics using fMRI and graph theoretical measures. Neuroimage 59: 1404–12.

35. Bassett DS, Bullmore E (2006) Small-world brain networks. Neuroscientist 12: 512–23.

36. Lopes da Silva F (2013) EEG and MEG: relevance to neuroscience. Neuron 80: 1112–28.

37. Whitham EM, Pope KJ, Fitzgibbon SP, Lewis T, Clark CR, et al. (2007) Scalp electrical recording during paralysis: quantitative evidence that EEG frequencies above 20 Hz are contaminated by EMG. Clin Neurophysiol 118: 1877–88.

38. Malmivuo J (2012) Comparison of the properties of EEG and MEG in detecting the electric activity of the brain. Brain Topogr 25: 1–19.

39. Okada Y, Lähteenmäki A, Xu C (1999) Comparison of MEG and EEG on the basis of somatic evoked responses elicited by stimulation of the snout in the juvenile swine. Clin Neurophysiol 110: 214–29.

40. Gong G, Rosa-Neto P, Carbonell F, Chen ZJ, He Y, et al. (2009) Age- and gender related differences in the cortical anatomical network. J Neurosci 29: 15684–15693.

41. Meunier D, Stamatakis EA, Tyler LK (2014) Age-related functional reorganization, structural changes, and preserved cognition. Neurobiol Aging 35: 42–54.

42. Kondacs A, Szabo M (1999) Long-term intra-individual variability of the background EEG in normal. Clin Neurophysiol 110: 170–1716.

43. Napflin M, Wildi M, Sarnthein J (2007) Test–retest reliability of resting EEG spectra validates a statistical signature of persons. Clin Neurophysiol 118: 2519–2524.

44. Smit DJA, Stam CJ, Posthuma D, Boomsma DI, de Geus EJC (2008) Heritability of "Small-World" Networks in the Brain: A Graph Theoretical Analysis of Resting-State EEG Functional Connectivity; Hum Brain Mapp 29: 1368–1378.

45. Schutte NM, Hansell NK, de Geus EJ, Martin NG, Wright MJ, et al. (2013) Heritability of resting state EEG functional connectivity patterns. Twin Res Hum Genet 16: 962–9.

46. Olde Dubbelink KT, Hillebrand A, Stoffers D, Deijen JB, Twisk JW, et al. (2014) Disrupted brain network topology in Parkinson's disease: a longitudinal magnetoencephalography study. Brain 137: 197–207.

47. Friston KJ (1994) Functional and effective connectivity in neuroimaging: A synthesis. Hum Brain Mapp 2: 56–78.

48. Mantini D, Perrucci MG, Del Gratta C, Romani GL, Corbetta M (2007) Electrophysiological signatures of resting state networks in the human brain. Proc Natl Acad Sci 104: 13170–5.

49. Laufs H (2008) Endogenous brain oscillations and related networks detected by surface EEG-combined fMRI. Hum Brain Mapp 29: 762–9.

50. Honey CJ, Sporns O, Cammoun L, Gigandet X, Thiran JP, et al. (2009) Predicting human resting-state functional connectivity from structural connectivity. Proc Natl Acad Sci 106: 2035–2040.

51. Mormann F, Fell J, Axmacher N, Weber B, Lehnertz K, et al. (2005) Phase/amplitude reset and theta-gamma interaction in the human medial temporal lobe during a continuous word recognition memory task. Hippocampus 15: 890–900.

52. Sauseng P, Griesmayr B, Freunberger R, Klimesch W (2010) Control mechanisms in working memory: a possible function of EEG theta oscillations. Neurosci Biobehav Rev 34: 1015–22.

53. Klimesch W, Sauseng P, Hanslmayr S (2007) EEG alpha oscillations: the inhibition-timing hypothesis. Brain Res Brain Res Rev 53: 63–88.

54. Jensen O, Mazaheri A (2010) Shaping functional architecture by oscillatory alpha activity: gating by inhibition. Front Hum Neurosci 4: 186.

55. Rouhinen S, Panula J, Palva JM, Palva S (2013) Load dependence of β and γ oscillations predicts individual capacity of visual attention. J Neurosci 33: 19023–33.

56. Hillebrand A, Barnes GR, Bosboom JL, Berendse HW, Stam CJ (2012) Frequency-dependent functional connectivity within resting-state networks: an atlas-based MEG beamformer solution. Neuroimage 59: 3909–21.

57. Markov NT, Ercsey-Ravasz M, Van Essen DC, Knoblauch K, Toroczkai Z, et al. (2013) Cortical high-density counterstream architectures. Science 342: 1238406.

58. Peraza LR, Asghar AU, Green G, Halliday DM (2012) Volume conduction effects in brain network inference from electroencephalographic recordings using phase lag index. J Neurosci Methods 207: 189–99.

59. Tewarie P, Hillebrand A, Schoonheim MM, van Dijk BW, Geurts JJ, et al. (2014) Functional brain network analysis using minimum spanning trees in Multiple Sclerosis: an MEG source-space study. Neuroimage 88: 308–18.

60. de Waal H, Stam CJ, Lansbergen MM, Wieggers RL, Kamphuis PJ, et al. (2014) The effect of souvenaid on functional brain network organisation in patients with mild Alzheimer's disease: a randomised controlled study. PLoS One 9: e86558.

20

Distinct Facial Processing Related Negative Cognitive Bias in First-Episode and Recurrent Major Depression: Evidence from the N170 ERP Component

Jiu Chen[1], Wentao Ma[2], Yan Zhang[2], Xingqu Wu[2], Dunhong Wei[2], Guangxiong Liu[2], Zihe Deng[2], Laiqi Yang[2]*, Zhijun Zhang[1]*

1 Neurologic Department of Affiliated ZhongDa Hospital, Neuropsychiatric Institute and Medical School of Southeast University, Nanjing, Jiangsu Province, China, 2 Center for Mental Disease Control and Prevention, Third Hospital of the People's Liberation Army, Baoji, Shaanxi Province, China

Abstract

Background: States of depression are associated with increased sensitivity to negative events. For this novel study, we have assessed the relationship between the number of depressive episodes and the dysfunctional processing of emotional facial expressions.

Methodology/Principal Findings: We used a visual emotional oddball paradigm to manipulate the processing of emotional information while event-related brain potentials were recorded in 45 patients with first episode major depression (F-MD), 40 patients with recurrent major depression (R-MD), and 46 healthy controls (HC). Compared with the HC group, F-MD patients had lower N170 amplitudes when identifying happy, neutral, and sad faces; R-MD patients had lower N170 amplitudes when identifying happy and neutral faces, but higher N170 amplitudes when identifying sad faces. F-MD patients had longer N170 latencies when identifying happy, neutral, and sad faces relative to the HC group, and R-MD patients had longer N170 latencies when identifying happy and neutral faces, but shorter N170 latencies when identifying sad faces compared with F-MD patients. Interestingly, a negative relationship was observed between N170 amplitude and the depressive severity score for identification of happy faces in R-MD patients while N170 amplitude was positively correlated with the depressive severity score for identification of sad faces in F-MD and R-MD patients. Additionally, the deficits of N170 amplitude for sad faces positively correlated with the number of depressive episodes in R-MD patients.

Conclusion/Significance: These results provide new evidence that having more recurrent depressive episodes and serious depressive states are likely to aggravate the already abnormal processing of emotional facial expressions in patients with depression. Moreover, it further suggests that the impaired processing as indexed by N170 amplitude for positive face identification may be a potentially useful biomarker for predicting propagation of depression while N170 amplitude for negative face identification could be a potential biomarker for depression recurrence.

Editor: Ulrich von Hecker, Cardiff University, United Kingdom

Funding: This study was supported by the Special Research Fund for Traditional Chinese Medicine in Chinese Army (Grant no. 10ZYX108); the Key Program for Clinical Medicine and Science and Tochnology: Jiangsu Provence Clinical Medical Research Center (Grant no. BL2013025); the National Natural Science Foundation of China (Grant no. 91132000). The funders had no role in study design, data collection and analysis, decision to publish, or preparation of the manuscript.

Competing Interests: The authors have declared that no competing interests exist.

* Email: yanglaiqi6666@163.com (LY); janemengzhang@vip.163.com (ZZ)

Introduction

Depression is a commonly occurring mental disease [1]. The first study of the cognitive theories of depression [2] indicated that cognitive processing can be affected by the unconscious negative or pessimistic schemata activated by stressful events, which include selection, encoding, perception, and interpretation of actual experiences [3,4]. The depressive effect is thought to be due to the negative schemata, which lies dormant until activated by stressful life events [2,4]. However, previous studies have demonstrated that negative cognition comes into being only during depressive episodes [5], and the cognitive processing bias for negative stimuli plays a key role in its onset [6]. Other

supporting evidence suggests that depressive states are classically related to increased sensitivity to negative events [7]. This hypersensitivity may be further enhanced with each recurrent depressive episode.

Gotlib and Neubauer have demonstrated that these negative schemata influence information processing by elevating the salience of negative events and by decreasing the salience of positive events [8]. Accordingly, for positive social stimuli, patients with major depression DISORDER (MDD) were less likely to identify mild happy expressions as more intense than neutral and negative expressions, relative to controls [9]. Using emotional stimuli, numerous studies have indicated that patients with MDD have an attentional bias that is specific to sad faces and an impaired inhibition of attending to negative social information [7,10,11]. However, little is known about how effective facial emotional stimuli are during perceptual processing and whether they may lead to a better understanding of mood-related attention bias in depression, particularly in recurrent depression. An in-depth understanding of the specific time course of cognitive processing during the perceptual processes of emotional stimuli can help to describe which specific cognitive processes are influenced by mood-related biases.

Recently, a study from the Canadian National Population Health Survey has reported that the recurrence of major depressive episodes strongly depends on the number of previous episodes [12]. Several pieces of neuroimaging evidence also suggest that the altered striatal connectivity may be affected by the number of depressive episodes, thus contributing to depressive recurrence risk [13]. First episode major depression patients (F-MD) had smaller left hippocampal volumes, left-right asymmetry [14] and larger amygdala volumes [15]. Numerous cross-sectional epidemiological studies have shown that the severity of depression is positively associated with the number of episodes, and that stressful life events during mild and long-term periods may reinforce depressive recurrent risk [16,17]. Previous studies have indicated that recurrent major depression patients (R-MD) have more serious cognitive impairment compared to F-MD patients. Examples of such cognitive impairment are autobiographical memory [18], verbal memory performance [19], executive function [20] and mental representation processing [21]. Also, recurrence chronically modifies access to emotive memories [18]. Moreover, previous studies have demonstrated that R-MD patients have an increased oxidative stress [22] and higher serum neopterin levels [23] compared to F-MD patients. Taken together, the evidence from these studies suggest that R-MD patients present with a more serious impairment compared with F-MD patients, and the recurrence of depressive episodes may reinforce the damage severity. Very little is known, however, about the relationship between the abnormal neural processing of emotional facial expressions and the number of depressive episodes. Furthermore, the differences between cognitive processing biases for negative faces between F-MD and R-MD patients are still poorly understood.

Event-related evoked potential (ERP) measurements, a powerful non-invasive approach that have a time resolution in the millisecond range and allow assessment of cognitive brain function, have been widely used to investigate individuals' information processing of different cognitive schemata [24]. ERP measurements are a type of long-latency evoked potentials extracted from ongoing electrical cerebral background activity by averaging related procedures to reflect human information processing [25]. In accordance with these experimental manipulations, the measurements can then identify and characterize impairments that may exist in pathological states. The amplitude of the electrophysiological response reflects the intensity of the internal information processing, while its latency represents the timing of that process.

Different electrophysiological components are considered to be associated with different cognitive functions. The N170 component, which is a negative-going component and arose from occipito-temporal brain generators, was first reported by Bentin et al. (1996) [26]. Subsequently, numerous ERP studies have demonstrated that the N170 component is sensitive to facial emotional expressions. For example, Batty and Taylor used unfamiliar faces expressing the six basic emotions and neutral faces, and showed that ERP measurements report global effects of

emotion from 90 ms, while latency and amplitude differences for emotional expressions are found from 140 ms. This suggests that the N170 component may represent rapid processing of emotional expressions [27]. Using an emotional faces task, Blau et al. and Japee et al. demonstrated that the N170 response shows a strong modulation by emotional facial expression [28,29]. Recently, Wronka and Walentowska used an emotional faces task to discriminate emotional expressions and also demonstrated that N170 amplitude was modulated by facial emotional expressions [30]. Furthermore, in these previous studies, all of the researchers have consistently indicated that if the faces are presented as the attentional focus and the subjects are required to direct their attention to the facial expressions, N170 amplitude is modulated by facial emotional expressions [31–34]. Taken together, the evidence from these studies shows that the N170 amplitude and latency modulation can be used as a neurophysiological indicator of the cognitive processing of emotional faces. Moreover, the onset of the N170 effect can be used as a chronopsychophysiological marker for the onset of the processing of emotional expressions. To sum, the N170 component is an ideal brain marker to assess possible cortical markers of emotional face processing in F-MD and R-MD patients.

The objective of our current study is to compare the neural processing of emotional facial expressions by patients with a first episode and recurrent depression to that of healthy control subjects using the ERP technique. Based on the previous studies, we predict that patients with MDD will present with an impairment of emotion processing. We also predict that there will be a difference between F-MD and R-MD patients. The F-MD group will likely have longer N170 latencies and lower N170 amplitudes to three emotional faces relative to the HC group. The R-MD group will likely have lower N170 amplitudes for happy and neutral faces, but higher N170 amplitudes for sad faces relative to the HC group. Moreover, we further predict that there will be a correlation between the number of depressive episodes and the altered processing of emotional faces. The new information we discover regarding the repeated physiopathologic mechanism for depression will be extremely valuable for clarifying diagnoses, advising disease treatments and planning clinical trials.

Materials and Methods

Ethics statement

All procedures were approved by the Human Participants Ethics Committee of the Baoji Third Hospital of the People's Liberation Army and written informed consent was obtained from all participants prior to entry into the study. Ability to provide informed consent was assessed first by the participant's referring clinician who was not associated with the study and an additional study physician prior to inclusion in the study. None of the participants had significant cognitive impairment which would interfere with their ability to provide informed consent. All potential participants who declined to participate or otherwise did not participate were eligible for treatment and were not disadvantaged in any other way by not participating in the study.

Subjects

From inpatients (all of whom were Chinese Han and right-handed) at Center for Mental disease Control and Prevention of Baoji Third Hospital of the People's Liberation Army in China, we recruited 45 F-MD patients (21 males and 24 females) and 40 R-MD patients (18 males and 22 females); see Table 1 (subjects were aged 18–65 years; mean age: F-MD group: 30.6 ± 11.3 years; R-MD group: 32.8 ± 13.6 years). Psychiatric diagnoses were

Table 1. Demographics and clinical measures of depressed patients and HC subjects.

Items	F-MD (N = 45)	R-MD (N = 40)	HC (N = 46)	F values (χ^2)	p values
Age (years)	30.6(11.3)	32.8(13.6)	31.1(10.8)	0.736	0.830
Gender (males/females)	21/24	18/22	22/24	0.043	0.214
Education (years)	12.6(3.0)	13.1(3.3)	13.8(2.1)	1.003	0.672
HDRS$_{17}$	22.6(7.9)[b]	23.8(8.9)[c]	2.5(1.3)	8.322	0.010*
MMSE scores	25.1(1.3)[a b]	21.5(2.5)[c]	29.0(2.2)	6.242	0.013*
AVLT-DR	3.8(1.2)[a b]	1.9(1.5)[c]	7.8(2.3)	7.660	0.007*
TMT-A (seconds)	78.3(32.6)[a b]	88.6(38.3)[c]	67.4(16.4)	9.603	0.000*
TMT-B (seconds)	212.4(121.4)[a b]	258.6(143.2)[c]	175.3(63.2)	10.312	0.000*
SDMT	34.8(12.3)[a b]	23.9(10.6)[c]	39.6(13.2)	9.328	0.000*
DST	11.3(2.2)[b]	10.0(2.1)[c]	12.5(2.6)	4.463	0.031*
CDT	7.3(1.7)[b]	7.2(1.3)[c]	9.1(1.4)	3.204	0.040*
Number of episode	1.0(0.0)	3.6(2.0)	NA	NA	NA
First	45(100%)	-			
Second	-	16(40.0%)			
Third	-	10(25.0%)			
Fourth	-	8(20.0%)			
Fifth	-	5(12. 5%)			
Sixth	-	1(2.5%)			
Age at onset (years)	28.1(2.1)	28.3(4.6)	NA	NA	NA
Duration of illness (years)	0.6(0.3)[a]	3.5(1.1)	NA	NA	NA
Duration of current episode (weeks)	28.2(6.2)[a]	31.0(8.1)	NA	NA	NA
Antidepressant comedication	38(84.4%)	40(100%)	NA	NA	NA

Notes: Abbreviation: F-MD: first episode of major depression; R-MD: recurrent episodes of major depression; HC: Healthy controls; NA: not applicable; HDRS$_{17}$: 17 items the Chinese Hamilton Depression Rating Scale; MMSE: Mini mental state exam; AVLT-DR: Auditory verbal learning test- delayed recall; TMT-A: Trail making test-A; TMT-B: Trail making test-B; SDMT: Symbol digit modalities test; DST: Digit span test; CDT: Clock drawing test.
*Significant differences were found among first episode depression patients and recurrent depression patients and HC subjects. P values were obtained by ANOVA analysis except for gender (chi square test). a–c: post-hoc analysis (LSD test for demographic information and Bonferroni correction for multiple comparison) further revealed the source of ANOVA difference (a: first episode patients vs. recurrent patients; b: first episode patients vs. HC subjects; c: recurrent patients vs. HC subjects).

determined by at least two psychiatrists who agreed on the diagnosis based on the DSM-V criteria [1] for major depression.

Illness durations ranged from 2 months to 30 years (mean illness duration: F-MD group: 0.6±0.3 years; R-MD group: 3.5±1.1 years). Patients' education ranged from 8 years to 22 years (mean years of education: F-MD group: 12.6±3.0 years; R-MD group: 13.1±3.3 years). The severity of depression was evaluated with the 17-item Hamilton Depression Rating Scale (HDRS) [35]. A minimum score of 22.4 was required to participate. All patients received the same antidepressant medication (serotoninergic antidepressive treatment) and the same psychological treatment (psychotherapy interviews and group therapy) [4]. All subjects were clinically stable at the time of testing.

For comparison, 46 healthy control subjects (HC, 22 males and 24 females) without any history of psychiatric illness were matched to the patients in the F-MD and R-MD groups according to age, gender and education (subjects were aged 18–65 years; mean age: 31.1±10.8 years). Exclusion criteria for the patients and the control subjects were a history of substantial head injury, seizures, neurological diseases, dementia, impaired thyroid function, corticoid use or alcohol or substance abuse or dependence. **Table 1** provided group information about age, gender, and education.

Procedures

The experiment was performed with E-Prime 2.0 software (Psychology Software Tools Inc., Pittsburgh, USA). The experimental procedure used an "emotional oddball paradigm" [24,25]. Stimuli consisted of six faces that were selected from a highly standardized set of pictures developed by the Psychology Department of the Chinese Academy of Sciences. The faces had neutral, happy and sad expressions [36]. Standard faces always presented neutral expressions, whereas deviant faces were either the same face displaying an emotion (happy or sad) or a different neutral face (change in identity).

Subjects were confronted with a total of 16 blocks that were defined by 100 stimuli (e.g., 80 frequent stimuli with face A neutral; five deviant face A happy, five deviant face A sad and 10 face B neutral). During the ERP recording, subjects sat on a chair in a quiet, dimly-lit, sound-proof room with their head restrained in a chin rest and placed at 1 m from the 17″ computer screen (refresh rate 75 Hz). Stimuli subtended a visual angle of 3°×4°. Similar to previous reports [37,38], faces were presented for 100 ms in order to assure conscious perception of the faces. A black screen was displayed as an intertribal interval and lasted randomly between 1300 and 1600 ms. The subjects had 1500 ms to answer after the stimulation onset [25]. The participants had to quickly point out the occurrence of a deviant face among the presentation of standard faces by pressing a button with their right index finger. The order of the 16 blocks varied across participants. Reaction time (RT) and accuracy were recorded automatically for each trial.

EEG acquisition and analysis

Electroencephalogram (EEG) data acquisition was carried out continuously throughout the experiment. The EEG data were acquired using a BrainAmp MR portable ERP system (Brain Products GmbH, Munich, Germany) with 32 scalp electrodes. Electrodes were placed according to the extended international 10–20 system [39]. Two ear electrodes served as reference electrodes in off-line analyses, and the AFz electrode was used for grounding. The vertical electro-oculogram (VEOG) and horizontal electro-oculogram (HEOG) were recorded with bipolar channels from sites above the midpoint of the left eye and 10 mm from the right lateral canthus in order to control the interference of eye blinks with the EEG-signal. The EEG was band-pass filtered from 0.1 to 100 Hz, amplified with a gain of 20 and data was stored on a computer disk at the sample rate of 500 Hz. The EEG signal was analyzed using Brain Vision Analyzer software (Brain Products GmbH, Munich, Germany). Offline, the signal was digitally filtered (high pass = 0.1 Hz, low pass = 30 Hz). EEG signals with amplitude larger than ± 70 µV were interpreted as artifacts and rejected. To calculate the ERP, epochs of EEG were averaged off–line, and time was locked to stimulus onset from 200 ms pre–stimulus to 800 ms post stimulus relative to a 200 ms pre–stimulus baseline. Only trials leading to correct responses were included. The mean number of epochs included in each ERP average varied between 73.2 and 128.6 for the various types of stimuli used.

Statistical analyses

The statistical analyses were conducted with SPSS 17.0 software (SPSS Inc., Chicago, IL, USA). The analysis of variance (ANOVA) and chi-square test were used to compare the demographic data and neuropsychological test performances between patients and HC subjects. Accuracy and RTs were also analyzed. After rejecting responses with RTs shorter than 200 ms and longer than 1200 ms, a mean RT of correct responses in each stimulus condition was calculated for each subject. The data for accuracy and RTs were analyzed by separate 3×3 ANOVAs with Group (F-MD, R-MD, and HC) as one between-subjects factor, target expression (happy, neutral, and sad) as within-subject factors.

The peak amplitude and peak latency of the N170 response were identified within a time window of 130–210 ms after the onset of the target stimulus [28,40]. The quantification was restricted to the data from the lateral occipital channels P7 and P8. All ERP data were analyzed by a $3 \times 3 \times 2$ repeated–measure ANOVA with Group (F-MD, R-MD, and HC) as one between-subjects factor, target expression (happy, neutral, and sad), and electrode location (P7 vs. P8 for N170) as within-subject factors. Post hoc comparisons were analyzed by Bonferroni test.

To investigate the behavioral significance of altered amplitude and latency of event-related N170 potential, the linear regression model with a step-wise analysis was used. This allowed us to examine the relationships between the amplitude and latency of N170, the HDRS$_{17}$ score and behavioral data in each group, and between the amplitude and latency of N170 and the number of episodes in the R-MD group. The statistical significance threshold was set at $P < 0.05$.

Results

Demographic and neuropsychological characteristics

Demographic characteristics were shown in **Table 1**. No significant differences in age, gender, and years of education were noted between all groups (all $Ps > 0.05$). Compared with HC subjects, the F-MD and R-MD groups showed the significant declines in muilt-domains of cognitive function, including episodic memory (i.e., AVLT -DR), executive function (i.e., TMT-A and -B), perceptual speed (i.e., SDMT), working memory (i.e., DST) and visuo-spatial cognition (i.e., CDT) (all $Ps < 0.05$). Compared with F-MD patients, R-MD patients showed significantly lower MMSE, AVLT -DR, SDMT, and higher TMT-A and -B scores (all $Ps < 0.05$).

Behavioral results

Reaction times. There was a significant main effect of group in F-MD patients (mean = 1026 ± 312 ms). The F-MD group was slower compared with both the R-MD (mean = 964 ± 362 ms) and HC groups (mean = 842 ± 252 ms) (F (2, 128) = 14.83, $P < 0.001$). A significant main effect of target expression was also observed (F (2, 128) = 8.26, $P = 0.030$). The interaction of group×target expression was significant (F (2, 128) = 24.62, $P < 0.001$).

Post hoc comparisons showed that F-MD patients had slower RTs for happy, neutral and sad faces relative to HC subjects (t's > 4.03, P's < 0.004). R-MD patients had slower RTs for happy and neutral faces, but shorter RTs for sad faces relative to HC subjects (t's > 6.23, P's < 0.001). R-MD patients also had shorter RTs for sad faces compared with F-MD patients (t(83) = 2.92, $P = 0.005$) (Figure 1).

Accuracy. There was a significant group effect on accuracy in R-MD patients (mean = $80.2 \pm 10.3\%$). Accuracy was lower than both the F-MD group (mean = $85.8 \pm 10.8\%$) and the HC group (mean = $92.7 \pm 5.2\%$) (F (2, 128) = 22.06, $P < 0.001$). No significant main effect of target expression was found (F (2, 128) = 1.64, $P = 0.063$). The interaction of group×target expression was significant (F (2, 128) = 3.25, $P = 0.024$).

Post hoc comparisons showed that the F-MD and R-MD groups had lower accuracy for happy and neutral faces relative to HC group (t's > 3.26, P's < 0.008). However, the R-MD group had greater accuracy for sad faces compared with the F-MD and HC groups (t's > 2.32, P's < 0.016).

Electrophysiological results

N170 amplitude. There was a significant main effect of group on lower amplitudes in the R-MD group (mean = -6.82 ± 2.40 µV). Amplitudes were lower when compared with those of the F-MD (mean = -7.65 ± 3.26 µV) and HC groups (mean = -10.16 ± 2.82 µV) (F (2, 124) = 12.38, $P < 0.001$). A significant main effect of target expression was observed (F (2, 124) = 9.63, $P < 0.001$). No significant main effect of electrode location was found (F (1, 124) = 1.22, $P = 0.096$). The interaction of group×target expression was highly significant (F (2, 124) = 13.02, $P < 0.001$).

Post hoc comparisons showed that the F-MD group had lower amplitudes for happy, neutral and sad faces relative to the HC group (t's > 3.26, P's < 0.005). The R-MD group had lower amplitudes for happy and neutral, but higher amplitudes for sad faces relative to the HC group (t's > 3.08, P's < 0.005). Also, the R-MD group had higher amplitudes for sad faces compared to the F-MD group (t(168) = 3.88, $P = 0.004$). In the HC subjects, amplitudes for happy faces were significantly higher than those of neutral and sad faces (t's > 2.73, P's < 0.008), and amplitudes for neutral faces were significantly higher than those for sad faces

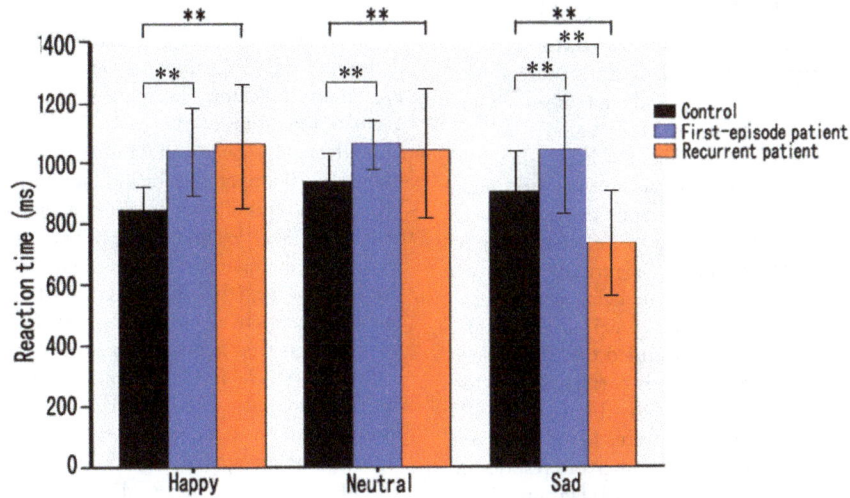

Figure 1. Mean reaction time (ms) for first episode and recurrent depression patients and healthy controls in happy, neutral, and sad face task.

($t(91) = 2.89$, $P = 0.007$). In both F-MD and R-MD groups, amplitudes for sad faces were significantly higher than those of happy and neutral faces (t's>3.65, P's<0.007), but no significant differences in amplitudes were found between happy and neutral faces (P's>0.05) (Figure 2).

N170 latency. There was a significant main effect of group on longer latencies in the R-MD patients (mean = 201.62 ± 28.16 ms). Latencies were longer when compared with those of the F-MD (mean = 192.07 ± 31.42 ms) and the HC groups (mean = 173.85 ± 21.09 ms) (F (2, 124) = 6.92, $P = 0.025$). A significant main effect of target expression was observed (F (2, 124) = 5.38, $p = 0.031$). No significant main effect of electrode location was found (F (1, 124) = 0.78, $P = 0.126$). The interaction of group×target expression was significant (F (2, 124) = 8.85, $P < 0.001$).

Post hoc comparisons showed that F-MD and R-MD groups had longer latencies for happy, neutral and sad faces relative to the HC group (t's>3.23, P's<0.008), and the R-MD group had longer latencies for happy and neutral faces but shorter for sad faces compared with the F-MD group (t's>3.60, P's<0.006). In HC subjects, latencies for happy faces were significantly shorter than those of neutral and sad faces (t's>3.02, P's<0.010). In F-MD patients, none of the within-group comparisons showed significant differences (P's>0.05). In R-MD patients, latencies for sad faces were significantly shorter than those of happy and neutral faces (t's>4.23, P's<0.004), but no significant differences in latencies were found between happy and neutral faces (P's>0.05) (Figure 2).

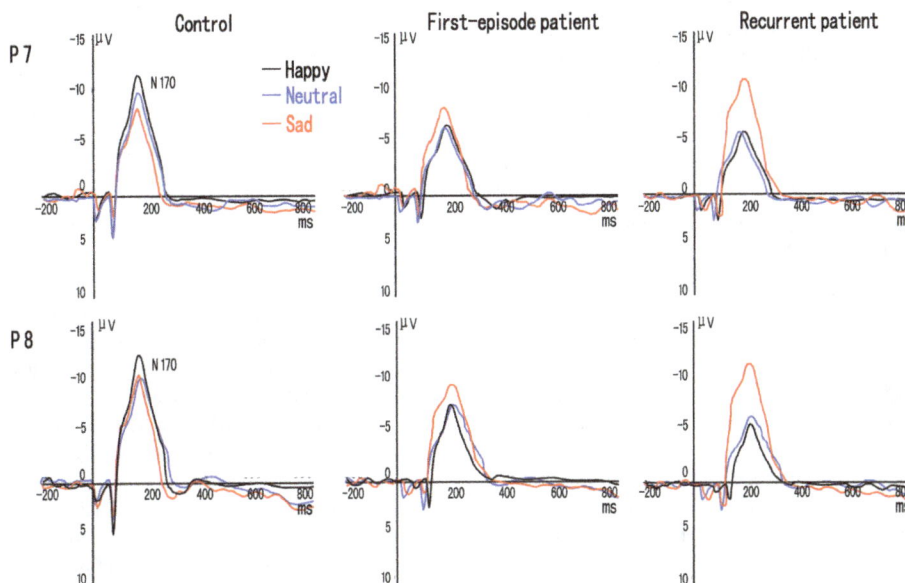

Figure 2. Grand-averaged event-related potential (ERP) waveforms of the N170 components elicited by happy (black line), neutral (blue line), and sad (red line) face pictures at P7 and P8 electrodes in first episode and recurrent depression patients and controls.

The relationship between HDRS$_{17}$, behavioral performance, number of episodes and ERP data

The multivariate regression analysis demonstrated that the deficits of N170 amplitude for happy and sad faces closely correlated with HDRS$_{17}$ scores in R-MD patients (F (1, 39) = 12.02, P<0.001, negative relationship for happy faces; F (1, 39) = 16.92, P<0.001, positive relationship for sad faces) (Figure 3). The correlation between N170 amplitude for sad faces and HDRS$_{17}$ score confirmed a markedly negative relationship in F-MD patients (F (1, 44) = 7.68, P<0.001) (Figure 3). However, no correlations were evident with respect to behavioral performance in the F-MD and R-MD groups (P's>0.05). Interestingly, the multivariate regression analysis demonstrated that the deficits of N170 amplitude for only sad faces positively correlated with the number of episodes in R-MD patients (F (1, 39) = 14.36, P<0.001) (Figure 3). Additionally, no correlations were found between HDRS$_{17}$ scores, behavioral performance, number of episodes or the deficits of N170 latency in the F-MD and R-MD groups (P's> 0.05). Furthermore, control subjects had no correlations between N170 index, behavioral performance or cognitive scores (all P's> 0.05).

Discussion

To our knowledge, our study is the first to investigate the relationship between the abnormal neural processing of emotional facial expressions and the number of depressive episodes in patients. Our study further confirms that the electrophysiological processing of emotional facial expressions is altered in patients with depressive disorders. Our new data also provides new insights into understanding the unconscious negative cognitive bias, which may be an important biomarker for depression recurrence.

Our study reports that F-MD and R-MD patients had slower RTs and lower accuracies for identifying happy and neutral faces relative to HC subjects. This data suggests that their processing for happy and neutral faces is impaired. These results corroborated and expanded the previously described emotional processing deficits in clinical depression [41–43]. A noticeable exception was that R-MD patients had shorter RTs and higher accuracies for sad faces compared with the F-MD and HC groups. These results suggest that R-MD patients employ specific processing schemata for negative faces and rely on different processing mechanisms for the happy and neutral faces. In fact, R-MD patients are more excited for sad faces and may exaggerate the negative emotion [9,44]. Taken together, the specific cognitive bias for sad faces by R-MD patients may be a consequence of focus on their inner world (negative emotion) [33], which may be strongly associated with interpersonal dysfunction in their clinical manifestation.

Our study also showed that F-MD and R-MD patients had reduced N170 amplitudes and longer N170 latencies for identification of happy and neutral faces. These data suggest dysfunctional emotional processing that includes the speed and strength of processing. These findings were also consistent with previous depression studies that showed impaired facial processing [4,7,45,46]. Depressed patients have impaired performance with only positive stimuli [18]. Furthermore, patients with depressive disorders show reduced intensity and frequency of facial expressions with positive hedonic stimuli or specific physiological reactivity [47]. Several neuroimaging studies have also indicated that reduced amygdala activation in response to positive stimuli in depression may be linked to anhedonic symptoms caused by inappropriate salience attribution to positive information [48,49]. Taken together, the evidence suggests that N170 impairment during facial processing may underlie one of the hallmark features

of depression - anhedonic symptoms. It may also lead to a better understanding of interpersonal difficulties that are related to depression [42,50], since patients utilize facial expressions as important indicators to manage their own behavior and to evaluate the attitudes of others.

Interestingly, our study indicated that R-MD patients had higher N170 amplitudes for sad faces compared to the F-MD and HC groups and shorter N170 latencies for sad faces compared with the F-MD group. This positive ERP in the R-MD group seems directly related to negative items and can be correlated with the bias for negative information [51,52]. These findings were similar to previous depression reports that suggest faces expressing more sadness tend to be chosen as displaying greater intensity than happy and neutral faces. This may be due to the fact that sad faces are more arousing to R-MD patients than faces expressing other emotions when compared with the two other groups [52]. However, the negative cognitive bias was not found in F-MD patients, opposite of the R-MD patients who processed different emotional faces with a remarkably unconscious cognitive bias. This result suggests that R-MD patients have a specific emotional processing mechanism for negative faces, distinguishing them from F-MD patients. It further suggests that the unconscious negative cognitive bias may predict a sequential progression in F-MD patients, which could be strongly associated with the neuropathologic spread of depression. However, additional longitudinal studies will be needed to determine whether the unconscious negative cognitive bias in F-MD patients is specifically associated with the disease's progression.

Our current study also investigated the relationship between HDRS$_{17}$ score, behavioral data and ERP indexes. The data revealed a negative relationship between N170 amplitude and severity of depression for happy face recognition, while N170 amplitude was positively correlated with severity of depression for sad face recognition in R-MD patients. Collectively, these findings suggest that propagation of depression may intensify reductions in happy emotions while reinforcing negative emotions in R-MD patients. It is possible that the heightened perception of negative events may lead depressed individuals to feel worse or worthless about themselves and the whole outer world. Simultaneously, their lower mood can hinder their perception of happy events. Thus, they focus more on their inner world, which may be strongly associated with interpersonal dysfunction in their clinical manifestation [53]. However, only a negative relationship for sad face recognition was found in F-MD patients, suggesting that repeated episodes of depression may aggravate the deficits in emotional processing for happy faces and eventually lead to a lower mood [43]. Impaired positive emotional processing as indexed by N170 amplitude may be a useful and important biomarker of potential progression of depression [54].

In this study, the relationship between the amplitude and latency of N170 and the number of depressive episodes was also examined to confirm whether the unconscious negative bias in depression is a marker for stable cognitive vulnerability and possibly related to the recurrence of depression. Our results indicated that the N170 amplitudes for sad face recognition were significantly positively correlated with the number of depressive episodes, indicating that the emotional processing of sad faces differs with episode occurrence [4,12]. As a result, it should be suggested that the hypersensitive perception of negative social stimuli is a stable cognitive vulnerability predictor associated with depression recurrence [7]. With episode repetition, patients generate specifically related mechanisms that result in negative bias reinforcement. The mechanisms can propagate depression through decreases in social reinforcement and social support that

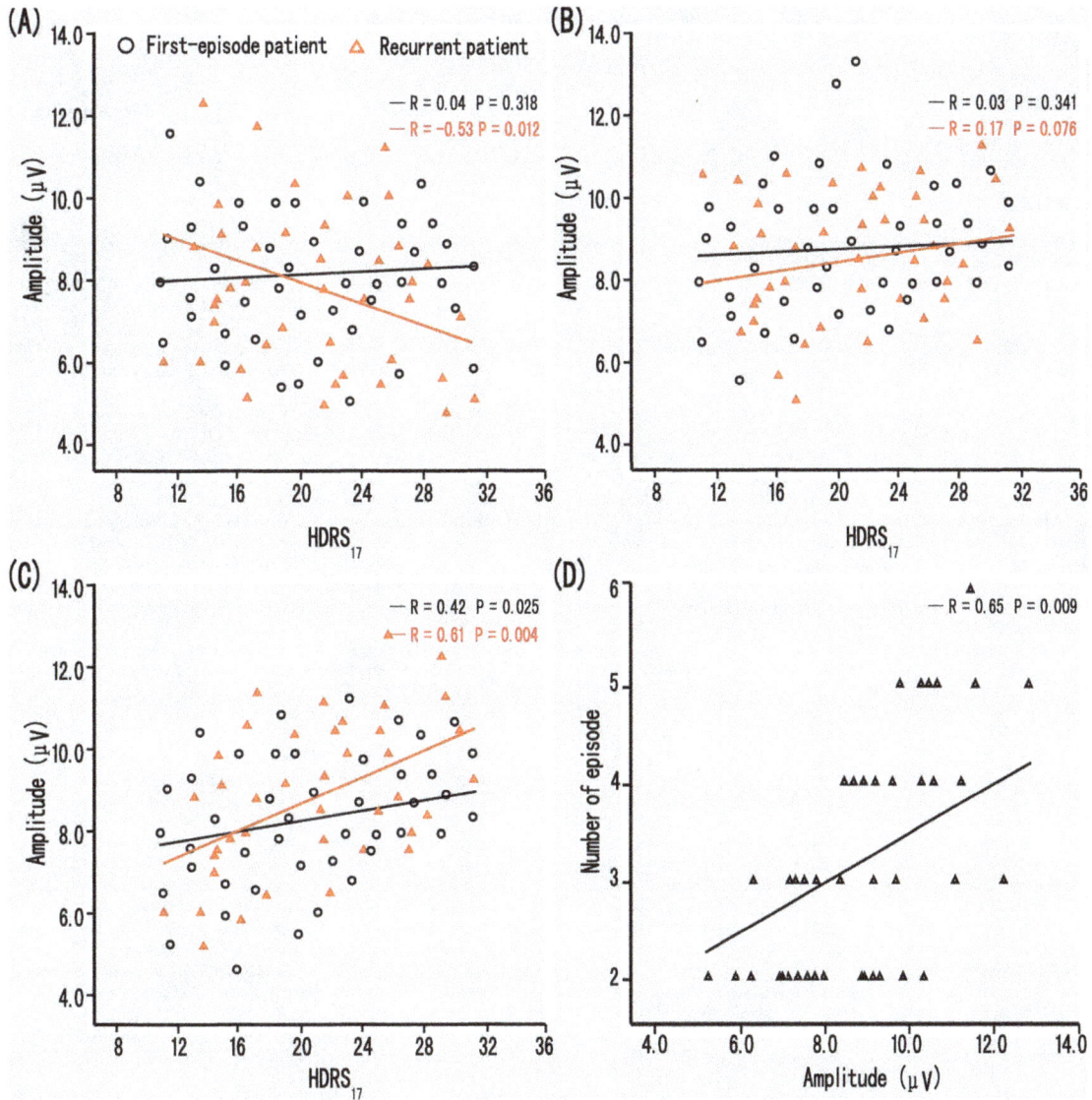

Figure 3. Correlation of clinical variables and the amplitude of event-related N170 potential in F-MD and R-MD patients. (A, B, C) Scattergrams representing the correlations between the groups and the N170 amplitude elicited by happy (A), neutral (B) and sad (C) facial pictures in F-MD (black line) and R-MD (red line) patients. (D) Scattergrams representing the correlations between the number of patient episodes and the N170 amplitude elicited by sad facial pictures in R-MD patients. Amplitude data are merged from P7 and P8 electrodes.

include negative feedback seeking, excessive reassurance seeking and interpersonal avoidance [4,50]. Taken together, the evidence suggests that the unconscious negative cognitive bias may predict the recurrence of depression, and that the impaired negative emotional processing indexed by N170 amplitude may be a useful and important biomarker of potential depression recurrence.

There are, of course, limitations to this study. First, the sample size is relatively small in this study, which could affect the explanation of our results. Second, some of the depressed patients had mild anxiety symptoms, which could have influenced the results. Additionally, all patients were receiving antidepressant medication during the task. This could have influenced the behavioral or ERP performances of the patient groups. Finally, there are limitations imposed by the cross-sectional design of this study. Prospective longitudinal studies that assess changes in these complex relationships over time are needed. These future studies will help determine whether or not the changes in these

parameters can be used as potential biomarkers for identifying individuals at high risk of recurrence and may clarify the diagnosis, or predict outcome in future studies.

Conclusion

The current study provides novel insight into the relationship between the abnormal neural processing of emotional facial expressions and the number of patients' depressive episodes. Our findings have important clinical implications for a more principled understanding of repeated physiopathological mechanisms of depression. Moreover, they further suggest that impaired emotional processing as indexed by N170 amplitude of positive and negative faces may be a useful biomarker for predicting the propagation and recurrence of depression. It will be a more significant and interesting contribution if future studies examine the relationship between the number of previous depressive episodes and the impaired emotional processing from the abnormal brain structure by functional magnetic resonance imaging technique.

Acknowledgments

We thank all psychiatric nurses and doctors for their help in this study.

References

1. American Psychiatric Association (APA) (2013) Diagnostic and Statistical Manual of Mental Disorders, 5th Edition, DSM-V. APA, Arlington, VA.
2. Beck A, Rush A, Shaw B, Emery G (1979) Cognitive therapy of depression. New York: Guilford Press.
3. Just N, Abramson L, Alloy L (2001) Remitted depression studies as tests of the cognitive vulnerability hypotheses of depression onset: a critique and conceptual analysis. Clin Psychol Rev 1: 63–83.
4. Nandrino JL, Dodin V, Martin P, Henniaux M (2004) Emotional information processing in first and recurrent major depressive episodes. J Psychiatr Res 5: 475–484.
5. Blackburn I, Roxborough H, Muir W, Glabus M, Blackwood D (1990) Perceptual and physiological dysfunction in depression. Psychol Med 1: 95–103.
6. Mathews A, MacLeod C (2005) Cognitive vulnerability to emotional disorders. Annu Rev Clin Psychol 1: 167–195.
7. Dai Q, Feng Z (2012) More excited for negative facial expressions in depression: evidence from an event-related potential study. Clin Neurophysiol 11: 2172–2179.
8. Gotlib IH, Neubauer DL (2000) Information processing approaches to the study of cognitive biases in depression. In: Johnson, S.L., Hayes, A.M. (Eds.), Stress, Coping and Depression. Erlbaum, Mahwah, pp. 117–143.
9. Yoon KL, Joormann J, Gotlib IH (2009) Judging the intensity of facial expressions of emotion, depression-related biases in the processing of positive affect. J Abnorm Psychol 181: 223–228.
10. Hankin BL, Gibb BE, Abela JRZ, Flory K (2010) Selective attention to affective stimuli and clinical depression among youths: role of anxiety and specificity of emotion. J Abnorm Psychol 119: 491–501.
11. Zhong MT, Zhu XZ, Yi JY, Yao SQ, Atchley AA (2011) Do the early attentional components of ERPs reflect attentional bias in depression? It depends on the stimulus presentation time. Clin Neurophysiol 122: 1371–1381.
12. Bulloch A, Williams J, Lavorato D, Patten S (2014) Recurrence of major depressive episodes is strongly dependent on the number of previous episodes. Depress Anxiety 1: 72–76.
13. Meng C, Brandl F, Tahmasian M, Shao J, Manoliu A, et al. (2014) Aberrant topology of striatum's connectivity is associated with the number of episodes in depression. BrainPt 2: 598–609.
14. Kronmüller KT, Schröder J, Köhler S, Götz B, Victor D, et al. (2009) Hippocampal volume in first episode and recurrent depression. Psychiatry Res 1: 62–66.
15. Frodl T, Meisenzahl EM, Zetzsche T, Born C, Jäger M, et al. (2003) Larger amygdala volumes in first depressive episode as compared to recurrent major depression and healthy control subjects. Biol Psychiatry 4: 338–344.
16. Roca M, Armengol S, García-García M, Rodriguez-Bayón A, Ballesta I, et al. (2011) Clinical differences between first and recurrent episodes in depressive patients. Compr Psychiatry 1: 26–32.
17. Mitchell PB, Parker GB, Gladstone GL, Wilhelm K, Austin MP (2003) Severity of stressful life events in first and subsequent episodes of depression: the relevance of depressive subtype. J Affect Disord 3: 245–252.
18. Nandrino JL, Pezard L, Posté A, Réveillère C, Beaune D (2002) Autobiographical Memory in Major Depression A Comparison between First-Episode and Recurrent Patients. Psychopathology 6: 335–340.
19. Fossati P, Harvey PO, Le Bastard G, Ergis AM, Jouvent R, et al. (2004) Verbal memory performance of patients with a first depressive episode and patients with unipolar and bipolar recurrent depression. J Psychiatr Res 2: 137–144.
20. Karabekiroğlu A, Topçuoğlu V, Gimzal Gönentür A, Karabekiroğlu K (2010) Executive function differences between first episode and recurrent major depression patients. Turk Psikiyatri Derg 4: 280–288.
21. Chen J, Yang LQ, Zhang ZJ, Ma WT, Wu XQ, et al. (2013) The association between the disruption of motor imagery and the number of depressive episodes of major depression. J Affect Disord 2: 337–343.
22. Stefanescu C, Ciobica A (2012) The relevance of oxidative stress status in first episode and recurrent depression. J Affect Disord 1–3: 34–38.
23. Celik C, Erdem M, Cayci T, Ozdemir B, Ozgur Akgul E, et al. (2010) The association between serum levels of neopterin and number of depressive episodes of major depression. Prog Neuropsychopharmacol Biol Psychiatry 2: 372–375.
24. Kim EY, Lee SH, Park G, Kim S, Kim I, et al. (2013) Gender Difference in Event Related Potentials to Masked Emotional Stimuli in the Oddball Task. Psychiatry Investig 2: 164–172.
25. Campanella S, Rossignol M, Mejias S, Joassin F, Maurage P, et al. (2004) Human gender differences in an emotional visual oddball task: an event-related potentials study. Neurosci Lett 1: 14–18.
26. Bentin S, Allison T, Puce A, Perez E, McCarthy G (1996) Electrophysiological Studies of Face Perception in Humans. J Cogn Neurosci 6: 551–565.
27. Batty M, Taylor MJ (2003) Early processing of the six basic facial emotional expressions. Cogn Brain Res 3: 613–20.
28. Blau VC, Maurer U, Tottenham N, McCandliss BD (2007) The face-specific N170 component is modulated by emotional facial expression. Behav Brain Funct 3: 7.
29. Japee S, Crocker L, Carver F, Pessoa L, Ungerleider LG (2009) Individual differences in valence modulation of face-selective M170 response. Emotion 9: 59–69.
30. Wronka R, Walentowska W (2011) Attention modulates emotional expression processing. Psychophysiology 48: 1047–1056.
31. Caharel S, Courtay N, Bernard C, Lalonde R, Rebai M (2005) Familiarity and emotional expression influence an early stage of face processing: an electrophysiological study. Brain Cogn 59: 96–100.
32. Ibáñez A, Gleichgerrcht E, Hurtado E, González R, Haye A, et al. (2010) Early neural markers of implicit attitudes: N170 modulated by intergroup and evaluative contexts in IAT. Front Hum Neurosci 4: 188.
33. Dai Q, Feng ZZ (2011) Deficient distracter inhibition and enhanced facilitation for emotional stimuli in depression: an ERP study. Int J Psychophysiol 79: 249–258.
34. Calvo MG, Beltrán D (2014) Brain lateralization of holistic versus analytic processing of emotional facial expressions. Neuroimage 92C: 237–247.
35. Zheng YP, Zhao JP, Phillips M, Liu JB, Cai MF, et al. (1988) Validity and reliability of the Chinese Hamilton Depression Rating Scale. Br J Psychiatry 152: 660–664.
36. Wang Y, Luo YJ (2005) Standardized and assessment of face expression of undergraduate students. Chin J Clin Psychol (in Chinese) 13: 396–398.
37. Hurtado E, Haye A, González R, Manes F, Ibáñez A (2009) Contextual blending of ingroup/outgroup face stimuli and word valence: LPP modulation and convergence of measures. BMC Neurosci 10: 69.
38. Ibáñez A, Hurtado E, Riveros R, Urquina H, Cardona JF, et al. (2011) Facial and semantic emotional interference: behavioral and cortical responses to the dual valence association task. Behav Brain Funct 7: 8.
39. Jasper HH (1958) The ten-twenty electrode system of the International Federation. Electroencephalogr Clin Neurophysiol 10: 371–375.
40. Hietanen JK, Astikainen P (2013) N170 response to facial expressions is modulated by the affective congruency between the emotional expression and preceding affective picture. Biol Psychol 2: 114–124.
41. Joormann J, Gotlib IH (2006) Is this happiness I see? Biases in the identification of emotional facial expressions in depression and social phobia. J Abnorm Psychol 115: 705–714.
42. Joormann J, Gotlib IH (2007) Selective attention to emotional faces following recovery from depression. J Abnorm Psychol 116: 80–85.
43. Demenescu LR, Kortekaas R, den Boer JA, Aleman A (2010) Impaired attribution of emotion to facial expressions in anxiety and major depression. PLoS ONE 12: e15058.
44. Leppanen JM (2006) Emotional information processing in mood disorders: a review of behavioral and neuroimaging findings. Curr Opin Psychiatry 19: 34–39.
45. Campanella S, Falbo L, Rossignol M, Grynberg D, Balconi M, et al. (2012) Sex differences on emotional processing are modulated by subclinical levels of alexithymia and depression: a preliminary assessment using event-related potentials. Psychiatry Res 1–2: 145–153.
46. Rossignol M, Philippot P, Crommelinck M, Campanella S (2008) Visual processing of emotional expressions in mixed anxious-depressed subclinical state: an event-related potential study on a female sample. Neurophysiol Clin 5: 267–275.
47. Sloan DM, Strauss ME, Wisner KL (2001) Diminished response to pleasant stimuli by depressed women. J Abnorm Psychol 3: 488–493.
48. Arnone D, McKie S, Elliott R, Thomas EJ, Downey D, et al. (2012) Increased amygdala responses to sad but not fearful faces in major depression: relation to mood state and pharmacological treatment. Am J Psychiatry 8: 841–850.
49. Stuhrmann A, Dohm K, Kugel H, Zwanzger P, Redlich R, et al. (2013) Mood-congruent amygdala responses to subliminally presented facial expressions in major depression: associations with anhedonia. J Psychiatry Neurosci 4: 249–258.
50. Joiner T (2000) Depression's vicious scree: self-propagatory and erosive factors in depression chronicity. Clin Psychol Sci Pract 7: 203–218.
51. Dietrich D, Emrich H, Waller C, Wieringa B, Johannes S, et al. (2000) Emotion/cognition-coupling in word recognition memory of depressive patients: an event-related potential study. Psychiatry Res 96: 15–29.
52. Vanderhasselt MA, De Raedt R, Dillon DG, Dutra SJ, Brooks N, et al. (2012) Decreased cognitive control in response to negative information in patients with

Author Contributions

Conceived and designed the experiments: JC LY ZZ. Performed the experiments: ZD YZ. Analyzed the data: JC WM DW. Contributed reagents/materials/analysis tools: XW GL. Contributed to the writing of the manuscript: JC.

21

Functional Cortical Network in Alpha Band Correlates with Social Bargaining

Pablo Billeke[1,2,3]*, **Francisco Zamorano**[1,2,3], **Mario Chavez**[5], **Diego Cosmelli**[2,4], **Francisco Aboitiz**[2,3]

1 División Neurociencia de la Conducta, Centro de Investigación en Complejidad Social (CICS), Facultad de Gobierno, Universidad del Desarrollo, Santiago, Chile, **2** Centro Interdisciplinario de Neurociencias, Pontificia Universidad Católica de Chile, Santiago, Chile, **3** Departamento de Psiquiatría, Escuela de Medicina, Pontificia Universidad Católica de Chile, Santiago, Chile, **4** Escuela de Psicología, Pontificia Universidad Católica de Chile, Santiago, Chile, **5** CNRS UMR-7225, Hôpital de la Salpêtrière, Paris, France

Abstract

Solving demanding tasks requires fast and flexible coordination among different brain areas. Everyday examples of this are the social dilemmas in which goals tend to clash, requiring one to weigh alternative courses of action in limited time. In spite of this fact, there are few studies that directly address the dynamics of flexible brain network integration during social interaction. To study the preceding, we carried out EEG recordings while subjects played a repeated version of the Ultimatum Game in both human (social) and computer (non-social) conditions. We found phase synchrony (inter-site-phase-clustering) modulation in alpha band that was specific to the human condition and independent of power modulation. The strength and patterns of the inter-site-phase-clustering of the cortical networks were also modulated, and these modulations were mainly in frontal and parietal regions. Moreover, changes in the individuals' alpha network structure correlated with the risk of the offers made only in social conditions. This correlation was independent of changes in power and inter-site-phase-clustering strength. Our results indicate that, when subjects believe they are participating in a social interaction, a specific modulation of functional cortical networks in alpha band takes place, suggesting that phase synchrony of alpha oscillations could serve as a mechanism by which different brain areas flexibly interact in order to adapt ongoing behavior in socially demanding contexts.

Editor: Sam Doesburg, Hospital for Sick Children, Canada

Funding: This work was supported by CONICYT [Grant number 791220014 to PB], Project "Anillo en Complejidad Social" [SOC-1101 to PB, DC and FZ] and by the Millennium Center for the Neuroscience of Memory, Chile [NC10-001-F], which is developed with funds from the Innovation for Competitivity from the Ministry for Economics, Fomentation and Tourism, Chile. MC is partially supported by the EU-LASAGNE Project [Contract no.318132 (STREP)]. The funders had no role in study design, data collection and analysis, decision to publish, or preparation of the manuscript.

Competing Interests: The authors have declared that no competing interests exist.

* Email: pbilleke@udd.cl

Introduction

In daily life, we spend an great deal of time dealing with social dilemmas [1]. A crucial characteristic of such situations is that goals that tend to clash can co-exist with the consequence of making an analytical approach non-trivial [2]. Naturally, then, when people face social dilemmas, several cognitive processes must be recruited. Neurobiological studies have identified several brain areas which underlie different functions supporting our capacity to maintain a social interaction and solve social dilemmas [3,4]. Rather than having specific and isolated functions, it has been proposed that these areas work as a network which requires a rapid, efficient, adaptive interaction among them and with other domain-general networks [5,6]. Thus social processing, like empathy [7] and imitation [8], has been shown to generate an increase in the connectivity among different brain areas. In spite of this evidence, it remains unknown whether specific changes in functional connectivity of the brain networks are related to social behavior. Indeed, a recent study shows that flexible organization in connectivity patterns of fronto-parietal network is related to our capacity to adapt our cognitive resources according to the task demands [9]. Thus, we hypothesize that during social interactions, a particular functional reorganization of brain functional connec-

tivity takes place, and that this reorganization is reflected in the dynamics of the cortical networks as estimated by inter-site-phase-clustering between brain sources.

Empirical studies have led to the hypothesis that functional neural assemblies are largely distributed and linked to form a web-like structure in the brain [10]. Within this framework, brain regions are conceived as partitioned into a collection of modules, representing functional units that are separable from -but related to- the functions of other modules. Detecting the modular brain structure may be crucial to understanding the structural and functional properties of neural systems during social interactions. To evaluate this possibility, we used Graph Theory analysis of the electroencephalographic (EEG) activity of human subjects while they played a standard behavioral economics game that recreates a social dilemma of bargaining, namely the repeated version of the Ultimatum Game (Figure 1) [11,12]. The game involves two players, namely the proposer and the responder. The proposer makes an offer as to how to split a certain amount of money between the two players. The responder can either accept or reject the offer. If the offer is accepted, the money is split as proposed, but if it is rejected, neither player receives any money. Crucially, during this repeated interaction, proposers have to predict the most probable behavior of the responders to estimate the risk of

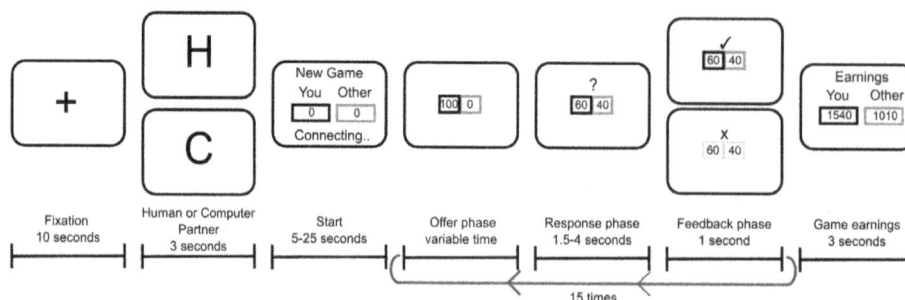

Figure 1. Timeline of a game. Proposers (black box) and responders (gray box, computational simulations, see Methods) played a repeated Ultimatum Game. The proposer makes an offer on how to split 100 Chilean pesos between the responder and himself/herself (offer phase). The responder decides to either accept or reject it (response phase). If the responder accepts the offer, the money is split as proposed, and if he/she rejects it, the money is lost. The response is shown on the screen during 1 s (feedback phase). Each game consists of 15 offers. At the beginning of each game, the proposer sees a cue that indicates if his/her partner is a human ("H") or computer ("PC").

their actions and adapt their own behavior accordingly [13]. To make this behavioral prediction, it is necessary to recruit brain networks that participate in social processing to figure out the other players' intentions (e.i., Mentalizing) [14].

Methods

Twenty-five individuals (11 women) participated for monetary compensation after online recruitment. Seventeen subject data were originally recollected for the control task of a previous work [15]. All the analyses presented here are new. All participants were right-handed Spanish speakers, aged from 20 to 37 years (M = 25.31, SEM = 0.71). All participants had normal or corrected-to-normal vision, no color-vision deficiency, no history of neurological diseases, and no current psychiatric diagnosis or psychotropic prescriptions. All participants provided their written informed consent to participate in this study and the Ethics Committee of the Pontificia Universidad Católica de Chile approved the experimental protocol. All experiments were performed at the Cognitive Neuroscience Laboratory of the Department of Psychiatry of the University.

Task

Participants played as proposers in a repeated version of the Ultimatum Game (see Figure 1). Subjects believed they were playing either with a human partner or a computer partner, but they were actually always playing with a computational simulation (see below). Participants began their participation by reading on-screen instructions describing the game. At the beginning of each game, participants watched the fixation cross (10 seconds, fixation phase). Then, a signal on the screen indicated whether the game was against a computer ("PC") or a human ("H") partner. Each game consisted of 15 rounds and each participant played as a proposer 32 times with different simulated responders (16 human games and 16 computer games, randomly distributed). For computer games, the experimenter explained to the participant that the computer simulation assigned a probability to accept the offer given the amount of money offered (a direct relation), and that this probability could change between different games but not during a game with the same computer partner. Importantly, the simulation used in human and computer games was the same. Each trial had three phases as follows: In the first (offer phase, variable duration), the proposer had to make the offer. In the second (anticipation phase, 1.5–4 seconds), the proposer waited for the response of the partner. In the last phase (feedback phase, 1 second), the response was revealed to the proposer. At the end of

each game, the earnings each player had made in the game were revealed. After the set of games concluded, the experimenter interviewed each participant individually in order to check whether they had understood the game correctly. The amount of money each participant received depended on his/her performance in one of the 32 games chosen randomly, and ranged from 6,000 to 12,000 Chilean pesos, 12 to 24 USD approximately.

Simulation

Simulations used in the tasks were based on a mixed logistic modeling of 33 people playing as receptors with other people (for more details see [13]). Using this model, we were able to create different virtual players. All participants played with the same simulated partners. Specifically, the simulation algorithm assigns a probability to reject or accept the offer given the following two equations:

for round (x) = 1,

$$logit(R_x) = (b_0 + r_0^i) + (b_1 + r_1^i)O_x$$

and for round (x) > 1,

$$logit(R_x) =$$
$$(b_0 + r_0^i) + (b_1 + r_1^i)O_x + (b_2 + r_2^i)\Delta O_x + b_2 Pr_x + b_3 \Delta O_x Pr_x$$

where $logit(R_x)$ is the logit transform of the probability of rejection for the round x, O_x the offer, ΔO_x the change of offer in relation to the preceding offer, and PR_x the preceding response. The coefficients for each regressor were composed by a population parameter (b_y) and a random effect for each simulated responder (r_y^i, y = regressor and i = simulated partner). The simulation and experimental setting generated a credible human interaction for the following reasons: (1) The distributions of acceptances and rejections, and the offering behaviors related to a rejection in the simulation game were similar to those obtained in a real human game [13], suggesting that simulated responders elicited comparable behaviors in proposers. (2) During post hoc interviews, experimenters asked participants whether they believed that they had played against a human counterpart. All participants indicated that they actually believed that they had played against another human and that they felt the human games different from the computer games. We used the $logit(R_x)$ to the quantification of the risk per each offer made.

Electrophysiological Recordings

Continuous EEG recordings were obtained with a 40-electrode NuAmps EEG System (Compumedics Neuroscan). All impedances were kept below 5 kΩ. Electrode impedance was retested during pauses to ensure stable values throughout the experiment. All electrodes were referenced to averaged mastoids during acquisition and the signal was digitized at 1 kHz. Electro-oculogram was obtained with four electrodes with both vertical and horizontal bipolar derivation. All recordings were acquired using Scan 4.3 (Compumedics Neuroscan) and stored for off-line treatment. At the end of each session, electrode position and head points were digitalized using a 3D tracking system (Polhemus Isotrak).

EEG Data Analysis

EEG signals were preprocessed using a 0.1–100 Hz band-pass Butterworth filter (third-order, forward and reverse filtering). Eye blinks were identified by a threshold criterion of ±100 μV, and their contribution was removed from each dataset using principal component analysis by singular value decomposition and spatial filter transform using Scan 4.3 (Compumedics Neuroscan). Other remaining artifacts (e.g., muscular artifacts) were detected by visual inspection of the signal and the trials that contained them were removed. After this procedure, we obtained 424±33 artifact-free trials across the subjects. Time frequency (TF) distributions were obtained by means of the wavelet transform, between −1.5 and 1.5s. We displayed the result only for −1 to 1 s over the segmented signals to avoid edged artifact. A signal x(t) was convolved with a complex Morlet's wavelet function defined as $w(t,f_0) = A e^{-t^2/2\sigma_t^2} e^{i2\pi f_0 t}$. Wavelets were normalized and thus $A = (\sigma_t\sqrt{\pi})^{-1/2}$ the width of each wavelet function $m = f_o/\sigma_t$ was chosen to be 7; where $\sigma_f = \frac{1}{2}\pi\sigma_t$. TF contents was represented as the energy of the convolved signal: $E(t,f_o) = |w(t,f_o) \otimes x(t)|^2$. Thus, we obtained the phase and amplitude per each temporal bin (in steps of 10 ms) and frequency (from 4 to 30 Hz in step of 1 Hz). We used for analysis only the 90 riskiest and the 90 safest offers per subject and condition, in order to ensure equal number of trials for statistical comparison. For all power spectrum analysis, we used the dB of power related to a baseline during the fixation phase (ten seconds at the beginning of each game, Figure 1).

Source Estimations

The neural current density time series at each elementary brain location was estimated by applying a weighted minimum norm estimate inverse solution [16] with unconstrained dipole orientations in single-trials. A tessellated cortical mesh template surface derived from the default anatomy of the Montreal Neurological Institute (MNI/Colin27) wrapped to the individual head shape (using ~300 headpoints per subject) was used as a brain model to estimate the current source distribution. We defined 3×390 sources constrained to the segmented cortical surface (3 orthogonal sources at each spatial location, avoiding deep and basal structures since the sensitivity of the EEG signal to the activity of those structures is poor), and computed a three-layer (scalp, inner skull, outer skull) boundary element conductivity model and the physical forward model [17]. The measured electrode level data $X(t) = [x_1(t), \cdots, x_{n\_electrode}(t)]$ is assumed to be linearly related to a set of cortical sources $Y(t) = [y_1(t), \cdots, y_{m\_source}(t)]$ and additive noise $N(t) : X(t) = LY(t) + N(t)$, where L is the physical forward

model. The inverse solution was then derived as $Y(t) = WX(t) = RL^T(LRL^T + \lambda^2 C)^{-1}X(t)$ where W is the inverse operator, R and C are the source and noise covariances respectively, the superscript T indicates the matrix transpose, and λ^2 is the regularization parameter. R was the identity matrix that was modified to implement depth-weighing (weighing exponent: 0.8 [18]), The regularization parameter λ was set to 1/3. To estimate cortical activity at the cortical sources, the recorded raw EEG time series at the sensors x(t) were multiplied by the inverse operator W to yield the estimated source current, as a function of time, at the cortical surface: $Y(t) = WX(t)$. Since this is a linear transformation, it does not modify the spectral content of the underlying sources. It is therefore possible to undertake time–frequency analysis on the source space directly. Finally, we reduced the number of sources by keeping a single source at each spatial location that pointed into the direction of maximal variance. To this end, we applied a principal component analysis to covariance matrix obtained from the 3 orthogonal time series estimated at each source location. This resulted in a single filter for each spatial location that was then applied to the complex valued data to derive frequency specific single trial source estimates. Since we used a small number of electrodes (40) and no individual anatomy for head model calculation, the spatial precision of the source estimations are limited. In order to minimize the possibility of erroneous results we only present source estimations if there are both statistically significant differences at the electrode level and the differences at the source levels survive a multiple comparison correction.

Functional Network

We consider the functional links in brain signals defined via the phase-locking value (PLV) computed between all pairs of electrodes or brain sources [19]. The PLV measures the inter-site-phase-clustering. To compute the PLVs, we used a complex Morlet's wavelet function of 7 cycles. By means of this complex wavelet transform, an instantaneous phase $\phi_i^{tr}(t,f)$ is obtained for each frequency component of signals i (electrodes or sources) at each trial (tr). The PLV between any pair of signals (i,k) is inversely related to the variability of phase differences across trials:

$$PLV_{ik}(t,f) = \frac{1}{N_{tr}}\left| \sum_{tr=1}^{N_{tr}} \exp^{j(\phi_i^{tr}(t,f) - \phi_k^{tr}(t,f))} \right|$$

where N_{tr} is the total number of trials. If the phase difference varies little across trials, its distribution is concentrated around a preferred value and PLV<1. In contrast, under the null hypothesis of a uniformity of phase distribution, PLV values are close to zero. Finally, to assess whether two different nodes are functionally connected, we calculated the significance probability of the PLVs by a Rayleigh test of uniformity of phase. According to this test, the significance of a PLV determined from N_{tr} can be calculated as $p = \exp^{(-N_{tr}PLV^2)}$ [20]. To correct for multiple testing, the False Discovery Rate (FDR, q<0.05) method was applied to each matrix of PLVs. In the construction of the networks, a functional connection between two brain sites was assumed as an undirected and weighted edge (functional connectivity strength between node $w_{ij} = PLV_{ij}$, for significant links and $w_{ij} = 0$ otherwise). We calculated the strength of inter-site-phase-clustering for each node (electrode or source) as the sum of all significant PLVs of that node.

Network partitions

To partition the functional networks in modules, we used a random walk-based algorithm [21]. This data-driven approach is based on the intuition that a random walker on a graph tends to remain into densely connected subsets corresponding to modules. To find the modular structure, the algorithm starts with a partition in which each node in the network is the sole member of a module. Modules are then merged by an agglomerative approach based on a hierarchical clustering method. At each step the algorithm evaluates the quality of partition Q, which compares the abundance of edges lying inside each community with respect to a null model. The modularity of a given partition is defined as, $Q = \sum_{s=1}^{M} \left[l_s/L - (k_s/2L)^2 \right]$ where M is the number of modules, L is the total number of connections in the network, l_s is the number of connections between vertices in module s, and k_s is the sum of the degrees of the vertices in modules. The partition that maximizes Q is considered as the partition that better captures the modular structure of the network. Further details can be found in [22,23].

To evaluate the agreement between community structures we use the Rand index [24], which is a traditional criterion for comparison of different results provided by classifiers and clustering algorithms, including partitions with different numbers of classes or clusters. For two partitions P and P', the Rand index is defined as $R = \dfrac{(a+d)}{(a+b+c+d)}$; where a is the number of pairs of data objects belonging to the same class in P and to the same class in P', b is the number of pairs of data objects belonging to the same class in P and to different classes in P', c is the number of pairs of data objects belonging to different classes in P and to the same class in P', and d is number of pairs of data objects belonging to different classes in P and to different classes in P'. The Rand index has a straightforward interpretation as a percentage of agreement between the two partitions and it yields values between 0 (if the two partitions are randomly drawn) and 1 (for identical partition structures).

Statistical analysis

For pair comparison and correlation, we used non-parametric tests (Wilcoxon and Spearman correlation). For multiple regressions, we used robust linear regression. To correct for multiple comparisons in time-frequency chart and sources, we used the Cluster-based permutation test for the EEG data [25]. In the latter method, clusters of significant areas were defined by pooling neighboring sites (in the time-frequency chart) that showed the same effect (p<0.05). The cluster-level statistics was computed as the sum of the statistics of all sites within the corresponding cluster. We evaluated the cluster-level significance under the permutation distribution of the cluster that had the largest cluster-level statistics. The permutation distribution was obtained by randomly permuting the original data. After each permutation, the original statistical test was computed (e.g., Wilcoxon), and the cluster-level statistics of the largest cluster resulting was used for the permutation distribution. After 1,000 permutations, the cluster-level significance for each observed cluster was estimated as the proportion of elements of the permutation distribution greater than the cluster-level statistics of the corresponding cluster.

Software

All behavioral statistical analyses were performed in R. The EEG signal processing was implemented in MATLAB using in-house scripts (LAN toolbox, available online at http://lantoolbox. wikispaces.com/, e.g. [26]). For the source estimation and head model, we used the BrainStorm [27] and openMEEG toolboxes [28].

Results

Behavior

Subjects in both human (HGs) and computer games (CGs) made comparable offers in the amount of money (HG = $42.5; CG = $42.3, Chilean pesos; Wilcoxon signed rank test; p = 0.78) and risk (measured as the logit of the probability to acceptance; HG = 0.89; CG = 0.86; p = 0.9). Like in our previous work, we found a strategic difference between HGs and CGs given by the evolution of the offer risk during a game. In CGs there was a stronger correlation between the offer risk and the round number (Spaerman's rho = 0.88, p<2e−16) than that of HG (rho = 0.61, p = 0.01), giving a difference in the interaction between conditions (HG and CG) and round number in the robust linear regression (Table 1). These results suggest that subjects use a learning strategy in CGs but a bargaining strategy in HGs [15].

EEG

We explored the oscillatory brain activity related to the anticipation of the other's response. We calculated the risk for each offer and compared the 90 riskiest with the 90 safest offers per subject. To explore changes in the global dynamics we first compared the overall power and inter-site-phase-clustering strength (by means of PLV) between risky and safe offers per condition, at the electrode level. For this, we explored for changes in the sum of the inter-site-phase-clustering strength or power across all electrodes. First we defined a time-window of interest (0 to 1 second after the subject made the offer) and calculated a repeated measure ANOVA. In this analysis we found that the interaction between conditions (Human and Computer games), offer risk (risky vs. safe offer) and frequency band (theta, 4–7 Hz, alpha, 8–12 Hz, beta 13–25 Hz) was significant ($F_2 = 3.25$, p = 0.0406, Table S1 in File S1). Then, we explored the entire time-frequency chart and, in those regions where we found significant modulations, we explored their topographies and the electrodes that showed significant effect (Figure 2).

Over occipital electrodes, we found a significant drop in alpha power before the subject made the offer in both HGs and CGs (main effect: 8–10 Hz; −0.8 to −0.2 s; O1 and O2 electrodes; Figure 2A–B). After the subjects made the offer and before they received the response (anticipatory phase), we found a drop in alpha band power over left posterior temporo-parietal electrodes only in HGs (main effect: 9–12 Hz; 0.5 to 1 s; TP8 electrode; Figure 2A, upper panel, Wilcoxon rank sum test and cluster based permutation test, p<0.01). During this anticipatory phase, we also found an increase of the alpha inter-site-phase-clustering strength prior to the difference in power (main effect: 7–10 Hz; 0.2 to 0.4 s; FC3, C3, CP3 and Pz electrode; Figure 2A, lower panel, note that the inter-site-phase-clustering strength was calculated based on all possible electrode pairs). This synchrony increase was mainly in risky offers made during HG (7–10 Hz, Figure 2C). Notably, we did not find any difference in inter-site-phase-clustering between risky and safe offers made during CGs (Figure 2B–D).

Since the volumetric conduction of distal sources can spuriously generate synchrony at the electrode level, we carried out the same analysis using both the current source density (CSD) at the electrode level and source reconstruction at cortical level. CSD analysis replicates the difference between human and computer games shown in Figure 2 (See Figure S1 in File S1). For source reconstruction, we calculated the electrical activity in 390 source nodes over the cortex (Figure 3A), avoiding subcortical structures where the sensitivity of EEG is poor. Then, we calculated the strength of inter-site-phase-clustering for each node in alpha band (7–10 Hz, where we found the main modulation at the electrode

Table 1. Model of the risk of offers.

	Scope	Std. Error	T-value	p-value
(Intercept)	0.3747	0.1136	3.2976	0.00002
Round	0.1021	0.0125	8.1701	0.00000001
Human Games	0.3101	0.1607	1.9296	0.06
Round×Human Games	−0.0686	0.0177	−3.8813	0.0006
degree of freedom = 26				

level), and found differences in the medial parietal and frontal nodes between safe and risky offers for HGs but not for CGs (Figure 3B). In order to evaluate if the strength change reflects a change in functional network, we calculated the community structure of the networks at group and individual levels for both conditions at cortical source level (see Methods).

In agreement with the above result, we found that the community structure changed between risky and safe offers in HGs but not in CGs, at group levels, in frontal and parietal regions (Figure 3C). We obtained seven communities per condition except for safe offers in HGs in which we obtained six. We found a bilateral module in dorsolateral prefrontal cortex, which was conserved across conditions (light-blue in Figure 3C). We observed two modules in inferior frontal gyrus and fronto-polar regions, which were joined only in safe offers in HGs (blue and red in Figure 3C). We also found a central module in sensory-motor cortex, which was greater especially in the left hemisphere in risky offers in HGs (Green). Finally, we detected one medial and two lateral modules in parietal and occipital regions, which changed in risky offers in HGs in comparison with the other conditions.

In order to evaluate whether this differential functional organization is specifically related to social interaction, we computed the individual differences in community structure between risky and safe offer networks using the rand index (at the cortical source level). Interestingly, the difference in community structure was significantly correlated with the differences in the risk of the offer only in HGs (rho = −0.44, p = 0.02), but not in CGs (rho = 0.2, p = 0.2). Indeed, using robust linear regression, the interaction between conditions (HGs and CGs) and risk differences was significant (t_{46} = −2.05, p = 0.045) even after correcting by power and inter-site-phase-clustering strength differences between risky and safe offers (Table 2). This indicates that functional network activation was specifically related to the behavior during HGs (t_{44} = −2.42, p = 0.02) independently of change of strength of inter-site-phase-clustering (p = 0.99) and possible influences of changes in power (p = 0.04, Table 2).

Discussion

It has been proposed that the complex and flexible behaviors that sustain human social interactions rely on the dynamic modulation of patterns of interaction among specialized large-scale brain systems [29]. Here, we explored such specific modulations of patterns in brain connectivity during two types of interaction. Crucially, we used two tasks that were exactly the same except by the context instructed to the subject (human *vs* computer partners), and we found a significant modulation in alpha power and inter-site-phase-clustering, depending on the social context. A recent work has shown that inter-site-phase-clustering in alpha band at the electrode level correlates with the activity of fronto-parietal networks [30]. In that work, using

concomitant EEG and fMRI recordings during rest, the authors found that the inter-site-phase-clustering of alpha band was specifically correlated with the BOLD signal of frontal pole, inferior parietal lobe and medial parietal lobe [30]. Interestingly, the activity of fronto-parietal networks is specifically correlated to alpha band, and does not show correlation with other frequency bands [30]. This specific correlation includes the anterior prefrontal cortex and the medial parietal cortex where we found inter-site-phase-clustering strength modulation at source level. Although other studies have found a correlation between alpha inter-site-phase-clustering with default mode network (see [31]), our results are in accordance with the correlation with fronto-parietal regions (compared Figure 2B with Figure 1 in [30]), and match the hypothesis that the fronto-parietal network participates in cognitive control, especially in a trial-by-trial high adaptive control situation [32]. Moreover, evidence from intracortical recording in monkeys, shows the existence of a prefronto-parietal network that shows phase synchrony at in 5–10 Hz [33]. This network increases its inter-site-phase-clustering strength during the anticipation of top-down controlled processes [33]. Indeed, cognitive control is highly required to solve difficult social situations like the dilemmas recreated by game theory tasks such as the one used here [34]. In the same line, it has been proposed that cognitive control is necessary for humans to develop pro-social behavior like mutual cooperation [35]. Thus, the increase in phase synchrony that we found probably reflects the higher cognitive demands required by the expectation of the partner's behavior in a repeated interaction with humans (e.g., integrating the other's intention, the previous interactions and the future consequences) than that required in a computer interaction.

An important limitation of our work concerns the interpretation of functional connectivity using EEG. Volume conduction may cause spurious connectivity by the fact that activity in one source can be represented in multiple measurement points [36]. In order to lessen erroneous results, we explored the synchrony in both electrode and source reconstruction levels, and studied global dynamics rather that local modulations. Additionally, our results indicated that inter-site-phase-clustering changes were dissociated from power changes, which argues against possible volume conduction effects. Finally, behavior was significantly related to network dynamics independently of its overall inter-site-phase-clustering strength and power.

It has been proposed that alpha power shows a negative correlation with cortical activity [37–40]. Alpha power has shown a negative correlation with the dorsal attention network and a positive correlation with the cingulo-opercular network, with no relation to the fronto-parietal network [41]. Works in focused attention suggest that phase locking during the processing of a stimulus can occur with concomitant amplitude reduction [42]. Additionally, it seems that oscillatory alpha activity operates in a phasic manner [43,44]. Thus, the phase of pre-stimulus alpha

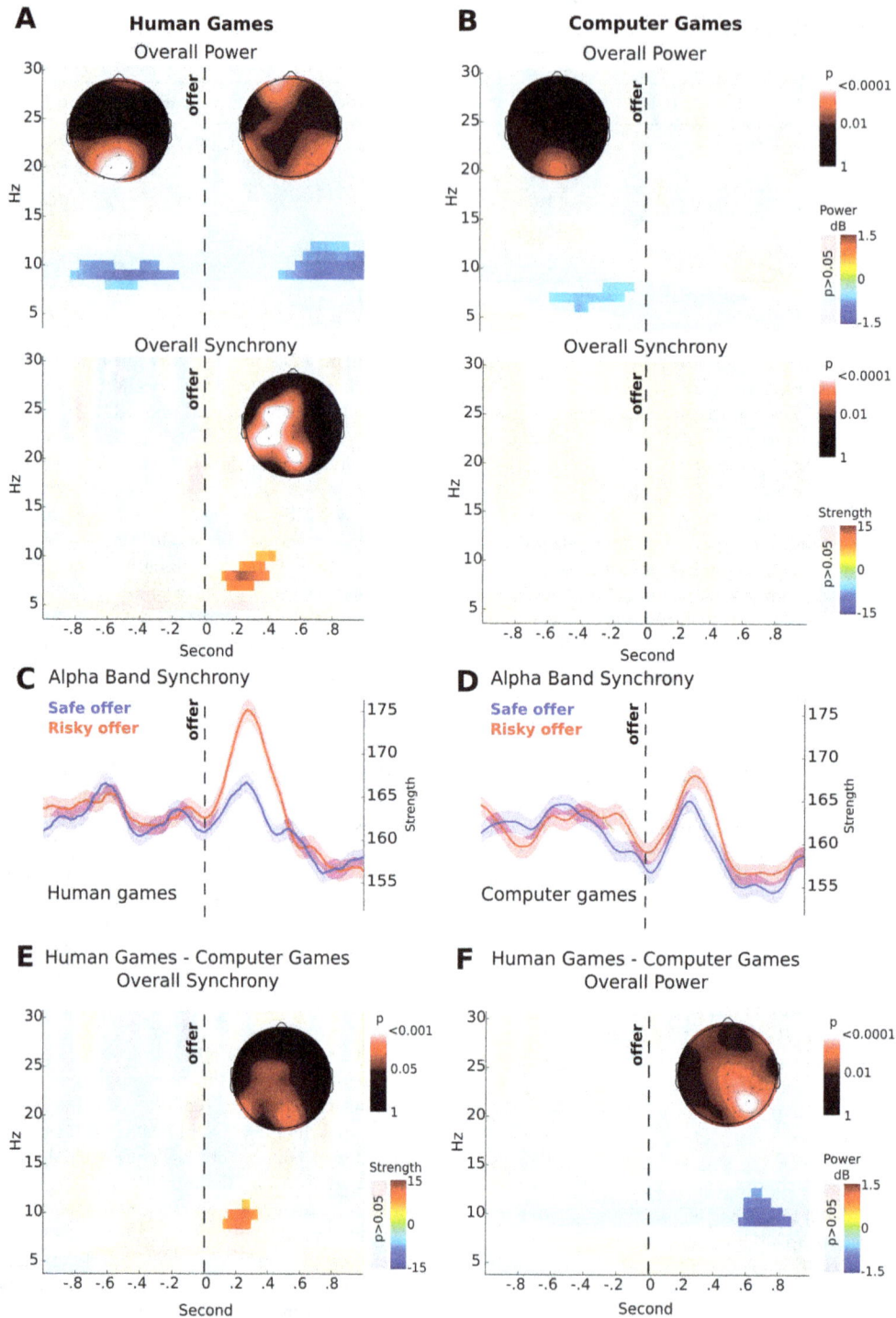

Figure 2. Scalp levels. A, B, Time-frequency charts of the difference between risky and save offers in human (**A**) and computer games (**B**). The upper panel shows differences in the overall power (dB) and the lower panel in strength of synchrony (inter-site-phase-clustering). **C, D** Inter-site-phase-clustering strength in alpha band (7–10 Hz) in safe (blue) and risky (red) offer in human (**C**) and computer (**D**) games. Areas represent the standard error of means. **E, F,** Difference between human and computer games in overall power (**E**) and synchrony (**F**). **A–F,** The non-significant areas are overshadowed and for each significant area, the scalp distribution of p-values is shown. Time-frequency charts and time line plots show the mean of the power or the sum of inter-site-phase-clustering strengths across all electrodes, and the topographic plots show the distribution of the significant time-frequency windows highlighted.

oscillations modulates visual detection [45]. Following this evidence, it has been proposed that alpha oscillation works as a pulsed inhibition and that its synchronized activity could have a important role in the change of network activity in the brain [46–

48]. In our experiment, alpha inter-site-phase-clustering modulation was temporally dissociated from power modulation (Figure 2). Using the same task but only considering games among actual human partners, we have previously shown that the power

A Nodes=390

Node Index
random

B Alpha synchrony in human games

Z value
7
0

C Clustering

Human games   Computer games

Safe offers

Risky offers

Communities:

D

Computer games
Human games

Rand index
between risky and safe offers

0.9
0.85
0.8
0.75
0.7

rho = 0.2 ;   p = 0.2;   robust model p = 0.64
rho = -0.44 ; p = 0.02; robust model p = 6e-4

-0.8 -0.7 -0.6 -0.5 -0.4 -0.3

Risk difference
between risky and safe offers

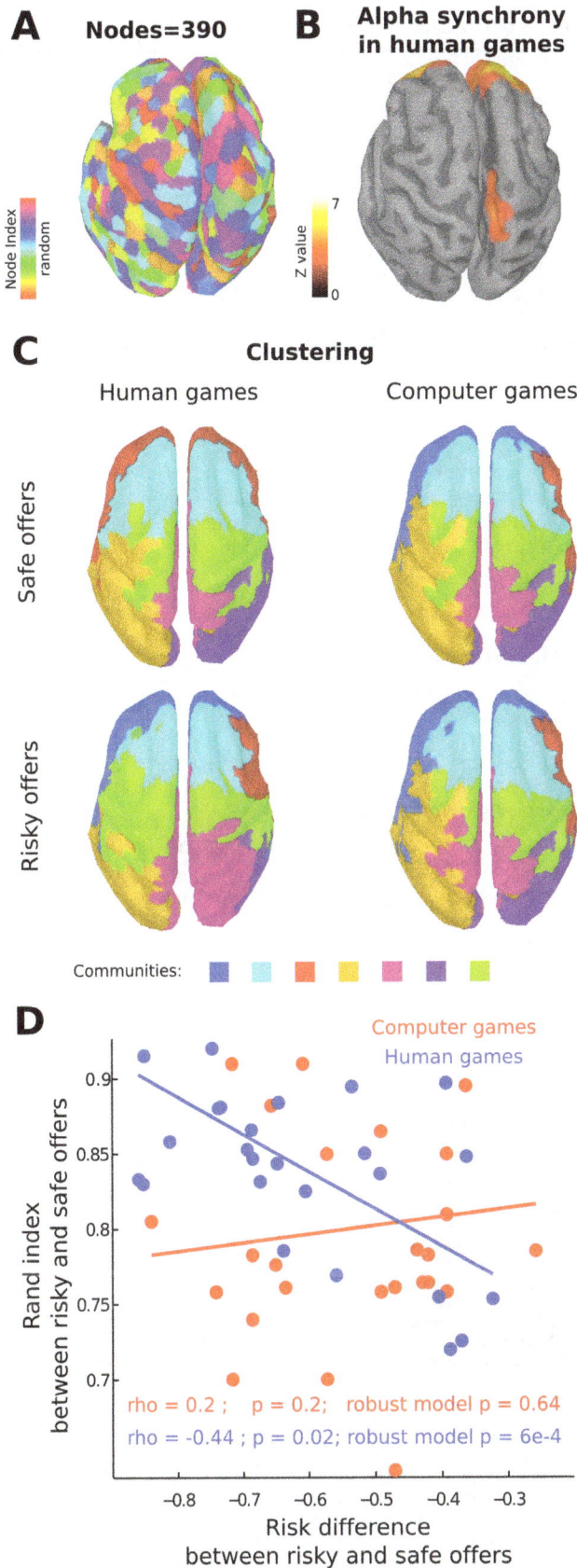

Figure 3. Source level. A, Cortical areas that represent each node in the global network (colors represent node indexes in random order). **B,** Areas where the synchrony (inter-site-phase-clustering) differences between risky and safe offers in human game were significant (FDR, q<0.05). **C,** Community structure of the population networks by conditions (colors represent de community index). Note that there are no main variations between risky and safe offers in the computer game, while there is a notorious variation in human games. **D,** Correlation between the differences in the risk of the offers made (logit of the probability to acceptance, risky offers – safe offers) and the change of the community structure per each subject. Note that only in human games there is a significant correlation. Blue depicts human games and red computer games.

modulation in alpha is associated with the risk of the offer in a temporo-parietal region compatible with social processing areas (such as the temporo-parietal junction and superior temporal sulcus), and the entropy of the offer in regions syndicated as part of the cingulo-opercular network [13]. Altogether, this evidence is compatible with a functional dissociation between phase and power modulation in the alpha band measure over the scalp [49].

Since cognitive control processes necessary to solve social dilemmas require flexible long-range communication and integration among brain areas [5], we finally explored changes in the cortical network structure using graph theory analysis. At the population level, the community structure between risky and safe offers did not differ in games with computer partners. Interestingly, in human games the community structure was different between conditions mainly in prefrontal and parietal cortex. Although a one-to-one assignment of anatomical brain regions to the retrieved modules is difficult to define, our results reveal an overlap between the modules and some well-known functional areas of the brain. The modules in inferior frontal gyrus are compatible with the frontal parts of the fronto-parietal control network [50]. As we mentioned above, cognitive control is an essential process that enables us to carry out social interaction [34]. In childhood, prefrontal cortex maturation correlates with both impulse control and cooperative behavior in social contexts [51]. In addition, alterations in cognitive control are an important factor underlying social impairments of several psychiatric diseases such as schizophrenia [52,53] and depression [54,55]. The notorious differences in frontal and parietal modules in HGs may therefore reflect the behavioral control required to carry out a social bargaining. Across the HGs, people tended to change less their offers, as if expecting that the others would also change their behaviors (Table 1, and [15]). Thus on the first rounds, people can tolerate rejection and do not change their behavior in order to obtain more acceptances on the later rounds [15,56]. However, to maintain this strategy, a greater cognitive control is required. In accordance with this interpretation, we found a specific correlation in HGs, where people who presented less difference between high-risk and low-risk offers showed a greater functional network differentiation (Figure 3D).

The functional networks that we found also include a central module in sensory-motor cortex. This module is compatible with the source of mu rhythms [57] whose power decreases (also called suppression or local desynchronization) has been related to mirror system activity during social games [58], motor coordination between humans [59] and the imagination of social interactions [60]. Moreover, recent work has shown that power in alpha range over sensory motor cortex is related to facial emotion recognition and it is negatively correlated with connectivity of the motor sensory cortex with other cortical areas [61]. In our experiment we found that the main modulation of global alpha synchrony was temporally dissociated from power modulation (Figure 2). However, the change in power was related to the community structure and not to the overall synchrony as the robust linear model shows

Table 2. Model of the difference in modularity between risky and safe offer (Rand Index).

	Scope	Std. Error.	T-value	p-value
(Intercept)	0.8329	0.0539	15.4663	0
Risk diff.	0.0639	0.0939	0.6801	0.5008
Strength diff.	0	0.0003	-0.0093	0.9926
Power diff.	0.5665	0,268	2.1138	0.0415
Human Games	-0.128	0.0711	-1.7992	0.0804
Risk diff.×Human Games	-0.2923	0.1203	-2.4295	0.0202
degree of freedom = 44				

(Table 2). This most likely reflects that the relations between phase synchrony and power is specific for each cortical area. Due to the low spatial resolution of our source reconstructions, we cannot accurately test these local differences. Finally, the spatial variations of the modules in lateral parietal region could be related to attentional and control networks that present nodes in this region [62,63]. Thus, the variation of community structure over these networks could reflect flexible changes in attentional and control processing during social interactions.

In conclusion, our results complement evidence that shows that during social interaction, humans establish flexible global interactions among different brain regions [6]. More specifically, we show that changes in the functional network in alpha band range takes place during social interaction, which could reflect cognitive control requirements to maintain an ongoing bargaining. Inter-site-phase-clustering (phase synchrony) of alpha oscillations could

therefore serve as a mechanism by which cognitive control areas exert modulation over and receive information from social specialized brain areas in order to adapt behavior to current demands and changing social contexts.

Acknowledgments

We want to thank Matías Morales and Marina Flores for proofreading the manuscript.

Author Contributions

Conceived and designed the experiments: PB DC FA. Performed the experiments: PB FZ. Analyzed the data: PB FZ MC. Contributed reagents/materials/analysis tools: PB FZ MC. Wrote the paper: PB MC DC FA.

References

1. Batson C (1990) How social an animal? The human capacity for caring. Am Psychol 45: 336–346. doi:10.1037/0003-066X.45.3.336.

2. Humphrey N (1976) The Social Function of intellect. In: Hinde PPGB& RA, editor. Growing points in ethology. Cambridge, England: Cambridge University Press.

3. Adolphs R (2009) The social brain: neural basis of social knowledge. Annu Rev Psychol 60: 693–716. doi:10.1146/annurev.psych.60.110707.163514.

4. Rilling JK, Sanfey AG (2011) The neuroscience of social decision-making. Annu Rev Psychol 62: 23–48. doi:10.1146/annurev.psych.121208.131647.

5. Kennedy DP, Adolphs R (2012) The social brain in psychiatric and neurological disorders. Trends Cogn Sci 16: 559–572. doi:10.1016/j.tics.2012.09.006.

6. Barrett LF, Satpute AB (2013) Large-scale brain networks in affective and social neuroscience: towards an integrative functional architecture of the brain. Curr Opin Neurobiol 23: 361–372. doi:10.1016/j.conb.2012.12.012.

7. Betti V, Zappasodi F, Rossini PM, Aglioti SM, Tecchio F (2009) Synchronous with your feelings: sensorimotor gamma band and empathy for pain. J Neurosci 29: 12384–12392. doi:10.1523/JNEUROSCI.2759-09.2009.

8. Dumas G, Nadel J, Soussignan R, Martinerie J, Garnero L (2010) Inter-brain synchronization during social interaction. PLoS One 5: e12166. doi:10.1371/journal.pone.0012166.

9. Cole MW, Reynolds JR, Power JD, Repovs G, Anticevic A, et al. (2013) Multi-task connectivity reveals flexible hubs for adaptive task control. Nat Neurosci 16. doi:10.1038/nn.3470.

10. Varela F, Lachaux JP, Rodriguez E, Martinerie J (2001) The brainweb: phase synchronization and large-scale integration. Nat Rev Neurosci 2: 229–239. doi:10.1038/35067550.

11. Güth W, Schmittberger R, Schwarze B (1982) An experimental analysis of ultimatum bargaining. J Econ Behav Organ 3: 367–388. doi:10.1016/0167-2681(82)90011-7.

12. Slembeck T (1999) Reputations and Fairness in Bargaining Experimental Evidence from a Repeated Ultimatum Game. Discuss Pap Dep Econ Univ St Gall 9904: 29.

13. Billeke P, Zamorano F, Cosmelli D, Aboitiz F (2013) Oscillatory Brain Activity Correlates with Risk Perception and Predicts Social Decisions. Cereb Cortex 23: 2872–2883. doi:10.1093/cercor/bhs269.

14. Koster-Hale J, Saxe R (2013) Theory of Mind: A Neural Prediction Problem. Neuron 79: 836–848. doi:10.1016/j.neuron.2013.08.020.

15. Billeke P, Zamorano F, López T, Rodriguez C, Cosmelli D, et al. (2014) Someone has to Give In: Theta Oscillations Correlate with Adaptive Behavior in Social Bargaining. Soc Cogn Affect Neurosci in press. doi:10.1093/scan/nsu012.

16. Baillet S, Mosher JC, Leahy RM (2001) Electromagnetic brain mapping. IEEE Signal Process Mag 18: 14–30.

17. Clerc M, Gramfort A, Olivi E, Papadopoulo T (2010) The symmetric BEM: bringing in more variables for better accuracy. In: Supek S, Sušac A, editors. 17th International Conference on Biomagnetism Advances in Biomagnetism – Biomag2010. Dubrovnik (Croatia): Springer Berlin Heidelberg, Vol. 28. 109–112. doi:10.1007/978-3-642-12197-5_21.

18. Lin F-H, Witzel T, Ahlfors SP, Stufflebeam SM, Belliveau JW, et al. (2006) Assessing and improving the spatial accuracy in MEG source localization by depth-weighted minimum-norm estimates. Neuroimage 31: 160–171. doi:10.1016/j.neuroimage.2005.11.054.

19. Lachaux JP, Rodriguez E, Martinerie J, Varela FJ (1999) Measuring phase synchrony in brain signals. Hum Brain Mapp 8: 194–208.

20. Fisher N (1995) Statistical analysis of circular data. Cambridge University Press.

21. Pons P, Latapy M (2005) Computing communities in large networks using random walks (long version). J Graph Algorith Appl 10: 191–218.

22. Newman MEJ (2006) Modularity and community structure in networks. Proc Natl Acad Sci U S A 103: 8577–8582. doi:10.1073/pnas.0601602103.

23. Valencia M, Pastor M a, Fernández-Seara M a, Artieda J, Martinerie J, et al. (2009) Complex modular structure of large-scale brain networks. Chaos 19: 023119. doi:10.1063/1.3129783.

24. Rand WM (1971) Objective Criteria for the Evaluation of Clustering Methods. J Am Stat Assoc 66: 846–850.

25. Maris E, Oostenveld R (2007) Nonparametric statistical testing of EEG- and MEG-data. J Neurosci Methods 164: 177–190. doi:10.1016/j.jneumeth.2007.03.024.

26. Zamorano F, Billeke P, Hurtado JM, López V, Carrasco X, et al. (2014) Temporal Constraints of Behavioral Inhibition: Relevance of Inter-stimulus Interval in a Go-Nogo Task. PLoS One 9: e87232. doi:10.1371/journal.pone.0087232.

27. Tadel F, Baillet S, Mosher JC, Pantazis D, Leahy RM (2011) Brainstorm: a user-friendly application for MEG/EEG analysis. Comput Intell Neurosci 2011: 879716. doi:10.1155/2011/879716.

28. Gramfort A, Papadopoulo T, Olivi E, Clerc M (2011) Forward field computation with OpenMEEG. Comput Intell Neurosci 2011: 923703. doi:10.1155/2011/923703.

29. Cocchi L, Zalesky A, Fornito A, Mattingley JB (2013) Dynamic cooperation and competition between brain systems during cognitive control. Trends Cogn Sci 17: 493–501. doi:10.1016/j.tics.2013.08.006.

30. Sadaghiani S, Scheeringa R, Lehongre K, Morillon B, Giraud A-L, et al. (2012) Alpha-Band Phase Synchrony Is Related To Activity in the Fronto-Parietal Adaptive Control Network. J Neurosci 32: 14305–14310. doi:10.1523/JNEUROSCI.1358-12.2012.

31. Jann K, Dierks T, Boesch C, Kottlow M, Strik W, et al. (2009) BOLD correlates of EEG alpha phase-locking and the fMRI default mode network. Neuroimage 45: 903–916. doi:10.1016/j.neuroimage.2009.01.001.

32. Dosenbach NUF, Fair D a, Cohen AL, Schlaggar BL, Petersen SE (2008) A dual-networks architecture of top-down control. Trends Cogn Sci 12: 99–105. doi:10.1016/j.tics.2008.01.001.

33. Phillips JM, Vinck M, Everling S, Womelsdorf T (2013) A Long-Range Fronto-Parietal 5- to 10-Hz Network Predicts "Top-Down" Controlled Guidance in a Task-Switch Paradigm. Cereb Cortex. doi:10.1093/cercor/bht050.

34. Declerck CH, Boone C, Emonds G (2013) When do people cooperate? The neuroeconomics of prosocial decision making. Brain Cogn 81: 95–117. doi:10.1016/j.bandc.2012.09.009.

35. Stevens JR, Hauser MD (2004) Why be nice? Psychological constraints on the evolution of cooperation. Trends Cogn Sci 8: 60–65. doi:10.1016/j.tics.2003.12.003.

36. Haufe S, Nikulin V V, Müller K-R, Nolte G (2013) A critical assessment of connectivity measures for EEG data: a simulation study. Neuroimage 64: 120–133. doi:10.1016/j.neuroimage.2012.09.036.

37. Gonçalves SI, de Munck JC, Pouwels PJW, Schoonhoven R, Kuijer JP a, et al. (2006) Correlating the alpha rhythm to BOLD using simultaneous EEG/fMRI: inter-subject variability. Neuroimage 30: 203–213. doi:10.1016/j.neuroimage.2005.09.062.

38. Laufs H, Kleinschmidt a, Beyerle a, Eger E, Salek-Haddadi a, et al. (2003) EEG-correlated fMRI of human alpha activity. Neuroimage 19: 1463–1476. doi:10.1016/S1053-8119(03)00286-6.

39. Laufs H, Holt JL, Elfont R, Krams M, Paul JS, et al. (2006) Where the BOLD signal goes when alpha EEG leaves. Neuroimage 31: 1408–1418. doi:10.1016/j.neuroimage.2006.02.002.

40. Cosmelli D, López V, Lachaux J-P, López-Calderón J, Renault B, et al. (2011) Shifting visual attention away from fixation is specifically associated with alpha band activity over ipsilateral parietal regions. Psychophysiology 48: 312–322. doi:10.1111/j.1469-8986.2010.01066.x.

41. Sadaghiani S, Scheeringa R, Lehongre K, Morillon B, Giraud A-L, et al. (2010) Intrinsic connectivity networks, alpha oscillations, and tonic alertness: a simultaneous electroencephalography/functional magnetic resonance imaging study. J Neurosci 30: 10243–10250. doi:10.1523/JNEUROSCI.1004-10.2010.

42. Hanslmayr S, Klimesch W, Sauseng P, Gruber W, Doppelmayr M, et al. (2005) Visual discrimination performance is related to decreased alpha amplitude but

43. increased phase locking. Neurosci Lett 375: 64–68. doi:10.1016/j.neulet.2004.10.092.

43. Varela F, Toro A, John ER, Schwartz E (1981) Perceptual framing and cortical alpha rhythm. Neuropsychologia 19: 675–686.

44. VanRullen R, Koch C (2003) Is perception discrete or continuous? Trends Cogn Sci 7: 207–213. doi:10.1016/S1364-6613(03)00095-0.

45. Busch N a, Dubois J, VanRullen R (2009) The phase of ongoing EEG oscillations predicts visual perception. J Neurosci 29: 7869–7876. doi:10.1523/JNEUROSCI.0113-09.2009.

46. Jensen O, Mazaheri A (2010) Shaping functional architecture by oscillatory alpha activity: gating by inhibition. Front Hum Neurosci 4: 186. doi:10.3389/fnhum.2010.00186.

47. Mazaheri A, Jensen O (2010) Rhythmic pulsing: linking ongoing brain activity with evoked responses. Front Hum Neurosci 4: 177. doi:10.3389/fnhum.2010.00177.

48. Klimesch W (2012) Alpha-band oscillations, attention, and controlled access to stored information. Trends Cogn Sci 16: 606–617. doi:10.1016/j.tics.2012.10.007.

49. Palva S, Palva JM (2011) Functional roles of alpha-band phase synchronization in local and large-scale cortical networks. Front Psychol 2: 204. doi:10.3389/fpsyg.2011.00204.

50. Power JDD, Cohen ALL, Nelson SMM, Wig GSS, Barnes KAA, et al. (2011) Functional Network Organization of the Human Brain. Neuron 72: 665–678. doi:10.1016/j.neuron.2011.09.006.

51. Steinbeis N, Bernhardt BC, Singer T (2012) Impulse Control and Underlying Functions of the Left DLPFC Mediate Age-Related and Age-Independent Individual Differences in Strategic Social Behavior. Neuron 73: 1040–1051. doi:10.1016/j.neuron.2011.12.027.

52. Couture SM, Granholm EL, Fish SC (2011) A path model investigation of neurocognition, theory of mind, social competence, negative symptoms and real-world functioning in schizophrenia. Schizophr Res 125: 152–160. doi:10.1016/j.schres.2010.09.020.

53. Billeke P, Aboitiz F (2013) Social Cognition in Schizophrenia: From Social Stimuli Processing to Social Engagement. Front Psychiatry 4: 1–12. doi:10.3389/fpsyt.2013.00004.

54. Cusi AM, Nazarov A, Holshausen K, Macqueen GM, McKinnon MC (2012) Systematic review of the neural basis of social cognition in patients with mood disorders. J Psychiatry Neurosci 37: 154–169. doi:10.1503/jpn.100179.

55. Billeke P, Boardman S, Doraiswamy PM (2013) Social cognition in major depressive disorder: A new paradigm? Transl Neurosci 4: 437–447. doi:10.2478/s13380-013-0147-9.

56. Avrahami J, Güth W, Hertwig R, Kareev Y, Otsubo H (2013) Learning (not) to yield: An experimental study of evolving ultimatum game behavior. J Socio Econ 47: 47–54. doi:10.1016/j.socec.2013.08.009.

57. Arroyo S, Lesser RP, Gordon B, Uematsu S, Jackson D, et al. (1993) Functional significance of the mu rhythm of human cortex: an electrophysiologic study with subdural electrodes. Electroencephalogr Clin Neurophysiol 87: 76–87. doi:10.1016/0013-4694(93)90114-B.

58. Perry A, Stein L, Bentin S (2011) Motor and attentional mechanisms involved in social interaction–evidence from mu and alpha EEG suppression. Neuroimage 58: 895–904. doi:10.1016/j.neuroimage.2011.06.060.

59. Naeem M, Prasad G, Watson DR, Kelso J a S (2012) Functional dissociation of brain rhythms in social coordination. Clin Neurophysiol 123: 1789–1797. doi:10.1016/j.clinph.2012.02.065.

60. Vanderwert RE, Fox N a, Ferrari PF (2013) The mirror mechanism and mu rhythm in social development. Neurosci Lett 540: 15–20. doi:10.1016/j.neulet.2012.10.006.

61. Popov T, Miller G a., Rockstroh B, Weisz N (2013) Modulation of α power and functional connectivity during facial affect recognition. J Neurosci 33: 6018–6026. doi:10.1523/JNEUROSCI.2763-12.2013.

62. Smith SM, Fox PT, Miller KL, Glahn DC, Fox PM, et al. (2009) Correspondence of the brain's functional architecture during activation and rest. Proc Natl Acad Sci U S A 106: 13040–13045. doi:10.1073/pnas.0905267106.

63. Corbetta M, Shulman GL (2002) Control of goal-directed and stimulus-driven attention in the brain. Nat Rev Neurosci 3: 201–215. doi:10.1038/nrn755.

22

Sustained Selective Attention to Competing Amplitude-Modulations in Human Auditory Cortex

Lars Riecke[1]*, Wolfgang Scharke[2], Giancarlo Valente[1], Alexander Gutschalk[3]

1 Department of Cognitive Neuroscience, Faculty of Psychology and Neuroscience, Maastricht University, Maastricht, The Netherlands, 2 Department of Child and Adolescent Psychiatry, Psychotherapy and Psychosomatics, University Hospital, RWTH Aachen University, Aachen, Germany, 3 Department of Neurology, Ruprecht-Karls-Universität Heidelberg, Heidelberg, Germany

Abstract

Auditory selective attention plays an essential role for identifying sounds of interest in a scene, but the neural underpinnings are still incompletely understood. Recent findings demonstrate that neural activity that is time-locked to a particular amplitude-modulation (AM) is enhanced in the auditory cortex when the modulated stream of sounds is selectively attended to under sensory competition with other streams. However, the target sounds used in the previous studies differed not only in their AM, but also in other sound features, such as carrier frequency or location. Thus, it remains uncertain whether the observed enhancements reflect AM-selective attention. The present study aims at dissociating the effect of AM frequency on response enhancement in auditory cortex by using an ongoing auditory stimulus that contains two competing targets differing exclusively in their AM frequency. Electroencephalography results showed a sustained response enhancement for auditory attention compared to visual attention, but not for AM-selective attention (attended AM frequency vs. ignored AM frequency). In contrast, the response to the ignored AM frequency was enhanced, although a brief trend toward response enhancement occurred during the initial 15 s. Together with the previous findings, these observations indicate that selective enhancement of attended AMs in auditory cortex is adaptive under sustained AM-selective attention. This finding has implications for our understanding of cortical mechanisms for feature-based attentional gain control.

Editor: Jyrki Ahveninen, Harvard Medical School/Massachusetts General Hospital, United States of America

Funding: This work was supported by Veni grant 451-11-014 to LR from the Netherlands Organization for Scientific Research (www.nwo.nl). The funder had no role in study design, data collection and analysis, decision to publish, or preparation of the manuscript.

Competing Interests: The authors have declared that no competing interests exist.

* Email: L.Riecke@MaastrichtUniversity.nl

Introduction

How can we hear out a sound in an auditory scene? According to contemporary views [1,2], the extraction of a sound of interest from a mixture is facilitated by directing one's attention toward a distinctive feature of that sound, as this leads to selective enhancement of that feature and temporally coherent features in the cortex relative to unattended features. Evidence for such a top-down, feature-based gain control mechanism comes from several human brain studies showing that selective attention to a specific tone frequency or a specific location enhances neural responses to sounds that comprise the attended frequency or originate from the attended location, respectively [3,4,5,6,7,8,9]. Thus, attentional gain control seems to operate on various sound features in the cortex, including tone frequency and sound location.

Recently, this idea has been extended to amplitude modulation (AM), i.e., the temporal envelope of the sound waveform. It has been shown that selective attention to an AM sound may enhance cortical responses synchronized with the AM (the auditory steady-state response, SSR), compared with selective attention to a differently modulated, competing sound [10,11,12,13] or to visual input [14,15,16,17,18,19,20]. Considering that AM has been suggested to be encoded in AM-frequency specific channels

[21,22] in the auditory cortex (AC) [23,24] and earlier processing stages [25,26,27,28], these findings may suggest that attentional gain control operates on temporal AM representations in AC.

A limitation of these studies is that the attended sound could be distinguished from the unattended sound based on not only AM, but also other sound features, such as carrier frequency or location. Thus, it remains unclear whether the observed response enhancements reflect selective attention to AM or to other sound features that may have been enhanced, e.g., through tonotopic or location-specific representations that were captured by the SSR due to their temporal coherence with the AMs [2]. Moreover, most studies used relatively short sounds in the range of a few seconds or less and did not investigate changes in response enhancement over time. Thus, it remains unclear whether AM-specific attentional gain control operates stably over intervals of several tens of seconds [18]. Finally, most studies focused on rapid AMs (AM frequencies of 20 Hz or higher), while comparatively little is known about gain control for slower AMs in the range of a few Hz [12,13] although the latter are crucial for speech comprehension [29]. The few studies that used relatively long speech sounds (spoken sentences) [30,31,32] found sustained speaker-selective attentional enhancement in AC, even when the competing sounds originated from the same location, had similar frequencies, or produced similar peripheral excitation patterns. As for the other studies, it is uncertain whether listeners in these studies attended exclusively to the slow AMs in the speech signals or to other distinctive sound features, such as the timbre of the voice or the size of the resonance body.

The goal of the present study was to address the previous limitations and to investigate gain control in human cortex based on attention to slow AM frequencies alone over a long interval. We tested whether selective listening to one of two competing periodic AM frequencies is accompanied by selective enhancement of the temporal representation of that AM frequency in AC (compared with the representation of the competing AM frequency, which was applied to the same tone carrier at the same location). To that end, we first identified the time-locked auditory cortical representation of the individual AM frequencies using the SSR measured with scalp electroencephalography (EEG). We then characterized this temporal AM-frequency representation together with participants' perception under different attentional (but otherwise similar) conditions induced by behavioral tasks that required either sustained selective listening to one or the other AM frequency, or visual attention.

Our principal finding is that sustained AM-selective attention does not induce sustained response enhancement for the attended AM compared with the ignored AM. Although we observed an initial trend toward AM-selective attentional response enhancement, overall the response to the ignored AM frequency was enhanced.

Materials and Methods

Participants

Fourteen paid volunteers (eight females, ages 18–39 years) with no reported hearing, vision, or motor problems participated in the study after providing written informed consent. Ethical approval was obtained from the local ethics committee (*Ethische Commissie Psychologie*) of the Faculty of Psychology and Neuroscience of Maastricht University.

Stimuli

Figure 1 illustrates the waveforms of the auditory stimuli. Stimulus duration was set to 55 s to allow studying changes of both perception and AM representation over a long interval. The stimuli contained either a single AM tone (single-AM stimuli; see Figure 1, upper two rows) or two AM tones of the same carrier frequency (dual-AM stimulus; see Figure 1, lower three rows) [33,34,35]. The single-AM stimuli were generated by multiplying a 930-Hz sinusoidal carrier with a full-wave rectified full-amplitude sinusoidal modulator (modulation depth: 100%). The frequency of the rectified modulator was set to 2.5 Hz (f_1) or 7 Hz (f_2) to create what we will refer to as "slow AM" or "fast AM", respectively. The dual-AM stimulus was generated by adding the slow AM and fast AM after setting amplitudes so that both AMs would appear equally salient (see below, section Procedure).

The specific modulation rates chosen had several advantages. Firstly, they allow studying neural correlates of syllable analysis [36] and speech comprehension [29]. Secondly, they evoke robust responses in the EEG power spectrum for pure tone carriers, i.e., strong and well-separated peaks at low harmonics [33,37,38,39,40,41]. Thirdly, they are sufficiently different from each other to provide robust temporal cues for auditory stream segregation (referred to as "streaming" in the following) [42]. Finally, they are sufficiently similar and sufficiently slow to reduce spectral cues and pitch cues for streaming, because the side-bands

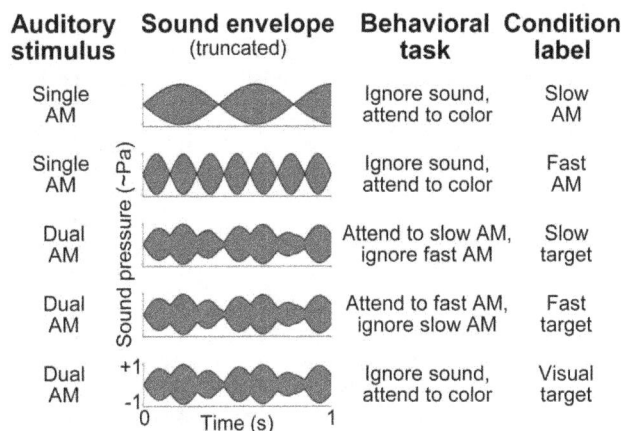

Figure 1. Auditory stimuli, behavioral tasks, and experimental design. Simple auditory rhythms were generated by applying either a slow or fast AM to a fixed pure tone carrier (rows 1, 2). A polyrhythm was generated by mixing these single rhythms, i.e., both AMs were applied to the same carrier and then added (rows 3–5). The stimuli had a duration of 55 s and were presented during selective auditory and visual attention tasks (third column), which served to draw participants' attention to the slow or fast rhythm (rows 3, 4) or away from auditory input (rows 1, 2, 5). The single-AM conditions were used to identify the time-locked neural representation of the individual AMs. The dual-AM conditions were used to test whether this temporal AM representation was selectively enhanced during sustained selective attention to/away from a specific AM (in the absence of acoustic stimulus differences and location or pitch cues for streaming).

that these modulations induce in the stimulus spectrum are not resolved in the excitation pattern of the auditory nerve [43].

The auditory stimuli were matched for peak amplitude. Starting phases of carrier and modulators were held constant throughout. Stimuli were sampled at a rate of 44.1 kHz with 16-bit resolution and presented binaurally at maximal 65 dB SPL using Presentation software (Neurobehavioral Systems), a Sound Blaster Live sound card (Creative Technology), a Soundcraft EXF8 mixer (Harman), a P4050 amplifier (Yamaha), and two JBL Control 25 loudspeakers (Harman). The speakers were located in front of the participant in the left and right upper corner of the EEG recording chamber. The speaker-ear distance was approximately 1.5 m.

Task and design

The experimental design involved the five conditions illustrated in Figure 1 (see labels in last column). They were defined by combining the three auditory stimuli (slow, fast, or dual AM) with selective auditory and visual attention tasks that served to draw the participants' attention either toward a specific AM or away from the auditory stimuli and keep participants in a stable alert state.

For the selective listening task, the dual AM was used as the auditory stimulus. Participants were instructed to focus their attention on either the slow or fast rhythm in the mixture, depending on the experimental condition ("slow target" condition or "fast target" condition, respectively), and ignore the concurrent "non-target" rhythm. They were further instructed to report their current percept whenever a rhythm became perceptually dominant over the other (when the initial percept had finished building up and, thereafter, in case a perceptual reversal occurred) by pressing a corresponding button. For the visual attention task, either one of the single AMs ("slow AM" condition or "fast AM" condition) or the dual AM ("visual target" condition) was used as the auditory stimulus, depending on the experimental condition.

Participants were instructed to ignore this stimulus and focus their attention on the color of a fixation cross. The cross was presented in white on a black screen throughout all auditory and visual tasks, and in the visual task, it further changed its color to green, red, or blue for 200 ms at irregular times. Participants were instructed to report whenever the cross turned green or red in the visual task by pressing a corresponding button. Participants performed the tasks using their two index fingers on two buttons of a button box. The labels of the two buttons were "*slow*" and "fast" (for the *slow* target condition), "slow" and "*fast*" (for the *fast* target condition), or "green" and "red" (for the visual target condition), and they were shown above the cross in the center of the screen.

Individual trials lasted 80 s and contained three consecutive intervals. The first 5 s comprised a preparation interval, during which the cross and the button labels indicating the upcoming task lighted up. The subsequent 55 s comprised the task interval, during which an auditory stimulus was presented and the participant performed the task as indicated, while the cross and button labels remained visible. The final 20 s comprised a rest interval, during which only the cross remained visible for another 10 s followed by a blank screen. The order of trials was pseudorandomized so that each combination of two successive conditions appeared equally often in order to counterbalance possible long-term perceptual aftereffects of preceding modulations [44,45,46].

Procedure

AM-saliency matching. Participants were seated in a comfortable chair in a sound-attenuating, electrically shielded booth. Saliency matches for the slow and fast AM were obtained using a sound level adjustment task as follows. Participants were presented with the dual-AM stimulus and asked to adjust the amplitude ratio of the slow and fast rhythm so that these rhythms would appear equally salient. The AM-saliency matches, defined as the average of ten measurements, revealed that participants scaled the amplitudes of the slow AM and fast AM on average to a ratio of 1:1.3, indicating that they perceived the slow AM in the original dual-AM stimulus as more salient, in line with results on modulation detection [47,48]. For the subsequent EEG experiments, the relative amplitudes in the dual-AM stimulus were set individually according to the obtained matches so that the two AMs would appear equally salient.

EEG experiments. Following AM-saliency matching, participants practiced the different tasks until they felt confident that they could perform them well. For the EEG measurements, they received further instructions to keep their gaze at the fixation cross, to relax, and to avoid motor activity other than button presses. They then underwent five blocks of EEG measurements, each comprising nine experimental trials and simultaneous EEG recordings, with self-terminated breaks in between blocks. In total, nine trials of each condition were presented and one hour of experimental EEG data was recorded. During debriefing, participants were asked to provide written report of their strategies for performing the tasks and rate their perception of a potential third "beating" rhythm in the dual AM conditions (f_2-f_1, the interaction of the individual AM rates in the peripheral auditory system) on a two-point scale.

EEG recording. EEG was recorded from 64 positions on the scalp in reference to the left mastoid, using Ag/AgCl electrodes (mounted in Easycaps, modified full 10%-system) and Neuroscan amplifiers that were decoupled from the audio system via optical fibers. Electrooculography was recorded below the left eye using an additional electrode. Interelectrode impedances were kept below 5 kΩ by abrading the skin. The EEG recordings were bandpass-filtered (cutoffs: 0.05 and 100 Hz, analog filter) and then digitized using a sampling rate of 250 Hz.

Behavioral data analysis

Button responses in the auditory task were re-sampled at a rate of 1 Hz to create a time series of participants' reported dominant percept (which alternated between the target and the non-target) for each trial. Two measures were extracted from these on/off-series for each participant: First, after concatenating the trials, a perceptual dominance index was defined as the proportion of overall time that the participant reportedly perceived the target as dominant. Second, for each time point, the probability of perceiving the target was computed for each target condition (slow target, fast target) as the proportion of trials that the participant reported perceiving the target as dominant. The time series of this latter measure was used to identify the endpoint of the interval during which perceptual dominance initially built up [49] (by averaging across the two target conditions and across participants, fitting a sixth-order polynomial, and extracting the time point of the earliest curve slope reversal). Button responses in the visual task were considered as hits or false alarms, depending on whether the reported color did or did not match the actual color, respectively. Hit rates and false alarm rates were computed and transformed into z-scores that were then subtracted to obtain the sensitivity index d' [50]. On average, participants made 2.1 ± 1.0, 2.4 ± 1.3, and 4.0 ± 0.02 button presses (mean ± s.d. across participants) per trial in the slow target, fast target, and visual target condition, respectively.

Neural data analysis

An overview of our EEG data analysis steps is provided in Figure 2.

EEG data preprocessing. EEG data were analyzed using the EEGLAB toolbox [51] and custom Matlab scripts. Data preprocessing involved band-pass filtering (cutoffs: 0.5 and 50 Hz, FIR filter), temporal resampling (sampling rate: 125 Hz), and re-referencing to an average reference (based on the mean activity of all channels). To reduce artifacts, the channel waveforms from each participant were first decomposed into a linear sum of 65 spatially fixed and maximally temporally independent components (ICs) using the extended Infomax ICA algorithm [52,53]; for details see Figure S1. The main advantage of the ICA-based artifact reduction is that it allows the removal of repetitive artifacts without the need to reject entire data epochs [54,55,56]. Next, ICs resembling brain activity were separated from ICs resembling artifacts using visual inspection and standard criteria: ICs primarily accounting for eye movements or blinks were identified based on their far-frontal scalp distributions and irregular occurrence/timing across trials. Other artifact-related ICs, including those accounting for motor activity, were identified based on their non-dipolar scalp maps, flat activity spectra, and irregular occurrence/timing across trials [54,56]. Finally, ICs deemed to resemble brain activity (on average 26 ± 4 ICs, mean ± s.d. across participants) were recomposed and back-projected to yield artifact-reduced EEG channel waveforms.

Extraction of normalized neural response. Neural responses to AM were assessed using the SSR, which captures the magnitude of neural activity fluctuating at the AM frequency. Our frequencies of interest included the first two harmonics of the slow AM (f_1: 2.5 Hz, $2f_1$: 5 Hz) and the fast AM (f_2: 7 Hz, $2f_2$: 14 Hz), and the beat frequency (f_2-f_1: 4.5 Hz). Two arbitrary, stimulus-unrelated frequencies (the first two harmonics of both 2.2 Hz and 6.7 Hz) were further chosen to serve as control frequencies.

1. Preprocessing (per participant)
•Band-pass filtering
•Temporal resampling
•Re-referencing

↓

2. Artifact reduction (per participant)
•Independent component analysis (ICA)
•IC classification based on visual inspection (Fig.S1)
•Removal of artifact-related ICs
•Back-projection of artifact-reduced IC data onto channels

↓

3. Extraction of AM response (per channel and participant)
•Extraction of power spectrum from interval of interest per trial
•Averaging of spectra across trials
•Extraction of neural response for selected frequencies (Fig.3)
•Averaging of neural responses associated with the same fundamental (f and $2f$)

↓

4. Channel selection based on single-AM conditions
•Averaging of slow AM condition (slow response) and fast AM condition (fast response)
•Averaging across participants
•Selection of channels showing strongest responses (Fig.5)

↓

5. Analysis for AM-selective attention effects (per participant)
•Averaging of neural response across the selected channels
•Definition of the 'targets' response: Average of attend slow condition (slow response) and attend fast condition (fast response)
•Definition of the 'non-targets' response: Average of attend slow condition (fast response) and attend fast condition (slow response)
•Definition of neural dominance index: targets response minus non-targets response
•Submit each participant's neural dominance index to random-effects statistical analysis (compare with zero)

↓

6. Analysis for audiovisual attention effects (per participant)
•Averaging of neural response across the selected channels
•Averaging of slow response and fast response in visual target condition
•Averaging of targets response and non-targets response
•Compare the two average measures using random-effects statistical analysis

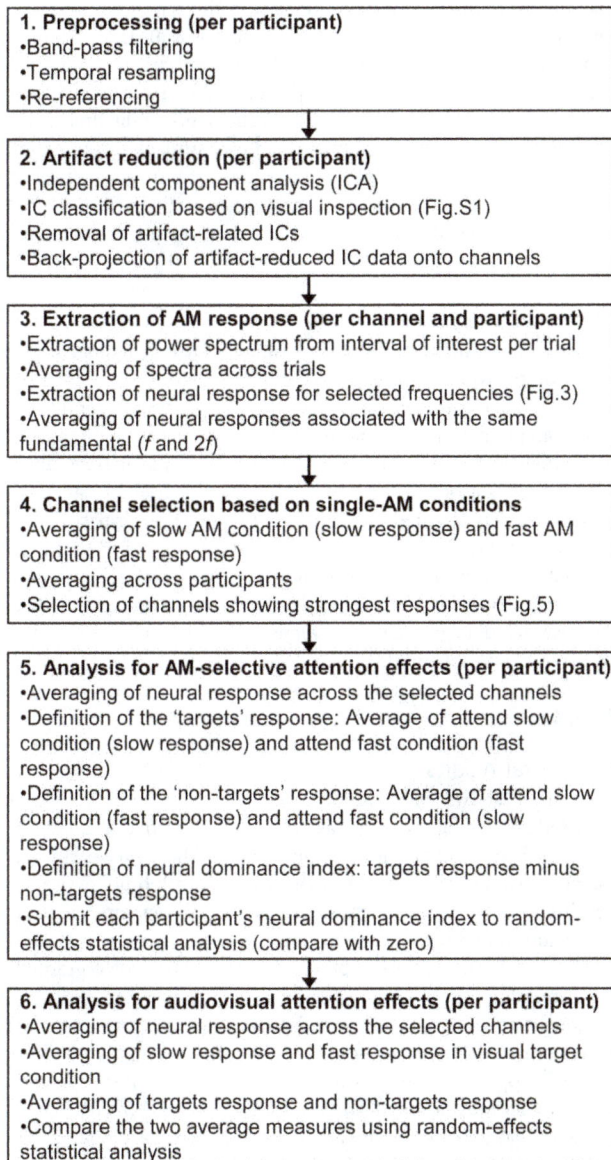

Figure 2. EEG data processing steps. The flowchart provides an overview of the main processing steps applied to the EEG data. Further details are provided in the main text (section Data analysis), Figure S1 (step 2), Figure 3 (step 3), and Figure 5 (step 4). Additional analyses are explained in the main text.

Following previous approaches for SSR measurement [57,58], a normalized measure of the neural response was used; see Figure 3A. This normalized neural response was computed separately for each participant, EEG channel, experimental condition, and frequency of interest as follows. First, for each EEG channel, single-trial EEG power spectral density was estimated by decomposing the channel waveform using the fast Fourier transform. Second, after averaging the single-trial spectra across trials belonging to the same experimental condition, then for each frequency of interest, squared magnitude was extracted for the frequency bin of interest and for "control" bins adjacent to that critical bin (excluding the nearest neighbor on each side of the critical bin to avoid potential leakage effects; see [58]). The adjacent bins were then averaged to define the baseline for the frequency of interest. Finally, for each frequency of interest, the

normalized neural response was computed by dividing the power of the frequency of interest by the power of its baseline minus one. This unit-free measure, which we will refer to as "neural response" for simplicity, is unbiased with respect to broad-band signals (e.g. ongoing brain rhythms in the low-frequency range, such as the alpha band visible in Figure 3B), facilitating its comparison across different frequencies and task conditions.

As shown by Figure 3B, initial EEG data exploration for the critical frequencies at scalp location Cz revealed robust neural responses (i.e., significantly larger than zero, the nominal baseline) for the first two harmonics of each AM frequency (statistical group analysis, $t_{13} = 4.21$, 4.29, 3.09, 2.69, $P < 0.0005$, 0.0005, 0.005, 0.001 for f_1, f_2, $2f_1$, and $2f_2$, respectively) and also the beat frequency ($t_{13} = 3.92$, $P < 0.0005$), in line with previous observations [34,35,37,38]. No significant response was observed for the control frequencies (all $t_{13} < 0.84$, $P > 0.22$). Based on this initial data quality check (and specifically the significant responses to the first two harmonics) and previous approaches [39], we focused subsequent analyses on the average of the first two harmonics. To that end, we averaged the neural response at f_1 with the neural response at $2f_1$, separately for each participant, EEG channel, and experimental condition (analogous for the neural responses associated with f_2 and $2f_2$). In the remainder of this text, we will refer to the averaged harmonics simply as f_1 (for the slow modulation) or f_2 (for the fast modulation).

Extraction of measures of interest. Our first goal was to identify neural activity that followed best the envelope of the

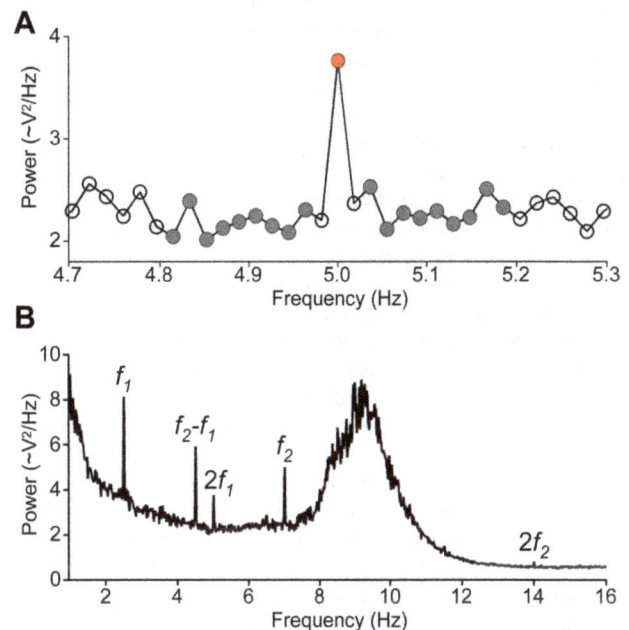

Figure 3. Definition of the neural response. Panel **A** shows group average EEG power spectral density in the dual-AM conditions at a scalp location presumed to reflect auditory-evoked activity (Cz). The magnitude of neural activity to the AMs was assessed using the SSR (which we will refer to as "neural response"), defined as the power ratio of an AM-specific frequency bin (illustrated here for $2f_1$, red circle) to the averaged neighboring bins (baseline, gray circles) minus one. Analyses of shorter time windows (see text, section Time windows of interest) involved fewer baseline bins to avoid overlap between baselines associated with neighboring critical frequencies. Panel **B** provides a larger view of the spectrum shown in panel A. The neural response to the dual AM was significantly stronger than zero for the frequencies of interest (f_1, f_2, $2f_1$, $2f_2$, f_2-f_1).

individual AMs (temporal AM-frequency representation). To that end, the neural response to the single AM stimuli was computed by averaging the response at f_1 in the slow AM condition with the response at f_2 in the fast AM condition; this was done separately for each participant and EEG channel. From the resulting frequency-averaged response, EEG channels showing the strongest responses were extracted for each participant. Our main goal was to test whether this temporal AM-frequency representation is sensitive to attention. Therefore, after averaging the selected channels, further attention-specific measures were extracted from the channel-averaged neural responses for each participant: Firstly, the neural response to the targets was extracted by averaging the response at f_1 in the slow target condition with the response at f_2 in the fast target condition. Secondly, the neural response to the non-targets was extracted analogously by averaging the response at f_2 in the slow target condition with the response at f_1 in the fast target condition. Thirdly, the neural response to the dual AM under visual attention was extracted by averaging the response at f_1 with the response at f_2 in the visual target condition. Finally, the effect of AM-selective attention was quantified using a neural dominance index computed by subtracting the response to the non-targets from the response to the targets. Positive values of this index thus indicate stronger neural responses to the target than to the non-target (i.e., neural dominance of the target), whereas negative values indicate the opposite.

Time windows of interest. The channel waveforms from which the aforementioned measures were initially extracted spanned either the whole task interval or consecutive portions thereof, both excluding the initial stimulus-onset-response interval (the first 1-s portion of the task interval). The purpose of the latter time-resolved analysis was to inspect slow temporal changes of the relevant measures across the task interval. This analysis was enabled by sliding an 11-s analysis window in 1-s steps across the task interval to create a series of 44 consecutive neural responses associated with partially overlapping time windows. In this way, time series of the aforementioned measures of interested could be generated, and slow changes in these measures could be assessed by fitting a line using least squares and extracting the line slope. This analysis was done separately for each participant, and the resulting individual slopes were then submitted to a statistical group analysis to test whether the slopes differed significantly from zero (i.e., no slow change across the task interval).

The different analysis window durations in the whole-interval analysis and time-resolved analysis inevitably induce different frequency resolutions (0.019 Hz and 0.091 Hz, respectively). To avoid overlap among baselines associated with neighboring frequencies of interest, a different number of baseline bins was used for the two analyses (18 bins and 2 bins, respectively).

Correlating neural and behavioral responses. To assess the link between neural and behavioral responses in the auditory task, we first extracted the time series of the neural response; this was done after averaging across the selected channels separately for each trial, each frequency of interest (f_1, f_2), each target condition (slow target, fast target), and each participant. From these single-trial series, a series of neural dominance indices (described above, see section Extraction of measures of interest) was computed; this was done separately for each target condition and each participant. Analogously, we extracted time series of the behavioral response: For each target condition and participant, a series of short-term perceptual dominance indices was computed by sliding an 11-s analysis window in 1-s steps across the behavioral time series (excluding the first 1-s portion of the task interval) and extracting from each window the proportion of time

that the participant reportedly perceived the target as dominant. Finally, after concatenating the index series of all trials from the two target conditions, linear dependence between the neural and perceptual indices was assessed for each participant using Pearson's correlation coefficient r. Participants' individual correlation coefficients were then submitted to statistical group analysis to test whether r differed significantly from zero (i.e., no correlation) after excluding data from four participants (P11-P14) who showed insufficient variance in their behavioral response (Figure S2).

Statistical analysis

The relevant measures that were obtained from each participant (the aforementioned measures of interest, neural and perceptual indices, Fisher transform of r, and line slope) were submitted to group analyses using nonparametric statistical tests [59]. Condition labels were randomly shuffled for each participant and a paired t-test statistic was computed from the shuffled data. This procedure was iterated 5000 times to create a distribution of permutation-based t-statistics. A permutation-based P-value was computed as the proportion of iterations for which the permutation-based t-statistic was larger than the t-statistic obtained from the original data (reported in section Results). The significance criterion α was set to 0.05.

Results

Behavioral results

Figure 4 shows the proportion of trials for which listeners reported perceiving the target as dominant, plotted as a function of time (see Figure S2 for single-subject data). The target dominated listeners' percept for 82±3% of the auditory task time (perceptual dominance index, mean ± s.e.m. across participants) with no significant difference between slow and fast targets ($t_{13} = 0.74$, $P = 0.47$). The initial target percept appeared to evolve gradually after stimulus onset, which has also been observed in studies on auditory streaming [60]. An analysis of curve slopes (see section Behavioral data analysis) revealed that this perceptual build-up finished approximately within the first 13 seconds. Excellent performance was observed in the visual task ($d' = 4.52±0.2$, mean ± s.e.m. across participants), suggesting that participants paid attention to the visual stimuli.

Temporal AM-frequency representation in cortex

To extract neural activity that follows best the individual AM frequencies, we first explored the scalp distribution of the average

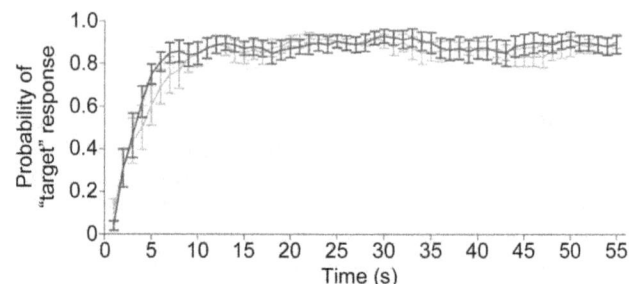

Figure 4. Behavioral results. The plot shows the average probability of perceiving the target as dominant, as a function of time separately for the slow target (dark gray) and fast target (light gray). Error bars represent s.e.m. across all participants. See Figure S2 for single-subject data.

neural response to the single AM stimuli. Consistent with previous data [58], Figures 5A–C show the strongest responses in fronto-central and temporo-posterior scalp regions (see red regions/crosses in Figure 5A; channels Fz, F1, F2, F3, F4, FCz, FC3, FC4, C3, TP9, TP10, P7, P9, P10, PO9, PO10, O9, O10; see Figure S3 for single-subject data). These regions, which we considered to reflect stimulus phase-locked activity of neuronal populations in bilateral AC based on previous EEG source analyses [40,61,62], were then selected for channel-averaged analyses testing for attention-related effects. Averaging across 10, 20, or 50 channels yielded similar results, suggesting that the specific number of selected channels played little role as in related studies [12,13]. The time-resolved analysis of the extracted neural response (i.e., the time course of the average neural response to the single AM stimuli, averaged across the selected channels) revealed that our single AM stimuli evoked robust phase-locking throughout the task interval (neural response>0, Figure 5D). Fitting a line and analyzing the line slope revealed adaptation, i.e., the neural response became weaker across the task interval (line slope <0: $t_{13} = -1.79$, $P = 0.049$, Figure 5D), consistent with previous ideas [37].

Effect of AM-frequency selective attention

Figure 6 illustrates our main result, the effect of AM-selective attention on the channel-averaged neural response. Whole-interval analysis revealed that this response differed significantly for targets vs. non-targets ($t_{13} = -2.38$, $P = 0.025$). Surprisingly, the response to *non-targets* was stronger (Figure 6A, neural dominance index < 0; see Figure S4 for single-subject data). No significant effect was observed for the stimulus-unrelated control frequencies ($t_{13} = 1.73$, $P = 0.11$). These results thus contradict our hypothesis of sustained AM-selective attentional enhancement.

In the following four analyses, we explored this result in more detail, i.e., for shorter time intervals (Figures 6B, C), in relation to listeners' perceptual reports (Figure S2), for separate AM frequencies (Figure 6D), and at individual scalp locations (Figure 6E).

Firstly, plotting the neural dominance index over time revealed negative values mostly during the late portions of the task interval (Figure 6B), which suggests that the observed effect arose only after some delay. This notion was supported by fitting a line to the time series and analyzing the line slope, which showed that the "negative" effect built up slowly (fitted line slope <0: $t_{13} = -1.78$, $P = 0.037$). Notably, the initial 15-s interval showed exclusively positive values. Within this early interval, the neural response exhibited a pattern across attention conditions (Figure 6C, left) that agrees qualitatively with our initial hypothesis of AM-selective attentional enhancement; however, the difference between responses to targets vs. non-targets was not statistically significant ($t_{13} = 1.15$, $P = 0.14$). For reference, Figure 6C (right) shows the average neural response during the final 15-s interval (targets vs. non-targets: $t_{13} = -1.16$, $P = 0.12$).

Secondly, correlation analysis of neural and behavioral dominance indices revealed no significant result ($t_9 = -1.54$, $P = 0.082$). However, the same analysis applied to a dataset that excluded the initial perceptual build-up interval (this interval contained no or only few changes in perception; see Behavioural results) revealed weak but significant coupling (average $r = -0.037 <0$: $t_9 = -1.78$, $P = 0.048$): the longer the target dominated the listener's percept during the analysis interval, the more the non-target dominated the average neural response during this interval. No statistically significant correlation was observed for the stimulus-unrelated control frequencies ($t_9 = -0.99$, $P = 0.17$).

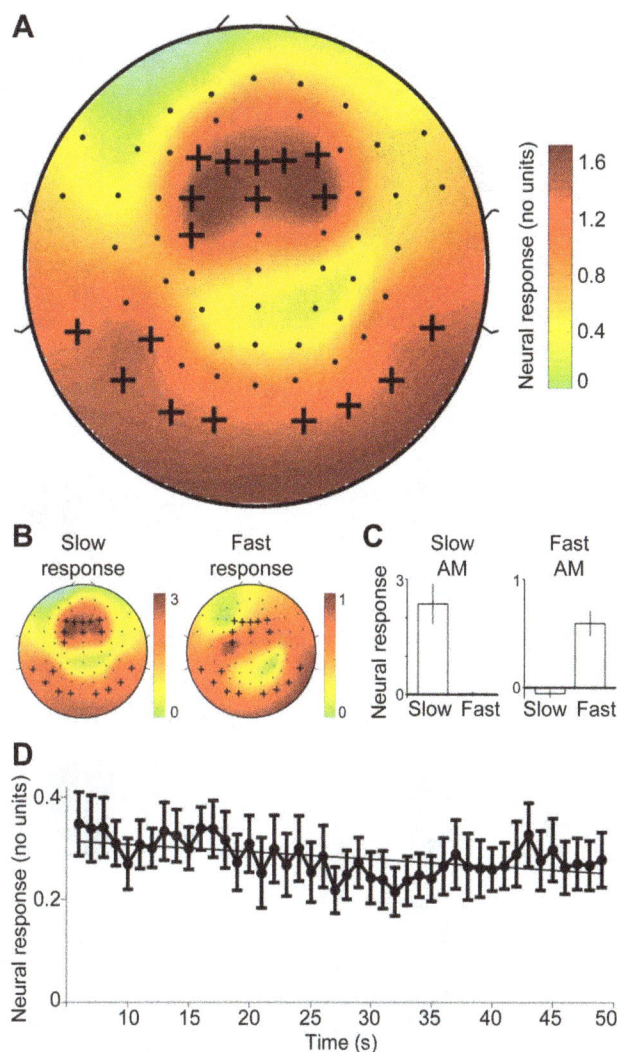

Figure 5. Temporal AM-frequency representation in cortex. Panel **A** shows the scalp distribution of the group average neural response to the single AMs, suggesting a neural origin in AC. EEG channels for which neural activity followed best the individual AM frequencies were selected (crosses), averaged, and further tested for attention-related effects (see Figure 6). See Figure S3 for single-subject data. Panel **B** shows scalp topographies analogously to panel A, but separately for the slow response and the fast response. Panel **C** shows the magnitude of the neural response in the slow AM condition (left plot) and fast AM condition (right plot), averaged across the channels selected in panel A. Within each plot, the left bar corresponds to the slow response (i.e., at f_1) and the right bar corresponds to the fast response (i.e., at f_2). Error bars represent s.e.m. across all participants. Panel **D** shows the magnitude of the neural response over time averaged across the channels selected in panel A. Error bars represent s.e.m. across all participants. The units are the same as in panel A, and the lower magnitudes result from using a shorter analysis window (see section Time windows of interest). The fitted line exhibits a significant negative slope, indicating that this response adapted across the task interval.

Thirdly, the neural response exhibited a similar pattern for each AM frequency (Figure 6D), i.e., there was no statistically significant interaction (f_1/f_2 × target/non-target: $t_{13} = 0.77$, $P = 0.24$), suggesting that slow targets and fast targets contributed similarly to the overall effect.

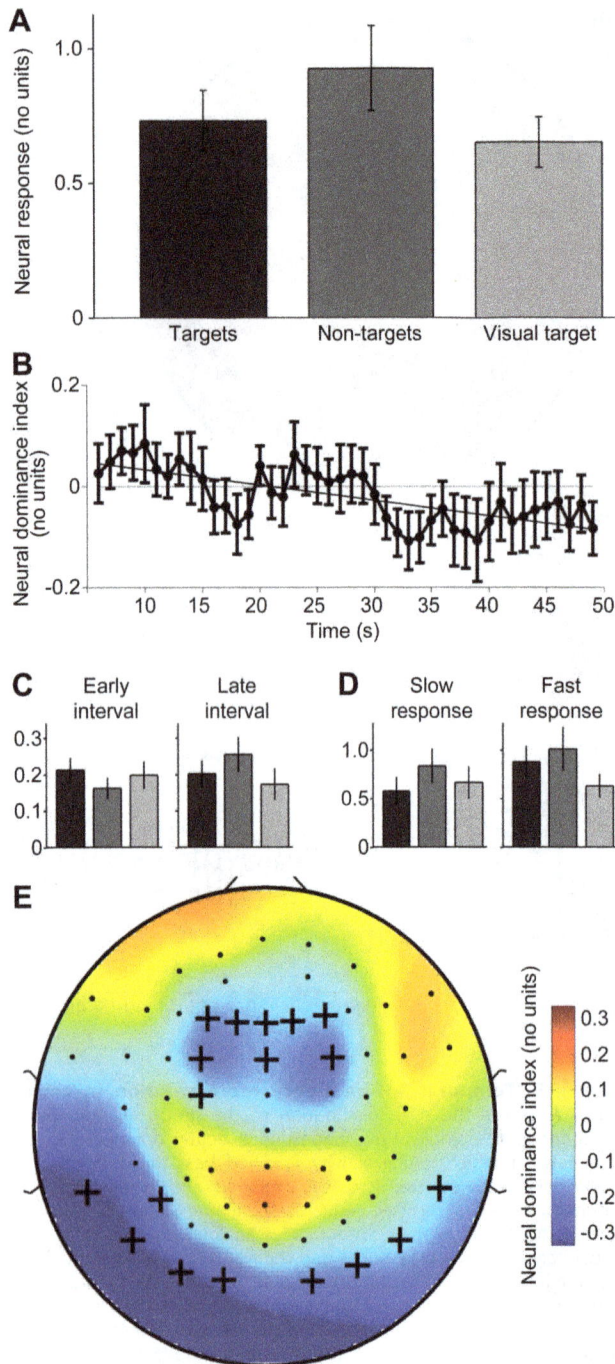

section Time windows of interest). Panel **D** also shows neural responses as in panel A, but separately for the slow neural response (left) and the fast neural response (right), revealing overall similar patterns. Panel **E** shows the spatial distribution of the neural dominance index. Blue and red hue indicates neural dominance of the non-targets and targets, respectively. Crosses indicate the channels from which the results in the other panels were obtained (same as in Figure 5A).

Finally, plotting the neural dominance index separately for each channel revealed a spatial distribution across the scalp highly complementary to that of the average response to the single AM stimuli ($r = -0.80$; compare Figure 6E vs. Figure 5A), thus providing no indication that neural generators outside AC were the source of the effect.

Effect of auditory vs. visual attention

Figure 6 further illustrates the effect of auditory attention relative to visual attention. Whole-interval analysis revealed that the neural response to the dual AM was significantly stronger in the auditory task than the visual task ($t_{13} = 2.22$, $P = 0.019$; Figure 6A; see Figure S4 for single-subject data), consistent with findings based on more rapidly modulated sounds [15,16,17]. As shown by Figure 6A, this enhancement relative to the visual task was driven mostly by the response to non-targets ($t_{13} = 2.71$, $P = 0.0024$) and to a smaller, non-significant extent by the response to targets ($t_{13} = 1.05$, $P = 0.15$). No effect was observed for the stimulus-unrelated control frequencies ($t_{13} = -1.35$, $P = 0.90$).

Beat frequency representation in cortex

Exploratory analysis of the neural response associated with the beat frequency (obtained after averaging the dual-AM conditions) revealed results similar to those obtained for the two AM-stimulus frequencies: The scalp distribution was highly similar ($r = 0.86$) to that observed before (compare Figures 7A, 5A). Channel-averaged analysis further revealed a positive effect of the auditory tasks compared with the visual task as before ($t_{13} = 1.84$, $P = 0.048$; Figure 7B). Finally, group comparison revealed that participants who reported hearing a third beating rhythm in the auditory task (participants P1, P7, P10, P11) produced stronger neural responses at the beat frequency (normalized with respect to the average of slow response and fast response) than participants who reported not hearing such a rhythm (Wilcoxon-Mann-Whitney Test, $U = 38$, $P = 0.0040$); see Figure 7C.

Discussion

Previous studies have shown that selective attention to an AM sound enhances the SSR evoked by the AM of that sound, compared with the SSR evoked by a competing, unattended AM sound with distinct tone frequency or location [10,11,12,13]. The main goal of our study was to test if similar selective attentional enhancement occurs in the absence of location and pitch cues, i.e., when attention is focused exclusively and continuously on a specific ongoing AM.

We observed an enhancement of temporal AM-frequency representations likely located in AC (as measured by the SSR) during sustained auditory attention relative to visual attention, consistent with previous findings [15,16,17,18]. In contrast to other findings based on shorter intervals [10,11,12,13], sustained AM-selective attention produced overall stronger neural enhancement for the *non-target* AM than the target AM. Thus, overall, this main result does not support the notion of sustained AM-selective attentional enhancement in AC.

Figure 6. Effects of attention on AM representation in cortex. Panel **A** shows the channel-averaged neural response to the dual AM stimulus in the different attention conditions. Overall, the response was significantly stronger for the non-targets than the targets. Furthermore, the response was substantially stronger during auditory attention than visual attention. Error bars represent s.e.m. across all participants. See Figure S4 for single-subject data. Panel **B** shows the time course of the neural dominance index (defined as the neural response to targets minus the neural response to non-targets) and fitted linear trend (oblique line), indicating that the observed dominance of non-targets (panel A) arose mostly late during the task interval. Error bars represent s.e.m. across all participants. Panel **C** shows time-averaged neural responses as in panel A limited to the initial 15-s interval (left) and the final 15-s interval (right), illustrating the change in neural dominance from early to late interval. The units are the same as in panel A, and the lower magnitudes result from using a shorter analysis window (see

A

B **C**

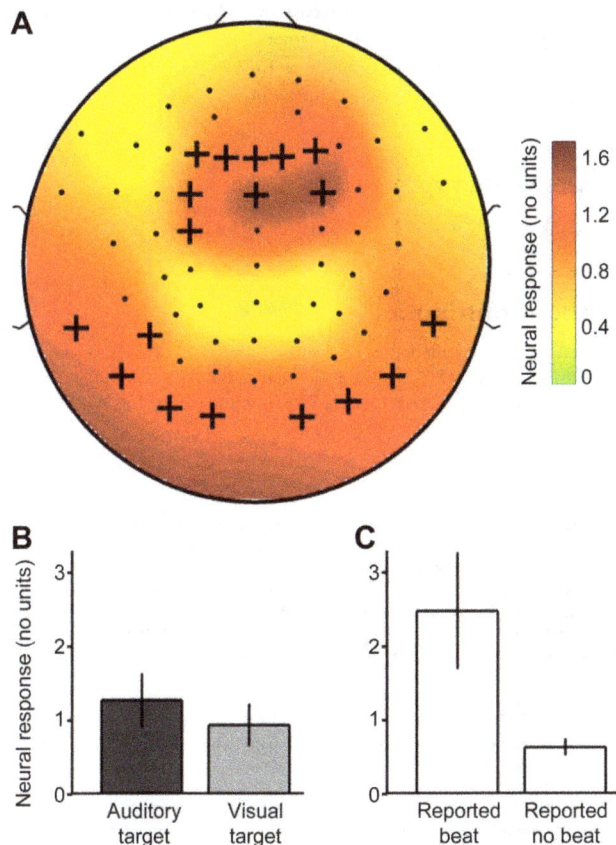

Figure 7. Beat frequency representation in cortex. Panel **A** shows the scalp distribution of the group average neural response associated with the beat frequency in the dual-AM conditions. Crosses indicate the channels from which the results in the other panels were obtained (same as in Figure 5A). Panel **B** shows the channel-averaged neural response associated with the beat frequency in the different attention conditions. The response was significantly stronger during auditory attention than visual attention. Error bars represent s.e.m. across all participants. Panel **C** shows the channel-averaged neural response associated with the beat frequency in the dual-AM conditions, separately for participants who reported hearing a beat and participants who reported hearing no beat. The response was significantly stronger for participants reporting a beat. Error bars represent s.e.m. across four and ten participants (left and right column respectively).

We found further that the neural dominance of the non-targets evolved rather slowly: the longer listeners had attempted to hear out a specific AM frequency, the less that AM frequency dominated the temporal AM representation. Because our AMs were invariant both within and between attention conditions, this adaptive effect of sustained AM-selective attention must be attributed to non-acoustic factors, such as the short-term history of the listener's perceptual state or potential transient learning effects [63] that influenced top-down attentional engagement. Perceptual AM-specific adaptation is known to apply to a range of AM frequencies including the ones used here [44,45,46,47]. A candidate mechanism underlying this perceptual phenomenon is AM-specific neural adaptation in AC, which has been observed in monkeys using AMs similar to the ones used here [64]. In our study, the neural response to single AMs attenuated significantly over the task interval (Figure 5D), showing that continuous exposure to these AMs rendered them less dominant in cortex. Furthermore, several participants in our study reported informally

that they perceived the target as slowly fainting until the percept switched toward the competing non-target, after which the desired target became more perceivable again. Considering findings of carrier frequency- and pitch-specific adaptation in AC [65,66], these observations suggest that our results reflect AM-specific adaptation that comprised response enhancement during sustained AM-selective attention. A possible purpose of this putative AM-specific adaptation could be to bias temporal processing in AC toward AM frequencies outside the listener's focus of sustained attention in order to support the auditory system in keeping track of task-irrelevant sound features [67] such as different AM frequencies.

Closer inspection of the initial sound interval revealed a trend that fits well with the previous findings of attentional response enhancement during this interval [10,11,12,13]. The fact that we could not detect a more robust (statistically significant) AM-selective attentional response enhancement during this interval may be due to the rather limited number of data points (i.e., few trials related to the long duration of our stimuli). Another potential explanation is that, in the absence of location and pitch cues, AM-selective attentional enhancement applies predominantly to non-temporal AM-frequency representations that were not captured by our SSR measure, for example, spatially segregated AM frequency channels (see Introduction) whose outputs exhibit no phase-locking. A final potential explanation is that robust selective attentional enhancement of temporal AM representations in AC requires the competing sounds to be distinguishable based on multiple distinct features, rather than AM frequency alone. In other words, the lack of a robust effect during the initial portion of our stimulus may be due to the absence of pitch and location cues, which compromised listeners' ability to perceptually segregate the competing AMs and thereby compromised attentional response enhancement. Further research is needed to disentangle these possibilities.

Conclusively, selective attentional cortical gain control based on AM frequency seems to operate adaptively under sustained attention and within an early interval. Furthermore, this mechanism seems to benefit from the presence of multiple distinct sound features, e.g., when the competing sounds differ not only in their AM, but also their location and pitch. These additional distinct features may facilitate performance in sustained attention tasks by allowing listeners to shift their attentional focus across these features, thereby enabling the feature-based cortical gain control mechanism to overcome adaptation to a specific feature.

A noteworthy side finding is that the cortical interaction of the competing AM frequencies (i.e., the beating frequency), which was already observed in a previous study [33], was enhanced both during auditory attention (compared with visual attention) and in listeners who reported hearing well the beating (compared with listeners who reported hearing no beating). These observations support the earlier suggestion [35] that the strength of the auditory cortical representation of the beating pattern determines the perceived salience of that beat.

Supporting Information

Figure S1 ICA-based artifact reduction. The figure shows for each participant (P1-P14) the centroid power spectral density, the centroid weights (scalp topography), and the IC weights underlying the centroid (from left to right). Furthermore, for each participant, the upper half shows data (centroid spectrum, centroid weights, individual IC weights) that were considered brain activity, and the lower half shows data considered artifacts. On average, ICs labeled as brain activity showed a more marked and dipole-like scalp topography (see centroid weights) and clearer harmonics in the frequency range of our AMs (see centroid spectrum), compared with ICs labeled as artifacts.

Figure S2 Behavioral results per participant. Analogous to Figure 4, the time series show for each participant the probability of perceiving the target as dominant, separately for the slow target (dark gray) and fast target (light gray).

Figure S3 Temporal AM-frequency representation in cortex per participant. Analogous to Figure 5A, the plots show for each participant the scalp distribution of the average neural response to the single AMs. Crosses indicate the channels from which the data in Figure S3 were obtained (same as in Figure 5A).

Figure S4 Effects of attention on AM representation in cortex per participant. Analogous to Figure 6A, the plots show for each participant the channel-averaged neural response to the dual AM stimulus in the attention conditions.

Acknowledgments

We thank three anonymous reviewers for useful comments on a previous version of the manuscript.

Author Contributions

Conceived and designed the experiments: LR AG WS. Performed the experiments: LR WS. Analyzed the data: LR WS GV. Contributed reagents/materials/analysis tools: GV. Wrote the paper: LR WS GV AG.

References

1. Alain C, Bernstein LJ (2008) From sounds to meaning: the role of attention during auditory scene analysis. Current Opinion in Otolaryngology & Head and Neck Surgery 16: 485-489.
2. Shamma SA, Elhilali M, Micheyl C (2011) Temporal coherence and attention in auditory scene analysis. Trends in Neurosciences 34: 114–123.
3. Hillyard SA, Hink RF, Schwent VL, Picton TW (1973) Electrical signs of selective attention in the human brain. Science 182: 177–180.
4. Woldorff MG, Gallen CC, Hampson SA, Hillyard SA, Pantev C, et al. (1993) Modulation of early sensory processing in human auditory cortex during auditory selective attention. Proceedings of the National Academy of Sciences of the United States of America 90: 8722–8726.
5. Hansen JC, Hillyard SA (1984) Effects of stimulation rate and attribute cuing on event-related potentials during selective auditory attention. Psychophysiology 21: 394–405.
6. Hansen JC, Hillyard SA (1988) Temporal dynamics of human auditory selective attention. Psychophysiology 25: 316–329.
7. Rif J, Hari R, Hamalainen MS, Sams M (1991) Auditory attention affects two different areas in the human supratemporal cortex. Electroencephalography and Clinical Neurophysiology 79: 464–472.
8. Alho K, Woods DL, Algazi A (1994) Processing of auditory stimuli during auditory and visual attention as revealed by event-related potentials. Psychophysiology 31: 469–479.
9. Tiitinen H, Sinkkonen J, Reinikainen K, Alho K, Lavikainen J, et al. (1993) Selective attention enhances the auditory 40-Hz transient response in humans. Nature 364: 59–60.
10. Bidet-Caulet A, Fischer C, Besle J, Aguera PE, Giard MH, et al. (2007) Effects of selective attention on the electrophysiological representation of concurrent sounds in the human auditory cortex. The Journal of Neuroscience 27: 9252–9261.
11. Muller N, Schlee W, Hartmann T, Lorenz I, Weisz N (2009) Top-down modulation of the auditory steady-state response in a task-switch paradigm. Frontiers in human neuroscience 3: 1.
12. Xiang J, Simon J, Elhilali M (2010) Competing streams at the cocktail party: exploring the mechanisms of attention and temporal integration. The Journal of Neuroscience 30: 12084–12093.
13. Elhilali M, Xiang J, Shamma SA, Simon JZ (2009) Interaction between attention and bottom-up saliency mediates the representation of foreground and background in an auditory scene. PLoS Biology 7: e1000129.
14. Lazzouni L, Ross B, Voss P, Lepore F (2010) Neuromagnetic auditory steady-state responses to amplitude modulated sounds following dichotic or monaural presentation. Clinical Neurophysiology 121: 200–207.
15. Ross B, Picton TW, Herdman AT, Pantev C (2004) The effect of attention on the auditory steady-state response. Neurology & Clinical Neurophysiology 2004: 22.
16. Saupe K, Widmann A, Bendixen A, Muller MM, Schroger E (2009) Effects of intermodal attention on the auditory steady-state response and the event-related potential. Psychophysiology 46: 321–327.
17. Okamoto H, Stracke H, Bermudez P, Pantev C (2011) Sound processing hierarchy within human auditory cortex. Journal of Cognitive Neuroscience 23: 1855–1863.
18. Gander PE, Bosnyak DJ, Roberts LE (2010) Evidence for modality-specific but not frequency-specific modulation of human primary auditory cortex by attention. Hearing Research 268: 213–226.
19. Linden RD, Picton TW, Hamel G, Campbell KB (1987) Human auditory steady-state evoked potentials during selective attention. Electroencephalography and Clinical Neurophysiology 66: 145–159.
20. de Jong R, Toffanin P, Harbers M (2010) Dynamic crossmodal links revealed by steady-state responses in auditory-visual divided attention. International Journal of Psychophysiology 75: 3–15.
21. Dau T, Kollmeier B, Kohlrausch A (1997) Modeling auditory processing of amplitude modulation. II. Spectral and temporal integration. The Journal of the Acoustical Society of America 102: 2906–2919.
22. Dau T, Kollmeier B, Kohlrausch A (1997) Modeling auditory processing of amplitude modulation. I. Detection and masking with narrow-band carriers. The Journal of the Acoustical Society of America 102: 2892–2905.
23. Herdener M, Esposito F, Scheffler K, Schneider P, Logothetis NK, et al. (2013) Spatial representations of temporal and spectral sound cues in human auditory cortex. Cortex 49: 2822–2833.
24. Barton B, Venezia JH, Saberi K, Hickok G, Brewer AA (2012) Orthogonal acoustic dimensions define auditory field maps in human cortex. Proceedings of the National Academy of Sciences of the United States of America 109: 20738–20743.
25. Baumann S, Griffiths TD, Sun L, Petkov CI, Thiele A, et al. (2011) Orthogonal representation of sound dimensions in the primate midbrain. Nature neuroscience 14: 423–425.
26. Schreiner CE, Langner G (1988) Periodicity coding in the inferior colliculus of the cat. II. Topographical organization. Journal of Neurophysiology 60: 1823–1840.
27. Langner G, Albert M, Briede T (2002) Temporal and spatial coding of periodicity information in the inferior colliculus of awake chinchilla (Chinchilla laniger). Hearing Research 168: 110–130.
28. McAlpine D (2004) Neural sensitivity to periodicity in the inferior colliculus: evidence for the role of cochlear distortions. Journal of neurophysiology 92: 1295–1311.
29. Kingsbury BED, Morgan N, Greenberg S (1998) Robust speech recognition using the modulation spectrogram. Speech Communication 25: 117–132.
30. Zion Golumbic EM, Ding N, Bickel S, Lakatos P, Schevon CA, et al. (2013) Mechanisms underlying selective neuronal tracking of attended speech at a "cocktail party". Neuron 77: 980–991.
31. Ding N, Simon JZ (2013) Adaptive temporal encoding leads to a background-insensitive cortical representation of speech. The Journal of Neuroscience 33: 5728–5735.
32. Ding N, Simon JZ (2012) Emergence of neural encoding of auditory objects while listening to competing speakers. Proceedings of the National Academy of Sciences of the United States of America 109: 11854–11859.
33. Xiang J, Poeppel D, Simon JZ (2013) Physiological evidence for auditory modulation filterbanks: cortical responses to concurrent modulations. The Journal of the Acoustical Society of America 133: EL7–12.
34. Lins OG, Picton TW (1995) Auditory steady-state responses to multiple simultaneous stimuli. Electroencephalography and Clinical Neurophysiology 96: 420–432.
35. Draganova R, Ross B, Borgmann C, Pantev C (2002) Auditory cortical response patterns to multiple rhythms of AM sound. Ear and hearing 23: 254–265.
36. Greenberg S, Carvey H, Hitchcock L, Chang S (2003) Temporal properties of spontaneous speech: A syllable-centric perspective. Journal of Phonetics 31: 465–485.
37. Picton TW, Skinner CR, Champagne SC, Kellett AJ, Maiste AC (1987) Potentials evoked by the sinusoidal modulation of the amplitude or frequency of a tone. The Journal of the Acoustical Society of America 82: 165–178.
38. Rees A, Green GG, Kay RH (1986) Steady-state evoked responses to sinusoidally amplitude-modulated sounds recorded in man. Hearing Research 23: 123–133.
39. Tlumak AI, Durrant JD, Delgado RE, Boston JR (2011) Steady-state analysis of auditory evoked potentials over a wide range of stimulus repetition rates: profile in adults. International Journal of Audiology 50: 448–458.
40. Wang Y, Ding N, Ahmar N, Xiang J, Poeppel D, et al. (2012) Sensitivity to temporal modulation rate and spectral bandwidth in the human auditory system: MEG evidence. Journal of Neurophysiology 107: 2033–2041.

41. Simpson MI, Woods WP, Prendergast G, Johnson SR, Green GG (2012) Stimulus variability affects the amplitude of the auditory steady-state response. PLoS One 7: e34668.

42. Grimault N, Bacon SP, Micheyl C (2002) Auditory stream segregation on the basis of amplitude-modulation rate. The Journal of the Acoustical Society of America 111: 1340–1348.

43. Joris PX, Schreiner CE, Rees A (2004) Neural processing of amplitude-modulated sounds. Physiological Reviews 84: 541–577.

44. Richards VM, Buss E, Tian L (1997) Effects of modulator phase for comodulation masking release and modulation detection interference. The Journal of the Acoustical Society of America 102: 468–476.

45. Wojtczak M, Viemeister NF (2003) Suprathreshold effects of adaptation produced by amplitude modulation. The Journal of the Acoustical Society of America 114: 991–997.

46. Gutschalk A, Micheyl C, Oxenham AJ (2008) The pulse-train auditory aftereffect and the perception of rapid amplitude modulations. The Journal of the Acoustical Society of America 123: 935–945.

47. Kay RH (1982) Hearing of modulation in sounds. Physiological Reviews 62: 894–975.

48. Houtgast T (1989) Frequency selectivity in amplitude-modulation detection. The Journal of the Acoustical Society of America 85: 1676–1680.

49. Bregman AS (1978) Auditory streaming is cumulative. Journal of Experimental Psychology: Human Perception and Performance 4: 380–387.

50. Macmillan NA, Creelman CD (1991) Detection theory: a user's guide. Cambridge: Cambridge UP.

51. Delorme A, Makeig S (2004) EEGLAB: an open source toolbox for analysis of single-trial EEG dynamics including independent component analysis. Journal of neuroscience methods 134: 9–21.

52. Lee TW, Girolami M, Bell AJ, Sejnowski TJ (2000) A unifying information-theoretic framework for independent component analysis. Computers & Mathematics with Applications 39: 1–21.

53. Bell AJ, Sejnowski TJ (1995) An information-maximization approach to blind separation and blind deconvolution. Neural Computation 7: 1129–1159.

54. Jung TP, Makeig S, Humphries C, Lee TW, McKeown MJ, et al. (2000) Removing electroencephalographic artifacts by blind source separation. Psychophysiology 37: 163–178.

55. Jung TP, Makeig S, Westerfield M, Townsend J, Courchesne E, et al. (2000) Removal of eye activity artifacts from visual event-related potentials in normal and clinical subjects. Clinical Neurophysiology 111: 1745–1758.

56. Delorme A, Sejnowski T, Makeig S (2007) Enhanced detection of artifacts in EEG data using higher-order statistics and independent component analysis. Neuroimage 34: 1443–1449.

57. Kay SM (1988) Modern Spectral Estimation: Theory and Application. Englewood Cliffs, NJ: Prentice Hall.

58. Picton TW, John MS, Dimitrijevic A, Purcell D (2003) Human auditory steady-state responses. International Journal of Audiology 42: 177–219.

59. Maris E, Oostenveld R (2007) Nonparametric statistical testing of EEG- and MEG-data. Journal of neuroscience methods 164: 177–190.

60. Deike S, Heil P, Bockmann-Barthel M, Brechmann A (2012) The Build-up of Auditory Stream Segregation: A Different Perspective. Frontiers in psychology 3: 461.

61. Liegeois-Chauvel C, Lorenzi C, Trebuchon A, Regis J, Chauvel P (2004) Temporal envelope processing in the human left and right auditory cortices. Cerebral Cortex 14: 731–740.

62. Herdman AT, Lins O, Van Roon P, Stapells DR, Scherg M, et al. (2002) Intracerebral sources of human auditory steady-state responses. Brain Topography 15: 69–86.

63. Fritz JB, Elhilali M, David SV, Shamma SA (2007) Auditory attention—focusing the searchlight on sound. Current Opinion in Neurobiology 17: 437–455.

64. Bartlett EL, Wang X (2005) Long-lasting modulation by stimulus context in primate auditory cortex. Journal of Neurophysiology 94: 83–104.

65. Gutschalk A, Patterson RD, Scherg M, Uppenkamp S, Rupp A (2007) The effect of temporal context on the sustained pitch response in human auditory cortex. Cerebral Cortex 17: 552–561.

66. Naatanen R, Sams M, Alho K, Paavilainen P, Reinikainen K, et al. (1988) Frequency and location specificity of the human vertex N1 wave. Electroencephalography and Clinical Neurophysiology 69: 523–531.

67. Winkler I, Teder-Salejarvi WA, Horvath J, Naatanen R, Sussman E (2003) Human auditory cortex tracks task-irrelevant sound sources. Neuroreport 14: 2053–2056.

Permissions

All chapters in this book were first published in PLOS ONE, by The Public Library of Science; hereby published with permission under the Creative Commons Attribution License or equivalent. Every chapter published in this book has been scrutinized by our experts. Their significance has been extensively debated. The topics covered herein carry significant findings which will fuel the growth of the discipline. They may even be implemented as practical applications or may be referred to as a beginning point for another development.

The contributors of this book come from diverse backgrounds, making this book a truly international effort. This book will bring forth new frontiers with its revolutionizing research information and detailed analysis of the nascent developments around the world.

We would like to thank all the contributing authors for lending their expertise to make the book truly unique. They have played a crucial role in the development of this book. Without their invaluable contributions this book wouldn't have been possible. They have made vital efforts to compile up to date information on the varied aspects of this subject to make this book a valuable addition to the collection of many professionals and students.

This book was conceptualized with the vision of imparting up-to-date information and advanced data in this field. To ensure the same, a matchless editorial board was set up. Every individual on the board went through rigorous rounds of assessment to prove their worth. After which they invested a large part of their time researching and compiling the most relevant data for our readers.

The editorial board has been involved in producing this book since its inception. They have spent rigorous hours researching and exploring the diverse topics which have resulted in the successful publishing of this book. They have passed on their knowledge of decades through this book. To expedite this challenging task, the publisher supported the team at every step. A small team of assistant editors was also appointed to further simplify the editing procedure and attain best results for the readers.

Apart from the editorial board, the designing team has also invested a significant amount of their time in understanding the subject and creating the most relevant covers. They scrutinized every image to scout for the most suitable representation of the subject and create an appropriate cover for the book.

The publishing team has been an ardent support to the editorial, designing and production team. Their endless efforts to recruit the best for this project, has resulted in the accomplishment of this book. They are a veteran in the field of academics and their pool of knowledge is as vast as their experience in printing. Their expertise and guidance has proved useful at every step. Their uncompromising quality standards have made this book an exceptional effort. Their encouragement from time to time has been an inspiration for everyone.

The publisher and the editorial board hope that this book will prove to be a valuable piece of knowledge for researchers, students, practitioners and scholars across the globe.

List of Contributors

Yu Jin, Begoña Díaz, Marc Colomer, Núria Sebastián-Gallés
Speech Acquisition and Perception Group, Center for Brain and Cognition, Department of Technology, Pompeu Fabra University, Barcelona, Spain

Thalía Fernández
Departamento de Neurobiología Conductual y Cognitiva, Instituto de Neurobiología, Universidad Nacional Autónoma de México, Juriquilla, Querétaro, México

Juan Silva-Pereyra, Belén Prieto-Corona and Mario Rodríguez-Camacho
Proyecto de Neurociencias, Facultad de Estudios Superiores (FES) Iztacala, Universidad Nacional Autónoma de México, Estado de México, México

Vicenta Reynoso-Alcántara
Facultad de Psicología, Universidad Veracruzana, Campus Xalapa, Veracruz, México

Prema Sriram
Australian School of Advanced Medicine, Macquarie University, Sydney, Australia

Stuart L. Graham, Hemamalini Arvind and Alexander Klistorner
Australian School of Advanced Medicine, Macquarie University, Sydney, Australia
Save Sight Institute, Department of Ophthalmology, University of Sydney, Sydney, Australia

Chenyu Wang and Michael Barnett
Brain and Mind Research Institute, University of Sydney, Sydney, Australia

Con Yiannikas
Concord Hospital, Sydney, Australia

Raymond Garrick
St Vincent's Hospital, Sydney, Australia

John Parratt
Royal North Shore Hospital, Sydney, Australia

Sheng Su
School of Computer Science and Engineering, University of Electronic Science and Technology of China, ChengDu, China

Zhenghua Wu
School of Computer Science and Engineering, University of Electronic Science and Technology of China, ChengDu, China
Key Laboratory for NeuroInformation of Ministry of Education, School of Life Science and Technology, University of Electronic Science and Technology of China, ChengDu, China

Giulia Righi
Department of Psychology, University of Massachusetts at Amherst, Amherst, Massachusetts, United States of America

Adrienne L. Tierney
Harvard College Writing Program, Harvard University, Cambridge, Massachusetts, United States of America

Helen Tager-Flusberg
Department of Psychological and Brain Sciences, Boston University, Boston, Massachusetts, United States of America

Charles A. Nelson
Division of Developmental Medicine, Boston Children's Hospital, Boston, Massachusetts, United States of America
Department of Pediatrics, Harvard Medical School, Boston, Massachusetts, United States of America
Harvard Graduate School of Education, Cambridge, Massachusetts, United States of America

Joshua L. Roffman, Donald C. Goff, Jennifer L. Greenberg and Sabine Wilhelm
Department of Psychiatry, Massachusetts General Hospital, Harvard Medical School, Boston, Massachusetts, United States of America

Yigal Agam and Dara S. Manoach
Department of Psychiatry, Massachusetts General Hospital, Harvard Medical School, Boston, Massachusetts, United States of America
Athinoula A. Martinos Center for Biomedical Imaging, Harvard Medical School, Charlestown, Massachusetts, United States of America

Jordan W. Smoller
Department of Psychiatry, Massachusetts General Hospital, Harvard Medical School, Boston, Massachusetts, United States of America

Center for Human Genetics Research, Massachusetts General Hospital, Harvard Medical School, Boston, Massachusetts, United States of America

Mark Vangel
Athinoula A. Martinos Center for Biomedical Imaging, Harvard Medical School, Charlestown, Massachusetts, United States of America

Patience J. Gallagher, Jonathan Chaponis and Stephen Haddad
Center for Human Genetics Research, Massachusetts General Hospital, Harvard Medical School, Boston, Massachusetts, United States of America

Charles J. Duffy
Department of Neurology and the Center for Visual Science, The University of Rochester Medical Center, Rochester, New York, United States of America

Michael S. Jacob
Department of Neurology and the Center for Visual Science, The University of Rochester Medical Center, Rochester, New York, United States of America
Department of Psychiatry, The University of California San Francisco Medical Center, San Francisco, California, United States of America

Johannes Höhne
Neurotechnology group, Berlin Institute of Technology, Berlin, Germany

Elisa Holz and Andrea Kübler
Department of Psychology I, University of Würzburg, Würzburg, Germany

Pit Staiger-Sälzer
Beratungsstelle für Unterstützte Kommunikation (BUK), Diakonie Bad Kreuznach, Bad Kreuznach, Germany

Klaus-Robert Müller
Machine Learning Laboratory, Berlin Institute of Technology, Berlin, Germany,
Bernstein Center for Computational Neuroscience, Berlin, Germany
Department of Brain and Cognitive Engineering, Korea University, Anam-dong, Seongbuk-gu, Seoul, Korea

Michael Tangermann
BrainLinks-BrainTools Excellence Cluster, University of Freiburg, Freiburg, Germany

Divya Chander
Department of Anesthesiology, Perioperative and Pain Medicine, Stanford University School of Medicine, Stanford, California, United States of America

S. García
Department of Anesthesiology, Atlanta VA Medical Center/Emory University, Atlanta, Georgia, United States of America

Jono N. MacColl, Sam Illing and Jamie W. Sleigh
Department of Anaesthesia, Waikato Clinical School, University of Auckland, Hamilton, New Zealand

Matthias J. Wieser and Paul Pauli
Department of Psychology, University of Würzburg, Würzburg, Germany

Tobias Flaisch
Department of Psychology, University of Konstanz, Konstanz, Germany

Yuming Chen and Yuejia Luo
Institute of Affective and Social Neuroscience, Shenzhen University, Shenzhen, China

Dandan Zhang
Institute of Affective and Social Neuroscience, Shenzhen University, Shenzhen, China
State Key Laboratory of Cognitive Neuroscience and Learning, Beijing Normal University, Beijing, China

Yunzhe Liu
State Key Laboratory of Cognitive Neuroscience and Learning, Beijing Normal University, Beijing, China

Chenglin Zhou
School of Kinesiology, Shanghai University of Sport, Shanghai, China

Sabah Mozafari and Javad Mirnajafi-Zadeh
Department of Physiology, Faculty of Medical Sciences, Tarbiat Modares University, Tehran, Iran

Fereshteh Pourabdolhossein
Department of Physiology, Faculty of Medical Sciences, Tarbiat Modares University, Tehran, Iran
UMR CNRS 7221, Evolution des Régulations Endocriniennes, Département Régulations, Développement et Diversité Moléculaire, Muséum National d'Histoire Naturelle, Paris, France

Mohammad Javan
Department of Physiology, Faculty of Medical Sciences, Tarbiat Modares University, Tehran, Iran
Department of Stem Cells and Developmental Biology at Cell Science Research Center, Royan Institute for Stem Cell Biology and Technology, ACECR, Tehran, Iran

Ghislaine Morvan-Dubois, Alejandra Lopez-Juarez, Jacqueline Pierre-Simons and Barbara A. Demeneix
UMR CNRS 7221, Evolution des Régulations Endocriniennes, Département Régulations, Développement et Diversité Moléculaire, Muséum National d'Histoire Naturelle, Paris, France

Ido Amihai
National University of Singapore, Psychology Department, Singapore, Singapore

Maria Kozhevnikov
National University of Singapore, Psychology Department, Singapore, Singapore
Martinos Center for Biomedical Imaging, MGH & Harvard Medical School, Charlestown, Massachusetts, United States of America

Lili Wu and Jianxin Zhang
Key Laboratory of Mental Health, Institute of Psychology, Chinese Academy of Sciences, Beijing, China

Huajian Cai, Ruolei Gu, Yu L. L. Luo, Jing Yang and Yuanyuan Shi
Key Laboratory of Behavioral Science, Institute of Psychology, Chinese Academy of Sciences, Beijing, China

Lei Ding
School of Electrical and Computer Engineering, University of Oklahoma, Norman, Oklahoma, United States of America

Carles Grau
Starlab Barcelona, Barcelona, Spain
Neurodynamics Laboratory, Department of Psychiatry and Clinical Psychobiology, Psychology and Medicine Faculties, University of Barcelona, Barcelona, Spain

Alejandro Riera and Giulio Ruffini
Starlab Barcelona, Barcelona, Spain
Neuroelectrics Barcelona, Barcelona, Spain

Romuald Ginhoux, Thanh Lam Nguyen, Hubert Chauvat and Michel Berg
Axilum Robotics, Strasbourg, France

Julià L. Amengual
Cognition and Brain Plasticity Unit, Department of Basic Psychology, University of Barcelona, Barcelona, Spain

Alvaro Pascual-Leone
Berenson Allen Center for Noninvasive Brain Stimulation, Beth Israel Deaconess Medical Center, Harvard Medical School, Boston, Massachusetts, United States of America

Xiaohong Yang, Weijun Li and Yufang Yang
Key Laboratory of Behavioral Science, Institute of Psychology, Chinese Academy of Sciences, Beijing, China

Xiangrong Shen
Key Laboratory of Behavioral Science, Institute of Psychology, Chinese Academy of Sciences, Beijing, China
College of Humanities and Communications, Shanghai Normal University, Shanghai, China

Mike Sharman and Katia Lehongre
Institut National de la Santé et de la Recherche Médicale (INSERM), Institut du Cerveau et de la Moelle Epiniére (ICM), Unité Mixte de Recherche 1127, PICNIC Lab, Paris, France
Centre National de la Recherche Scientifique (CNRS), Institut du Cerveau et de la Moelle Epiniére (ICM), Unité 7225, PICNIC Lab, Paris, France

Cécile Gallea
Institut National de la Santé et de la Recherche Médicale (INSERM), Institut du Cerveau et de la Moelle Epiniére (ICM), Unité Mixte de Recherche 1127, (CENIR), Paris, France

Thomas Similowski
Université Pierre et Marie Curie-Paris 6, Faculté de Médecine Pitié-Salpêtrié re, Paris, France
Assistance Publique–Hôpitaux de Paris, Groupe Hospitalier Pitié-Salpêtrière Charles Foix, Service de Pneumologie et Réanimation Médicale (Département "R3S"), Paris, France
Sorbonne Universités, Université Pierre et Marie Curie-Paris 6, Unité Mixte de Recherche 1158 "Neurophysiologie Respiratoire Expérimentale et Clinique", Paris, France
Institut National de la Santé et de la Recherche Me´dicale (INSERM), Unité Mixte de Recherche 1158 "Neurophysiologie Respiratoire Expérimentale et Clinique", Paris, France

Christian Straus
Université Pierre et Marie Curie-Paris 6, Faculté de Médecine Pitié-Salpêtrié re, Paris, France
Assistance Publique–Hôpitaux de Paris, Groupe Hospitalier Pitié-Salpêtrière Charles Foix, Service de Pneumologie et Réanimation Médicale (Département "R3S"), Paris, France
Sorbonne Universités, Université Pierre et Marie Curie-Paris 6, Unité Mixte de Recherche 1158 "Neurophysiologie Respiratoire Expérimentale et Clinique", Paris, France

Institut National de la Santé et de la Recherche Me´dicale (INSERM), Unité Mixte de Recherche 1158 "Neurophysiologie Respiratoire Expérimentale et Clinique", Paris, France
Assistance Publique–Hôpitaux de Paris, Groupe Hospitalier Pitié-Salpêtrière Charles Foix, Service des Explorations Fonctionnelles de la Respiration, de l'Exercice et de la Dyspnée (Département "R3S"), Paris, France
Assistance Publique–Hôpitaux de Paris, Groupe Hospitalier Pitié-Salpêtrière Charles Foix, Centre de Référence Maladies Rares "syndrome d'Ondine", Paris, France

Anupreet K. Tumber, Nichole E. Scheerer and Jeffery A. Jones
Psychology Department and Laurier Centre for Cognitive Neuroscience, Wilfrid Laurier University, Waterloo, Ontario, Canada

Martin Hardmeier, Florian Hatz and Peter Fuhr
Department of Neurology, Hospital of the University of Basel, Basel, Switzerland

Habib Bousleiman
Department of Neurology, Hospital of the University of Basel, Basel, Switzerland
Swiss Tropical and Public Health Institute, University of Basel, Basel, Switzerland,

Christian Schindler
Swiss Tropical and Public Health Institute, University of Basel, Basel, Switzerland,

Cornelis Jan Stam
Department of Clinical Neurophysiology and Magnetoencephalography, VU University Medical Center, Amsterdam, The Netherlands

Jiu Chen and Zhijun Zhang
Neurologic Department of Affiliated ZhongDa Hospital, Neuropsychiatric Institute and Medical School of Southeast University, Nanjing, Jiangsu Province, China

Wentao Ma, Yan Zhang, Xingqu Wu, Dunhong Wei, Guangxiong Liu, Zihe Deng and Laiqi Yang
Center for Mental Disease Control and Prevention, Third Hospital of the People's Liberation Army, Baoji, Shaanxi Province, China

Pablo Billeke and Francisco Zamorano
División Neurociencia de la Conducta, Centro de Investigación en Complejidad Social (CICS), Facultad de Gobierno, Universidad del Desarrollo, Santiago, Chile

Centro Interdisciplinario de Neurociencias, Pontificia Universidad Católica de Chile, Santiago, Chile
Departamento de Psiquiatría, Escuela de Medicina, Pontificia Universidad Católica de Chile, Santiago, Chile

Diego Cosmelli
Centro Interdisciplinario de Neurociencias, Pontificia Universidad Católica de Chile, Santiago, Chile
Escuela de Psicología, Pontificia Universidad Católica de Chile, Santiago, Chile

Francisco Aboitiz
Centro Interdisciplinario de Neurociencias, Pontificia Universidad Católica de Chile, Santiago, Chile
Departamento de Psiquiatría, Escuela de Medicina, Pontificia Universidad Católica de Chile, Santiago, Chile

Mario Chavez
CNRS UMR-7225, Hôpital de la Salpêtriére, Paris, France

Lars Riecke and Giancarlo Valente
Department of Cognitive Neuroscience, Faculty of Psychology and Neuroscience, Maastricht University, Maastricht, The Netherlands

Wolfgang Schark
Department of Child and Adolescent Psychiatry, Psychotherapy and Psychosomatics, University Hospital, RWTH Aachen University, Aachen, Germany

Alexander Gutschalk
Department of Neurology, Ruprecht-Karls- Universität Heidelberg, Heidelberg, Germany

Index